CLINICAL ASSESSMENT TOOLS
FOR USE WITH NURSING DIAGNOSES

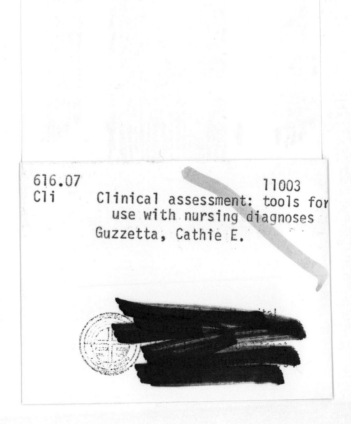

CLINICAL ASSESSMENT TOOLS
FOR USE WITH
NURSING DIAGNOSES

CATHIE E. GUZZETTA, RN, CCRN, PhD, FAAN

Associate Professor and Chair, Cardiovascular Nursing
The Catholic University of America
Washington, D.C.

SHELIA D. BUNTON, RN, MSN

Major, Army Nurse Corp
Clinical Head Nurse, Surgical-Thoracic Intensive Care Unit
Tripler Army Medical Center
Honolulu, Hawaii

LINDA A. PRINKEY, RN, MSN, CCRN

Director of Nursing Care, Cardiac Surgical Unit
Alexandria Hospital, Alexandria, Virginia

ANITA P. SHERER, RN, MSN, CCRN

Clinical Specialist, Cardiology
Moses H. Cone Memorial Hospital
Greensboro, North Carolina

PATRICIA C. SEIFERT, RN, MSN, CNOR

Administrative Director, Perioperative Nursing Specialty
The Washington Hospital Center, Washington, D.C.;
Formerly Assistant Nursing Coordinator
Cardiac Surgery, The Fairfax Hospital
Falls Church, Virginia

The C. V. Mosby Company

ST. LOUIS • BALTIMORE • PHILADELPHIA • TORONTO   1989

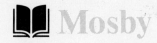 Mosby

Editor: William Grayson Brottmiller
Senior developmental editor: Sally Adkisson
Project manager: Carol Sullivan Wiseman
Production editor: Pat Joiner
Book and cover design: Gail Morey Hudson

The opinons expressed herein are those of the authors and do not
necessarily reflect those of the U.S. Army or any of its component parts.

Printed in the United States of America

The C.V. Mosby Company
11830 Westline Industrial Drive, St. Louis, Missouri 63146

Library of Congress Cataloging in Publication Data

Clinical assessment tools for use with nursing
  diagnoses.

  Includes bibliographies and index.
  1. Nursing assessment. 2. Diagnosis. I. Guzzetta,
Cathie E. [DNLM: 1. Information Systems. 2. Nursing
Assessment. WY 100 C6402]
RT48.C58 1989   610.73   88-32949
ISBN 0-8016-2840-7

C/VH/VH 9 8 7 6 5 4 3 2 1

CONTRIBUTORS

LYNELLE N. BABA, RN, MS, CCRN

Clinical Nurse Specialist, Trauma/Critical Care Unit, Washington Hospital Center, Washington, D.C.

CHAROLD L. BAER, RN, PhD

Professor, Department of Adult Health and Illness, The Oregon Health Sciences University, Portland, Oregon

CORNELIA BECK, RN, PhD

Professor, College of Nursing, Assistant Professor, Department of Psychiatry, College of Medicine, University of Arkansas for Medical Sciences, Little Rock, Arkansas

PATRICIA A. BOHANNON, RN, OCN, PhD

Associate Professor, Clinical Nurse Specialist, School of Nursing, University of Texas Health Science Center, Houston, Texas

HELEN A. BOZZO, RN, MS, CRRN

Rehabilitation Clinical Specialist, Washington Hospital Center, Washington, D.C.

SUSAN M. BRADY, RN, MSN

Clinical Nurse Specialist, Morristown Memorial Hospital, Morristown, New Jersey

CYNTHIA A. GOLDBERG, RN, MSN

Major, Army Nurse Corps, Medical-Surgical Clinical Nurse Specialist, Walter Reed Army Medical Center, Washington, D.C.

MARY FRAN HAZINSKI, RN, MSN

Clinical Specialist, Pediatric Intensive Care, Vanderbilt University Medical Center, Nashville, Tennessee

ANN MARIE JANEK, RN, MSN

Assistant Patient Care Director, Surgical Unit, Fair Oaks Hospital, Fairfax, Virginia

CHRISTINE A. KESSLER, RN, MN

Clinical Specialist, Surgery/Post-Trauma Unit, The Fairfax Hospital, Falls Church, Virginia; Formerly Assistant Professor of Nursing, Seattle Pacific University, Seattle, Washington

MARIE LOOBY, MSN, RN, C

Clinical Nurse Specialist, Gerontology, The Fairfax Hospital, Falls Church, Virginia

THOMAS G. O'DONNELL, RN, BSN

Nursing Service Coordinator, Whitman-Walker Clinic, Washington, D.C.

SANDRA O'SULLIVAN, RN, CCRN, BSN

Cardiac Nurse Specialist, Moffitt, Pease, Lim Associates, Consultant Cardiologists, Harrisburg, Pennsylvania

JANE C. ROTHROCK, RN, DNSc, CNOR

Professor, Perioperative Nursing, Delaware County Community College, Media, Pennsylvania

POLLY RYAN, RN, MSN

Doctoral Student, School of Nursing, University of Wisconsin-Milwaukee, Milwaukee, Wisconsin

JULIE A. SHINN, RN, MA, CCRN

Educational Coordinator, Critical Care, Stanford University Medical Center, Stanford, California

CANDICE J. SULLIVAN, RN, MSN

Major, Army Nurse Corps, Head Nurse, Labor, Delivery and Postpartum Unit, Ireland Army Hospital, Fort Knox, Kentucky

MARY TERHAAR, RN, DNSc

Clinical Specialist, Maternal-Child Nursing, The Fairfax Hospital, Falls Church, Virginia

SUSAN FICKERTT WILSON, RN, PhD

Associate Professor, Harris College of Nursing, Texas Christian University, Forth Worth, Texas

REVIEWERS

We gratefully acknowledge the expertise, interest, and assistance of the following individuals who reviewed chapters in this book and assisted in the clinical testing of the assessment tools.

URSULA ALAO-RATHBONE, RN

Staff Nurse, Critical Care Unit, Arlington Hospital, Arlington, Virginia

JUNE K. AMLING, RN, MSN, CNRN

Pediatric Neurosurgical Clinical Nurse Specialist, Hermann Hospital/University of Texas Medical School, Houston, Texas

LYNELLE N. BABA, RN, MS, CCRN

Clinical Nurse Specialist, Washington Hospital Center, Washington, D.C.

CHRISTINE BABICKI, MSN, RN, CS

Clinical Nurse Specialist, National Rehabilitation Hospital, Washington, D.C.

NANCY DICKSON BAIR, RN, MSN, CCRN

Clinical Practitioner Teacher, Medical Intensive Care, The Methodist Hospital, Houston, Texas

CYNTHIA ANN BRAY, MS, RN, CNOR

Clinical Specialist/Education Director, Perioperative Nursing, Hahnemann University Hospital, Philadelphia, Pennsylvania

BETH ANN BRISCOE, RN, BSN

Staff Nurse IV, Stanford University Medical Center, Stanford, California

KATHLEEN BYINGTON, RN, MSN

Pediatric Clinical Specialist, Vanderbilt University Medical Center, Nashville, Tennessee

CAROL M. CALLAHAN, RN, MS, CCRN

Cardiac Rehabilitation Nurse Coordinator, Milwaukee County Medical Complex, Milwaukee, Wisconsin

SUSAN L. CARLSON, RN, MSN

Education Coordinator, The Fairfax Hospital, Falls Church, Virginia

DEIRDRE M. CAROLAN, BSN, Med/Surg Certification

Clinician IV, The Fairfax Hospital, Falls Church, Virginia

VINCE CASSANI III, RN, MSN

Captain, Army Nurse Corps, Headnurse, Neonatal ICU and Newborn Nursery, Letterman Army Hospital, San Francisco, California

SANDY CISNEROS, RN

Staff Nurse, Orthopedics, Fair Oaks Hospital, Fairfax, Virginia

JEANNE DAHL, RN, C

Clinical Nurse II, Admission Nursery, The Fairfax Hospital, Falls Church, Virginia

DENICE A. DAVIS, RN, BSN

Nursing Instructor, Garland County Community College, Hot Springs, Arkansas; Masters candidate, Graduate Program, College of Nursing, University of Arkansas for Medical Sciences, Little Rock, Arkansas

BRENDA DEREFIELD-JONES, RN, BSN, MEd

Associate Nurse, Surgical Intensive Care, Washington Hospital Center, Washington, D.C.

DEBRA M. DERICKSON, RN, BA, CRRN

Assistant Nursing Coordinator, George Washingon University Hospital, Washington, D.C.

CAROLYN DOBBINS, RN, BSN, RNP

Charge Nurse, Jefferson Regional Medical Center, Pine Bluff, Arkansas; Masters candidate, Graduate Program, College of Nursing, University of Arkansas for Medical Sciences, Little Rock, Arkansas

ANDREA E. DORY, RN

Head Nurse, Spinal Cord Injury Unit, Bronx Veterans Administration Medical Center, Bronx, New York

JOY DUTTON, RN

Staff Nurse IV, Stanford University Medical Center, Stanford, California

SUSAN KILEY ECKERT, RN, MSN, CCRN

Clinical Specialist, Washington Hospital Center, Washington, D.C.

DEBORAH ANNE GALLEHER, BSN

Clinician II, The Fairfax Hospital, Falls Church, Virginia

CAROL ANNE GERSON, RN, MS

Major, Army Nurse Corps, Medical-Surgical Clinical Specialist, Walter Reed Army Medical Center, Washington, D.C.

TOBY GIBERSTONE, MA, RN, CRRN

Supervisor, Patient Management Services, Sinai Rehabilitation Center, Sinai Hospital of Baltimore, Baltimore, Maryland

TONNIE GLICK, RN, BS, MICP, CCRN, MEd

Spinal Cord Injury Coordinator, Kessler Institute, West Orange, New Jersey

SUZANNE K. GOETSCHIUS, MSN, RN, C

Director, Senior Citizens Health Center, Lawrence Memorial Hospital of Medford, Medford, Massachusetts

CECELIA A. GRAMSKY, RN, CCRN

Primary Nurse, Surgical Intensive Care, Washington Hospital Center, Washington, D.C.

BARBARA HALL, RN, NNP

Neonatal Nurse Practitioner, Neonatal Intensive Care Unit, The Fairfax Hospital, Falls Church, Virginia

LuANN HALL, RN, MSN

Clinical Nurse Specialist, Neonatal Intensive Care Unit, The Fairfax Hospital, Falls Church, Virginia

JUDITH A. HEADLEY, RN, MSN

Clinical Nurse Specialist, Division of Medicine, University of Texas, M.D. Anderson Cancer Center, Houston, Texas

NINA M. HEPPE, MSN, RN

Clinical Educator, Surgical Services, The Bryn Mawr Hospital, Bryn Mawr, Pennsylvania

MARILYN HICKMAN, RN, BSN

Assistant Head Nurse, The Oregon Health Sciences University Hospital, Portland, Oregon

JANE H. JOHNSON, RN, MSN, CNOR

Perioperative Nursing Faculty, Delaware County Community College, Media, Pennsylvania; Nursing Faculty, Neumann College, Aston, Pennsylvania

MARYANNE H. JOHNSON, RN, MSN

Hospital Education Instructor, Medical Critical Care, Coronary Care, Hermann Hospital/University of Texas Medical School, Houston, Texas

ANNE KELLY, RN, MSN

Medical Oncology Nurse Specialist, University of Texas, M.D. Anderson Cancer Center, Houston, Texas

PATTI KENNEY, RN, MSN

Assistant Professor, School of Nursing, Cardinal Stritch College, Milwaukee, Wisconsin

KATHLEEN KILBANE, RN, MSN

Pediatric Clinical Specialist, Vanderbilt University Medical Center, Nashville, Tennessee

SUSAN V. M. KLEINBECK, RN, MS

Nurse Consultant/Educator, Neodesha, Kansas

JANE KOERNER, RN

Clinical Nurse IV, Neonatal Intensive Care Unit, The Fairfax Hospital, Falls Church, Virginia

EMILY LIEBSCHER, RN, NNP

Neonatal Nurse Practitioner, Neonatal Intensive Care Unit, The Fairfax Hospital, Falls Church, Virginia

PATRICIA MANNING-HOUDE, MSN, RN, C

Gerontological Nurse Practitioner, Private Practice, Danvers, Massachusetts

SUSAN McGEE, RN

Clinical Nurse II, Neonatal Intensive Care Unit, The Fairfax Hospital, Falls Church, Virginia

NORMA D. McNAIR, RN, MSN, CCRN, CNRN

Neurosurgical Clinical Nurse Specialist, Hermann Hospital/University of Texas Medical School, Houston, Texas

JULIE ANN MINICH-CASTRO, RN, BSN

First Lieutenant, Army Nurse Corps, Assistant Head Nurse, Labor, Delivery, and Postpartum Unit, Ireland Army Hospital, Fort Knox, Kentucky

PATRICE B. OLIN, RN, BSN

Clinical Nurse III, St. Joseph's Hospital, Milwaukee, Wisconsin

SHARON OWENS, RN, BSN

Clinical Nurse III, Neonatal Intensive Care Unit, The Fairfax Hospital, Falls Church, Virginia

ROSEMARY PEREZ, RN, BSN

Assistant Nursing Coordinator, Neonatal Intensive Care Unit, The Fairfax Hospital, Falls Church, Virginia

TERESA M. PETRUCCI, RN, BSN

Captain, Army Nurse Corps, Clinical Staff Nurse, Medical-Surgical Unit, Walter Reed Army Medical Center, Washington, D.C.

MICHELLE RENAUD, RN, MS

Major, Army Nurse Corps, Headnurse, Neonatal Intensive Care, Darnell Army Community Hospital, Fort Hood, Texas

ANNE B. SCOTT, RN, BSN, CRRN

Clinical Coordinator, Department of Rehabilitation Medicine, Mount Sinai Hospital, New York, New York

ORLANDO SEGARRA, RN, BSN

Captain, Army Nurse Corps, Clinical Staff Nurse, Medical Intensive Care, William Beaumont Army Medical Center, El Paso, Texas

RHONDA L. STEPHENSON, RN, BSN

First Lieutenant, Army Nurse Corps, Head Nurse, OB-GYN Clinic, Ireland Army Hospital, Fort Knox, Kentucky

JEAN C. STEWART, RN, MSN, CNRN, CEN

Continuing Education Instructor, Ben Taub General Hospital Emergency Center, Houston, Texas

AMY SUMMERS, RN, BSN

Clinical Nurse III, Neonatal Intensive Care Unit, The Fairfax Hospital, Falls Church, Virginia

PAMELA SUTHERLAND, RN

Clinical Nurse III, Neonatal Intensive Care Unit, The Fairfax Hospital, Falls Church, Virginia

ANNE LEISERING TOY, RN, BSN, MS

Cardiac Rehabilitation Program Coordinator, St. Joseph's Hospital, Milwaukee, Wisconsin

BARBARA TURNER, RN, DNSc, FAAN

Lieutenant Colonel, Army Nurse Corps, Consultant, Nursing Research to the Surgeon General, Madigan Army Medical Center, Tacoma, Washington

NAOMI BELLE WADE, RN, BSN

Captain, Army Nurse Corps, Clinical Staff Nurse, Medical-Surgical Unit, Walter Reed Army Medical Center, Washington, D.C.

CHRIS GORMAN WALTON, RN, BSN

Masters candidate, Graduate Program, College of Nursing, University of Arkansas for Medical Sciences, Little Rock, Arkansas

JULIA B. WILLIAMS, RN, MSN

Major, Army Nurse Corps, Head Nurse, Medical Intensive Care, William Beaumont Army Medical Center, El Paso, Texas

LORI WILLIAMS, RN, MSN, OCN

Medical Oncology Nurse Specialist, Bone Marrow Transplant, University of Texas, M.D. Anderson Cancer Center, Houston, Texas

BETTY WOLFINGER, RN, BSN

Staff Nurse, The Oregon Health Sciences University Hospital, Portland, Oregon

BRIAN L. VOTAVA, RN, BSN

Clinical Staff Nurse, Medical Intensive Care, William Beaumont Army Medical Center, El Paso, Texas

FOREWORD

The basic cognitive skills that registered nurses bring to assessment and diagnostic processes are pattern recognition, validation of judgments, and interpretation of meaning within a particular context. Assessment is an ongoing process of cue and pattern recognition; cues serve to trigger pattern recognition and/or to validate an already recognized pattern. The format for assessment then plays a key role in the diagnostic process by focusing attention on a cue or cluster of cues. A Unitary Person Assessment Tool for patients with cardiovascular problems[3] served as the prototype for this book, which represents a major effort by practicing nurses in general and specialty practices to translate the Unitary Person Framework into meaningful categories for assessment.

The relevance of the Unitary Person Framework for practicing nurses has been a concern since it was presented at the third conference on classification of nursing diagnoses.[11] At the fourth conference, nurse theorists working with the North American Nursing Diagnosis Association (NANDA) responded to the concern by proposing assessment factors and empirical indicators for the nine patterns.[11] Participants at the fifth conference, working in small groups, attempted to increase their understanding of the Unitary Person Framework by categorizing each defining characteristic for approved diagnoses into the nine patterns.[5] Individual elaborations and use for practice were presented at the conferences by nurse scholars and clinical nurse specialists.[1,7,8] A standardized assessment format based on the nine patterns has yet to be developed.

The need for standardized assessment tools for nursing practice has long been recognized by nurse leaders and theorists. Many of the latter have proposed original frameworks for practice[6,9,10] that direct the nurse to widely divergent categories for assessment. Johnson[4] urged greater concentration on a smaller number of conceptual schemata so nurses and society might agree on the precise nature of nursing practice. Gordon[2] has been a strong advocate for adopting a standardized structure for assessment and proposed eleven functional health patterns as a typology of assessment categories. The merging of the Unitary Person Framework with elements of a biomedical format for specialty areas pursued by Guzzetta and her colleagues in this book could serve as a stimulus for wide-scale testing and eventual consensus on a structure for assessment.

The ongoing collaboration among theorists, clinicians, educators, and researchers, a hallmark of the classification conferences, merits continuation in the genesis, testing, and refinement of a format for assessment. Guzzetta and her colleagues have laid the foundation for such collaboration. It is up to the rest of us to use their work to contribute to the elaboration of the Unitary Person Framework.

References on p. xiv.

Audrey M. McLane, PhD, RN

Hendersonville, North Carolina
Professor Emerita, Marquette University
Milwaukee, Wisconsin

REFERENCES

1. Feild L and Newman M: Clinical application of the unitary man framework: case study analysis. In Kim MJ and Moritz DA: Classification of nursing diagnoses: proceedings of the Third and Fourth conferences, New York, 1982, McGraw-Hill Book Co.
2. Gordon M: Nursing diagnosis: process and application, New York, 1982, 1987, McGraw-Hill Book Co.
3. Guzzetta CE et al: Unitary person assessment tool: easing problems with nursing diagnoses, Focus Crit Care 15(2):12, 1988.
4. Johnson DE: State of the art of theory development in nursing. In Theory development: what, why, how? New York, 1978, National League for Nursing.
5. Kim MJ, McFarland GK, and McLane AM: Classification of nursing diagnoses: proceedings of the Fifth Conference, St Louis, 1984, The CV Mosby Co.
6. King IM: A theory for nursing: systems, concepts, process, New York, 1981, John Wiley & Sons.
7. Kirk LW: The design for relevance, revisited: an elaboration of the conceptual framework for nursing diagnosis. In Hurley ME, editor: Classification of nursing diagnoses: proceedings of the Sixth Conference, St Louis, 1986, The CV Mosby Co.
8. Newman MA: Nursing's emerging paradigm: the diagnosis of pattern. In McLane AM, editor: Classification of nursing diagnoses: proceedings of the Seventh Conference, St Louis, 1987, The CV Mosby Co.
9. Orem DE: Nursing: concepts of practice, New York, 1971, 1980, 1985, McGraw-Hill Book Co.
10. Roy C: Introduction to nursing: an adaptation model, Englewood Cliffs, NJ, 1976, Prentice-Hall, Inc.
11. Roy C: Theoretical framework for classification of nursing diagnoses. In Kim MJ and Moritz DE, editors: Classification of nursing diagnoses: proceedings of the Third and Fourth Conferences, New York, 1982, McGraw-Hill Book Co.

PREFACE

Many nurses are uncomfortable using nursing diagnoses. This discomfort can be traced to a fundamental gap between assessment and formulation of nursing diagnoses. The assessment tools used in clinical practice create many of these problems. If an assessment tool does not have a nursing perspective, nursing diagnoses are difficult to identify. Most nurses throughout the United States use a traditional medical data base with psychosocial questions added to the beginning or the end to lend a nursing perspective. Because the patient is assessed primarily from a medical point of view, a holistic assessment does not take place. As a result, nurses have trouble identifying nursing diagnoses because they have been collecting only part of the data they need. In effect, nurses have difficulty using nursing diagnoses because the first step of the nursing process, the assessment phase, has been largely ignored and inadequately developed.

Over the past 15 years, however, much work has been done to formalize, standardize, and research diagnostic statements related to patient problems. Yet, very little effort has been made in developing a nursing data base for measuring appropriate signs and symptoms to formulate nursing diagnoses. Thus, nurses have worked on nursing diagnoses while ignoring the most preliminary step: assessment. As a result of the work on diagnoses, the assessment phase must be restructured and standardized from a nursing perspective before problems with nursing diagnoses (and the remaining steps of the nursing process) can be resolved.

Nurses have not standardized their data base, probably because of the recommendation that a conceptual model or framework of nursing be used to guide the development of a nursing data base. Nurses may be reluctant to follow this recommendation because they are not sure how to translate conceptual theory into bedside practice. In addition, the many conceptual models currently available to nursing have made it difficult to standardize a nursing data base across the country because the models and assessment tools derived from them are very different.

The nursing diagnostic process could be enhanced if an assessment tool were developed from a more standardized framework designed to incorporate nursing diagnoses. Such a nursing conceptual framework, called the Unitary Person Framework, has been developed by the North American Nursing Diagnosis Association (NANDA). The framework was created to guide the development of nursing diagnoses. It views the health of the individual as manifested by nine human response patterns (exchanging, communicating, relating, valuing, choosing, moving, perceiving, knowing, and feeling) that are reflective of the *whole* person. Within the Unitary Person Framework, a nursing diagnosis is a "judgment about the health of the person based on the data collected from the nine human response patterns." If nurses are to formulate judgments based on data collected from human response patterns, construction of a data base that incorporates the signs and symptoms necessary to make such judgments is not only logical but fundamental.

Several years after this framework was developed, a new classification system for organizing nursing diagnoses, Taxonomy I, was created. The nine human response patterns of the Unitary Person Framework serve as the major category headings for Taxonomy I. All nursing diagnoses approved by NANDA are organized under the nine human response patterns of Taxonomy I. The authors hypothesized that it might be possible to use the nine human response patterns and the sublevel categories of Taxonomy I as the foundation for creating a holistic data base that would be compatible with nursing diagnoses.

From these ideas, a nursing data base prototype based on the Unitary Person Framework was developed. The prototype was organized according to the nine human response patterns of Taxonomy I to facilitate identification of nursing diagnoses.

The results of this work were exciting. After developing, refining, and clinically testing the prototype, it was discovered that the data were so rich that nursing diagnoses appeared to "fall out" after assessment. Because the variables in the tool measure human response patterns, the data collected are pertinent to nursing diagnoses and are collected from a holistic point of view. Thus, the prototype facilitates evaluation of specific signs and symptoms necessary to validate a particular nursing diagnosis.

The data obtained from the nursing data base prototype are the same as those elicited from the traditional assessment tools nurses use, including data derived from physical examination. The only difference lies in the way the resulting data are formatted and the addition of patterns necessary for assessing the whole patient. As a result, a holistic assessment is easily accomplished, and nursing diagnoses are logically and accurately identified.

The nursing data base prototype, which focuses on the cardiovascular patient, was then used to develop assessment tools for a variety of other patient populations. Thus, 22 other assessment tools, all created from the prototype, have been developed and clinically tested and are presented in this book.

Although the tools in this book differ from one another because they assess the unique needs of particular patient groups, they are all based on NANDA's Unitary Person Framework and Taxonomy I. Therefore, the theory, process, structure, and outcome of all the tools offer a model for standardization of nursing data bases across the county.

This book is divided into five units. Unit I contains information related to the development of the prototype. Because the tools in this book are very different from traditional assessment tools, it is essential that the nurse be thoroughly familiar with the content in Chapter 1 (discussing the need for a nursing data base) and Chapter 2 (how the prototype was developed from the Unitary Person Framework and Taxonomy I). The chapters contain information that must be understood to use the tools effectively.

The more experienced nurse may wish to skim Chapter 3, which deals with suggested focus questions and parameters to elicit appropriate data when using the prototype. Nurses with less clinical experience may wish to become more familiar with this material. All readers will find Chapter 4 (practical applications) particularly helpful when trying to translate conceptual theory into bedside practice. This chapter presents a filled-in version of the prototype from a case study. It also contains a sample care plan that illustrates how nursing diagnoses flow from the nursing assessment and direct the remaining steps of the nursing process. This chapter outlines how the prototype, as well as all other tools in this book, can be adapted for use in clinical practice. Finally, it also describes how the tools can be revised, shortened, and used as screening tools.

After thoroughly reviewing the first four chapters, the reader should have a solid understanding of the approach used in the remaining chapters. Units II, III, IV, and V present nursing assessment tools for specific patient populations. Standards of nursing care, if available, have been incorporated into the framework of each tool. Within each chapter, there is a discussion of the way the tool was developed and refined, the patient populations and settings to which the tool applies, the way to use the tool, a copy of the tool, and a filled-in version based on a case study.

Although the ideas in this book have the potential not only to standardize but also to revolutionize the approach to nursing assessment, it is realized that changing traditional methods of assessment is not an easy task. The authors have only one request of their readers—that they approach the ideas in this book with an open mind and a willingness to stretch and expand traditional ways of thinking. Nurses function within the healing environment and have the ability and responsibility to holistically assess and care for patients. It is hoped that nurses will find this book a challenge in expanding their scope of nursing practice.

COVER DESIGN

The coxcomb is a symbol used by Florence Nightingale in early nursing research. Nine coxcombs are depicted here, each representing a pattern of the whole person. Each coxcomb represents a multidimensional and interconnected pattern containing within itself opposite yet complementary forces. The arrangement is asymmetrical, suggesting that each coxcomb is capable of shifting and changing its emphasis for each person at any point in space and time. The outward rotational design interrelated with the coxcombs represents the forceful, continual, and cyclic movement capturing the concept of psychophysiologic unity—the endless exchange of body-mind-spirit elements of living things with the universe.

CEG
SDB
LAP
APS
PCS

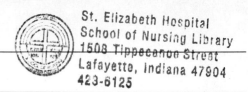

CONTENTS

UNIT I

DEVELOPING A NURSING DATA BASE PROTOTYPE

1 Need for a Nursing Data Base, 3

2 Developing a Nursing Data Base Prototype from the Unitary Person Framework, 6

3 General Focus Questions and Parameters for Eliciting Appropriate Data, 23

4 Practical Applications: Cardiovascular Assessment Tool, 40

UNIT II

ASSESSING PATIENTS WITH MAJOR SYSTEMS DYSFUNCTIONS

5 Pulmonary Assessment Tool, 59

6 Neurologic Assessment Tool, 75

7 Renal Assessment Tool, 92

8 Endocrine Assessment Tool, 108

UNIT III

ASSESSING PATIENTS WITH MAJOR SPECIALTY DYSFUNCTIONS

9 Medical-Surgical Assessment Tool, 129

10 Gynecologic Assessment Tool, 145

11 Psychiatric Assessment Tool, 161

12 Critical Care Assessment Tool, 179

13 Perioperative Assessment Tool, 198

14 Transplant Assessment Tool, 223

15 Trauma Assessment Tool, 239

16 Orthopedic Assessment Tool, 256

17 Oncologic Assessment Tool, 272

18 Acquired Immunodeficiency Syndrome Assessment Tool, 288

UNIT IV

ASSESSING PATIENTS THROUGHOUT THE LIFE SPAN

19 Labor-Delivery Assessment Tool, 307

20 Neonatal Assessment Tool, 328

21 Pediatric Assessment Tool, 343

22 Adolescent Assessment Tool, 357

23 Gerontologic Assessment Tool, 372

UNIT V

ASSESSING REHABILITATION PATIENTS

24 Cardiac Rehabilitation Assessment Tool, 393

25 Stroke Rehabilitation Assessment Tool, 407

26 Spinal Cord Injury Rehabilitation Assessment Tool, 423

Appendix I Taxonomy I Revised, 437

Appendix II Selected Normal Laboratory Values, 440

Index, 448

CLINICAL ASSESSMENT TOOLS
FOR USE WITH NURSING DIAGNOSES

■ UNIT I ■
DEVELOPING A NURSING DATA BASE PROTOTYPE

CHAPTER 1

NEED FOR A NURSING DATA BASE

CATHIE E. GUZZETTA

Many nurses have problems using nursing diagnoses because the first step in the nursing process, the nursing assessment phase, has been largely ignored. Many problems encountered by nurses can be linked to the assessment tools used in nursing practice. If nurses collect the wrong data, they will continue to have problems with nursing diagnoses. Before these problems can be solved, the assessment phase must be restructured and standardized from a holistic and nursing point of view.

This chapter includes:

- *An examination of the problems encountered when using traditional nursing assessment tools*
- *Reasons it is necessary to develop assessment tools based on nursing models*

Chapter 2 presents a new nursing data base prototype that facilitates the identification of nursing diagnoses from a holistic and nursing viewpoint. Chapter 3 discusses focus questions and parameters needed to elicit appropriate data when assessing patients using this data base. Chapter 4 illustrates a case study and practical applications of the nursing data base prototype tool. The remainder of the book presents 22 other assessment tools, developed from the nursing data base prototype, that can be used to evaluate patients. To use this book effectively, a thorough reading of Chapters 1 and 2 and a familiarity with Chapters 3 and 4 are urged.

TRADITIONAL NURSING DATA BASE

The kind of data base commonly used by nurses throughout the country includes pertinent demographic data, the patient's past medical history, a review of systems, and a physical examination. It also usually includes some psychosocial questions at the beginning or end. Such

a format is comfortable and most nurses believe it provides the appropriate categories of information necessary to assess patients. The data base published only a few years ago by Kenner, Guzzetta, and Dossey was similar to those used by nurses nationwide.[9]

If such an assessment tool is evaluated, however, it is found to be nothing more than a traditional medical data base with some psychosocial questions tacked on to lend a nursing perspective. The problem with using a medical data base in nursing practice is that nurses do not collect all the appropriate data necessary to holistically assess patients. If all appropriate data are not obtained, it is impossible to support the existence of nursing diagnoses.[5]

To fully understand why a medical data base does not provide the necessary data to formulate nursing diagnoses, nurses must examine the goals and concerns of medicine. Traditionally, medicine has been guided by the biomedical model, which asserts that all disease is caused by the malfunction of specific molecules or organs.[2,4,6] This model asserts that if enough sophisticated equipment and testing techniques were available it would be possible to discover the molecular causes and cures for all diseases (e.g., the common cold, acquired immunodeficiency syndrome [AIDS], and essential hypertension). As a result, medicine is concerned with the pathology, diagnosis, and treatment of disease. The resultant medical data base has been logically developed and structured to serve this medical point of view.

In contrast, nursing is concerned with the way the patient responds, physiologically and psychologically, to disease or illness. As a result, nurses view the patient differently than physicians. A medical data base does not allow nurses to collect all data pertinent to the practice of nursing. Therefore when nurses use a medical data base, they cannot assess the patient holistically because they collect only a part of the necessary data.

Yet, since the inception of the nursing diagnosis movement, nurses have attempted to identify and formulate nursing diagnoses from an inadequate data base. Therefore nurses have struggled with nursing diagnoses and their related problems[8] because they have not been collecting all the data they need.

The psychosocial questions frequently added to the traditional medical data base represent attempts to achieve a more holistic assessment (e.g., how has the patient coped with previous illness? What support systems are available to the patient? What does the patient perceive or understand about the illness? What are the patient's usual sleep or exercise patterns?). However, why were the psychosocial questions that appear on your nursing data base chosen? Who selected them? Are you confident that other questions necessary for assessing the whole patient are *not* missing? What approach can be used to determine what data *are* missing? If a hundred nursing data bases across the country were compared, a hundred types of psychosocial questions without any consistency or logic for inclusion would be found. The inclusion of psychosocial questions is usually based on the perceived importance of certain psychosocial categories by the person or group developing the data base.

The medical data base fails to guide the collection of data from the psychosocial realm. It does not provide nurses with a direction for deciding what psychosocial data should be collected to provide a holistic assessment. Most important, the medical data base provides no guidelines for how psychosocial data are interrelated with the physiologic realm.[7]

OVERVIEW OF NURSING MODELS USED TO GUIDE ASSESSMENT

The nursing diagnosis movement formally emerged as an organized process in 1973 with the formation of the North American Nursing Diagnosis Association (NANDA). Over 15 years, enormous work has been accomplished in formalizing, refining, standardizing, and researching diagnostic statements related to patient problems encountered by nurses. Yet, very little effort has been directed toward formalizing, refining, standardizing, and researching a nursing data base that could be used to measure signs and symptoms necessary to formulate such diagnoses.

Physicians have standardized a data base, but nurses have not.[6] One reason may be related to the recommendation by nurse theorists that a conceptual model of nursing be used to guide the development of a nursing data base.[3] Because of the many conceptual models available to nursing, it is impossible to standardize a nursing data base across the country because the conceptual models and resultant assessment tools are different.

In general, nurses have also been reluctant to use a conceptual model of nursing to structure a nursing data base because it is difficult to translate conceptual theory into bedside practice. Although information about conceptual models can be easily located in the literature, the application of such theory is not easily retrieved. In addition, for many nurses, theoretic terminology is confusing and associated with abstract and impractical ideas.

The terms, *conceptual framework, conceptual model,* and *theory,* often used interchangeably in the literature although their precise meanings differ, add to this confusion. A conceptual framework is a loosely organized set of ideas providing an overall structure to practice. When a conceptual framework becomes well organized and tested in practice, it becomes a conceptual model, which is viewed as a precursor to theory. Theory organizes scientific truths into patterns that reveal meaningful wholes. Theory, then, can be developed from models. Extensive testing and use in clinical practice are necessary, however, before a model is sufficiently developed and refined to become a theory.

Nurses should be concerned with conceptual frameworks or models because they serve as a guide to tie nursing actions together to meet a common goal, that of quality patient care. Frameworks and models provide the central focus for developing an organized, systematic approach to patient care. Nurses use conceptual frameworks and models to describe, explain, predict, and control the outcomes of nursing practice. These frameworks and models emphasize humanness and holism. Concern for the mind and concern for the body therefore assume equal importance.[2] Thus nursing frameworks and models help to assess unrelated and fragmented signs, symptoms, and parts.

Nurses can use the terminology and structure of a conceptual framework or model to develop a nursing data base. The framework or model helps to identify the assessment variables that should be included in the data base. It gives the structure necessary to understand how the data are interrelated. Ideally, it guides the organization of data, the formulation of nursing diagnoses, and the development of patient outcomes, plans, interventions, and evaluations.[3]

Many conceptual models of nursing can be used to develop a nursing data base. Examples are Roy's adaptation model,[15] Rogers' unitary man model,[13] King's systems model,[10] Orem's self-care model,[12] Yura and Walsh's human needs model,[17] Chrisman and Fowler's systems-in-change model,[1] Watson's human care model,[16] and Newman's health as expanding consciousness model.[11] Some nurses use a nursing data base developed from one of these models. Likewise, some institutions have chosen Gordon's functional health patterns as a guide to structure their data base.[14] Functional health patterns serve as a guide to organize assessment data but are not derived from a conceptual framework or model that guides nursing practice. As nurses become more familiar with nursing models and test them in clinical practice, they tend to choose a model that is realistic, useful, and in concert with their values and philosophy of nursing. All these nursing models view the individual from a holistic perspective and enhance the probability of integrated assessment. However, the use of such diverse models negates the possibility of standardizing a nursing data base across the country. Moreover, none of these conceptual models of nursing were specifically developed to enhance the identification of nursing diagnoses.

Chapter 2 discusses some solutions to these problems and presents a nursing data base prototype developed from a nursing framework that enhances the identification of nursing diagnoses.

REFERENCES

1. Chrisman MK and Fowler MD: The systems-in-change model for nursing practice. In Riehl J and Roy C, editors: Conceptual models for nursing practice, New York, 1980, Appleton-Century-Crofts.
2. Dossey BM and Guzzetta CE: Person-centered caring and the nursing process. In Guzzetta CE and Dossey BM: Cardiovascular nursing: bodymind tapestry, St Louis, 1984, The CV Mosby Co.
3. Guzzetta CE: Nursing diagnosis in nursing education: effect on the profession, Heart Lung 16:629, 1987.
4. Guzzetta CE, Bunton SD, Prinkey LA, Sherer AP, and Seifert PC: Unitary person assessment tool prototype. In Dossey BM, Keegan L, Guzzetta CE, and Kolkmeier L: Holistic nursing: a handbook for practice, Rockville, Md, 1988, Aspen Publishers, Inc.
5. Guzzetta CE, Bunton SD, Prinkey LA, Sherer AP, Seifert PC: Unitary person assessment tool: easing problems with nursing diagnosis, Focus Crit Care 15:12, 1988.
6. Guzzetta CE and Dossey BM: Nursing diagnosis: framework-process-problems, Heart Lung 12:281, 1983.
7. Guzzetta CE, Dossey BM, and Kenner CV: Nursing assessment and diagnosis. In Kenner CV, Guzzetta CE, and Dossey BM: Critial care nursing: body-mind-spirit, ed 2, Boston, 1985, Little, Brown & Co, Inc.
8. Guzzetta CE and Kinney MR: Mastering the transition from medical to nursing diagnosis, Prog Cardiovasc Nurs 1:41, 1986.
9. Kenner CV, Guzzetta CE, and Dossey BM: Critical care nursing: body-mind-spirit, ed 1, Boston, 1981, Little, Brown & Co, Inc.
10. King I: Toward a theory of nursing, Boston, 1971, Little, Brown & Co, Inc.
11. Newman MA: Health as expanding consciousness, St Louis, 1986, The CV Mosby Co.
12. Orem DE: Nursing: concepts of practice, ed 3, New York, 1985, McGraw-Hill Inc.
13. Rogers M: Introduction to the theoretical basis of nursing, New York, 1969, FA Davis Co.
14. Ross L: Organizing data for nursing diagnoses using functional health patterns. In McLane AM, editor: Classification of nursing diagnoses: proceedings of the Seventh Conference (NANDA), St Louis, 1987, The CV Mosby Co.
15. Roy C: Introduction to nursing: an adaptation model, Englewood Cliffs, NJ, 1976, Prentice Hall.
16. Watson J: Nursing: human science and human care, Norwalk, Conn, 1985, Appleton-Century-Crofts.
17. Yura H and Walsh MD: Human needs and the nursing process, New York, 1983, Appleton-Century-Crofts.

CHAPTER 2

DEVELOPING A NURSING DATA BASE
PROTOTYPE FROM THE UNITARY
PERSON FRAMEWORK

CATHIE E. GUZZETTA

Applying nursing diagnoses to the clinical setting has created problems. This chapter discusses how some of these problems have been solved by the following:

■ *Developing a nursing data base prototype tool from the Unitary Person Framework and Taxonomy I that eases the identification of nursing diagnoses*

■ *Refining and testing the nursing data base prototype tool in clinical practice*

■ *Determining the patient populations and settings for which the tool is applicable*

In addition, the emphasis areas incorporated in the tool, how to use the tool, and the benefits of the prototype are explained.

OVERVIEW OF THE NURSING DATA BASE PROTOTYPE

There are various problems in using nursing diagnoses. First, nursing assessments performed using a medical data base do not provide the necessary data to support the existence of nursing diagnoses.[9] Because nurses collect only part of the data needed, a holistic assessment cannot take place. Second, although nursing leaders have recommended the use of a conceptual framework or model of nursing to guide the assessment phase,[5,10] most nursing data bases are not developed from such frameworks or models[4] because of the difficulty in translating theory into bedside practice. Third, the existence of multiple conceptual frameworks and models precludes any possibility of standardizing a nursing data base. In addition, none of the frameworks or models was specifically created to be compatible with NANDA's accepted list of nursing diagnoses.

Recognizing these problems, NANDA developed a framework for nursing diagnoses (the Unitary Person Framework) and a system to classify them (Taxonomy I). Many problems encountered with nursing diagnoses could be solved by creating a nursing data base prototype tool from NANDA's work.

Unitary Person Framework

The Unitary Person Framework was created by a NANDA subcommittee of 14 nursing theorists charged with developing a conceptual framework for nursing diagnoses. This framework is *not* Martha Rogers' Unitary Man model (see Chapter 1). Although it uses some of Rogers' concepts, the Unitary Person Framework incorporates concepts and synthesizes ideas from all members of NANDA's subcommittee.

The highest level of the Unitary Person Framework is the health of the person—the most relevant area to nursing. From this framework, a person is an open system in mutual interaction with the environment. Moreover, the person is in a process of continuous development toward increasing complexity and diversity; in other words, a person's roles, function, structure, and services can become more complex and diverse.[14] This process is observed in persons progressing through the life span and from generation to generation. Each person is also characterized by a unique pattern and organization. The uniqueness of each person's pattern and organization is manifested by nine human response patterns[14] (see box on p. 7).

In this framework, health signifies a pattern of energy exchange enhancing the integrity of the person to move towards life's potential. Each person's health is also manifested by the nine human response patterns[14] (see box).

NINE HUMAN RESPONSE PATTERNS OF THE UNITARY PERSON FRAMEWORK

Exchanging: a human response pattern involving mutual giving and receiving

Communicating: a human response pattern involving sending messages

Relating: a human response pattern involving establishing bonds

Valuing: a human response pattern involving the assigning of relative worth

Choosing: a human response pattern involving the selection of alternatives

Moving: a human response pattern involving activity

Perceiving: a human response pattern involving the reception of information

Knowing: a human response pattern involving the meaning associated with information

Feeling: a human response pattern involving the subjective awareness of information

---

From the North American Nursing Diagnosis Association, St. Louis, 1986.

These patterns reflect the whole person.[14] If nurses evaluate the nine patterns composing the whole person, they can achieve a holistic assessment, and thus can be assured that they are not omitting anything from the assessment. The nine patterns provide the practical categories for developing a holistic nursing data base. They have also been used to develop the nursing diagnosis classification system (see next section).

Taxonomy I

Taxonomy I was developed from the Unitary Person Framework and represents a new classification system for nursing diagnoses that are developed and approved by NANDA.[3,11,12] Until Taxonomy I, NANDA alphabetically organized its accepted list of nursing diagnoses. Taxonomy I was developed to replace the old system and to better classify the diagnoses.

The major categories of Taxonomy I are the human response patterns of the Unitary Person Framework. All diagnoses approved by NANDA are organized under these nine major categories (see box on pp. 8-9). The diagnoses are placed within lower-level categories, depending on their degree of specificity. First- and second-level categories tend to be more abstract (e.g., second level categories include "altered" response patterns such as "altered nutrition." An alteration is the "process or state of becoming or being made different without changing into something else."[11,12]) Third-level categories define the specific area to be assessed (e.g., cellular, immune, bowel, role perfor-

mance, or individual versus family). Fourth- and fifth-level categories are more specific in defining the particular problem (e.g., a fourth-level category is "altered systemic nutrition: more than body requirements").

Parenthetical items were added by NANDA's Taxonomy Committee to clarify the schema. Blank spaces were added to emphasize the provisional nature and incompleteness of Taxonomy I. The blank spaces and parenthetical items are areas that remain to be defined and approved by NANDA. In addition, definitions for diagnostic qualifiers were approved to provide a standardized terminology for developing new and revising old diagnoses (see box on p. 10). Taxonomy I has been endorsed by NANDA for testing, revision, and expansion.[11,12]

Taxonomy I was revised in 1988 (see Appendix I) and reflects new diagnostic categories, revised diagnostic categories, and categories in which diagnostic terms have been modified. Taxonomy II has already been developed, although it has not been formally examined, voted on, or accepted by NANDA membership.

NURSING DATA BASE PROTOTYPE: CARDIOVASCULAR ASSESSMENT TOOL

The nursing data base prototype project was an outgrowth of NANDA's work. Within the Unitary Person Framework, a nursing diagnosis is *"a judgment about the health of the unitary person based on the data collected from the nine human response patterns."*[14] If nurses are to make judgments based on data from human response patterns, *"then construction of a data base that incorporates the signs and symptoms necessary to make these judgments is not only logical but fundamental."*[7]

The challenge encountered in developing the nursing data base prototype was to translate theory into bedside, clinical practice. The concepts of the Unitary Person Framework had to be put into effect to create a data base that would be practical and realistic in measuring human response patterns. The creation of NANDA's Taxonomy I, however, provided the necessary parameters to put the theoretical concepts into practice. Because the authors' clinical area of expertise was cardiovascular critical care nursing, the prototype was developed to assess the problems of critically ill cardiovascular patients. Thus the objectives of the project were to develop a nursing data base prototype that would:[7]

1. Be based on the Unitary Person Framework
2. Be organized according to the classification schema of Taxonomy I
3. Focus on critically ill cardiovascular patients
4. Include the standards of cardiovascular nursing practice[2] and the process standards of critical care nursing[1]
5. Be tested and refined in clinical practice

Three stages of development were necessary for the

NANDA NURSING DIAGNOSIS TAXONOMY I

1. Exchanging: a human response pattern involving mutual giving and receiving
   1.1 Alterations in nutrition
       1.1.1 (Cellular)
       1.1.2 (Systemic)
           1.1.2.1 More than body requirements
           1.1.2.2 Less than body requirements
           1.1.2.3 Potential for more than body requirements
           1.1.2.4 _____
   1.2 (Alterations in physical regulation)
       1.2.1 (Immune)
           1.2.1.1 Potential for infection
           1.2.1.2 _____
       1.2.2 Alteration in body temperature
           1.2.2.1 Potential
           1.2.2.2 Hypothermia
           1.2.2.3 Hyperthermia
           1.2.2.4 Ineffective thermoregulation
           1.2.2.5 _____
   1.3 Alterations in elimination
       1.3.1 Bowel
           1.3.1.1 Constipation
           1.3.1.2 Diarrhea
           1.3.1.3 Incontinence
       1.3.2 Urinary patterns
           1.3.2.1 Incontinence
               1.3.2.1.1 Stress
               1.3.2.1.2 Reflex
               1.3.2.1.3 Urge
               1.3.2.1.4 Functional
               1.3.2.1.5 Total
           1.3.2.2 Retention
       1.3.3 (Skin)
           1.3.3.1 _____
           1.3.3.2 _____
   1.4 (Alterations in circulation)
       1.4.1 (Vascular)
           1.4.1.1 Tissue perfusion
               1.4.1.1.1 Renal
               1.4.1.1.2 Cerebral
               1.4.1.1.3 Cardiopulmonary
               1.4.1.1.4 Gastrointestinal
               1.4.1.1.5 Peripheral
           1.4.1.2 Fluid volume
               1.4.1.2.1 Excess
               1.4.1.2.2 Deficit
                   1.4.1.2.2.1 Actual
                   1.4.1.2.2.2 Potential
           1.4.1.3 _____
       1.4.2 (Cardiac)
           1.4.2.1 Decreased cardiac output
           1.4.2.2 _____
   1.5 (Alterations in oxygenation)
       1.5.1 (Respiration)
           1.5.1.1 Impaired gas exchange
           1.5.1.2 Ineffective airway clearance
           1.5.1.3 Ineffective breathing pattern
       1.5.2 _____

1.6 (Alterations in physical integrity)
    1.6.1 Potential for injury
        1.6.1.1 Potential for suffocating
        1.6.1.2 Potential for poisoning
        1.6.1.3 Potential for trauma
    1.6.2 Impairment
        1.6.2.1 Skin integrity
            1.6.2.1.1 Actual
            1.6.2.1.2 Potential
        1.6.2.2 Tissue integrity
            1.6.2.2.1 Oral mucous membrane
            1.6.2.2.2 _____
            1.6.2.2.3 _____
        1.6.2.3 _____

2. Communicating: a human response pattern involving sending messages
   2.1 Alterations in communication
       2.1.1 Verbal
           2.1.1.1 Impaired
           2.1.1.2 _____
           2.1.1.3 _____
       2.1.2 (Nonverbal)
   2.2 _____
   2.3 _____
       2.3.1 _____
       2.3.2 _____

3. Relating: a human response pattern involving establishing bonds
   3.1 (Alterations in socialization)
       3.1.1 Impaired social interaction
       3.1.2 Social isolation
       3.1.3 _____
   3.2 (Alterations in role)
       3.2.1 (Role performance)
           3.2.1.1 Parenting
               3.2.1.1.1 Actual
               3.2.1.1.2 Potential
           3.2.1.2 Sexual
               3.2.1.2.1 Dysfunction
               3.2.1.2.2 _____
               3.2.1.2.3 _____
           3.2.1.3 (Work)
       3.2.2 Family processes
       3.2.3 _____
   3.3 Altered sexuality patterns
   3.4 _____

4. Valuing: a human response pattern involving the assigning of relative worth
   4.1 Alterations in spiritual state
       4.1.1 Distress
       4.1.2 _____
       4.1.3 _____
   4.2 _____
       4.2.1 _____
       4.2.2 _____

5. Choosing: a human response pattern involving the selection of alternatives
    5.1 Alterations in coping
        5.1.1 Individual
            5.1.1.1 Ineffective
                5.1.1.1.1 Impaired adjustment
                5.1.1.1.2 _____
            5.1.1.2 _____
        5.1.2 Family
            5.1.2.1 Ineffective
                5.1.2.1.1 Disabled
                5.1.2.1.2 Compromised
            5.1.2.2 Potential for growth
            5.1.2.3 _____
        5.1.3 (Community)
    5.2 (Alterations in participation)
        5.2.1 (Individual)
            5.2.1.1 Noncompliance
            5.2.1.2 _____
            5.2.1.3 _____
        5.2.2 (Family)
        5.2.3 (Community)
6. Moving: a human response pattern involving activity
    6.1 (Alterations in activity)
        6.1.1 Physical mobility
            6.1.1.1 Impaired
            6.1.1.2 Activity intolerance
            6.1.1.3 Potential activity intolerance
            6.1.1.4 _____
        6.1.2 (Social mobility)
            6.1.2.1 _____
            6.1.2.2 _____
    6.2 (Alterations in rest)
        6.2.1 Sleep pattern disturbance
        6.2.2 _____
    6.3 (Alterations in recreation)
        6.3.1 Diversional activity
            6.3.1.1 Deficit
            6.3.1.2 _____
        6.3.2 _____
    6.4 (Alterations in activities of daily living)
        6.4.1 Home maintenance management
            6.4.1.1 Impaired
            6.4.1.2 _____
        6.4.2 Health maintenance
        6.4.3 _____
    6.5 Alterations in self-care
        6.5.1 Feeding
            6.5.1.1 Impaired swallowing
            6.5.1.2 _____
            6.5.1.3 _____
        6.5.2 Bathing/hygiene
        6.5.3 Dressing/grooming
        6.5.4 Toileting
    6.6 Altered growth and development
        6.6.1 _____
        6.6.2 _____

7. Perceiving: a human response pattern involving the reception of information
    7.1 Alterations in self-concept
        7.1.1 Disturbance in body image
        7.1.2 Disturbance in self-esteem
        7.1.3 Disturbance in personal identity
        7.1.4 _____
    7.2 Sensory/perceptual alteration
        7.2.1 Visual
            7.2.1.1 Unilateral neglect
            7.2.1.2 _____
        7.2.2 Auditory
        7.2.3 Kinesthetic
        7.2.4 Gustatory
        7.2.5 Tactile
        7.2.6 Olfactory
    7.3 (Alterations in meaningfulness)
        7.3.1 Hopelessness
        7.3.2 Powerlessness
        7.3.3 _____
8. Knowing: a human response pattern involving the meaning associated with information
    8.1 Alterations in knowledge
        8.1.1 Deficit
        8.1.2 _____
        8.1.3 _____
    8.2 (Alterations in learning)
        8.2.1 _____
        8.2.2 _____
    8.3 Alterations in thought processes
        8.3.1 (Confusion)
        8.3.2 _____
        8.3.3 _____
9. Feeling: a human response pattern involving the subjective awareness of information
    9.1 Alterations in comfort
        9.1.1 Pain
            9.1.1.1 Chronic
            9.1.1.2 (Acute)
            9.1.1.3 _____
        9.1.2 (Discomfort)
    9.2 (Alterations in emotional integrity)
        9.2.1 Anxiety
        9.2.2 Grieving
            9.2.2.1 Dysfunctional
            9.2.2.2 Anticipatory
            9.2.2.3 _____
        9.2.3 Potential for violence
        9.2.4 Fear
        9.2.5 Post trauma response
            9.2.5.1 Rape trauma syndrome
                9.2.5.1.1 Rape trauma
                9.2.5.1.2 Compound reaction
                9.2.5.1.3 Silent reaction
            9.2.5.2 _____
        9.2.6 _____
        9.2.7 _____
    9.3 _____

From the North American Nursing Diagnosis Association, St. Louis, 1986.

NANDA DIAGNOSIS QUALIFIERS

CATEGORY 1

Actual: existing at the present moment; existing in reality

Potential: can, but has not yet, come into being; possible

CATEGORY 2

Ineffective: not producing the desired effect; not capable of performing satisfactorily

Decreased: smaller, lessened; diminished; lesser in size, amount, or degree

Increased: greater in size, amount or degree; larger, enlarged

Impaired: made worse, weakened; damaged, reduced, deteriorated

Depleted: emptied wholly or partially; exhausted of

Deficient: inadequate in amount, quality, or degree; defective; not sufficient; incomplete

Excessive: characterized by an amount or quantity that is greater than necessary, desirable, or usable

Dysfunctional: abnormal; impaired or incompletely functioning

Disturbed: agitated, interrupted, interfered with

Acute: severe but of short duration

Chronic: lasting a long time; recurring; habitual; constant

Intermittent: stopping and starting again at intervals; periodic; cyclic

---

From the North American Nursing Diagnosis Association, St. Louis, 1986.

Cardiovascular Assessment Tool. During the first stage, the nine human response patterns were used as the framework or skeleton for the prototype (Fig. 2-1). The order of the nine human response patterns was rearranged to allow pertinent historical data to be collected before specific physiologic data. Thus the "exchanging pattern" normally presented first in Taxonomy I was moved to a latter part of the tool.

In the second stage, the *Standards of Cardiovascular Nursing Practice*[2] and the process *Standards for Nursing Care of the Critically Ill*[1] were incorporated into the appropriate areas of the tool's skeleton (Fig. 2-2) These standards of practice serve as guides for the nurse when providing and evaluating the quality of nursing care.

During the third stage, specific assessment variables (signs and symptoms) pertinent to most of the nursing diagnoses were included (Fig. 2-3). When available, NANDA's defining characteristics were used.[13]

The tool clusters assessment variables for a particular

patient problem so a judgment can be formulated about whether the problem actually exists. Thus, for each category on the tool, subjective variables are included, followed by objective variables that need to be assessed and synthesized.

Detailed assessment variables necessary to adequately evaluate critically ill cardiovascular patients were also added. A holistic assessment includes the collection of detailed data from *all* the human response patterns. Thus a holistic assessment incorporates detailed physiologic data.[8] The "exchanging pattern," for example, reflects complex physiologic data and is as important to a thorough assessment as the other response patterns.[7]

The lower-level categories in the "exchanging pattern" were rearranged to provide a logical head-to-toe assessment. Furthermore, assessment variables were organized to prevent repetition of information. The vascular and cardiac categories (under altered circulation) were combined because, from a clinical viewpoint, it was not logical to separate them. Other assessment variables were added because they were highly relevant to the patient population being assessed (e.g., knowledge and perception of coronary artery disease risk factors). Some lower-level variables were deleted because they were not relevant for cardiovascular patients (e.g., potential for violence). However, the data base does offer enough flexibility to uncover such diagnoses if the signs and symptoms are present.

Varying levels of abstractness are found in the assessment variables in the tool. To minimize the tool's length, not all possible assessment variables related to each diagnosis are included. In many cases, summary assessment variables are provided. Questions and physical assessment parameters that should be used to elicit appropriate data are presented in Chapter 3. To facilitate formulation of appropriate nursing diagnoses, diagnoses associated with the variables have been placed in the right-hand column of the tool (see section on how to use the tool).

Fig. 2-3 shows the outcome of the nursing data base prototype, the Cardiovascular Assessment Tool. To fully explain the development of the data base, stars and brackets have been inserted in the tool in this chapter (Fig. 2-3). Items with brackets indicate diagnoses added by NANDA's Taxonomy Committee to enhance the clarity of the subcategories under a particular pattern. These items have not been formally accepted by NANDA's membership. Items with brackets and stars pertain to diagnoses informally added to Taxonomy II but not formally presented to or voted on by the NANDA membership. Those items have been included in the data base, however, because they were judged to be clinically useful to a holistic assessment.

After the Cardiovascular Assessment Tool was developed, many questions about how it might be adapted for other patient populations were received. Chapters 5 to 26 present other assessment tools, all developed from this prototype.

REFINING AND TESTING THE NURSING DATA BASE PROTOTYPE IN CLINICAL PRACTICE

After the Cardiovascular Assessment Tool was developed, it was clinically refined and tested on 10 critically ill cardiovascular patients by nurse experts and clinical nurse specialists in cardiovascular disease. The testing evaluated the adequacy of the tool in terms of flow, space for recording data, and completeness of assessment variables. Based on the results of the testing, the tool was revised.

The tools in this book are *clinical* rather than *research* tools. Research tools are measurement tools and techniques used to evaluate the results of scientific research. Reliability and validity testing must be conducted on research tools before the results from a study can be accepted. The *reliability* of a research tool refers to how consistently or dependably it measures what it was designed to measure. Its *validity* refers to the degree to which it measures what it is supposed to measure.

All tools in this book have been clinically tested and refined by nurse experts across the country. The term *clinically tested,* however, does not imply strict reliability and validity testing, as would be done with research tools. Most clinical assessment tools used by nurses have probably never undergone rigorous testing.

No attempts were made to obtain reliability estimates of any of the tools in this book because they were developed primarily as clinical tools and not as tools to evaluate scientific research. Reliability testing of a tool could be accomplished, however, through interrater reliability testing, wherein two nurse experts simultaneously assess the same patient and then independently record the data on the tool. The findings from both tools are compared to determine the percent agreement regarding the data recorded and the nursing diagnoses identified. This process is performed on the simultaneous testing of at least 10 patients, and the scores are averaged. If the tool is reliable, the recordings will be comparable, and the averaged percent agreement scores will be high (i.e., >70%). The equivalence of the results will indicate the reliability of the tool.

Validity testing of the tools has been done by panels of content experts (e.g., content validity). A panel was identified for each tool, and each panel reviewed, critiqued, and made recommendations for changing its tool and clinically tested it. Such validity testing was done to ensure that each tool adequately gauged what it was supposed to measure. Nurses who use and revise the tools in practice will strengthen the tools' validity.

PATIENT POPULATION AND SETTING

The Cardiovascular Assessment Tool was developed to assess the needs and problems of adult cardiovascular patients. It is designed for use in any critical care unit where cardiovascular patients are admitted (e.g., coronary care units, open heart surgical intensive care units). The tool is intended for use with stable adult cardiovascular patients but can also be used with unstable patients. When assessing unstable patients, however, a rapid evaluation of the patient according to the ABCs of basic life support and a rapid head-to-toe assessment takes precedence. Data for this quick evaluation are found under the "exchanging pattern," beginning with oxygenation and circulation. (During a rapid evaluation of the patient, the nurse assesses the patient's airway, breathing, and circulatory status and does not follow the sequential ordering under the "exchanging pattern"). The other response patterns (i.e., "communicating," "valuing," and "relating") can then be assessed when the patient has become more stable.

If the critically ill cardiovascular patient is admitted to a critical care unit with more than one major medical diagnosis (e.g., a cardiovascular problem and a metabolic problem), the Cardiovascular Assessment Tool can still be used to assess this patient. All tools in this book that are intended for adults, contain enough information to ensure an adequate assessment for any type of adult patient. However, to achieve the most complete assessment, the tool most appropriate for the patient's major presenting problem should be used because each tool contains detailed assessment variables pertaining to its focus area. The neonatal, pediatric, and adolescent tools in this book, however, are very different from the other adult tools and cannot be used interchangeably unless major adaptations are made (see Chapter 4). Chapters 5 to 26 describe the specific population and setting intended for the use of each tool.

CARDIOVASCULAR EMPHASIS AREAS

Critically ill cardiovascular patients have unique problems and needs, so the Cardiovascular Assessment Tool includes assessment variables related to prevalent problems among these patients within each of the human response patterns of the Unitary Person Framework. Table 2-1 contains the assessment areas of greatest concern when evaluating cardiovascular patients. These are *emphasis areas.* Emphasis areas pertinent to each tool are outlined in the chapter describing the use of that tool. For example, Chapter 5, which describes the Pulmonary Assessment Tool, includes a table outlining pulmonary emphasis areas.

HOW TO USE THE TOOL

To use the Cardiovascular Assessment Tool effectively, nurses must be thoroughly familiar with the Unitary Person Framework and Taxonomy I (see the previous sections). Nurses must also realize that the Cardiovascular Assessment Tool is different from most conventional assessment tools. As a result, they may encounter some initial difficulty in using the tool because it was not designed

Table 2-1

Cardiovascular emphasis areas

Pattern	Emphasis areas to determine
Communicating	Whether the patient is intubated
	Speech impairment
Valuing	Spiritual despair related to illness
	Family members' cultural practices related to illness
Relating	Support systems
	Physical/mental energy expenditures related to job, activities at home, and volunteer work
	Effects of illness related to roles and sexual relationships
Knowing	Knowledge of current health status, illness, and therapy
	Knowledge/perception of coronary artery disease and associated risk factors
	Knowledge/perception of illness/test/ surgery
	Expectations of therapy
	Misconceptions regarding illness/ therapy
	Readiness to learn
Feeling	Comprehensive data related to cardiovascular pain
	Recent stressful life events
	Verbalization and physical manifestations related to grief, anxiety, fear, anger, guilt, shame, sadness
Moving	Effects of illness on daily activities
	Effects of illness on ability to independently perform activities of daily living
	Effects of illness on environmental and home maintenance
Perceiving	Effects of illness/surgery on self-concept
	Perceived loss of control
Exchanging	Glasgow Coma Scale score
	Status of cardiovascular and hemodynamic variables
	Status of respiratory variables and ventilatory equipment
	Status of skin/tissue integrity
	Changes in nutritional status, elimination, and weight gain/loss
Choosing	Patient's and family's problem-solving methods
	Patient's and family's methods of dealing with stress
	Compliance with past health care regimen
	Willingness to comply with future health care regimen
	Patient's decision-making ability

to follow the organization or content of a traditional medical data base. The tool does not elicit information that solely reflects medical patterns. Rather, this tool is used to elicit data about holistic patterns in ways not traditionally used by nurses. It provides a new method of collecting and synthesizing data. Most important, this tool represents a nursing data base developed from a nursing framework that permits a holistic assessment to take place so nursing diagnoses can be identified.

Although most nurses probably agree that a holistic nursing data base is desirable, changing traditional assessment methods is not an easy task. For this reason, a trial usage period is recommended before conclusions regarding the usefulness of the tool are drawn. During this period, assessment of 10 critically ill cardiovascular patients using the Cardiovascular Assessment Tool is recommended.

Throughout the trial period, nurses will become familiar and more comfortable with the tool's organization and data-collection methods. With experience, they will become accustomed to new ways of clustering and processing information. With continued use, the time necessary to complete the tool will be reduced. Most important, the nurses' ability to identify appropriate signs and symptoms when using the tool will be enhanced. Finally, nurses using this tool will discover that nursing diagnoses are easily identified.

It is not necessary to complete this tool in one session. Nurses can designate priority sections that must be completed during the initial assessment. Other sections can be completed later, within a time frame acceptable to the institution. For example, the section dealing with sexuality (i.e., under the "relating pattern" regarding sexual relationships) is not a major priority when initially assessing a critically ill cardiovascular patient. Even though this section is found on the first page of the tool, the information related to it may be more appropriately assessed at a later time.

When assessing for specific signs and symptoms indicating a particular diagnosis, nurses should circle the diagnosis in the right-hand column of the tool when deviations from normal are found. A circled diagnosis does not necessarily confirm the existence of a problem but simply alerts health care givers to a possible problem or alteration. This tool is intended as a primary assessment; if a particular problem is suspected, a more complete evaluation or a secondary assessment based on the critical defining characteristics of the specific diagnosis under consideration will need to be done.

Certain signs and symptoms can indicate a number of diagnoses. For example, tachycardia can indicate altered cardiac output or anxiety. To avoid unnecessary repetition of assessment parameters, variables are arranged with the diagnosis most likely to result from the data assessed. However, data to support a specific diagnosis may occasionally be found in other patterns (i.e., tachycardia identified under the "exchanging pattern" may support the diagnosis of anxiety found under the "feeling pattern"). Therefore synthesis of all data is essential.

Some diagnoses are repeated several times in the right-hand column. These repetitions occur only within the appropriate response pattern and are designed for the convenience of identifying certain data directly with a corresponding nursing diagnosis. These diagnoses are not absolute but are intended to focus thinking and direct more detailed attention to a possible problem.

After completing the assessment, nurses should scan the circled problems, synthesize the data to determine whether other clusters of signs and symptoms also support the existence of a particular problem, and make a decision as to whether the actual diagnosis is present. If a potential problem rather than an acutal problem is suspected, write *potential* or *P* next to the diagnosis before circling it.

Nurses should not feel limited, however, by the diagnoses appearing in the column because other, unlisted diagnoses related to data collected may exist. Nurses should also note that the accepted list of nursing diagnoses does not consist of all possible problems encountered and dealt with by nurses. Many clinical problems are missing from the list. Because the list is incomplete, some data gathered from the assessment will not support the existence of one of NANDA's accepted diagnoses. In such a case, synthesize the data and label the new problem identified. Thus, if the patient exhibits observable signs and symptoms indicating a new diagnosis, word the problem concisely and identify the probable cause. If the new diagnosis seems clinically useful in defining a patient problem, submit it to NANDA for consideration to be added to Taxonomy I.

After synthesizing data, nurses might judge that all the nursing diagnoses circled in the right-hand column do not actually exist but that they indicate clusters of signs and symptoms pinpointing a more global nursing diagnosis. The data identified for fear and social isolation, when synthesized, for example, may actually support the diagnosis of altered self-concept related to effects of chronic illness. Thus, all diagnoses initially circled in the right-hand column may not appear on the problem list at the end of the tool.

After formulating a judgment about which problems actually exist, the nursing diagnoses and probable etiologies should be written on the nursing diagnosis/problem list at the end of the tool. The diagnoses should be prioritized, with the most critical diagnoses first. If a long list of nursing diagnoses is identified, nurses should not feel that they must solve all problems immediately, particularly if contact with the patient is short. Patient outcomes, outcome criteria, a plan for intervention, and a method of evaluating the outcome criteria should be identified for critical nursing diagnoses. The diagnoses judged not to be as crit-

ical can be considered at a later date or can be referred to other health team members for assistance (e.g., referral to the dietitian for a patient with a diagnosis of altered nutrition: more than body requirements).

The Cardiovascular Assessment Tool is not intended to be the standardized and final format for assessing critically ill cardiovascular patients. An assessment tool must meet the needs of individual institutions and the nurses using it. It is simply a working demonstration tool expected to be changed and revised by nurses in clinical practice. Further evaluation and refinement are necessary before adopting the tool for use within an institution. Nurses interested in changing, revising, and adopting this tool to a specific clinical setting should refer to Chapter 4. Chapter 4 also includes a completed version of the Cardiovascular Assessment Tool based on a case study. The Cardiovascular Assessment Tool and all tools found in Chapters 5 to 26 can also be reduced in length or adapted as screening tools for rapid patient evaluation (see Chapter 4).

HOW TO ELICIT APPROPRIATE DATA

Because the Unitary Person Framework and the Cardiovascular Assessment Tool contain some terminology that may be unfamiliar to nurses, general focus questions and parameters were developed and refined to elicit appropriate information when assessing cardiovascular patients. Nurses unfamiliar with the variables that should be assessed for any section of the tool should refer to Chapter 3.

Many of the questions and parameters in Chapter 3 are generic areas applicable to all tools in the book. For example, the same focus question can be used when collecting data related to cultural orientation (under the "valuing pattern") for any tool in this book. However, questions and parameters addressing the special concerns of the patient population being assessed have been developed for each tool. For example, in the Gerontologic Assessment Tool (see Chapter 23), specific gerontologic focus questions and parameters emphasizing the unique problems of the elderly are outlined (e.g., under "exchanging pattern," a focus question was added to assess the patient's history of falls, accidents, and injuries). Focus questions and parameters are included in each chapter to assist the nurse in eliciting the necessary data to comprehensively assess patients' problems.

BENEFITS OF THE NURSING DATA BASE PROTOTYPE DEVELOPED FROM THE UNITARY PERSON FRAMEWORK

There are many benefits of using the prototype or any tool in this book. Because the data measure human response patterns, they are pertinent to nursing diagnoses and are collected from a holistic and nursing point of view. The tools permit evaluation of specific signs and symptoms to assist in validating a diagnosis. When the tools are used in practice, the data are so rich that nursing diagnoses appear to "fall out" after the assessment. Continued use of these tools will be beneficial in easing problems with nursing diagnoses and in refining the Unitary Person Framework and Taxonomy I. Although the tools differ because they were developed to assess the unique needs of particular patient groups, they are all based on NANDA's Unitary Person Framework and Taxonomy I. Thus, the theory, process, structure, and outcome of the tools are the same, thereby offering a model for the standardization of nursing data bases across the country. The authors invite correspondence related to the use or further refinement of this work.*

REFERENCES

1. American Association of Critical-Care Nurses: Standards for nursing care of the critically ill, Reston, Va, 1981, Reston Publishing Co.
2. American Nurses' Association Division of Medical-Surgical Nursing Practice and American Heart Association Council on Cardiovascular Nursing: Standards of cardiovascular nursing practice, Kansas City, Mo, 1981, American Nurses' Association.
3. Aydelotte MK and Peterson KH: Keynote address: nursing taxonomics—state of the art. In McLane AM, editor: Classification of nursing diagnoses: proceedings of the Seventh Conference (NANDA), St Louis, 1987, The CV Mosby Co.
4. Dossey BM and Guzzetta CE: Person-centered caring and the nursing process. In Guzzetta CE and Dossey BM: Cardiovascular nursing: bodymind tapestry, St Louis, 1984, The CV Mosby Co.
5. Guzzetta CE: Nursing diagnosis in nursing education: effect on the profession, Heart Lung 16:629, 1987.
6. Guzzetta CE, Bunton SD, Prinkey LA, Sherer AP, and Seifert PC: Unitary person assessment tool prototype. In Dossey BM, Keegan L, Guzzetta CE, and Kolkmeier L: Holistic nursing: a handbook for practice, Rockville, Md, 1988, Aspen Publishers.
7. Guzzetta CE, Bunton SD, Prinkey LA, Sherer AP, and Seifert PC: Unitary person assessment tool: easing problems with nursing diagnosis, Focus Crit Care 15:12, 1988.
8. Guzzetta CE and Dossey BM: Nursing diagnosis: framework-process-problems, Heart Lung 12:281, 1983.
9. Guzzetta CE, Dossey BM, and Kenner CV: Nursing assessment and diagnosis. In Kenner CV, Guzzetta CE, and Dossey BM: Critical care nursing: body-mind-spirit, ed. 2, Boston, 1985, Little, Brown & Co.
10. Guzzetta CE and Kinney MR: Mastering the transition from medical to nursing diagnosis, Prog Cardiovasc Nurs 1:41, 1986.
11. Kritek PB: Report of the group work on taxonomics. In Kim MJ, McFarland GK, and McLane AM, editors: Classification of nursing diagnoses: proceedings of the Fifth Conference (NANDA), St Louis, 1984, The CV Mosby Co.
12. Kritek PB: Development of a taxonomic structure for nursing diagnoses: a review and update. In Hurley M, editor: Classification of nursing diagnoses: proceedings of the Sixth Conference (NANDA), St Louis, 1986, The CV Mosby Co.
13. McLane AM, editor: Classification of nursing diagnoses: proceedings of the Seventh Conference (NANDA), St Louis, 1987, The CV Mosby Co.
14. Roy C: Framework for classification systems development: progress and issues. In Kim MJ, McFarland GK, and McLane AM, editors: Classification of nursing diagnoses: proceedings of the Fifth Conference (NANDA), St Louis, 1984, The CV Mosby Co.

*Direct correspondence to Anita P. Sherer, RN, MSN, CCRN, 2063 Cooper Road, Graham, NC 27253.

NURSING DATA BASE PROTOTYPE (STAGE I)

Name _____ Age _____ Sex _____

Address _____ Telephone _____

Significant other _____ Telephone _____

Date of admission _____ Medical diagnosis _____

Allergies _____

Nursing Diagnosis
(Potential or Altered)

COMMUNICATING ▪ A pattern involving sending messages

Communication
   Verbal
   Nonverbal

VALUING ▪ A pattern involving the assigning of relative worth

Spiritual state
   Distress
   Despair

RELATING ▪ A pattern involving establishing bonds

Role performance
   Parenting
   Sexual dysfunction
   Work
   Family
   Social/leisure
Family processes

Sexuality patterns

Impaired social interaction
Social isolation
Social withdrawal

Fig. 2-1

NURSING DATA BASE PROTOTYPE (STAGE II)

Name _____ Age _____ Sex _____
Address _____ Telephone _____
Significant other _____ Telephone _____
Date of admission _____ Medical diagnosis _____
Allergies _____

Nursing Diagnosis
(Potential or Altered)

COMMUNICATING ▪ A pattern involving sending messages
Read, write, understand English (circle) _____ Communication
Other languages _____   Verbal
  Nonverbal

VALUING ▪ A pattern involving the assigning of relative worth
Religious preference _____ Spiritual state
Cultural orientation _____   Distress
  Despair

RELATING ▪ A pattern involving establishing bonds
Role
  Marital status _____ Role performance
  Age & health of significant other _____   Parenting
  _____   Sexual dysfunction
  _____   Work
Number of children _____ Ages _____   Family
  Financial support _____   Social/leisure
  Occupation _____ Family processes
    Job satisfaction/concerns _____
    Physical/mental energy expenditures _____ Sexuality patterns

Socialization
  Quality of relationships with others _____ Impaired social interaction
    Patient's description _____
    Significant others' descriptions _____ Social isolation
    Staff observations _____ Social withdrawal

Fig. 2-2

NURSING DATA BASE PROTOTYPE (STAGE III):
CARDIOVASCULAR ASSESSMENT TOOL

Name _____ Age _____ Sex _____
Address _____ Telephone _____
Significant other _____ Telephone _____
Date of admission _____ Medical diagnosis _____
Allergies _____

Nursing Diagnosis
(Potential or Altered)

COMMUNICATING ▪ A pattern involving sending messages
Read, write, understand English (circle) _____ Communication
Other languages _____   Verbal
Intubated _____ Speech impaired _____   Nonverbal
Alternate form of communication _____

VALUING ▪ A pattern involving the assigning of relative worth
Religious preference _____ Spiritual state
Important religious practices _____   Distress
Spiritual concerns _____   [Despair]*
Cultural orientation _____
Cultural practices _____

RELATING ▪ A pattern involving establishing bonds
Role
　Marital status _____ [Role performance]
　Age & health of significant other _____   Parenting
　_____   Sexual dysfunction
　Number of children _____ Ages _____   [Work]
　Role in home _____   [Family]*
　Financial support _____   [Social/leisure]*
　Occupation _____ Family processes
　　Job satisfaction/concerns _____
　　Physical/mental energy expenditures _____
　Sexual relationships (satisfactory/unsatisfactory) _____ Sexuality patterns
　　Physical difficulties/effects of illness related to sex _____
　　_____

Socialization
　Quality of relationships with others _____ Impaired social interaction
　　Patient's description _____
　　Significant others' descriptions _____
　　Staff observations _____
　Verbalizes feelings of being alone _____ Social isolation
　　Attributed to _____ [Social withdrawal]*

KNOWING ▪ A pattern involving the meaning associated with information
Current health problems _____
_____
Previous illnesses/hospitalizations/surgeries _____
_____
_____

Fig. 2-3

Continued.

History of the following problems: Knowledge deficit
   Heart _____
   Peripheral vascular _____
   Lung _____
   Liver _____ Kidney _____
   Cerebrovascular _____ Rheumatic fever _____
   Thyroid _____ Other _____
   Current medications _____

Risk factors   Present   Perceptions/knowledge of
  1. Hypertension   _____   _____
  2. Hyperlipidemia   _____   _____
  3. Smoking   _____   _____
  4. Obesity   _____   _____
  5. Diabetes   _____   _____
  6. Sedentary living   _____   _____
  7. Stress   _____   _____
  8. Alcohol use   _____   _____
  9. Oral contraceptives _____   _____
 10. Family history _____
_____

Perception/knowledge of illness/tests/surgery _____
_____

Expectations of therapy _____
Misconceptions _____
Readiness to learn _____
   Requests information concerning _____
   Educational level _____   Thought processes
   Learning impeded by _____

[Orientation]*
Level of alertness _____   [Orientation]*
Orientation: Person _____ Place _____ Time _____   [Confusion]*
Appropriate behavior/communication _____

[Memory]*
Memory intact: Yes _____ No _____ Recent _____ Remote _____   [Memory]*

FEELING ▪ A pattern involving the subjective awareness of information
Comfort
   Pain/discomfort: Yes _____ No _____   Comfort
      Onset _____ Duration _____
      Location _____ Quality _____ Radiation _____   Pain/chronic
      Associated factors _____   Pain/acute
      Aggravating factors _____   Discomfort
      Alleviating factors _____

[Emotional Integrity/States]
Recent stressful life events _____   Grieving
_____   Anxiety
Verbalizes feelings of _____   Fear
   Source _____   [Anger]*
_____   [Guilt]*
   Physical manifestations _____   [Shame]*
_____   [Sadness]*

Fig. 2-3, cont'd

MOVING ▪ A pattern involving activity
[Activity]
History of physical disability _____ Impaired physical mobility
_____ Activity intolerance
Limitations in daily activities _____
_____
Verbal report of fatigue/weakness _____
Exercise habits _____

[Rest]
Hours slept/night _____ Feels rested: Yes _____ No _____ Sleep pattern disturbances
Sleep aids (pillows, meds, food) _____ [Hypersomnia]*
Difficulty falling/remaining asleep _____ [Insomnia]*
 [Nightmares]*

[Recreation]
Leisure activities _____ Deficit in diversional activity
Social activities _____

[Environmental Maintenance]*
Home maintenance management Impaired home maintenance
 Size & arrangement of home (stairs, bathroom) _____ management
 _____ Safety needs _____ [Safety hazards]*
 Home responsibilities _____
_____

[Health Maintenance]*
Health insurance _____ Health maintenance
Regular physical checkups _____

Self-Care
Ability to perform ADLs: Independent _____ Dependent _____ Self-care
Specify deficits _____ Feeding
Discharge planning needs _____ Bathing/hygiene
 Dressing/grooming
 Toileting

PERCEIVING ▪ A pattern involving the reception of information
Self-Concept
Patient's description of self _____ Self-concept
Effects of illness/surgery on self-concept _____ Body image
_____ Self-esteem
 Personal identity

[Meaningfulness]
Verbalizes hopelessness _____ Hopelessness
Verbalizes/perceives loss of control _____ Powerlessness

Sensory/Perception Sensory/perception
History of restricted environment _____
Vision impaired _____ Glasses _____ Visual
Auditory impaired _____ Hearing aid _____ Auditory
Kinesthetics impaired _____ Kinesthetic
Gustatory impaired _____ Gustatory
Tactile impaired _____ Tactile
Olfactory impaired _____ Olfactory
Reflexes: Biceps R _____ L _____ Triceps R _____ L _____
  Brachioradialis R _____ L _____ Knee R _____ L _____
  Ankle   R _____ L _____ Plantar R _____ L _____

Fig. 2-3, cont'd

Continued.

EXCHANGING ▪ A pattern involving mutual giving and receiving

[Circulation]

Cerebral

Neurologic changes/symptoms _____ Cerebral tissue perfusion

Pupils	Eye Opening
L 2 3 4 5 6 mm	None (1)
R 2 3 4 5 6 mm	To pain (2)
Reaction: Brisk _____	To speech (3)
Sluggish _____ Nonreactive _____	Spontaneous (4)

Fluid volume
   Deficit
   Excess

Best Verbal	Best Motor
No sound (1)	Flaccid (1)
Incomprehensible sound (2)	Extensor response (2)
Inappropriate words (3)	Flexor response (3)
Confused conversation (4)	Semipurposeful (4)
Oriented (5)	Localized to pain (5)
	Obeys commands (6)

Cardiac output

Glasgow Coma Scale total _____

Cardiac

PMI _____ Pacemaker _____ Cardiopulmonary tissue

Apical rate & rhythm _____ perfusion

Heart sounds/murmurs _____

Dysrhythmias _____ Fluid volume

BP:	Sitting	Lying	Standing	Deficit
	R ___ L ___	R ___ L ___	R ___ L ___	Excess

A-Line reading _____

Cardiac index _____ Cardiac output _____ Cardiac output

CVP _____ PAP _____ PCWP _____

IV fluids _____

IV cardiac medications _____

_____

Serum enzymes _____

Peripheral   Peripheral tissue perfusion

Jugular venous distention R _____ L _____

Pulses: A = absent   B = bruits   D = doppler
     +3 = bounding   +2 = palpable   +1 = faintly palpable

Carotid R ___ L ___	Popliteal R ___ L ___	
Brachial R ___ L ___	Posterior tibial R ___ L ___	Fluid volume
Radial R ___ L ___	Dorsalis pedis R ___ L ___	Deficit
Femoral R ___ L ___		Excess

Skin temp _____ Color _____

Capillary refill _____ Clubbing _____ Cardiac output

Edema _____

[Physical Integrity]

Tissue integrity _____ Impaired tissue integrity

Skin integrity _____ Impaired skin integrity

Rashes _____ Lesions _____

Petechiae _____ Bruises _____

Abrasions _____ Surgical incisions _____

Other _____

Fig. 2-3, cont'd

[Oxygenation]
 Complaints of dyspnea _____ Precipitated by _____
 Orthopnea _____
 Rate _____ Rhythm _____ Depth _____   Ineffective breathing patterns
 Labored/unlabored (circle) Use of accessory muscles _____   Ineffective airway clearance
 Chest expansion _____ Splinting _____   Impaired gas exchange
 Cough: productive/nonproductive _____
 Sputum: Color _____ Amount _____ Consistency _____
 Breath sounds _____
 Arterial blood gases _____
 Oxygen percent and device _____
 Ventilator _____

[Physical Regulation]   Infection
 Immune   Hypothermia
  Lymph nodes enlarged _____ Location _____   Hyperthermia
  WBC count _____ Differential _____   Body temperature
  Temperature _____ Route _____   Ineffective thermoregulation

Nutrition   Nutrition
 Eating patterns
  Number of meals per day _____
  Special diet _____
  Where eaten _____
  Food preferences/intolerances _____
  Food allergies _____
  Caffeine intake (coffee, tea, soft drinks)

  _____
  Appetite changes _____
  Nausea/vomiting _____
 Condition of mouth/throat _____

 _____   Oral mucous membrane
 Height _____ Weight _____ Ideal body weight _____   More than body
                                                                            requirements
 Current therapy   Less than body requirements
  NPO _____ NG suction _____
  Tube feeding _____
  TPN _____
 Labs
  Na _____ K _____ CL _____ Glucose _____
  Cholesterol _____ Triglycerides _____ Fasting _____
  Hct _____ Hgb _____

Elimination
 Gastrointestinal/bowel   Bowel elimination
  Usual bowel habits _____   Constipation
  Alterations from normal _____   Diarrhea
  Abdominal physical examination _____   Incontinence
                                                                            GI tissue perfusion

 Renal/Urinary
  Usual urinary pattern _____   Urinary elimination
  Alterations from normal _____   Incontinence
  Color _____ Catheter _____   Retention
  Urine output: 24 hour _____ Average hourly _____   Renal tissue perfusion
  Bladder distention _____
  BUN _____ Creatinine _____ Specific gravity _____
  Urine studies _____

Fig. 2-3, cont'd

Continued.

CHOOSING ▪ A pattern involving the selection of alternatives
Coping

Patient's usual problem-solving methods _____   Ineffective individual coping
_____   Ineffective family coping

Family's usual problem-solving methods _____
_____

Patient's method of dealing with stress _____
_____

Family's method of dealing with stress _____
_____

Patient's affect _____
Physical manifestations _____
Support systems available _____
_____

[Participation]

Compliance with past/current health care regimens _____   Noncompliance
_____   [Ineffective participation]*

Willingness to comply with future health care regimen _____
_____

*[Judgment]**

Decision-making ability   [Judgment]*
    Patient's perspective _____   [Indecisiveness]*
    Others' perspectives _____

Prioritized nursing diagnosis/problem list

1. _____
2. _____
3. _____
4. _____
5. _____

Signature _____   Date _____

[ ] = Added by NANDA's Taxonomy Committee.
[ ]* = Added by authors from Taxonomy II. See also text p. 10.

Fig. 2-3, cont'd

CHAPTER 3

GENERAL FOCUS QUESTIONS
AND PARAMETERS FOR ELICITING
APPROPRIATE DATA

CATHIE E. GUZZETTA

This chapter provides general focus questions and parameters that can be used to elicit data when using the Cardiovascular Assessment Tool. It also provides generic information that can be applied to most of the other tools in this book. This chapter includes:

- *The way to use the general focus questions and parameters*
- *Suggested questions to ask or parameters to evaluate when assessing the nine human response patterns using the Cardiovascular Assessment Tool*
- *Ways to apply the questions and parameters*

HOW TO USE THE GENERAL FOCUS QUESTIONS AND PARAMETERS

The Unitary Person Framework and the Cardiovascular Assessment Tool contain terminology that may be unfamiliar to nurses. Focus questions and parameters were developed and refined to assist the nurse in directing a line of questioning. The questions and parameters follow the content of the tool and were developed to clarify assessment variables when eliciting data. These questions are not all inclusive, and nurses should not feel confined by them. There are many other ways to elicit the appropriate information based on the patient's situation and condition and the skill of the nurse.

Many of the questions and parameters are generic areas applicable to all the tools. For example, the alternate form of communication variable under the "communicating pattern" in the Cardiovascular Assessment Tool is a generic variable found in most tools in the book. To elicit the necessary information about this variable, nurses should refer to the focus questions and parameters in this chapter. Thus when using any of the assessment tools, nurses may refer to this chapter for these generic questions and parameters.

Specific questions and parameters that address the special concerns of the patient population being assessed have also been developed for each tool found in Chapters 5 to 26. For example, in Chapter 6, which includes the Neurologic Assessment Tool, specific neurologic focus questions and parameters emphasizing the unique problems of the neurologic patient are presented (e.g., under the "communicating pattern," focus questions were added to assess whether the patient demonstrates expressive or receptive aphasia). Focus questions and parameters are included in each chapter to assist in eliciting the necessary data to assess unique variables.

Performing a holistic assessment demands clustering and synthesizing the subjective and objective data reflecting the patient's psychophysiologic responses to illness. Thus, for all tools in this book, the assessment variables designed to elicit information about a particular problem are clustered to assist the nurse in synthesizing the data necessary to judge whether a specific patient problem actually exists. For all tools in this book, subjective variables, followed by the appropriate objective variables, are included under each tool's category. For recording subjective data, it is recommended that information taken verbatim from the patient's family or significant other should be placed in quotation marks with the name or relationship of the person giving the information included in parentheses (e.g., "I have always trusted his judgment" [wife]). All data not in quotation marks can be assumed to be the observation or interpretation of the nurse performing the assessment.

The remainder of this chapter presents suggested questions to ask or parameters to evaluate when assessing the patient's nine human response patterns using the Cardiovascular Assessment Tool.

COMMUNICATING PATTERN FOCUS QUESTIONS AND PARAMETERS
Read, write, understand English

"Do you have any difficulty reading or writing English? Do you have any difficulty understanding English? Speaking English? How well?" Does the patient have a physiologic reason for not understanding English (i.e., reduced circulation to the brain, stroke, brain tumor, oral anatomic defect)? Does the patient have a psychologic reason (i.e., psychosis, lack of stimuli)?

Other languages

"What language do you speak at home? Most of the day? Do you speak any other languages?" Is anyone available to act as the patient's interpreter or provide flash cards?

Intubated

Is the patient intubated? How long has the patient been intubated?

Speech impaired

Is the patient able to speak? Does the patient have a tracheostomy or laryngectomy? Does the patient have a talking tracheostomy? Use esophageal talking? Does the patient stutter or have slurred speech? Does the patient have difficulty speaking because of shortness of breath? Does the patient have facial paralysis? Is the patient able to modulate speech? Is the patient able to find words, name words, identify objects, and speak in sentences?[1,4]

Alternate form of communication

Does the patient have difficulty with phonation? What other forms of communication does the patient use (i.e., sign language, writing, typewriter, computer, or sign board)?[4]

VALUING PATTERN FOCUS QUESTIONS AND PARAMETERS
Religious preference

"What is your religion? Do you practice your religion? Is religion important to you? Do your religious practices provide support for you?"

Important religious practices

"Is it important for you to be able to attend your church or synagogue services? Would you like to talk to a priest, rabbi, or minister? What religious items are important for you to have while you are here (e.g., Bible, rosary, or candles)? Do your religious beliefs and practices affect how you will be treated for your illness? Are there any treatments that are forbidden by your religion? During your hospitalization, how can we assist you to maintain religious practices important to you?"

Spiritual concerns

Does the patient show excessive concern for the meaning of life or death? Does the patient express anger toward God? Inner conflicts about beliefs? Concern about relationship with God? Inability to decide whether to participate in regular religious practices? Does the patient question the meaning of suffering or existence? Does the patient displace anger toward a religious representative? Does the patient regard illness as a form of punishment?

Cultural orientation

"What is your cultural background or heritage? Were you born in another country? When did you come to the United States? Is your family from another country? Do you have strong ties to the customs of your country? Are you a member of any particular cultural or ethnic group?"

Cultural practices

"Do you practice any special customs? How closely are you tied to them? How does your family usually react when a family member becomes sick? Are family members usually with you when you are sick? Are there any foods you are not permitted to eat? Are there any medical treatments you will not accept because of your beliefs? How does your illness (or desire for health) affect your ability to participate in your usual customs?"

RELATING PATTERN FOCUS QUESTIONS AND PARAMETERS
Role
Marital status

Is the patient married, divorced, widowed, single, separated, or have a nonmarital or common-law partner?

Age and health of significant other

Self-explanatory.

Number of children and ages

Self-explanatory.

Role in home

"Are you the major decision maker in your home? Major provider of child care? Provider of discipline for children? Person responsible for other siblings or parents?" (Also refer to home responsibilities under the "moving pattern" for other questions.) "How has this illness changed your responsibilities in your home and your role as a spouse or parent? Do you feel you are able to carry out the tasks normally expected of you at home? How do you feel about these changes?"

Financial support

"Are you the major breadwinner in the family? Do you have enough money to meet your expenses? Do you need assistance with your finances?"

Occupation

"What kind of work do you do? How many hours do you work per week? Do you take work home with you? Are you retired? Are you involved in volunteer work?"

Job satisfaction/concerns

"Do you like your job? Retirement? Do you have any major concerns or problems related to your job?"

Physical/mental energy expenditures

"Do your job, activities at home, and volunteer work involve strenuous physical activity? Do they involve intense concentration or mental energy? Do you feel your work is very stressful? Does it require most of your energy and efforts? Do your job and activities leave you feeling physically or emotionally exhausted?"

Sexual relationships

(Circle satisfactory or unsatisfactory). If unsatisfactory, does the patient report difficulties, limitations, or changes in sexual behaviors or activities? Does the patient verbalize a change of interest in self or others?

Physical difficulties/effects of illness related to sex

Does the patient describe an actual or perceived limitation in sexual activity imposed by disease, illness, or therapy? Does the patient verbalize some form of altered body structure or function such as pregnancy, recent childbirth, drugs, surgery, physical anomalies, paralysis, disease processes, trauma, or radiation that might interfere with sexual functioning?[1,4]

Socialization
Quality of relationship with others

"How do you and _____ get along? Any problems?" (Also ask the family the same questions.) "In general, how do you get along with other people?"

Staff observations

Do the patient and significant other appear to get along? Are they supportive of each other? Do they constantly fight or upset each other? How does the patient interact with the staff?

Verbalizes feeling of being alone: attributed to

"Do you feel comfortable when talking to your peers and family or others? Do you feel comfortable in social situations? In most social situations, do you feel a sense of belonging? Interest? Caring? Do you feel that your family and friends are supportive of the things you do and the things about which you think and care? Do you prefer to be alone most of the time? Do you feel your physical condition isolates you from people? Do you feel alone? Rejected? Different from others? Why?[4] (Also refer to social activities, under the "moving pattern.")

KNOWING PATTERN FOCUS QUESTIONS AND PARAMETERS
Current health problems

"What brought you to the hospital?" (This line of questioning should include a description of the patient's current problems.) Attempt to elicit the signs, symptoms, and problems in the order in which they occurred. This information will provide a focus for collecting more specific data in the associated pattern of concern (e.g., for a patient who was admitted to a critical care unit for syncope, the nurse performs a comprehensive assessment of the neurologic and cardiac categories under the "exchanging pattern"). For each sign and symptom identified in the pattern of concern, determine when, where, and under what circumstances the sign and symptom occurred. Also determine its location, quality, quantity, duration, and aggravating, alleviating, and associated factors. Within each pattern, also state pertinent "negatives" or absences of certain signs or symptoms that might generally be involved with the problem (e.g., absence of pedal edema, sudden weight gain, or dyspnea in a patient suspected of having decreased cardiac output).

Previous illnesses/hospitalizations/surgeries

Summarize all the patient's major and minor health and illness problems. Summarize past hospitalizations (chronological dates and, if appropriate, attending physicians). Summarize past surgical procedures (chronological dates, attending physicians, and complications, if appropriate).

History of the following problems
Heart

"Have you had any history of heart disease, heart attack, heart murmur, heart infection, chest pain, or palpitations?"

Peripheral vascular

"Have you had any leg problems?" Does the patient complain of intermittent claudication (i.e., calf cramping and fatigue, which is precipitated by exercise and relieved by rest)? Determine the location of the pain, its quality, duration, and precipitating and alleviating factors.

Lung

"Have you had a history of lung disease, tuberculosis, lung infections, asthma, bronchitis, or asbestos exposure?"

Liver

"Have you had any liver problems or liver enlargement? Have you ever had infectious mononucleosis? Hepatitis?"

Kidney

"Have you had any kidney problems, kidney infections, or kidney stones?"

Cerebrovascular

"Have you had any dizziness, blackouts, strokes, or high blood pressure?"

Rheumatic fever

"Have you ever had rheumatic fever?"

Thyroid

"Have you ever had any thyroid problems (i.e., hyperthyroid or hypothyroid problems)?"

Other

"Have you ever had any gallbladder, gastrointestinal, or genitourinary problems?

Current medications

"What medications are you taking? How long have you been taking this medication?" (Determine the name of the medication, dosage, frequency, and side effects.) "What medications did you take yesterday before you came to the hospital? Were there any medications you should have taken yesterday but omitted?" If the patient has brought any medications to the hospital, identify the names of the drugs, dosages, and frequencies of administration. If the patient is not sure of the names of the medications, the family should bring the bottles to the hospital to be checked by the nurse. Determine if the patient is taking any over-the-counter medications such as aspirin, acetaminophen, ibuprofen, laxatives, sleeping pills, or diet pills. Also determine if the patient is taking narcotics, insulin, digitalis, or steroid hormone replacement.[2]

Risk factors

Determine whether the patient has any of the subsequent coronary artery disease risk factors, and determine the patient's perception and level of knowledge about each. Is the patient aware of how the risk factors (if present) affect the heart? Does the patient consider the risk factor to be a true risk to health?[2,11]

1. Hypertension: When diagnosed? (Refer to current medications, diet, and rest for how hypertension is treated. Refer to health maintenance for how problem is followed up.)
2. Hyperlipidemia: When diagnosed? (Refer to current medications, diet, and rest regimen for how hyperlipidemia is treated. Refer to health maintenance in the "moving pattern" for how problem is followed up.)
3. Smoking: Type of tobacco (e.g., cigarettes, cigars, pipe, chewing tobacco); amount per day or per week; age began smoking; age smoking habit increased, decreased, ceased?
4. Obesity: How much overweight? How long overweight? How treated? (Refer to diet and ideal body weight under nutrition in the "exchanging pattern.")

5. Diabetes: When diagnosed? At what age? (Refer to current medications and diet for how it is treated. Refer to health maintenance for how problem is followed up.)
6. Sedentary living: Are daily activities associated with any form of exercise or activity? (Also refer to the "moving pattern.")
7. Stress: What kind of stressors are in the patient's life? Are home life, work, and family interaction highly stressful? (Refer to recent stressful life events under the "feeling pattern.")
8. Alcohol use: How much does the patient drink (average daily, weekend, or social consumption)? Type of alcohol (e.g., whiskey, gin, beer, wine; include amounts). Has alcohol consumption interferred with the patient's marriage, job, or health? Has the patient ever been hospitalized for alcoholism?
9. Oral contraceptives: Does the patient take any oral contraceptives? What kind? How long? (Refer to current medications.)
10. Family history: Determine the age, sex, and health status of living family members, including parents, siblings, children, and spouse. Determine the age, sex, and cause of death of deceased family members. Determine any family history associated with the above risk factors (No. 1 to 9). Also determine any familial disease history related to cancer, heart disease, peripheral vascular disease, cerebrovascular disease, stroke, migraine headaches, respiratory disease, tuberculosis, nervous or mental conditions, epilepsy, kidney disease, arthritic conditions, hematologic abnormalities, rheumatic fever, sickle cell anemia, or thyroid disease.

Perception/knowledge of illness/tests/surgery

"What is your biggest health problem? Can you tell me what you know about this problem? What do you think causes this problem? Can you tell me about the tests you are about to undergo? Can you tell me what you know about the surgery you are about to have?"

Expectations of therapy

"How do you expect your health problem to be treated while you are here? What has been planned to help you while you are here? What do you think will be the results of this therapy?"

Misconceptions

"Have you heard anything about your illness that puzzles you? Have you received any especially disturbing information from staff, family, or friends? Do you have any questions about your illness and treatment?" (Also assess the above answers given by the patient or family under risk factors, perception/knowledge of illness/tests/surgery, and expectations of therapy, and determine if information is correct and realistic.)

Readiness to learn

Does the patient ask questions about the therapy, treatment, illness, or prognosis? Does the patient deny that a problem exists? Does the patient acknowledge the illness but express a desire not to know details about tests, therapy, surgery, or prognosis?[2,3] Does the patient demonstrate readiness to learn by good eye contact, body language, and motivation to listen?

Requests information concerning

Indicates readiness to learn; specify what information is requested.

Educational level

"How many years of education do you have?"

Learning impeded by

Does the patient's current physical condition permit or prohibit learning to take place (i.e., barriers such as pain, distractions, and confusion)? Does the patient's emotional and psychologic status permit or prohibit learning to take place?

Orientation
Level of alertness

Is the patient alert? Lethargic? Comatose? Does the patient attend to events occurring in the room or in close proximity to the bed?

Orientation

Is the patient oriented to person, place, and time?

Appropriate behavior/communication

Is the patient confused? Is the patient's behavior appropriate for the situation? Is the patient's verbal and nonverbal form of communication appropriate for the situation?

Memory
Memory intact

(Circle yes or no.)

Recent

"What day, month, and year is it? Where do you live? What is your telephone number? What kind of clothes did you wear to the hospital? What did you eat for dinner last night? Breakfast this morning?"

Remote

"Can you recall the holidays we celebrated last month? In the month of _____? Tell me about your childhood (i.e., where did you live? go to school?)."

FEELING PATTERN FOCUS QUESTIONS AND PARAMETERS
Comfort
Pain/discomfort

"Do you have any pain or discomfort?" (Circle yes or no.) For each source of pain or discomfort, determine:[2,3]

Onset

"When did the pain begin? Was it gradual or sudden? Have you ever had it before?"

Duration

"How long did it last?"

Location

"Where is the pain or discomfort? Please point to the area or areas."

Quality

"Is the pain sharp, dull, continuous, intermittent? Is it mild or severe?"

Radiation

"Does the pain go to other areas of the body? Does it travel?"

Associated factors

"Because of the pain, have you noticed any other problems (i.e., nausea or vomiting, shortness of breath, sweating, or dizziness)?"

Aggravating factors

"What makes the pain worse (e.g., deep breathing, moving, or eating)?"

Alleviating factors

"What makes the pain better (e.g., antacids, medication, eating, changing positions, or shallow breathing)?"

Emotional integrity/states
Recent stressful life events

"Within the last year, have you experienced any stressful events (e.g., family, financial, or work-related problems such as death or serious illness of a spouse or child, loss of job, retirement, loss or change of home, major financial burdens)? Has anything upset you recently?"

Verbalizes feelings and source

"How are you feeling about yourself? Your situation? Do you have feelings of anxiety, fear, anger, guilt, shame, or sadness?"

Does the patient verbalize a conflict about values and goals of life? Does the patient verbalize anxiety related to a threat to self-concept? A threat of death? A threat or change in health status, socioeconomic status, role functioning, environment, or interactional patterns? Does the patient express a feeling of increased tension, apprehension, uncertainty, inadequacy, or shakiness? Does the patient verbalize feeling jittery, distressed, rattled, overexcited, scared, or fearful?[4]

Physical manifestations

Does the patient exhibit symptoms and behavior consistent with anxiety (e.g., elevated heart rate or blood pressure above normal; cool extremities; darting eye movements; continuous nonpurposeful activity [such as picking at sheets, nails, hair, or constant leg motion]; verbose, nondirected conversation; startle reflex to normal sounds)? Does the patient exhibit symptoms and behavior consistent with other feelings such as depression (e.g., lack of eye contact, withdrawn behavior, constant weeping or crying, loss of appetite, interrupted sleep patterns, unusually long sleep patterns, nonengagement, or sad facial expressions)?[4]

MOVING PATTERN FOCUS QUESTIONS AND PARAMETERS
Activity
History of physical disability

"Do you have any difficulty moving or walking? Do you have any limitations in your movement (e.g., unable to raise your arm above your head)? Have you noticed any decrease in muscle strength, muscle control, or muscle size?[4] Have restrictions been imposed on your activities or movement because of medical recommendations?" Does the patient have any perceptual, cognitive, neuromuscular, or musculoskeletal impairments? Does the patient use crutches or a cane, walker, or wheelchair?

Limitations in daily activities

"Have you noticed any pain, discomfort, or shortness of breath when you perform your normal daily activities? Have you noticed any decreased strength or endurance in your normal daily activities? Are there any activities you once did that you cannot do any more or at present? Why?" What is the patient's response to activity (i.e., do heart rate and blood pressure return to preactivity levels within 3 minutes after the activity)? Can the patient ambulate without symptoms (i.e., pain or shortness of breath)?

Verbal report of fatigue/weakness

"Have you found yourself feeling constantly tired, having no energy, or feeling too weak to accomplish daily activities?"

Exercise habits

"Are you involved in any type of exercise program?" (Determine type, duration, and frequency.) "Can you tell me what kind of exercise is involved in your job, outside activities, and sports and during household activities?"

Rest
Hours slept/night

"When do you usually sleep (i.e., during the day, evening, or night)? Can you tell me how many hours you generally sleep at a time (not necessarily at night)? Do you take any rest periods during the day for naps, relaxation, or meditation? What is the length, time, and reason for these rest periods?"

Feels rested

"Do you usually feel rested after sleeping?" (Circle yes or no.)

Sleep aids

"Do you use any aids to help you to sleep (e.g., pillows, tranquilizers, hypnotics, alcohol, hot milk, warm bath or shower, music, or food)?"

Difficulties falling/remaining asleep

"Do you have any difficulties falling asleep? Staying asleep? Going back to sleep once you are awake? Do you have frequent or recurrent nightmares that awaken you?"

Recreation
Leisure activities

"What fun or relaxing things do you do in your leisure time? Do you have any hobbies? Do you enjoy any sports? Do you enjoy reading, listening to music, painting, playing cards, sewing, and so forth?"

Social activities

"Are you involved in any social activities (e.g., church groups, clubs, or organizations)? Were social activities important to you before this hospitalization?"

Environmental maintenance
Size and arrangement of home (stairs, bathroom)

"Do you have any difficulties in your home regarding the location of your bedroom or bathroom, or do you have any stairs to climb? Where are the kitchen and bathrooms in relation to the bedrooms (i.e., upstairs or downstairs? Same level)? Does the entry to the house or apartment require climbing stairs? If so, how many? Are there any alternate access routes? Do you have the necessary cooking equipment, linens, cloths, and hygienic aids? Are you familiar with your neighborhood resources (e.g., neighbors, grocery store, laundry, and pharmacy)?"

Safety needs

"Can you describe any safety devices that you may need (e.g., railing in bathtub) or safety hazards (e.g., torn carpet or frayed electrical cords) in your home?"[4]

Home responsibilities

"Tell me what your typical day is like concerning meal planning and preparation, shopping, cleaning, child care, bill paying, and household chores?"

Health maintenance
Health insurance

"Do you have health insurance? Do you receive any financial medical assistance (i.e., Medicare? Medicaid)?"

Regular physical checkups

"Do you see a physician for regular checkups? Do you see other physicians or nurse practitioners for any other reason? How often do you visit a dentist?"[4]

Does the patient demonstrate a lack of knowledge about basic health practices? Does the patient indicate a lack of responsibility for meeting basic health practices? Does the patient express an interest in improving health behaviors? Does the patient report a lack of equipment or financial or personal resources?[4]

Self-care
Ability to perform activities of daily living (ADLs)

Independent or dependent with regard to the subsequent actions:

Feeding

Is the patient able to feed self and drink without assistance?

Bathing/hygiene

"What is your usual form of bathing? When? How often? Are you able to wash your body, get in and out of the bath or shower, and regulate the water flow and temperature? Do you require a special rail or stool in the tub? Are you able to wash your hair and brush your teeth?"[4]

Dressing/grooming

Is the patient able to put on and take off necessary items of clothing? Is the patient able to fasten clothing? Is the patient able to maintain a satisfactory appearance (e.g., brush hair or apply makeup)?[4]

Toileting

"Are you able to get to the toilet or commode? Are you able to sit on and rise from the toilet or commode? Are you able to manipulate your clothing for toileting? Are you able to carry out proper toilet hygiene? Are you able to flush the toilet or empty the commode?"[4]

Specify deficits

From above list.

Discharge planning needs

Based on the above list, do any of the self-care deficits indicate a need for a home referral for assistance (i.e., visiting nurse or companion)? Will the patient need special training or assistive devices to be independent (or less dependent) at home?

PERCEIVING PATTERN FOCUS QUESTIONS AND PARAMETERS
Self-concept
Patient's description of self

"If you could describe what kind of person you are, what would you say? Can you make a statement describing yourself? How do you feel about yourself as a person? Are you comfortable about the way you look, feel, and function?" Does the patient verbally or nonverbally express an actual or perceived change in body structure or functioning?[4]

Effects of illness/surgery on self-concept

"What does this illness or surgery mean to you? And your family? How serious do you think your condition is?" Does the patient express negative feelings about self-image? Is the patient preoccupied with a change or loss of body parts? Does the patient demonstrate responsibility for self-care, or does the patient demonstrate self-neglect? Does the patient ignore, neglect, or traumatize a specific body part?[4] Does the patient refuse to look in a mirror or at a body part? Does the patient refuse to discuss the illness, injury, or surgery?[1]

Meaningfulness
Verbalizes hopelessness

"What are your attitudes and feelings about the future? Do you believe there is a possible solution to your problem? What are your plans for the future?" Does the patient demonstrate negative feelings, passivity, decreased verbalization, flat affect, a lack of initiative, decreased response to stimuli, decreased appetite, increased sleep, lack of involvement in care, and sighing and verbal cues such as "I can't"?[4] (Also see emotional integrity states under the "feeling pattern.")

Verbalizes/perceives loss of control

"What do you think that you can do to change, improve, or help your current situation or problem?" Does the patient perceive a loss of control regarding the outcomes of care? Or over self-care? Is the patient depressed or apathetic about physical deterioration despite compliance with medical regimen? Does the patient choose not to participate in decision making even when opportunities are provided? Does the patient express dissatisfaction or frustration over an inability to perform previous tasks or activities?[4]

Sensory/perception
History of restricted environment

Has the patient experienced any restricted environments (e.g., isolation, intensive care, bed rest, traction, confining illness, or incubator)? Has the patient experienced any socially restricted environments (e.g., institutionalization, home-bound, chronic illness, dying, or infant deprivation)?[4]

Vision impaired

"Do you have difficulty seeing? How is your near vision? Far vision?" Can the patient see the nurse, newsprint, or objects across the room? Does the patient have cataracts or a false eye?

Glasses

"Do you wear glasses or contact lenses? How well do they correct your vision?"

Auditory impaired

"Do you have any difficulty hearing?" Can the patient hear normal conversation?

Hearing aid

Does the patient use a hearing aid? Which ear? Does the patient like to use it? Does it improve hearing?

Kinesthetics impaired

Can the patient walk across the room appropriately? Can the patient maintain a sense of balance? Does the patient complain of dizziness? Does the patient demonstrate a lack of coordination?

Gustatory impaired

Does the patient complain of loss of taste? Does the patient complain of metallic or unusual tastes?

Tactile impaired

Does the patient complain of any loss in the sense of touch? Is the patient able to distinguish between dull, sharp, and light touches? Does the patient complain of numbness, tingling, or a prickly feeling?

Olfactory impaired

Does the patient complain of a loss of smell? Can the patient recognize the smell of rubbing alcohol after closing the eyes?

Reflexes

Test each deep tendon reflex (see box); compare the responses on corresponding sides, and grade the responses using the following scale:[6,8]

0	No response
1+	Sluggish or diminished
2+	Active or expected response
3+	More brisk than usual
4+	Brisk or hyperactive

TESTING FOR DEEP TENDON REFLEXES

Biceps: The patient's arm is flexed at a 45-degree angle at the elbow. Palpate the biceps tendon in the antecubital fossa. Place your fingers over the biceps muscle and your thumb over the tendon. With the reflex hammer, strike your thumb. Flexion of the elbow should occur.

Brachioradialis: The patient's arm is flexed up to a 45-degree angle and rests on your arm with the hand slightly pronated. With the reflex hammer, directly strike the brachioradialis tendon. Observe for flexion and supination of the forearm.

Triceps: The patient's arm is flexed up to a 90-degree angle, with the patient's hand resting against the side of your body. Palpate the triceps tendon and strike it directly with the reflex hammer just above the elbow. Contraction of the triceps muscle causes extension of the elbow.

Knee: The patient's knee is flexed up to a 90-degree angle, with the lower leg loosely hung. Support the patient's upper leg with your hand without allowing it to rest against the side of the table. With the reflex hammer, strike the patellar tendon just below the patella. The lower leg will extend when the quadriceps contract.

Ankle: With the patient sitting, flex the knee and dorsiflex the ankle up to a 90-degree angle holding the heel of the foot in your hands. Strike the Achilles tendon at the level of the ankle malleoli. Contraction of the gastrocnemius muscle causes plantar flexion of the foot at the ankle. Note also the speed of relaxation after muscular contraction.

Plantar: The patient's ankle is held in one hand while a sharp object is stroked from the lateral surface of the sole, starting at the heel of the foot and going to the base of the foot, curving medially across the ball and ending beneath the great toe. The normal response is flexion of all toes (negative Babinski's reflex). Extension or dorsiflexion of the great toe and fanning of the others represents a positive Babinski's reflex, which may reflect upper motor neuron disease.[6,8]

EXCHANGING PATTERN FOCUS QUESTIONS AND PARAMETERS
Circulation
Cerebral
Neurologic changes/symptoms

Does the patient complain of seizures, convulsions, difficulty in walking, vertigo, dizziness, loss of balance, falls, weakness or numbness, difficulty in swallowing, development of tremors, confusion, or forgetfulness? Does the family or patient report any changes in personality?[3]

Pupils

Assess pupillary size, shape, and equality. Determine reactions to light (i.e., brisk, sluggish, or nonreactive). When determining reaction to light, determine direct-light pupillary reflex (constriction of lighted eye) and consensual pupillary reflex (constriction of unlighted eye).[3]

Glasgow Coma Scale

Determine the patient's level of consciousness using the Glasgow Coma Scale, which consists of three categories (eye opening, best verbal response, and best motor response). Each category is scored, and the total is the Glasgow Coma Scale score.[3] The highest possible score is 15 (Table 3-1).

Cardiac
Point of maximum impulse

Determine the point of maximum impulse (PMI), which is produced at the onset of ventricular systole and is normally found near the fifth intercostal space midclavicular line. The PMI is assessed by placing the hand over the anterior precordium and shifting the second and third fingers until the PMI is found. It is normally the size of a penny or nickel.[2,11]

Pacemaker

Observe for an external or internal pacemaker. If internal, record the type and how it is functioning. If external, record the type, settings, and how it is functioning.

Apical rate and rhythm

What is the patient's apical heart rate? Is the rhythm regular or irregular? If irregular, is it regularly irregular or totally irregular?

Heart sounds/murmurs

Listen for the first and second heart sounds, and determine whether there is a third or fourth heart sound or whether the patient has any ejection sounds, midsystolic clicks, opening snaps, or murmurs as follows:[2,3]

FIRST HEART SOUND

The first heart sound (S_1) is heard with the diaphragm of the stethoscope over the entire precordium. It is due to the closure of the tricuspid and mitral valves.

SECOND HEART SOUND

The second heart sound (S_2) is heard with the diaphragm of the stethoscope and is loudest over the right and left second intercostal spaces. It is due to the closure of the pulmonic and aortic valves.

THIRD HEART SOUND

The third heart sound (S_3) or a ventricular gallop is heard with the bell of the stethoscope over the entire precordium (apex). S_3 occurs immediately after S_2. The third heart sound is usually pathological and is caused by the vibrations of a noncompliant ventricle occurring during rapid ventricular filling in early diastole after the opening of the mitral and tricuspid valves. It is associated with any condition that increases early diastolic pressures or rapid ventricular filling. It is generally an early sign of congestive heart failure. The rhythm and pattern of S_1, S_2, and S_3 somewhat resemble the sounds produced by saying "Kentuck-ky."

FOURTH HEART SOUND

The fourth heart sound (S_4) or atrial gallop is heard with the bell of the stethoscope over the apex. The fourth heart sound is an abnormal finding in the adult and may indicate increased resistance to ventricular filling. It is produced after atrial contraction as a result of the forceful ejection of blood from the atria into an overdistended ventricle. It is caused by any condition that impairs ventricular compliance such as hypertensive cardiovascular disease, coronary artery disease, or aortic stenosis. S_4 closely precedes S_1 so that the cadence of S_4, S_1, and S_2 is similar to the sound produced by saying "Ten-nes-see".

QUADRUPLE RHYTHMS

Quadruple rhythms refer to the cadence of a normal S_1, and S_2, plus S_3 and S_4. When the heart rate is slow, all four components may be heard separately, and they have been described as sounding like a cogwheel or a locomotive. With a fast heart rate, S_3 and S_4 may fuse together to form a single sound almost as loud as S_1 or S_2. Instead of a quadruple rhythm, a triple rhythm or *summation gallop*, which sounds like horses cantering down a dirt track, is heard.

EJECTION SOUNDS

Ejection sounds (ESs) are heard with the diaphragm of the stethoscope at the second right or left intercostal space or the apex. They are heard during the onset of early ventricular systole and commonly in association with pul-

Table 3-1
Glasgow Coma Scale*

Scale	Score	Explanation
EYE OPENING		
No eye opening	1	No eye opening. If the patient cannot open the eyes because of bandaging or swelling, the letter *E* is recorded after the total score. The nurse determines the minimum stimulus to cause opening of one or both eyes.
To pain	2	Eye opening only to pain. A noxious stimulus is used. It may be the same stimulus used to determine the best motor response.
To speech	3	Eye opening only to speech. The nurse may call the patient by name or may command the patient to open the eyes.
Spontaneous	4	Spontaneous eye opening.
BEST VERBAL RESPONSE		
No response	1	No verbal response. No sound or vocalization is made even after stimulation with a noxious stimulus.
Incomprehensible sounds	2	The sounds made are not comprehensible. The patient makes groans or moans not discernible as words.
Inappropriate words	3	The patient is not able to use words appropriately and can speak words but make no intelligent sentences. The patient often utters curses or disorganized ramblings but cannot enter into conversation.
Confused conversation	4	The patient can form sentences and group words, but the manner is confused. The patient is not fully oriented.
Oriented	5	The patient is appropriate and oriented to time, place, and person and can carry on a conversation.
BEST MOTOR RESPONSE		
Flaccid	1	The patient demonstrates no motor response. Arms and legs are lax and weak. The nurse must be sure that the stimulus is noxious and there is no spinal cord injury.
Extensor response	2	The patient exhibits decerebrate rigidity. Legs and arms are extended and in internal rotation. The wrists are flexed, and the patient makes a fist. The patient assumes this position in response to a noxious stimulus. If there is a question between the upper and lower extremities, the position of the upper extremities is used.
Flexor response	3	On stimulation, the patient flexes the upper extremities, but the lower extremities remain in extension. The wrist is flexed and the patient makes a fist. The patient exhibits decorticate rigidity.
Semipurposeful	4	The patient has a generalized flexion withdrawal to pain. The patient briskly flexes either or both arms or may grimace or frown. There is no manual and purposeful attempt to stop the stimulus.
Localizes to pain	5	The patient withdraws from the pain or tries to locate and stop the stimulus. The patient does not follow commands but tends to move the arms towards the stimulus. The stimulus should be maximal and the site used should be changed.
Obeys commands	6	The patient can follow commands. The patient will raise a certain number of fingers, hold up an arm, or release a grip.

Adapted from Cornelia Vanderstaay Kenner, Cathie E. Guzzetta, and Barbara Montgomery Dossey, *Critical Care Nursing: Body-Mind-Spirit*, 2nd ed., [p. 671]. Copyright © 1985 by Cornelia Vanderstaay Kenner, Cathie E. Guzzetta, and Barbara Montgomery Dossey. Reprinted by permission of Scott, Foresman and Company.
*Glasgow Coma Scale total. the patient who is completely awake will score 15.

monic or aortic stenosis and in pulmonary or systemic hypertension. They are heard immediately after S_1.

MIDSYSTOLIC CLICKS

Midsystolic clicks (MSCs) are heard with the diaphragm of the stethoscope over the apex and are commonly associated with prolapse of the mitral valve leaflet into the left atrium in a patient with Barlow syndrome. They are middle-to-late systolic sounds (heard after S_1) and are often followed by a systolic murmur.

OPENING SNAPS

Opening snaps (OSs) are heard with the diaphragm of the stethoscope at the lower left sternal border. OSs are heard because of the abrupt recoil or cessation of opening movement of the mitral or tricuspid valve during ventricular diastole when stenosis of one of these valves is present. OSs are heard shortly after S_2, and because the timing frequently overlaps with S_3, it is sometimes difficult to distinguish these two sounds without the aid of a phonocardiogram.

MURMURS

Murmurs should be assessed in regard to their timing, configuration, pitch, quality, intensity, location, and radiation.[2,3]

Timing. Murmurs are classified as systolic, diastolic, or continuous. A systolic murmur begins with or after S_1 and ends at or before S_2. A diastolic murmur begins with or after S_2 and ends at or before S_1. A continuous murmur begins in systole and extends through S_2 into part or all of diastole.

Configuration. Murmurs frequently have an identifiable configuration. A crescendo murmur progressively increases in loudness. A decrescendo murmur progressively decreases in loudness. A crescendo-decrescendo or diamond-shaped murmur peaks to intensify and then progressively decreases in sound. A holosystolic murmur (pansystolic, sustained, or plateau) murmur remains constant throughout systole.

Pitch and quality. Murmurs may be classified as high, medium, or low pitched. A high- or medium-pitched murmur is heard best with the diaphragm of the stethoscope, whereas a low-pitched murmur is heard best with the bell. Murmurs are also described in terms of their quality, such as harsh, rumbling, blowing, or whooping.

Intensity (grading). Murmurs are generally graded on a scale of 1 to 6 according to the intensity of the sound. A grade 1 murmur is barely audible with a stethoscope; a grade 2 murmur is faint but audible, and a grade 3 murmur is moderately loud. A grade 4 murmur is a loud murmur associated with a thrill; a grade 5 murmur is the loudest murmur heard requiring the use of a stethoscope, and a grade 6 murmur is so loud it can be heard with the stethoscope slightly removed from the chest.

Location and radiation. Each murmur is generally heard the loudest at a specific area or location over the precordium. These areas should be noted. Radiation of a murmur refers to the transmission of the sound to sites other than the primary location. It is also important to note the direction of the radiation.

Types of murmurs. The box on p. 34 classifies the types of murmurs associated with the A-V valves or semilunar valves, according to cause, timing, configuration, pitch, quality, location, and radiation.[3]

Dysrhythmias

Does the patient have dysrhythmias (i.e., tachydysrhythmias, bradydysrhythmias; atrial, junctional, or ventricular dysrhythmias; first-, second-, or third-degree heart blocks; premature atrial, junctional, or ventricular beats? Note any hemodynamic symptoms associated with the dysrhythmia (i.e., hypotension, dizziness, confusion, low urinary output, or decreased cardiac output).

Blood pressure

What is the patient's blood pressure (BP) in the right and left arm while sitting, lying, and standing? For any severe decreases in blood pressure from lying to sitting or standing, which indicate postural hypotension, assess the patient for the cause (i.e., dehydration, medications, neurologic impairment, prolonged bed rest with associated decrease in muscle tone).

A-line reading

What is the arterial blood pressure as measured by the arterial line? Is there a palpable femoral or carotid pulse?

Cardiac index

What is the patient's cardiac index? (Normal is 3.5 L/minute/m^2; it ranges from 2.5 to 4.5 L/minute/m^2. The cardiac index is derived by dividing the cardiac output by the body surface area.)[11]

Cardiac output

What is the cardiac output? (Normal is 5 L/minute.)[2]

Central venous pressure

What is the patient's central venous pressure (CVP)? (Normal is 4 to 15 cm H_2O or 3 to 11 mm Hg.)[2]

Pulmonary artery pressure

What is the patient's pulmonary artery pressure (PAP)? (Normal is less than 25 mm Hg systolic and 5 to 10 mm Hg diastolic, with a mean pulmonary artery pressure of less than 13 mm Hg.)[2]

Pulmonary capillary wedge pressure

What is the patient's pulmonary capillary wedge pressure (PCWP)? (Normal ranges from 4 to 12 mm Hg.)[12]

CLASSIFICATION OF HEART MURMURS

AORTIC STENOSIS

Cause: Forward flow of blood from the left ventricle to the aorta through an obstructed aortic valve
Timing: Systole
Configuration: Crescendo-decrescendo
Quality and pitch: Harsh and low pitched
Location: Aortic auscultatory area (second intercostal space, right sternal border)
Radiation: Into the neck or carotid vessels

AORTIC INSUFFICIENCY

Cause: Backward flow of blood from the aorta to the left ventricle through an incompetent (leaky) aortic valve
Timing: Diastole
Configuration: Decrescendo
Quality and pitch: Blowing and high pitched
Location: Aortic auscultatory area (second intercostal space, right sternal border)
Radiation: Left sternal border

MITRAL STENOSIS

Cause: Forward flow of blood from the left atrium to the left ventricle through an obstructed mitral valve
Timing: Diastole
Configuration: Crescendo-decrescendo
Quality and pitch: Rumbling and low pitched
Location: Apex
Radiation: Usually none

MITRAL REGURGITATION

Cause: Backward flow of blood from the left ventricle to the left atrium through an incompetent mitral valve
Timing: Systole
Configuration: Holosystolic
Quality and pitch: Blowing and high pitched
Location: Apex
Radiation: Left axillary line

PULMONARY STENOSIS

Cause: Forward flow of blood from the right ventricle to the pulmonary artery through an obstructed pulmonic valve
Timing: Systole
Configuration: Crescendo-decrescendo
Quality and pitch: Harsh and medium pitched
Location: Pulmonary auscultatory area (second intercostal space, left sternal border)
Radiation: Usually none

PULMONARY REGURGITATION

Cause: Backward flow of blood from the pulmonary artery to the right ventricle through an incompetent pulmonic valve
Timing: Diastole
Configuration: Decrescendo; increases in intensity with inspiration
Quality and pitch: Blowing and high (or low) pitched
Location: Third and fourth left intercostal spaces
Radiation: Usually none

TRICUSPID STENOSIS

Cause: Forward flow of blood from the right atrium to the right ventricle through an obstructed tricuspid valve
Timing: Diastole
Configuration: Crescendo-decrescendo
Quality and pitch: Rumbling and low pitched
Location: Lower left sternal border and tricuspid auscultatory area (fifth intercostal space, lower left sternal border)
Radiation: Usually none

TRICUSPID REGURGITATION

Cause: Backward flow of blood from the right ventricle to the right atrium through an incompetent tricuspid valve
Timing: Systole
Configuration: Holosystolic; increases in intensity with inspiration
Quality and pitch: Blowing and high pitched
Location: Tricuspid auscultatory area (fifth intercostal space, lower left sternal border)
Radiation: Usually none

PERICARDIAL FRICTION RUB

Pericardial friction rubs sound similar to and may be confused with heart murmurs. Rubs are characterized by the following:
Cause: Roughening and irritation of pericardial surface
Timing: Systole, diastole, or both (may have systolic, early diastolic, and presystolic components)
Quality and pitch: Usually loud, leathery, scratchy, and high pitched
Location: Third intercostal space at left sternal border
Radiation: Usually none

IV fluids

What type of IV fluids is the patient receiving? What is the amount and rate of administration?

IV cardiac medications

Is the patient receiving any vasoactive IV medications? What is the name, dosage, and rate of administration?

Serum enzymes

What are the levels of the patient's serum cardiac enzymes (i.e., creatine phosphokinase [CPK] rises within 6 hours of cell destruction and peaks in 16 to 30 hours; CPK-MB isoenzyme is predominant in cardiac muscle tissue; lactate dehydrogenase [LDH] levels elevate 8 to 12 hours after acute myocardial infarction and peak at 3 to 4 days; LDH-1 and LDH-2 isoenzymes are specific for cardiac cell damage. Higher-than-normal levels of LDH-1 and LDH-2 are referred to as an LDH isoenzyme flip; and serum glutamic oxaloacetic transaminase [SGOT])[7,9,10] (see Appendix II). Note that individual values for these laboratory studies vary from institution to institution. Refer to your institution's designated normal values.

Peripheral
Jugular venous distension

Does the patient have distended venous neck veins? (Normally, the neck veins will become distended when the patient is lying down. When the patient is placed at a 45-degree angle, the neck veins should collapse or become visible only 1 to 2 cm above the clavicle. Pressures greater than 3 cm above the sternal angle are elevated. Increased jugular venous pressure is observed during inspiration in congestive heart failure, cardiac tamponade, and restrictive cardiomyopathies.)[2,3]

Pulses

For each set of pulses, if they are present by palpation, determine if they are 3+ (bounding), 2+ (palpable), or 1+ (faintly palpable). If the presence of a pulse is questionable, a Doppler ultrasonic anemometer can be used to determine its audible amplification. Each pulse should be evaluated for its quality, symmetry, and the presence of an audible bruit.[6,8]

Skin temperature

Is the patient's skin temperature normal, warm, hot, cool, clammy, or moist?

Color

Does the patient exhibit pink, pale, or red coloring? Does the patient exhibit pallor, jaundice, mottling, increased pigmentation, blanching, or cyanosis (note degree and location of cyanosis: eyes, ears, nose, mouth, tongue, neck, chest, legs, extremities, hands, fingers, and toes)?

Capillary refill

Does the patient have normal capillary refill? Capillary refill is assessed by pressing the nail bed, earlobe, or forehead so it blanches, releasing the pressure, and observing whether the skin color returns to normal within 2 seconds.[5]

Clubbing

Does the patient exhibit clubbing of the nail beds? (In clubbing, the skin proximal to the nail bed feels spongy, and in some cases the fingertips pulsate and flush. The proximal nail beds are convex and rise above the flat plane of the finger.)[2]

Edema

Does the patient have edema? Is the edema pitting, nonpitting, or dependent?

Physical integrity
Tissue integrity

Does the patient have any corneal, mucous membrane, integumentary, or subcutaneous tissue damage (e.g., a crushing injury or intravenous infiltration)?

Skin integrity

What is the general assessment of the skin in terms of hydration, vascularity, elasticity, texture, turgor, mobility, and thickness?

Does the patient have any disruption of skin surfaces or skin layers (e.g., rashes, lesions, petechiae, bruises, abrasions, moles, tumors, bullae, papules, blisters, pustules, vesicles, ulcerations, erosions, nodules, cysts, scales, crusts, fissures, calluses, bites, scars, keloids, hives, excoriations, plaques, bleeding, pruritus, dermatitis, or intravenous drug "track" marks)?

Does the patient have any invasion of body structures (e.g., surgical incisions, invasive hemodynamic lines, intravenous lines, stomas, tracheostomy tube, or gastric tube)?[6,8]

What is the condition, shape, texture, color, and thickness of the nails? What is the color of the nail beds? Does the patient have any nail lesions or splinter hemorrhages?

What is the color, distribution, quantity, and texture of the hair? What is the pattern of hair loss?

Oxygenation
Complaints of dyspnea: precipitated by

Does the patient complain of dyspnea? When does it occur? What precipitates the feeling? What alleviates it? What is the body position associated with it? Is the dyspnea exertional (i.e., does it occur with exertion or exercise)? Or is it paroxysmal nocturnal dyspnea (i.e., the patient characteristically goes to sleep in the recumbent position but is awakened 1 to 2 hours later with severe shortness of breath)?[2]

Orthopnea

Does the patient complain of orthopnea (i.e., the patient is unable to breathe normally in the recumbent position and usually sleeps with 2 to 3 pillows to improve breathing)?[2]

Rate/rhythm/depth

What is the patient's rate, rhythm, and depth of respirations? Is the patient's breathing regular? Is the depth shallow, moderate, or deep? Does the patient exhibit abnormal breathing patterns (i.e., asymmetric, obstructive, or restrictive)?

Labored/unlabored

Does the patient appear to be using a great deal of energy during breathing? Does the patient perceive that it takes a lot of work to breathe?

Use of accessory muscles

Does the patient use accessory muscles (i.e., costal or abdominal) for respiration? (List group used.)

Chest expansion

Does the patient's chest expand normally and symmetrically? (Describe abnormal movements.)

Splinting

Does the patient minimize coughing or avoid deep breathing to reduce pain (i.e., from a surgical incision)?

Cough

Does the patient have a productive or nonproductive cough? Is the patient's cough effort effective or ineffective? Weak or strong?

Sputum

What is the color, amount, odor, and consistency of the sputum?

Breath sounds

Does the patient have normal vesicular, bronchovesicular, and bronchial breath sounds? Does the patient have adventitious sounds (i.e., rales, crackles, wheezes, or pleural friction rubs)? Does the patient have vocal resonance (i.e., bronchophony, egophony, or whispered pectoriloquy)?

Arterial blood gases

Does the patient have normal arterial blood gases? (See Appendix II.)

Oxygen percent and device

If the patient is receiving oxygen, what is the percentage of oxygen delivered? What type of device is used to deliver it (i.e., nasal cannula, face mask, or catheter)?

Ventilator

What type of ventilator is used? What are the settings? How does the patient react to it (i.e., permitting the ventilator to do the work or fighting it)?

Physical regulation
Immune
Lymph nodes enlarged

Determine the size, shape, mobility, tenderness, and enlargement of the lymph nodes.

Location

Assess lymph nodes in the head, neck, axillae, and inguinal and pelvic areas.

WBC count/differential

Elevation of the total white blood cell count (leukocytes) usually indicates infection. The differential count is performed to determine the percentage of the types of leukocytes (i.e., neutrophils, lymphocytes, monocytes, eosinophils, and basophils) in the blood. Elevation of the neutrophils commonly indicates bacterial infections. Elevation of lymphocytes can indicate bacterial or viral infections or lymphocytic leukemia; elevations of monocytes can indicate bacterial or viral infections, and elevations of eosinophils can indicate allergic disorders or parasitic disease. Elevations of basophils are rare but can indicate some kind of myeloproliferative disease such as myelofibrosis or polycythemia vera[7,9,10] (see Appendix II). The normal values for the WBC count and differential vary from institution to institution. Refer to your institution's designated normal values.

Temperature

Normal rectal temperature is 36.1° C (97° F) to 37.0° C (99.6° F).

Route

Was the temperature taken orally, rectally, or axillary? The rectal route is 2° F higher than the axillary route, and 1° F higher than the oral route. The rectal temperature is considered the most accurate.

Nutrition
Eating patterns
Number of meals per day

"How many meals do you usually eat each day? Can you tell me what you eat and drink in a typical day?" (Prompt by naming food groups, specific meals, time of day, and probe regarding snacks.)

Special diet

"Do you have any fluid or dietary needs or restrictions (e.g., low-sodium, low-fat, low-calorie, low-sugar, or low-protein diet)?"

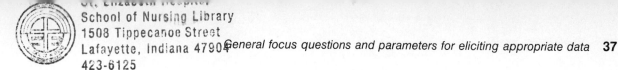

Where eaten

"Do you eat most of your meals at home or out?"

Food preferences/intolerances

"What kinds of food do you prefer? Are there any foods that do not agree with you (i.e., that you do not tolerate)?"

Food allergies

"Do you have any food allergies (i.e., dairy products, seafood, or fruits, or are you allergic to monosodium glutamate?"

Caffeine intake

"Can you tell me how many caffeinated beverages you drink each day (i.e., caffeinated coffee, tea, or soft drinks)? Do you eat a lot of chocolate?"

Appetite changes

"Have you noticed any change in your appetite lately (i.e., have you found yourself eating more, eating less, or drinking more or less)?" (NOTE: ask the patient specifically what was consumed the day before coming to the hospital. The patient may have been quite ill before admission, and the oral intake the day before admission may not reflect usual dietary and fluid habits. Also, the information may be helpful in determining specific nutritional and hydration problems that may have been precipitated by the acute illness.)

Presence of nausea/vomiting

Self-explanatory.

Condition of mouth/throat

Assess the condition and function of the patient's mouth, lips, buccal mucosa, teeth, tongue, hard and soft palate, and throat.[6,8]

General assessment

Is the patient able to bite, chew, taste, and swallow? Does the patient have any oral pain or odor?

Lips

What is the color, symmetry, and hydration of the lips? Does the patient have any crusting, fever blisters (herpes simplex), cracking, swelling, numbness, drooling, or ulcerations?

Buccal mucosa

What is the color, hydration, and pigmentation of the buccal mucosa? Does the patient have any ulcerations, nodules, white patches, plaques, dryness, excess saliva, or hemorrage? What is the color and condition of the gums? Does the patient have any inflammation, edema, bleeding, lesions, retraction, discoloration, or pain?

Teeth

What is the condition of the teeth? Does the patient have any missing, dark, or loose teeth; caries; pain; or sensitivity to heat or cold? Does the patient have a bridge or dentures (should be removed for examination)?

Tongue

What is the symmetry, color, mobility, size, hydration, and marking of the tongue? Does the patient have pain, soreness, ulcerations, burning, edema, fasciculations, nodules, abnormal smoothness, midline protrusion, or tumors under the tongue?

Hard palate

Does the patient have lesions, ulcers, or cysts?

Soft palate

What is the color and symmetry of the uvula, anterior and posterior pillars, tonsils, and posterior pharynx? Is there edema, exudate, inflammation, ulceration, tonsillar enlargement, pain, or tenderness? When patient says "ah," note the rise of the soft palate and uvula.

Throat

Does the patient complain of difficulty swallowing? Sore throat? Is the trachea midline? Deviated?

Height

Self-explanatory.

Weight

Self-explanatory.

Ideal body weight

Calculate ideal body weight: For men, 5 ft equals 106 lb; for each additional inch, add 6 lb (e.g., for a man 5 feet 2 inches, the ideal weight is 118 lb). For women, 5 ft equals 100 lb; for each additional inch add 5 lb (e.g., for a woman 5 feet 5 inches, the ideal weight is 125 lb).

Current therapy

Is the patient receiving nothing by mouth? Is the patient receiving nasogastric suctioning? Tube feedings (what type, amount, and frequency)? Total parenteral nutrition (what type, additives, and rate)?

Laboratory information

Assess the patient's blood sodium, potassium, chloride, hemoglobin, hematocrit, glucose, cholesterol, and triglycerides test results. (Were glucose, cholesterol and triglyceride tests performed when the patient was fasting? Circle yes or no.) (See Appendix II.) (Refer to your institution's designated normal values.)

Elimination
Gastrointestinal/bowel
Usual bowel habits

What are the patient's usual bowel habits? Does the patient use any laxatives, bran, fruits, or fruit juices to regulate bowel movements?

Alterations from normal

Does the patient have any difficulty with constipation, bowel cramping, diarrhea, or bowel incontinence? Does the patient strain or have pain or rectal bleeding with defecation?[1]

Abdominal physical examination

Observe the abdominal surface for rashes, scars, lesions, striae, or dilated veins. Does the patient have ascites (i.e., edema of the abdominal cavity)? Note the size, shape, contour, and symmetry of the abdomen. With the diaphragm of the stethoscope, determine the frequency, quality, and pitch of bowel sounds. (Do auscultation before palpation or percussion so bowel sounds will not be altered.) Bowel sounds are scored as 0 if they are absent, 1+ if hypoactive, 2+ if normal, and 3+ if hyperactive. Percuss the abdomen to determine liver borders, gastric air bubbles (in left upper quadrant), splenic dullness, air, fluid, or masses. Palpate the abdomen to determine organ enlargement, muscle spasm or rigidity, masses (note the location, size, shape, mobility, tenderness, consistency, pulsations), involuntary guarding, rebound tenderness, and pain.[3]

Renal/urinary
Usual urinary pattern

How many times per day does the patient urinate?

Alteration from normal

Does the patient have any alterations from normal such as incontinence or retention of urine? Does the patient describe any frequency, burning, pain, dribbling, urgency, hematuria, nocturia, oliguria, or polyuria?

Color

What is the color of the urine? Is there any blood?

Catheter

Does the patient have a urinary catheter? What type? How long? Any problems?

Urine output: 24 hour and average hourly

What is the patient's 24-hour urinary output? Hourly output?

Bladder distension

Is the bladder distended? Does the patient complain of bladder discomfort?

BUN/creatinine/specific gravity

What are the patient's blood urea nitrogen (BUN) and creatinine levels? What is the specific gravity of the urine? (See Appendix II.)

Urine studies

Assess the results of any urine studies (renal scan or urine culture) or other urine values (i.e., acetone, glucose, blood, or protein is abnormal), and pH (see Appendix II).[3,7,9]

CHOOSING PATTERN FOCUS QUESTIONS AND PARAMETERS
Coping
Patient's/family's usual problem-solving methods

"Do you believe that you solve problems well? Who helps you to solve problems? Is it easy or hard for you to accept help from others even if you might need it?" How does the patient view dependence on others? (Also see self-concept under the "perceiving pattern"). Does the patient or family verbalize an inability to meet basic needs? Does the family report that the patient is unable to ask others for help?

Patient's/family's method of dealing with stress

"When you have a really big problem, how do you deal with it? Do you get depressed? Cry? Become nervous? Drink alcohol? Eat extra food? Smoke? Take drugs? Ask someone for help? Call your family? Try to put it out of your mind? Try to solve the problem?" Does the patient inappropriately use defense mechanisms? What does the patient do to reduce stress (e.g., listen to music, use relaxation techniques, exercise, or go for a walk)?

Patient's affect

Does the patient demonstrate appropriate or inappropriate affect (feeling, mood, or emotion)? Is the patient's affect depressive or hostile?[1] Does the patient demonstrate little or no overt emotional expression? If little emotional expression is demonstrated, does the patient verbalize thoughts linked directly or indirectly to the physical symptoms or bodily functions? (The patient may be unaware of such associations. Also see emotional/integrity states under the "feeling pattern" and hopelessness/powerlessness under the "perceiving pattern.") Does the patient demonstrate inappropriate mood swings?[1]

Physical manifestations

Does the patient demonstrate physical manifestations of anxiety, rage, or withdrawal? (Even if the patient demonstrates little emotional expression, physical manifestations such as tachycardia, tachypnea, tremors, vomiting, urinary frequency, and/or impotence[1] may still be present.)

Support systems available

What support systems (e.g., spouse, children, family, relatives, and friends) are available to help the patient solve problems and deal with stress or crisis? Is the patient able to accept support from the clergy, a social worker, a psychologist, or community resources?

Participation
Compliance with past/current health care regimen

"In the past, have you had difficulty remembering to take your medications? Do you usually take all the medications the physician prescribes for you? Have you had any problems following your diet? Exercise program? Other activities or treatments prescribed by your physician? What problems have you had? Why do you think you have had problems with these areas?" Does the family or physician report that the patient has missed medical appointments or has deviated from previous health care instructions?

Willingness to comply with future health care regimen

"In the future, do you think you will have problems following your diet? Exercise program? Taking your medications? Following other prescribed activities or treatments? Do you plan to follow the physician's instructions? Do you foresee any problems with following these instructions? Is there anything that is particularly unpleasant or difficult for you regarding these instructions? Can you think of anything that will interfere with your ability to _____?"[4]

Does the patient have any disturbances in memory, problem-solving ability, concentration, or psychopathology that could interfere with performance of the prescribed regimen? Does the patient have the motivation to comply with the regimen? Is the patient undergoing emotional reactions (i.e., denial, anger, and anxiety) that would interfere with the regimen?

What are the family's or significant others' predictions about the patient's future compliance? Do the significant others understand the illness and treatment? Believe in the treatment? Have the time, energy, and resources to help the patient comply with the regimen? View their support and assistance as part of their role and responsibilities?

Judgment
Decision-making ability
Patient's perspective

"Do you believe you usually make sound judgments? Under what circumstances would you say you have difficulty making decisions? When faced with a big decision, do you ever find it difficult to make up your mind as to what to do?"

Others' perspectives

What is the family's or significant others' opinions about the soundness of the patient's judgments? And the ability of the patient to make timely decisions?

APPLYING THE GENERAL FOCUS QUESTIONS AND PARAMETERS

Chapter 4 applies the general focus questions and parameters using the Cardiovascular Assessment Tool via a case study and demonstrates how the appropriate data are used to formulate nursing diagnoses. It also provides a care plan for two of the identified nursing diagnoses to illustrate each step of the nursing process.

REFERENCES

1. Carpenito LJ: Nursing diagnosis: application to clinical practice, Philadelphia, 1983, JB Lippincott Co.
2. Guzzetta CE and Dossey BM: Cardiovascular nursing: bodymind tapestry, St Louis, 1984, The CV Mosby Co.
3. Kenner CV, Guzzetta CE, and Dossey BM: Critical care nursing: body-mind-spirit, Boston, ed 2, 1985, Little, Brown & Co, Inc.
4. Kim MJ, McFarland GK, and McLane AM: Pocket guide to nursing diagnoses, ed 2, St Louis, 1987, The CV Mosby Co.
5. Kinney MR, Packa DR, and Dunbar SB, editors: AACN's clinical reference for critical care nursing, ed 2, New York, 1988, McGraw-Hill Inc.
6. Malasanos L, Barkanskas V, Moss M, and Stoltenberg-Allen K: Health assessment, ed 3, St Louis, 1986, The CV Mosby Co.
7. Massachusetts General Hospital: Normal reference laboratory values, N Engl J Med 314:39, 1986.
8. Seidel HM, Ball JW, Dains JE, and Benedict GW: Mosby's guide to physical examination, St Louis, 1987, The CV Mosby Co.
9. Tilkian SM, Conover MB, and Tilkian AG: Clinical implications of laboratory tests, ed 4, St Louis, 1987, The CV Mosby Co.
10. Thompson J, McFarland G, Hirsh J, Tucker S, and Bowers A: Clinical nursing, St Louis, 1986, The CV Mosby Co.
11. Underhill SL, Woods SL, Sivarajan E, and Halpenny CJ: Cardiac nursing, Philadelphia, 1982, JB Lippincott Co.

PRACTICAL APPLICATIONS:

CARDIOVASCULAR ASSESSMENT TOOL

CATHIE E. GUZZETTA
SANDRA O'SULLIVAN

This chapter discusses the practical applications of the Cardiovascular Assessment Tool and includes:

- *A cardiovascular case study*
- *A completed version of the Cardiovascular Assessment Tool based on the case study*
- *A care plan based on the case study*
- *The way to adapt the tool in the practice setting*
- *The way to adapt the tool as a screening tool*

PRACTICAL APPLICATIONS

The Cardiovascular Assessment Tool, discussed in Chapter 2, was used as the prototype for developing all the tools in this book. (Refer to the blank version of the Cardiovascular Assessment Tool on pp. 17 to 22.) The case study that follows illustrates the way the nursing data base prototype: Cardiovascular Assessment Tool is used at the bedside to derive nursing diagnoses. Based on the information obtained from a cardiovascular patient admitted to the coronary care unit, the data was documented on the assessment tool, and the information was synthesized.

The data documented on the Cardiovascular Assessment Tool in Fig. 4-1 provide the necessary supportive information to confirm the existence of specific *nursing diagnoses*. After the diagnoses were identified, they were prioritized and written on the nursing diagnoses/problem list at the end of the tool. An example of a care plan (Table 4-1) for two nursing diagnoses derived from the case study illustrates the way the nursing diagnoses guide the remaining steps of the nursing process. The care plan illustrates one nursing diagnosis from the "exchanging pattern" and another from the "knowing pattern." For both diagnoses, patient outcomes, outcome criteria, nursing orders, and a

method of evaluation were developed. *Patient outcomes* provide a direct statement of the end the patient will reach with regard to the nursing diagnosis. *Outcome criteria* are then developed for each patient outcome. Outcome criteria are the parameters or tools used to measure whether the patient outcome has been achieved. The nursing plan is then developed in terms of *nursing orders*. Nursing orders are specific actions the nurse performs that are appropriate for helping the patient resolve problems and are designed to achieve effective patient outcomes. Nursing orders are the plan that guides the nurse in *implementing care*. After implementation of care, the patient outcomes and outcome criteria are *evaluated* to determine whether they have been successfully achieved and to what extent.

CASE STUDY

Mr. J.R., a 46-year-old newspaper reporter, was admitted to the coronary care unit with substernal chest pain lasting 15 to 20 minutes and associated with chills, elevated temperature, and conjunctival petechiae. He remembered that, as a child, he had been told that he had a heart murmur. He had remained asymptomatic throughout his life without any restrictions in activity. A month before admission, he had visited the dentist for a gingivectomy but had not received prophylactic antibiotics before or after the procedure.

The patient had a sinus tachycardia of 110 beats per minute and a blood pressure of 128/80 mm Hg. He had normal first and second heart sounds and a grade 3/6 holosystolic murmur at the lower left sternal border with radiation to the left axilla. Echocardiography later confirmed the diagnosis of acute mitral regurgitation. The initial electro-

Text continued on p. 45.

Table 4-1
Care plan: Mr. J.R.

Nursing Diagnosis: infection (cardiac value) related to invasive dental work and insufficient knowledge to avoid exposure to pathogen

Patient outcome	Outcome criteria	Nursing orders	Evaluation
The patient's infecting organism will be identified from blood culture studies	The patient will verbalize: • A general description of the procedure • The need for blood culture studies • The frequency of the studies • The amount of blood drawn	Explain the procedure to the patient: • Serial blood cultures are drawn to demonstrate a sustained rather than transient bacteremia. • Blood cultures are drawn so the appropriate effective drug therapy can be selected. • Three to six samples are drawn. • The amount of blood drawn during each venipuncture is generally not more than 1 tablespoon.	The patient verbalized the following points related to the procedure: • The general description • The need for blood cultures studies • The frequency • The amount of blood drawn
	The patient will practice relaxation and imagery techniques during the procedure and will not exhibit a high level of anxiety related to the drawing of blood cultures.	Teach the patient a relaxation technique to practice during the procedure. Assess the patient's reaction and level of relaxation during the procedure.	The patient practiced relaxation and imagery techniques during the procedure and did not demonstrate a high level of anxiety.
The patient will not experience any complications from the procedure.	The patient will not experience any complications such as redness, swelling, induration, bleeding, or discomfort at the venipuncture site and will verbalize the need to report any complications.	Evaluate the venipuncture site for signs and symptoms of complications. Also instruct the patient to report any swelling, redness, bleeding, or discomfort around the venipuncture area. Supervise the drawing of blood samples for culturing *before* antibiotic therapy is administered.	The patient did not experience any complications from the procedure and was able to verbalize the need to report any complications.
The patient will demonstrate symptomatic improvement as a result of effective antibiotic therapy.	The patient will verbalize: • The rationale for therapy • A general description of the therapy • The frequency of therapy • The duration of therapy	Teach the patient about: • The need to sterilize the endocardial vegetations • General information related to therapy • The frequency of therapy • The need for a 28-day course (or longer) of continuous intravenous antibiotic therapy	The patient verbalized the following points related to therapy: • The rationale • Description of the therapy • The frequency • The duration

Continued

Table 4-1—cont'd
Care plan: Mr. J.R.

Nursing Diagnosis: infection (cardiac value) related to invasive dental work and insufficient knowledge to avoid exposure to pathogen			
Patient outcome	Outcome criteria	Nursing orders	Evaluation
		Administer the antibiotic therapy as ordered by the physician immediately *after* all blood culture samples have been drawn.	
		Assess the response to the antibiotic therapy.	
	The patient's temperature will return to normal in 4 to 5 days.	Take the patient's temperature every 4 hours.	The patient's temperature returned to normal in 4 days.
	The patient's appetite will improve in 10 days.	Evaluate appetite and offer favorite foods.	The patient's appetite improved in 1 week.
	The patient's complaints of weakness and fatigue will decrease in 1 week.	Evaluate level of fatigue related to daily activites.	The patient's general complaints related to the infection disappeared in 3 days.
	The patient's blood culture studies will be negative within 1 week.	Evaluate the results of blood culture studies.	The patient's blood culture studies were negative 1 week after the administration of antibiotic therapy.
	The patient's rheumatoid factor will disappear.		The patient's rheumatoid factor disappeared.
	The patient will not experience a worsening of the heart murmur, heart failure, rhythm or conduction disturbances embolic manifestations, or hypersensitivity reaction.	Assess the patient carefully for clinical manifestations (such as worsening of the heart murmur, heart failure, rhythm or conduction disturbances, embolic manifestations, and hypersensitivity reactions such as petechiae) that may persist or develop despite effective antibiotic therapy.	The patient did not experience a worsening of the heart murmur, heart failure, rhythm or conduction disturbances, embolic manifestations, or hypersensitivity reactions.
The patient will not experience any adverse reactions or complications from therapy.	The patient will not demonstrate an allergic reaction such as rash, urticaria, diarrhea, anaphylactic reactions, or other adverse reactions to the therapy.	Determine whether the patient has a history of allergic reactions to antibiotic therapy. Assess the patient for any allergic reactions to the antibiotic therapy.	The patient did not experience any allergic reactions related to the antibiotic therapy.
	The patient will verbalize the need to report any leakage, pain, or discomfort at the venipuncture site.	Explain that the patient should report any complications.	The patient verbalized the need to report any leakage, pain, or discomfort from the venipuncture site. No complications were reported or observed.

Table 4-1—cont'd
Care plan: Mr. J.R.

Nursing diagnosis: knowledge deficit related to acute illness and prophylactic prevention of reinfection			
Patient outcome	**Outcome criteria**	**Nursing orders**	**Evaluation**
The patient will verbalize knowledge of endocarditis and methods of prophylactic care to prevent reinfection.	The patient will:	Teach the patient (and family) about endocarditis,* including the following:	The patient:
	• Verbalize the normal function of the heart, heart valves, and circulation	• The normal functioning of the heart, the heart valves (use heart model and drawings), and circulation	• Verbalized the function of the heart, heart valves, and circulation
	• Define the term *endocarditis* and why he was susceptible to infection.	• The definitions of endocarditis and why he was susceptible to infection	• Defined endocarditis and explained that his susceptibility was related to his abnormal heart valve
	• Identify which valve is infected	• The mitral valve was infected	• Identified that the mitral valve was infected
	• Describe valvular changes that occur with endocarditis	• The pathophysiologic changes associated with endocarditis	• Described the valvular changes that occur with endocarditis
	• Describe the signs and symptoms that occur with endocarditis	• The signs and symptoms of endocarditis	• Described the signs and symptoms of endocarditis
	• List the possible portals of entry for a reinfecting organism	• The possible portals of entry for reinfection	• Listed the portals of entry for a reinfecting organism
	The patient will demonstrate how to take his own temperature.	Demonstrate proper temperature-taking techniques.	The patient successfully demonstrated how to take his own temperature.
	The patient will state the need for daily temperature taking and recording for 1 month after discharge.	Give directions for recording daily temperatures for 1 month.	The patient stated the need for daily temperature taking and recording for 1 month after discharge.
	The patient will state the need to contact his physician at the first sign of fever or reinfection.	Explain the necessity of contacting the physician at the first sign of fever or reinfection.	The patient stated the need to contact his physician at the first sign of fever or reinfection.
	The patient will describe his inpatient and outpatient progressive activity schedule.	Provide the patient with a written inpatient and outpatient progressive activity schedule. Explain the schedule.	The patient described his inpatient and outpatient activity schedule.
	The patient will state reasons for no strenuous work, sports, or activities for 1 month after discharge.	Explain the need to restrict activities for 1 month after discharge to promote endocardial healing.	The patient stated the reasons for no work, sports, or strenuous activities for 1 month after discharge.

*Footnotes 1, 2, 3, 6, 7, and 8.

Continued

Table 4-1—cont'd
Care plan: Mr. J.R.

	Nursing diagnosis: knowledge deficit related to acute illness and prophylactic prevention of reinfection		
Patient outcome	**Outcome criteria**	**Nursing orders**	**Evaluation**
	The patient will demonstrate techniques of good oral hygiene.	Explain good oral hygiene: brushing with a soft-bristled toothbrush twice a day, using firm, gentle motion, and avoiding trauma to the gums	The patient demonstrated techniques of good oral hygiene.
	The patient will describe devices that cause gum trauma, which should be avoided.	Direct the patient not to use a Water-Pik, toothpicks, or other devices that might cause the gums to bleed.	The patient described devices that cause gum trauma that should be avoided.
	The patient will state the importance of regular dental checkups.	Explain the importance of regular dental examinations.	The patient stated the importance of regular dental checkups.
	The patient will state the need for informing his dentist or physicians about his history of endocarditis and need for prophylactic antibiotic medications before and after surgical or dental manipulations and procedures.	Explain the need for the patient to tell his dentist or physicians about his history of endocarditis and the need for prophylactic antibiotics before and after invasive surgical or dental manipulations or procedures.	The patient stated the importance of informing his dentist and physicians about his history of endocarditis and the need for prophylactic antibiotic therapy before and after surgical or dental manipulations or procedures.
	The patient will be able to read and verbalize correct information about the prophylactic use of antibiotic medications.	Provide the patient with the American Heart Association's *Prevention of Bacterial Endocarditis*.[1] Explain appropriate prophylactic use of antibiotics.	The patient read and adequately verbalized the correct information about prophylactic use of antibiotic medications.
	The patient will state the importance of continuing relaxation and imagery techniques after discharge.	Explain the importance of continuing relaxation and imagery techniques to reduce stress and promote healing.	The patient stated the importance of continuing relaxation and imagery techniques after discharge.
	The patient will state where and when to return for blood tests.	Explain the necessity of returning for follow-up blood cultures every 2 weeks for 6 weeks after completing antibiotic therapy to ensure sterile blood cultures.	The patient stated where and when he would return for blood tests.
	The patient will state names and telephone numbers of primary care nurse, cardiologist, and clinic.	Provide the patient with the names and phone numbers of the attending cardiologist, clinic, and primary care nurse. Encourage him to call with questions.	The patient stated the names and telephone numbers of his primary care nurse, cardiologist, and clinic.

cardiogram suggested that the patient had anteroseptal myocardial ischemia. Cardiac serum enzyme values were all normal. The presumptive diagnosis of subacute infective endocarditis was made during the first day of admission. Within the next few days, serial aerobic and anaerobic blood cultures revealed a heavy growth of *S. viridans.* The patient was medically treated with penicillin, streptomycin, and bed rest.[2,3]

The Cardiovascular Assessment Tool (Fig. 4-1) was used to guide and document data collected during Mr. J.R.'s assessment. Based on the results of this assessment, a care plan for two of the identified nursing diagnoses is presented (Table 4-1).

ADAPTING THE CARDIOVASCULAR ASSESSMENT TOOL IN THE PRACTICE SETTING

The Cardiovascular Assessment Tool was never intended to be the standardized and final format for assessing critically ill cardiovascular patients across the country because an assessment tool must meet the needs of individual institutions and the nurses using it. The tool is simply a working demonstration tool expected to be changed and revised by nurses in clinical practice.[4,5]

If the use of one of the tools in this book within an institution or practice is being considered, further evaluation and refinement are necessary. All nurses who will use the tool should have the opportunity to evaluate it and make suggestions about its refinement. Thus, copies of the tool should be made available so each nurse can assess several patients, evaluate the tool's adequacy, and recommend changes. Permission to evaluate the tool should be sought from the appropriate administrators.

Before beginning evaluation and refinement, the nurses must be familiar with Taxonomy I and the rationale for the development of the tool. Thus, in-service classes may be necessary to provide a common knowledge base before attempts to evaluate the tool are made.

During evaluation, the flow of the tool and the adequacy of the data collected should be assessed. From this evaluation, the ordering of the tool can be rearranged, and additions, deletions, or clarification of assessment variables can be made as needed. In evaluating the Cardiovascular Assessment Tool, for example, a critical care unit may primarily admit cardiovascular patients but may also admit many patients with chronic obstructive pulmonary disease. As a result, nurses evaluating the Cardiovascular Assessment Tool may decide to add more extensive variables to the "exchanging pattern" under oxygenation so these patients can be more comprehensively assessed. Likewise, if it is believed that data collected from the "choosing pattern" should be identified earlier in the assessment, then this pattern can be placed earlier in the tool. If it is believed that the length of the tool is too long for assessing patients in a particular institution, it may be shortened by deleting some variables. For example, it may be decided that deep tendon reflexes are not routinely assessed by nurses in the unit and therefore the variable should be deleted.

After this evaluation, all the nurses involved should submit recommendations for revisions and reorganization. The tool should then be revised and reevaluated to ensure that it has been sufficiently refined to everyone's satisfaction. This final revision can then be submitted to the appropriate committee or administrative individual for hospital approval, printing, and reproduction. For information on validity and reliability testing of the tools, refer to Chapter 2.

ADAPTING THE CARDIOVASCULAR ASSESSMENT TOOL AS A SCREENING TOOL

The tools in this book can be easily adapted as short screening tools for rapid assessment of patients. The subsequent sections describe the purpose of the screening tool, the places it might be used, the necessity of collecting adequate data during a screening assessment, the way to use the tool to facilitate identification of nursing diagnoses, and additional suggestions for developing screening tools.

Purpose of the screening tools

The Cardiovascular Screening Tool (Fig. 4-2) was developed for use in settings outside the acute care environment. The screening assessment helps to rapidly collect the patient data necessary for identifying nursing diagnoses. Appropriate health care referrals, acute care intervention, or preventative measures can then be initiated. The variables included in the Cardiovascular Screening Tool were identified and selected to be the critical variables necessary to assess the nine human response patterns holistically.

Population and settings

The Cardiovascular Screening Tool can be used by nurses working in cardiac rehabilitation settings, collaborative practice settings (with physicians), and community health care settings; by nurse practitioners in private practice; by nurses conducting support groups for cardiac patients; by nurses screening patients in an emergency room setting or walk-in clinic.

In the cardiac rehabilitation setting, for example, nurses deal with patients recovering from a cardiac event (either medical or surgical) who are unsure of their potential for recovery. The Cardiovascular Screening Tool can be used to guide the identification of the patient's potential for recovery in all nine human response patterns. Identifying the correct nursing diagnoses will assist nurses to plan a patient rehabilitation program appropriately geared to the problems and strengths of the individual. All nine human response patterns are equally important during an assessment of a patient undergoing rehabilitation because an alteration or deficit in one pattern will ultimately impair progress in another. Nurses in such settings can use the Cardiovascular Screening Tool during initial contact and then update the tool periodically during rehabilitation.

In another example, clinical nurse specialists in collaborative practice with physicians dealing with cardiovascular patients or nurses in community health settings can use the tool to rapidly screen patient complaints or problems so the patients can be directed to the proper health care professional for treatment. Additionally, the tool can be used by nurses in such settings to document the signs and symptoms necessary to support the existence of specific nursing diagnoses requiring referral to support groups such as smoke-enders groups, weight- and diet-counseling programs, relaxation therapy, or exercise programs.

Collecting sufficient data

Identification of nursing diagnoses is made easier when using the Cardiovascular Screening Tool because assessment focuses on the human responses to problems as assessed in patterns rather than on the medical diagnosis and subsequent medical care. In creating the Cardiovascular Screening Tool, many of the assessment variables originally found in the prototype tool were deleted. The variables remaining in each of the patterns are needed to provide enough information and flexibility to identify major problems confronting a cardiovascular patient population in an outpatient setting. The defining characteristics from NANDA for each nursing diagnosis were also considered.

Sufficient data from each pattern must be collected, clustered, and synthesized to identify appropriate nursing diagnoses when using both tools, even though the screening tool is much shorter than the assessment tool. In the "communicating pattern," for example, the nurse collects enough information to sufficiently assess how the patient communicates with others. Thus the nurse, while collecting data related to speech and language, also pays attention to the patient's verbal and nonverbal communication (i.e., voice character) and observes whether the patient's behavior is appropriate for the situation.

In the "valuing pattern," the nurse collects adequate data to determine patient values and whether problems exist. Spiritual concerns or cultural problems may not be freely verbalized during assessment, but if they do exist, they will surface if discussed.

In the "relating pattern," the nurse needs enough information to evaluate how the patient relates to others and whether an alteration in this pattern exists. The assessment focuses on the areas of role performance and sexual and social relationships. Many cardiovascular patients have acute problems that must be identified so appropriate inter-

vention strategies or health care referrals can be planned.

From the "knowing pattern," the nurse collects sufficient data to determine what the patient knows about the current health care status. Assessment guides the collection of data about knowledge and perception of risk factors, illness, tests, surgery, medications, physical activities, prognosis, and misconceptions. Nursing diagnoses related to knowing are then identified to plan appropriate teaching, exercise, behavior-modification, and relaxation programs.

To assess the "feeling pattern" adequately, the nurse needs to evaluate how the patient feels physically and psychologically. Alterations often motivate patients to seek health care services. Patients experiencing pain or discomfort, heart irregularities, palpitations, fluid accumulation, dyspnea, acute stress, or depression, will often seek advice to determine whether acute intervention is necessary.

Within the "moving pattern," the nurse evaluates how well and independently the patient moves or performs activities of daily living. The screening tool focuses on performance of daily activities, exercise capabilities, sleep abilities, and boredom about decreased social or leisure activities. Alterations in this pattern also motivate patients to seek health care services. For example, the cardiac patient unable to walk around the house without chest pain or dyspnea is likely to call on the nurse to evaluate whether these problems require referral.

Within the "perceiving pattern," the nurse collects sufficient data to evaluate the patient's self-perception and perception of the situation. Assessment focuses on self-concept, body image, self-esteem, personal identity, hopelessness, and powerlessness. This is the area where the meaningfulness of information is translated by the patient. This pattern may be difficult to evaluate during a screening assessment because the patient may often be unaware or unable to verbalize some of these perceptions. Data from this area are essential to collect, however, because the patient's perception of a situation will profoundly affect the responses in the other eight patterns. For example, if hopelessness is perceived toward the situation, the patient will probably not be motivated to learn about the illness or will not comply with the recommended medical regimen.

In the "exchanging pattern," nurses collect enough data to assess the patient's physical condition. They will need to use physical assessment and interviewing, questioning, and listening skills. The tool focuses on assessment of neurologic, cardiovascular, respiratory, nutritional, gastrointestinal, and urinary variables, as well as laboratory values. The complete physical assessment is not usually necessary in the screening setting because the patient is known to have a primary cardiovascular medical diagnosis. Therefore the physical assessment is limited but directed toward identifying new problems related to the medical diagnosis or recently developed complications or documenting the current status of the primary medical problem. Problems can be quickly identified from the screening tool. The nurse then can decide whether there is a need for an acute care referral and whether the patient should be directed to another facility for appropriate care.

Within the "choosing pattern," the nurse determines whether the patient is successfully selecting alternatives consistent with health-promoting and wellness behaviors. The tool guides the collection of data in the areas of problem solving and coping related to the illness, surgery, or situations and information about the patient's past and future willingness to comply with the health care regimen. If the patient has not been compliant with the past medical regimen, the current problem may be a direct result of this noncompliance. Efforts are then directed toward planning strategies acceptable to the patient to improve compliance behaviors.

How to use the screening tool

When using the Cardiovascular Screening Tool to assess cardiovascular patients, nurses should collect the appropriate data from each of the nine patterns. Many of the tool variables require yes or no answers or a checkmark to indicate the presence of a specific variable. Circle the possible nursing diagnosis in the right-hand column of the tool when data to support it are identified. After assessment, synthesize the data to determine whether other clusters of signs and symptoms also support the existence of a particular diagnosis and make a judgment as to whether the actual diagnosis is present. If a patient is suspected to have a potential problem, write *potential* or *p* next to the diagnosis before circling it.

After synthesizing the data and judging that certain diagnoses actually exist, write the diagnoses and probable etiologies on the nursing diagnoses/problem list at the end of the tool. The diagnoses should be set in order of priority, with the most critical diagnoses first. Nurses then decide, for each problem, whether to refer the patient to an acute care facility or other health care professionals or to plan intervention themselves.

Additional suggestions for developing screening tools

The Cardiovascular Screening Tool can be adapted in many ways. In some settings it may be beneficial to rede-

sign the tool so many of the pertinent variables can be answered through a questionnaire completed by the patient. The remaining data would then be completed by the nurse. It may be decided after evaluating the screening tool that more variables should be added under the "exchanging pattern" or that less information should be included in the "moving pattern." Thus it is possible to adapt the tool by changing, deleting, or adding variables to meet the needs of the particular setting and patient population.

The Cardiovascular Screening Tool can also be used as a working prototype by changing it to assess other types of patients (i.e., those who have a primary pulmonary or neurologic medical diagnosis). Under the "exchanging pattern," for example, variables can be added or changed (i.e., related to pulmonary or neurologic assessment parameters) to assess the system associated with the patient's primary medical diagnosis. The other eight patterns in the screening tool generally are adaptable to other medical diagnoses with little or no change. It is also possible to adapt any other tool in this book to create a screening tool for other settings and patient populations.

REFERENCES

1. American Heart Association: Prevention of bacterial endocarditis, Dallas, 1985, American Heart Association.
2. Guzzetta CE: The person with infective endocarditis. In Guzzetta CE and Dossey BM: Cardiovascular nursing: bodymind tapestry, St Louis, 1984, The CV Mosby Co.
3. Guzzetta CE: Subacute and acute infective endocarditis. In Kenner CV Guzzetta CE, and Dossey BM: Critical care nursing: body-mind-spirit, ed 2, Boston, 1985, Little, Brown & Co, Inc.
4. Guzzetta CE, Bunton SD, Prinkey LA, Sherer AP, and Seifert PC: Unitary person assessment tool prototype. In Dossey BM, Keegan L, Guzzetta CE, and Kolkmeier L: Holistic nursing: a handbook for practice, Rockville, Md, 1988, Aspen Publishers, Inc.
5. Guzzetta CE, Bunton SD, Prinkey LA, Sherer AP, and Seifert PC: Unitary person assessment tool: easing problems with nursing diagnosis, Focus Crit Care 15:12, 1988.
6. Marrie TJ: Infective endocarditis: a serious and changing disease, Crit Care Nurs 7:31, 1987.
7. Scrima DA: Infective endocarditis: nursing considerations, Crit Care Nurs 7:46, 1987.
8. Wingate S: Rehabilitation of the patient with valvular heart disease, J Cardiovasc Nurs 1:52, 1987.

CARDIOVASCULAR ASSESSMENT TOOL

Name _Mr. J.R._   Age _46_   Sex _Male_
Address _620 Michigan, N.W., Washington DC 20006_   Telephone _555-1212_
Significant other _Mrs. S. R. (Wife)_   Telephone _Same_
Date of admission _1/23_   Medical diagnosis _Chest pain 1/23; S. viridans endocarditis 1/24_
Allergies _NKA_

Nursing Diagnosis
(Potential or Altered)

COMMUNICATING ▪ A pattern involving sending messages
(Read) (write,) (understand) English (circle) _____   Communication
Other languages _None_   Verbal
Intubated _No_ Speech impaired _No_   Nonverbal
Alternate form of communication _____

VALUING ▪ A pattern involving the assigning of relative worth
Religious preference _Active Baptist_   Spiritual state
Important religious practices _Church on Sundays_   Distress
Spiritual concerns _None_   Despair
Cultural orientation _Caucasian, American_
Cultural practices _None_

RELATING ▪ A pattern involving establishing bonds
Role
   Marital status _Married 20 years_   Role performance
   Age & health of significant other _Wife 44 y/o in good health_   Parenting
     Sexual dysfunction
   Number of children _2_ Ages _16 y/o boy; 18 y/o girl (Scott/Julie)_   Work
   Role in home _Major breadwinner and decision maker_   Family
   Financial support _Has enough money to meet expenses_   Social/leisure
   Occupation _Newspaper reporter; works 40h/wk; takes work home_   Family processes
     Job satisfaction/concerns _Enjoys busy active job_
     Physical/mental energy expenditures _Job involves some mental stress_
   Sexual relationships ((satisfactory) unsatisfactory) _____   Sexuality patterns
     Physical difficulties/effects of illness related to sex _None_

Socialization
   Quality of relationships with others _Gets along well with people_   Impaired social interaction
     Patient's description _Relationship with wife, children & coworkers good_
     Significant others' descriptions _Wife states they get along well_
     Staff observations _Pt. & wife communicate well & support each other_
   Verbalizes feelings of being alone _No; many friends & full social life_   Social isolation
   Attributed to _____   Social withdrawal

KNOWING ▪ A pattern involving the meaning associated with information
Current health problems _Substernal chest pain this morning (lasting 15-20 min.) without radiation._
No associated diaphoresis, SOB, or N/V. Also complains of flu-like symptoms for 2 weeks. (Chills,
fever, fatigue)
Previous illnesses/hospitalizations/surgeries _Told he had a heart murmur as_
a child but has never had symptoms or been treated for murmur.
No restrictions in activity. Had a gingivectomy one month ago. No previous hospitalizations
or surgery.

Fig. 4-1

History of the following problems:

Heart *HEART MURMUR; NO HISTORY OF PREVIOUS CHEST PAIN OR CAD*

Peripheral vascular *NONE*

Lung *NONE*

Liver *NONE* Kidney *NONE*

Cerebrovascular *NONE* Rheumatic fever *YES—AS A CHILD WITH DEVELOPMENT OF MURMUR*

Thyroid *NONE* Other *NONE*

Current medications *TYLENOL FOR FEVER*

Risk factors	Present	Perceptions/knowledge of
1. Hypertension	*No*	
2. Hyperlipidemia	*No*	
3. Smoking	*No*	
4. Obesity	*No*	
5. Diabetes	*No*	
6. Sedentary living	*No*	*ACTIVE IN JOB AND HOBBIES*
7. Stress	*SOME*	*SOME DAYS JOB IS STRESSFUL*
8. Alcohol use	*YES*	*1-2 BEERS/DAY*
9. Oral contraceptives	–	

10. Family history *MOTHER, WIFE, & CHILDREN ALL IN GOOD HEALTH; FATHER HAD hx OF RHEUMATIC FEVER AND DIED OF AMI AT AGE 52.*

Perception/knowledge of illness/tests/surgery *PT. WORRIED HE HAS HAD AMI LIKE HIS FATHER; UNAWARE OF NEED FOR PROPHYLACTIC ANTIBIOTICS BEFORE ANY INVASIVE PROCEDURE WITH hx OF HEART MURMUR.*

Expectations of therapy *TO FIND OUT WHAT IS WRONG; GET BETTER & GO HOME*

Misconceptions *CONCERNED THAT HIS HISTORY IS VERY SIMILAR TO HIS FATHER'S*

Readiness to learn *ASKING QUESTIONS ABOUT HOW AMI IS DIAGNOSED & TREATED*

Requests information concerning *AS ABOVE*

Educational level *COLLEGE GRADUATE IN JOURNALISM*

Learning impeded by ———

(Knowledge deficit) *(circled, top right)*

Thought processes

Orientation

Level of alertness *FULLY ALERT*

Orientation: Person *YES* Place *YES* Time *YES*

Appropriate behavior/communication *YES*

Orientation

Confusion

Memory

Memory intact: Yes *X* No ——— Recent *YES* Remote *YES*

Memory

FEELING ▪ A pattern involving the subjective awareness of information

Comfort

Pain/discomfort: Yes ——— No *NONE AT PRESENT*

Onset – Duration –

Location – Quality – Radiation –

Associated factors –

Aggravating factors –

Alleviating factors –

Comfort

Pain/chronic

Pain/acute

Discomfort

Emotional Integrity/States

Recent stressful life events *NONE*

_____

Verbalizes feelings of *ANXIETY*

Source *CONCERNED ABOUT SIMILARITIES OF HIS FATHER'S HISTORY WITH HIS OWN.*

Physical manifestations *DARTING EYE MOVEMENTS, STARTLE REFLEX TO NORMAL SOUNDS, CONTINUOUS NON PURPOSEFUL FOOT ACTIVITY*

Grieving

(Anxiety) *(circled)*

Fear

Anger

Guilt

Shame

Sadness

Fig. 4-1, cont'd

Continued.

MOVING ▪ A pattern involving activity
Activity

History of physical disability _____ _____ | Impaired physical mobility
_____ | Activity intolerance

Limitations in daily activities _____ _____
_____

Verbal report of fatigue/weakness *LAST 2 WEEKS — BOTH FATIGUE & WEAKNESS*
Exercise habits *MUCH WALKING INVOLVED WITH JOB; EXERCISE WITH YARD WORK*

Rest

Hours slept/night _____*8 h*_____ Feels rested: Yes _*X*_ No _____ | Sleep pattern disturbances
Sleep aids (pillows, meds, food) _____*SHOWER BEFORE BEDTIME*_____ | Hypersomnia
Difficulty falling/remaining asleep _____*NONE*_____ | Insomnial
| Nightmares

Recreation

Leisure activities *FISHING/BOWLING ō WEEKENDS; YARDWORK* | Deficit in diversional activity
Social activities *SINGS IN CHURCH CHOIR WEEKLY*

Environmental Maintenance

Home maintenance management | Impaired home maintenance
 Size & arrangement of home (stairs, bathroom) *No PROBLEMS* | management
_____ Safety needs *NONE* | Safety hazards
 Home responsibilities *INVOLVED WITH BILL PAYING; ASSISTS WIFE*
WITH FOOD SHOPPING; YARDWORK

Health Maintenance

Health insurance *YES FROM WORK* | (Health maintenance)
Regular physical checkups *HAS NOT SEEN A PHYSICIAN IN YEARS; VISITED*
DENTIST ONE MONTH AGO

Self-Care

Ability to perform ADLs: Independent _____*X*_____ Dependent _____ | Self-care
Specify deficits *NONE* | Feeding
Discharge planning needs *NONE IDENTIFIED RELATED TO SELF-CARE* | Bathing/hygiene
| Dressing/grooming
| Toileting

PERCEIVING ▪ A pattern involving the reception of information
Self-Concept

Patient's description of self *"I AM A HARDWORKING GUY WITH A GOOD FAMILY "* | Self-concept
Effects of illness/surgery on self-concept *"I AM NOT SURE HOW THIS WILL* | Body image
AFFECT MY FUTURE JOB, FINANCES, & FAMILY. I GUESS I NEED TO | Self-esteem
FIND OUT WHATEVER THE PROBLEM IS FIRST BEFORE I WORRY ABOUT THAT." | Personal identity
Meaningfulness

Verbalizes hopelessness *NO — HOPES TO RETURN TO HOME & JOB* | Hopelessness
Verbalizes/perceives loss of control *No* | Powerlessness

Sensory/Perception | Sensory/perception

History of restricted environment *NONE*
Vision impaired *No* Glasses *No* | Visual
Auditory impaired *No* Hearing aid *No* | Auditory
Kinesthetics impaired *No* | Kinesthetic
Gustatory impaired *No* | Gustatory
Tactile impaired *No* | Tactile
Olfactory impaired *No* | Olfactory

Reflexes: Biceps R *2+* L *2+*   Triceps R *2+* L *2+*
    Brachioradialis R *2+* L *2+*   Knee R *2+* L *2+*
    Ankle R *2+* L *2+*   Plantar R *2+* L *2+*

Fig. 4-1, cont'd

EXCHANGING ▪ A pattern involving mutual giving and receiving
Circulation
Cerebral
Neurologic changes/symptoms *NONE NOTED* — Cerebral tissue perfusion

Pupils   Eye Opening
L 2 ③ 4 5 6 mm   None (1)
R 2 ③ 4 5 6 mm   To pain (2)
Reaction: Brisk *X*   To speech (3)   Fluid volume
Sluggish ___ Nonreactive ___   Spontaneous ④   Deficit
     Excess

Best Verbal   Best Motor
No response (1)   Flaccid (1)
Incomprehensible sound (2)   Extensor response (2)   Cardiac output
Inappropriate words (3)   Flexor response (3)
Confused conversation (4)   Semipurposeful (4)
Oriented ⑤   Localized to pain (5)
         Obeys commands ⑥

Glasgow Coma Scale total *15*
Cardiac
PMI *5ICS, MCL* Pacemaker —   Cardiopulmonary tissue
Apical rate & rhythm *110 AND REGULAR*   perfusion
Heart sounds/murmurs *NORMAL S₁ & S₂; NO S₃ OR S₄ OR RUBS; GRADE III/VI HOLOSYSTOLIC MURMUR*
Dysrhythmias *SINUS TACHYCARDIA*   *AT LLSB WITH RADIATION TO* Fluid volume
BP: Sitting   Lying *LEFT AXILLA* Standing   Deficit
R*124/78* L*126/78*   R*128/80* L*128/80*   R*126/78* L*126/80*   Excess
A-Line reading —
Cardiac index — Cardiac output —   (Cardiac output)
CVP — PAP — PCWP —   (POTENTIAL)
IV fluids *D5W TKO*
IV cardiac medications —

Serum enzymes *NORMAL CPK & LDH*
Peripheral   Peripheral tissue perfusion
Jugular venous distension R *No*   L *No*
Pulses: A = absent   B = bruits   D = doppler
    +3 = bounding   +2 = palpable   +1 = faintly palpable
Carotid R *2+* L *2+*   Popliteal   R *2+* L *2+*
Brachial R *2+* L *2+*   Posterior tibial R *2+* L *2+*   Fluid volume
Radial   R *2+* L *2+*   Dorsalis pedis R *2+* L *2+*   Deficit
Femoral R *2+* L *2+*   Excess
Skin temp *WARM/HOT* Color *PALE*
Capillary refill *2 SECONDS* Clubbing *NONE*   Cardiac output
Edema *NONE*

Physical Integrity
Tissue integrity *GUMS HEALING FROM GINGIVECTOMY*   Impaired tissue integrity
Skin integrity *NORMAL HYDRATION, ELASTICITY, & TURGOR*   Impaired skin integrity
Rashes *NONE*   Lesions *NONE*
Petechiae *BILATERAL CONJUNCTIVAL* Bruises *NONE*
Abrasions *NONE*   Surgical incisions *NONE*
Other *SPLINTER HEMORRHAGES ON DISTAL ⅓ OF NAIL ON INDEX AND*
     RING FINGER OF (RT) HAND

Fig. 4-1, cont'd

Continued.

Oxygenation

Complaints of dyspnea *NONE* Precipitated by ———

Orthopnea *NONE*

Rate *16* Rhythm *REGULAR* Depth *NORMAL*   Ineffective breathing patterns

Labored/(unlabored) (circle) Use of accessory muscles *NONE*   Ineffective airway clearance

Chest expansion *SYMMETRICAL* Splinting *NONE*   Impaired gas exchange

Cough: productive/nonproductive *NONE*

Sputum: Color ——— Amount ——— Consistency ———

Breath sounds *NORMAL BREATH SOUNDS; NO RALES, CRACKLES, OR WHEEZES*

Arterial blood gases ———

Oxygen percent and device ———

Ventilator ———

Physical Regulation *ESR ELEVATED; POSITIVE RHEUMATIC FACTOR*   (Infection)

Immune   Hypothermia

    Lymph nodes enlarged *NONE* Location ———   Hyperthermia

    WBC count *24,000* Differential *65% SEGS/15% BANDS*   (Body temperature)

    Temperature *101.4°F* Route *ORAL*   Ineffective thermoregulation

Nutrition   Nutrition

Eating patterns

    Number of meals per day *3 MEALS WITH SNACK BEFORE BEDTIME*

    Special diet *NONE*

    Where eaten *NONE*

    Food preferences/intolerances *DISLIKES FISH; INTOLERANCE TO CITRUS*

    Food allergies *NONE*

    Caffeine intake (coffee, tea, soft drinks)

    2 CUPS COFFEE/DAY; 2 COKES/DAY

    Appetite changes *POOR APPETITE LAST 2 WEEKS BUT DRINKING FLUIDS NORMALLY*

    Nausea/vomiting *NONE*

Condition of mouth/throat *LIPS HYDRATED; GUMS INFLAMMED; GOOD DENTAL HYGIENE; NO DENTURES*

OR MISSING TEETH; TONGUE HYDRATED; NORMAL HARD & SOFT PALATE   Oral mucous membrane

Height *5'9"* Weight *165* Ideal body weight *160*   More than body
        requirements

Current therapy   Less than body requirements

    NPO ——— NG suction ———

    Tube feeding ———

    TPN ———

Labs

    Na *140 mEq/L* K *4.2 mEq/L* CL *100 mEq/L* Glucose *106 mg/dl*

    Cholesterol *185 mg/dl* Triglycerides *150 mg/dl* Fasting *YES*

    Hct *44%* Hgb *13.5 g/dl*

Elimination

Gastrointestinal/bowel   Bowel elimination

    Usual bowel habits *DAILY BOWEL MOVEMENT*   Constipation

    Alterations from normal ———   Diarrhea

    Abdominal physical examination *NORMAL SIZE, SHAPE, & SYMMETRY; 2+*   Incontinence

BOWEL SOUNDS; NO MASSES, PAIN, OR ORGAN ENLARGEMENT   GI tissue perfusion

Renal/Urinary

    Usual urinary pattern *VOIDS WITHOUT DIFFICULTY*   Urinary elimination

    Alterations from normal *NONE*   Incontinence

    Color *YELLOW* Catheter ———   Retention

    Urine output: 24 hour ——— Average hourly *60 CC*   Renal tissue perfusion

    Bladder distention *NONE*

    BUN *22 mg/dl* Creatinine *0.7 mg/dl* Specific gravity *1.009*

    Urine studies *NONE*

Fig. 4-1, cont'd

CHOOSING ▪ A pattern involving the selection of alternatives

Coping

Patient's usual problem-solving methods _BELIEVES HE SOLVES PROBLEMS WELL; DISCUSSES PROBLEMS AND SOLUTIONS WITH WIFE_ — Ineffective individual coping

Family's usual problem-solving methods _WIFE USUALLY ASKS HUSBAND FOR HELP IN SOLVING BIG PROBLEMS_ — Ineffective family coping

Patient's method of dealing with stress _GETS EXTRA SLEEP AND TRIES TO FACE PROBLEM/STRESS & LOOK FOR SOLUTIONS_

Family's method of dealing with stress _WIFE TENDS TO EAT MORE; CHILDREN SOMETIMES GET ANGRY & CRY_

Patient's affect _NORMAL_

Physical manifestations _NONE_

Support systems available _PATIENT HAS A LARGE GROUP OF SOCIAL AND CHURCH FRIENDS WHO HAVE ASSISTED HIM IN PAST WITH PROBLEMS_

Participation

Compliance with past/current health care regimens _NO PAST EXPERIENCE WITH HEALTH CARE REGIMEN_ — Noncompliance

Willingness to comply with future health care regimen _ALTHOUGH PT. IS NOT SURE WHAT FUTURE REGIMEN WILL BE, HE STATES HE WILL GLADLY FOLLOW ADVICE GIVEN BY HEALTH CARE MEMBERS_ — Ineffective participation

Judgment

Decision-making ability — Judgment

   Patient's perspective _BELIEVES HIS ABILITY TO MAKE DECISIONS IS GOOD_ — Indecisiveness

   Others' perspectives _WIFE TRUSTS HIS JUDGMENT_

Prioritized nursing diagnosis/problem list _TO PATHOGEN_
1. _INFECTION (CARDIAC VALVE) R/TO INVASIVE DENTAL WORK & INSUFFICIENT KNOWLEDGE TO AVOID EXPOSURE_
2. _POTENTIAL DECREASED CARDIAC OUTPUT R/TO TACHYDYSRHYTHMIAS & DESTRUCTION OF MITRAL VALVE_
3. _KNOWLEDGE DEFICIT R/TO ACUTE ILLNESS AND PROPHYLACTIC PREVENTION OF REINFECTION_
4. _ANXIETY R/TO ACUTE ILLNESS, HOSPITALIZATION, & SIMILARITY OF HISTORY WITH FATHER'S_
5. _ALTERED HEALTH MAINTENANCE R/TO LACK OF HEALTH-SEEKING BEHAVIOR_

Signature _Cathie E. Guzzetta, RN_   Date _1/24_

Fig. 4-1, cont'd

CARDIOVASCULAR SCREENING TOOL

Name _____ Age _____ Sex _____
Address _____ Telephone _____
Significant other _____ Telephone _____
Date of admission _____ Medical diagnosis _____
Allergies _____

Nursing Diagnosis
(Potential or Altered)

COMMUNICATING ▪ A pattern involving sending messages
Read, write, understand English (circle)   Communication
Speech impaired: yes/no   Verbal
Character of voice _____   Nonverbal

VALUING ▪ A pattern involving the assigning of relative worth   Spiritual state
Spiritual concerns _____   Distress
                                                                                              Despair

RELATING ▪ A pattern involving establishing bonds
Predominant role in home _____   Role performance
    Problems _____   Family processes
Family situation: stable/unstable
Job satisfaction concerns _____
Sexual relationships intact: yes/no   Sexuality patterns
Social relationships: functional/dysfunctional   Impaired social interaction
    Prefers to be alone/with family/with friends   Social isolation
                                                                                              Social withdrawal

KNOWING ▪ A pattern involving the meaning associated with information
Risk factor analysis: (Designate + or −)
    1. Hypertension _____ 6. Sedentary living _____   Knowledge deficit
    2. Hyperlipidemia _____ 7. Stress _____
    3. Smoking _____ 8. Alcohol use _____
    4. Obesity _____ 9. Oral contraceptives _____
    5. Diabetes _____ 10. Family history _____

Perception/knowledge of:	Appropriate	Inappropriate
Illness/disease	_____	_____
Test/surgery	_____	_____
Medications	_____	_____
Physical activity	_____	_____
Prognosis	_____	_____

Misconceptions _____   Impaired thought processes
Orientation: Person _____ Place _____ Time _____   Orientation
Memory intact: yes/no   Recent _____ Remote _____   Memory

FEELING ▪ A pattern involving the subjective awareness of information
Presence of pain/discomfort: yes/no
    Onset _____ Location _____ Duration _____   Comfort
    Quality _____ Radiation: back/jaw/arm/other _____   Pain
    Associated factors: nausea/vomiting/headache/other _____   Discomfort
    Aggravating factors: activity/emotions/exposure/eating/other _____
Alleviating factors: rest/medication/position change/other _____
Patient's heart awareness: present/absent
    Irregularities _____ Palpitations _____
    Fluid accumulation _____ Dyspnea _____

Fig. 4-2

Recent stressful life events _____ Anxiety
   Verbalizes feelings of: Anxiety _____ Fear _____ Guilt _____ Fear
   Depression _____ Shame _____ Sadness _____ Anger _____ Guilt
      Other

MOVING: ▪ A pattern involving activity

Ability to perform daily activities/exercise habits: yes/no   Impaired physical mobility
   Verbal report of fatigue or weakness: yes/no   Activity intolerance
Verbalizes rest/sleep as: not restful _____ Sleep pattern disturbances
   Characterized by inability to fall or remain asleep _____
Verbalizes boredom over lack/decreased social/leisure activities   Deficit in diversional activities
Size and arrangement of home _____
   Home responsibilities: Shopping _____ Cooking _____ Impaired home maintenance
     Cleaning _____ Finance management _____ Transportation _____   management
Ability to perform activities of daily living independently: yes/no
   Specify deficits _____ Self-care

PERCEIVING: ▪ A pattern involving mutual giving and receiving

Verbalizes change in feelings about self due to: Self-concept
   Diagnosis _____ Illness _____ Surgery _____ Other _____   Body image
Verbalizes hopelessness/loss of control (circle)   Self-esteem
      Personal identity
      Hopelessness
      Powerlessness

EXCHANGING: ▪ A pattern involving mutual giving and receiving

Syncopal episodes: yes/no   Carotid bruits: positive/negative   Cerebral tissue perfusion
Pacemaker (brand, model, mode) _____ Cardiopulmonary tissue
Apical rate _____ Rhythm _____ Heart sounds_____   perfusion
Dysrhythmias _____ Cardiac output
Blood pressure _____ Position _____
Jugular venous distension: yes/no   Right _____ Left _____   Peripheral tissue perfusion
Capillary refill _____ Clubbing _____ Edema _____
Complaints of dyspnea: yes/no   Precipitated by _____ Ineffective breathing patterns
Rate _____ Rhythm _____ Depth _____Labored/unlabored   Ineffective airway clearance
Cough: productive/nonproductive   Describe sputum _____ Impaired gas exchange
Breath sounds: clear/rales/rhonchi/wheezes/other _____
Eating pattern: changed/unchanged
Caffeine intake: coffee/tea/soda/chocolate Food allergies _____ Nutrition
Height _____ Weight _____ Recent weight change _____   More/less than body
Labs: Cholesterol _____ HDL _____LDL _____ Triglycerides _____   requirements
Gastrointestinal changes _____ Bowel elimination
Urinary changes _____ Urinary elimination

CHOOSING: ▪ A pattern involving the selection of alternatives

Verbalizes individual/family inability to problem solve/cope with illness/   Ineffective coping
   surgery/situation _____
Compliance with past/current health care regimen: yes/no   Noncompliance
Willingness to comply with future health care regimen: yes/no   Ineffective participation
Verbalizes ability to make sound judgment: yes/no   Judgment
      Indecisiveness

Prioritized nursing diagnosis/problem list
1. _____
2. _____
3. _____

Signature _____ Date _____

Fig. 4-2, cont'd

■ UNIT II ■
ASSESSING PATIENTS WITH MAJOR SYSTEMS DYSFUNCTIONS

CHAPTER 5

PULMONARY ASSESSMENT TOOL

SHELIA D. BUNTON
SUSAN FICKERTT WILSON

The Pulmonary Assessment Tool was designed to assess pulmonary patients with unique biopsychosocial assessment needs. The tool incorporates specific signs and symptoms pertinent to the pulmonary patient that support and facilitate the identification of nursing diagnoses. This chapter includes:

- *The way the tool was developed and refined*
- *The patient population and setting to which it applies*
- *Selected pulmonary emphasis areas*
- *The way to use the tool*
- *Specific pulmonary focus questions and parameters to assist the nurse in eliciting appropriate data*
- *The Pulmonary Assessment Tool*
- *A case study*
- *A completed version of the tool based on the case study*

DEVELOPMENT AND REFINEMENT OF THE TOOL

The Pulmonary Assessment Tool was developed from the nursing data base prototype (see Chapter 2). Many of the hemodynamic monitoring and critical care variables originally incorporated in the prototype were retained, and pulmonary specific variables were added to facilitate its use in various settings. The content of this tool, supported by pulmonary and respiratory care books and reference articles, was then presented to a team of experienced pulmonary nurses.

Nurses with masters and doctoral degrees clinically tested the tool on eight adult patients in intensive care or acute medical units. These patients, varying in age from 28 to 71 years, had pulmonary oriented diagnoses that in-

cluded chronic obstructive pulmonary disease (COPD) and acute respiratory distress syndrome (ARDS). The testing evaluated the adequacy of the tool in terms of flow, space for documenting data, and completeness of assessment variables. Based on the results of the testing, the tool was revised.

PATIENT POPULATION AND SETTING

The tool was developed to assess the needs and problems of adult patients who might have respiratory related problems or diagnoses. For patients whose pulmonary disease is compounded by surgical or medical problems, use of the Critical Care Assessment Tool (see Chapter 12), which incorporates in-depth system parameters for assessing patients with multiple systems failure, is recommended.

The Pulmonary Assessment Tool can be used in both acute and chronic settings in hospitals, for presurgery screening, and in the clinic with stable or unstable pulmonary patients. To prevent increased dyspnea, air hunger, and anxiety in the patient, the nurse may complete the tool over two sessions, preferably within the first 24 hours after admission. The data in the tool may also require revision as the patient's condition changes from acute care toward rehabilitation and discharge. Depending on the patient's degree of orientation, family members or significant others may help in providing some of the data necessary to complete the assessment.

PULMONARY EMPHASIS AREAS

Pulmonary patients have specialized problems and needs. The Pulmonary Assessment Tool, developed to include assessment variables within the nine human response patterns, focuses on prevalent problems of the respiratory patient. Table 5-1 outlines these emphasis areas.

HOW TO USE THE TOOL

For effective use of the Pulmonary Assessment Tool, several factors must be considered. First, nurses must familiarize themselves with the nine human response patterns of the Unitary Person Framework (see Chapter 2), which provides the underlying framework for Taxonomy I. The human response patterns serve as the major category headings for Taxonomy I and the tool. The sequence of the response patterns, as it appears in Taxonomy I, has been changed in this tool to permit better ordering of assessment variables. Nursing diagnoses pertinent to respiratory patients along with the signs and symptoms necessary to identify them, have been added to the appropriate response patterns in the tool.

Second, nurses must realize that this tool is very different from conventional pulmonary assessment tools. As a result, nurses may encounter some initial difficulty in using it. They should remember, however, that this tool was not designed to follow the organization or content of the traditional medical data base; the data collected do not solely reflect medical patterns. Rather, this tool elicits information about holistic patterns in ways not traditionally assessed by nurses. It represents a new way of collecting and synthesizing data that requires new thinking when processing data. This tool represents a nursing data base developed from a nursing model that permits a holistic nursing assessment to take place so nursing diagnoses can be identified.

Although nurses would probably agree that a holistic nursing data base would help practice, it is realized that changing traditional assessment methods is not an easy task. For this reason, a trial usage period is recommended before nurses make any decisions about the merits of the tool. During this period, nurses should assess 10 pulmonary patients using the tool to become familiar and progressively more comfortable with its organization and data-collection methods. With experience, nurses will become accustomed to new ways of clustering and processing information. With continued use, the time necessary to complete the tool will be reduced. Most important, nurses will recognize the unique ability of the tool to elicit appropriate signs and symptoms. They will discover that nursing diagnoses are easily identified when using the tool.

It is not necessary to complete the entire tool in one session. Priority sections can be designated for initial assessment. Other sections or patterns can be completed later, within a time frame acceptable to the institution. To elicit appropriate data, the nurse should be familiar with the associated focus questions and parameters (see next section). When assessing specific signs and symptoms that may affirm a diagnosis, the nurse circles the diagnosis in the right-hand column. The circled diagnosis does not confirm the existence of a problem, but simply alerts the nurse to the possibility that it may exist. After completing the assessment, the nurse visually scans the circled potential problems, synthesizes the data to determine whether other clusters of signs and symptoms also support the existence of a particular problem, and then judges whether the actual diagnosis is present. Some diagnoses may be repeated in more than one place. These repetitions occur only within the appropriate response pattern and are convenient for identifying data directly with their corresponding nursing diagnoses. These diagnoses are not absolute but are intended to focus thinking and direct more detailed attention to collecting data concerning a possible problem.

Certain signs and symptoms can indicate any number of diagnoses. For example, fever can indicate infection and ineffective thermoregulation. To avoid unnecessary repetition of assessment parameters, variables are arranged with the diagnosis most likely to result from the data assessed. Thus, data to support a specific diagnosis may occasionally be found in other patterns or arranged with other diagnoses. Therefore, synthesis of all data is essential.

The Pulmonary Assessment Tool is not intended to be the standardized and final format for assessing pulmonary patients nationwide. An assessment tool must meet the needs of the individual institutions and nurses using it. It is a working demonstration tool that is expected to be changed and revised by nurses in clinical practice. Further evaluation and refinement of the tool are necessary before adopting it for use within a particular institution. Nurses interested in changing, revising, and adapting the tool to a specific clinical setting should refer to Chapter 4.

Table 5-1

Selected pulmonary emphasis areas

Patterns	Emphasis areas to determine
Communicating	Speech impairment
Knowing	Comprehensive history of lung-related illnesses
	Exposure to environmental irritants
	Perception of relationship between history and illness
Moving	Limitations in daily activities
	Verbal report of fatigue or weakness
Exchanging	Alterations in oxygenation, expanded to include in-depth physical assessment, laboratory data, pulmonary function tests, and bronchoscopy
	In-depth WBC differential
	Dyspnea while eating

HOW TO ELICIT APPROPRIATE DATA

Because the Unitary Person Framework and the Pulmonary Assessment Tool contain some terminology that may be unfamiliar to nurses, specific respiratory focus questions and parameters were developed and refined to help the nurse in eliciting appropriate information. These focus questions and parameters are outlined in Table 5-2, which is ordered to follow the content of the Pulmonary Assessment Tool (Fig. 5-1). The data in bold type in the tool are described more fully in the focus questions and parameters in Table 5-2. For example, the variable about exposure to environmental irritants under the "knowing pattern" is in bold type; if nurses are unsure what questions should be asked to elicit appropriate information about environmental irritants, they can use the questions and parameters in Table 5-2 to direct the line of questioning. These questions and parameters are only suggestions intended to assist the nurse in focusing content when collecting data; they are

Table 5-2
Pulmonary assessment tool: focus questions and parameters

Variables	Focus questions and parameters
COMMUNICATING	
Speech imparied	Does the patient have difficulty talking?
	Does the patient frequently pause while talking to take a breath?
	Is the work of breathing so great that the patient cannot speak?
	Is the work of breathing so great that the patient must whisper?
KNOWING	
Exposure to environmental/chemical irritants	"Do you work in an area where chemicals, cleaning agents, smoke, dust, or other irritants might be inhaled?"
	"Do you have allergies to cats, dogs, flowers, or pollen?"
	"Is the air in your home or work place extremely hot or cold? Humid or dry?"
	"Are there areas in your neighborhood or work place where you find it difficult to breath?"
	"If so, what do you suspect is the source?"
Recognizes relationship between history and illness	"Is there anything in your past history that you feel may have led to your illness?"
	"Can you tell me how your history of _____ is related to your illness?"
MOVING	
Limitations in daily activities	"Do you find you become short of breath while participating in your daily routine?"
Report of fatigue or weakness	"Do you find you are too weak or fatigued to accomplish your daily activities?"
EXCHANGING	
Complaints of dyspnea	"Do you ever notice you are unable to catch your breath or take in enough air?"
	"Do you ever feel faint or dizzy?"
	"Do you ever have tingling in your fingers?"
Orthopnea	Is the patient sitting upright, hunched forward, and supported on elbows (three-point position)?
Rhythm	Are the patient's respirations regular or irregular?
	Are the respirations smooth or even?
Depth	Are the respirations shallow or deep?
	Are the respirations symmetrical or asymmetrical?
Pursed lips	Does the patient exhale with lips in "O" shape?
	Does the patient have a prolonged expiratory phase?
Breath sounds	On auscultation, are sounds diminished, absent, or abnormal?
	If so, where? Upper, middle, or lower lobes?
	Are rales (crackles), rhonchi (wheezes), or rubs (squeaks) present? If so, where?
Dyspnea while eating	"Do you find it more difficult to breath while you are eating?"
	"Do you feel you are not getting enough air while you are eating?"

not static or absolute. Nurses should not feel they must ask only these questions or assess only these parameters because there are many other ways to elicit the appropriate information based on the situation or condition and the skill of the nurse. Focus questions and parameters for most other data not in bold type were presented in Chapter 3.

CASE STUDY

The case study models the process a nurse uses when assessing a patient. Then, based on the clustering of information obtained during the assessment, nursing diagnoses are formulated.

Sixty-two-year-old Mr. P.D. was admitted for exacerbation of COPD. He is married, recently retired, and has a lengthy history of respiratory illness. The Pulmonary Assessment Tool (Fig. 5-2) was used to assess Mr. P.D.

BIBLIOGRAPHY

Bates B: A guide to physical examination and history taking, ed 4, Philadelphia, 1987, JB Lippincott Co.

Gettrust KV, Ryan SC, and Engelman DS, editors: Applied nursing diagnosis, New York, 1985, John Wiley & Sons, Inc.

Glennon S, Matus V, and Bryan-Brown C: Respiratory disorders. In Kinney M, editor: AACN's clinical reference for critical care nursing, New York, 1981, McGraw-Hill Inc.

Kim MJ, editor: Ineffective airway clearance and breathing patterns, Nurs Clin North Am 22:1, 1987.

Seidel HM, Ball JW, Dains JE, and Benedict GW: Mosby's guide to physical examination, St Louis, 1987, The CV Mosby Co.

Taylor CM and Cress SS: Nursing diagnosis cards, Springhouse, Pa, 1987, Springhouse Corp.

Thompson J, McFarland GK, Hirsch JE, Tucker SM, and Bowers AC: Clinical nursing, St Louis, 1986, The CV Mosby Co.

Wade J: Comprehensive respiratory care, ed 3, St Louis, 1982, The CV Mosby Co.

PULMONARY ASSESSMENT TOOL

Name _____ Age _____ Sex _____

Address _____ Telephone _____

Significant other _____ Telephone _____

Date of admission _____ Medical diagnosis _____

Allergies _____

Nursing Diagnosis
(Potential or Altered)

COMMUNICATING ■ A pattern involving sending messages

Read, write, understand English (circle)_____ Communication

Other languages _____ Verbal

Intubated _____**Speech impaired** _____ Nonverbal

Alternate form of communication _____

VALUING ■ A pattern involving the assigning of relative worth

Religious preference _____ Spiritual state

Important religious practices/concerns _____ Distress

_____ Despair

Cultural orientation _____

Cultural practices _____

RELATING ■ A pattern involving establishing bonds

Role

Marital status _____ Role performance

Age & health of significant other _____ Parenting

_____ Sexual dysfunction

Number of children _____ Ages _____ Work

Role in home _____ Social/leisure

Financial support _____

Occupation _____

Job satisfaction/concerns _____ Family processes

Sexual relationships (satisfactory/unsatisfactory) _____ Sexuality patterns

Socialization

Quality of relationships with others _____ Impaired social interaction

Patient's description _____

Significant others' descriptions _____

Staff observations _____

Verbalizes feelings of being alone _____ Social isolation

Attributed to _____ Social withdrawal

KNOWING ■ A pattern involving the meaning associated with information

Current health problems _____ Knowledge deficit

_____

Current medications _____

_____

Previous illness/hospitalizations/surgeries _____

_____

Fig. 5-1

Continued.

History of the following problems:

Heart _____ Hypertension _____

Kidney _____ Liver _____

Diabetes _____ Cancer _____

Anemia _____

Lung: Asthma _____ Bronchitis _____ Emphysema _____

Fibrocystic disease _____ Pneumonia _____

Pneumothorax _____ Pulmonary edema/embolus _____

Tuberculosis _____ Smoking _____

Exposure to environmental/chemical irritants _____
_____

Perception/knowledge of illness/tests/surgery _____
_____

Recognizes relationship between history and illness _____
_____

Misconceptions _____

Readiness to learn _____

Requesting information concerning _____

Educational level _____

Learning impeded by _____

Orientation

Level of alertness _____

Orientation: Person _____ Place _____ Time _____

Appropriate behavior/communication _____

Memory

Memory intact: yes/no   Recent _____ Remote _____

FEELING ▪ A pattern involving the subjective awareness of information

Comfort

Pain/discomfort: yes/no

Onset _____ Duration _____

Location _____

Quality _____ Radiation _____

Aggravating factors _____

Alleviating factors _____

Emotional Integrity/States

Recent stressful life events _____
_____

Verbalizes feelings of _____

Source _____
_____

Physical manifestations _____

MOVING ▪ A pattern involving activity

Activity

History of physical disability _____

Use of device (cane, walker) _____

Limitations in daily activities _____
_____

Verbal report of fatigue or weakness _____
_____

Exercise habits _____

Exercise tolerance (treadmill) _____

Right column labels:

Knowledge deficit

Thought processes

Orientation
  Confusion
  Level of consciousness

Memory

Comfort
Pain/chronic
Pain/acute

Discomfort

Anxiety
Fear
Grieving
Anger
Shame
Sadness
Guilt

Impaired physical mobility
Activity intolerance

Fig. 5-1, cont'd

Self-Care

Ability to perform ADLs: Independent   Dependent   Self-care

    Feeding _____   _____   Feeding

    Bathing _____   _____   Bathing/hygiene

    Dressing _____   _____   Dressing/grooming

    Toileting _____   _____   Toileting

Discharge planning needs _____

_____

Rest   Sleep pattern disturbances

Hours slept/night _____ Feels rested: yes/no   Hypersomnia

Sleep aids (pillows, meds, food) _____   Insomnia

Difficulty falling/remaining asleep _____   Nightmares

Recreation

Leisure/social activities _____   Deficit in diversional activity

_____

Environmental Maintenance

Home maintenance management

    Size & arrangement of home (stairs, bathroom) _____   Impaired home maintenance

    _____ Safety needs _____   management

    Home responsibilities _____   Safety hazards

    _____

    Neighborhood pollutants/pets _____   Sanitation hazards

Health Maintenance

    Health insurance _____   Health maintenance

    Regular physical checkups _____

PERCEIVING ▪ A pattern involving the reception of information

Self-Concept   Self-concept

Presenting appearance _____

Patient's description of self _____   Body image

Effects of illness/surgery _____   Self-esteem

_____   Personal identity

Meaningfulness   Hopelessness

Verbalizes hopelessness _____   Powerlessness

Perceives/verbalizes loss of control _____   Loneliness

_____

Sensory/Perception   Sensory perception

History of restrictive environment _____

Vision impaired _____ Glasses _____   Visual

Auditory impaired _____ Hearing aid _____   Auditory

Kinesthetic impaired _____   Kinesthetic

Gustatory impaired _____   Gustatory

Tactile impaired _____   Tactile

Olfactory impaired _____   Olfactory

Reflexes: Biceps   R ____ L ____   Triceps R ____ L ____

         Brachioradialis R ____ L ____   Knee   R ____ L ____

         Ankle   R ____ L ____   Plantar R ____ L ____

Fig. 5-1, cont'd

Continued.

EXCHANGING ▪ A pattern involving mutual giving and receiving
Circulation

Neurologic changes/symptoms _____

Cerebral (circle appropriate response)   Cerebral tissue perfusion

    Pupils   Eye Opening

      L 2 3 4 5 6 mm   None (1)

      R 2 3 4 5 6 mm   To pain (2)

      Reaction: Brisk _____   To speech (3)   Fluid volume

      Sluggish _____ Nonreactive _____   Spontaneous (4)   Deficit

                                                Excess

    Best verbal   Best Motor

      No response (1)   Flaccid (1)

      Incomprehensible sounds (2)   Extensor response (2)

      Inappropriate words (3)   Flexor response (3)

      Confused conversation (4)   Semipurposeful (4)

      Oriented (5)   Localized to pain (5)

                              Obeys commands (6)

    Glasgow Coma Scale total _____

Cardiac

    Pacemaker _____ Apical rate & rhythm _____   Cardiopulmonary tissue

    Heart sounds/murmurs _____   perfusion

    Dysrhythmias _____   Fluid volume

    BP: Sitting   Lying

            R _____ L _____   R _____ L _____   Decreased cardiac output

    IV fluids _____

Peripheral   Peripheral tissue perfusion

    Jugular venous distention: yes/no   Right _____ Left _____ Fluid volume

    Pulses: _____   Deficit

    Skin temp _____ Color _____   Excess

    Capillary refill _____ Clubbing _____   Decreased cardiac output

    Edema _____

Physical Integrity

Tissue integrity _____ Rashes _____   Impaired skin integrity

    Lesions _____ Petechiae _____   Impaired tissue integrity

    Erythematous _____

    Surgical incision _____

    Other_____

Oxygenation

Thoracic examination: Pectus excavatum _____ Pectus carinatum _____ Ineffective airway clearance

    Barrel _____ Scoliosis _____ Other _____

Complaints of dyspnea _____ Precipitated by _____

Orthopnea _____

Rate _____ **Rhythm** _____ **Depth** _____

Labored/unlabored (circle) _____

Use of accessory muscles _____   Ineffective breathing patterns

Pursed lips _____ Nasal flaring _____   Impaired gas exchange

Cough: productive/nonproductive _____

Sputum: Color _____ Amount _____

        Character _____ Odor _____

Breath sounds _____

Arterial blood gases: pH _____ Po_2 _____ Pco_2 _____

O_2 saturation _____ Bicarbonate _____ BE _____

Hemoglobin _____ Hematocrit _____

Pulmonary function tests _____

Fig. 5-1, cont'd

CXR _____
Bronchoscopy _____
Oxygen percent and device _____
Ventilator settings _____

Physical Regulation
Immune
   Lymph nodes enlarged _____ Location _____   Infection
   WBC count _____
   Differential: Neutrophils _____   Hypothermia
     Lymphocytes _____ Basophils _____   Hyperthermia
     Monocytes _____ Eosinophils _____   Body temperature
   PT _____ PTT _____ Platelets _____   Ineffective thermoregulation
   Temperature _____ Route _____

Nutrition   Nutrition
Eating patterns
   Number of meals per day _____
   Special diet/supplements _____
   Food preferences/intolerances _____
   Food allergies _____
   Fluid intake _____
   Appetite changes _____
   Difficulty swallowing _____   Impaired swallowing
   History of ulcers _____ Heartburn _____
   Anorexia/nausea/vomiting _____
   Dyspnea while eating _____
Condition of mouth/throat _____   Oral mucous membrane
_____

Height _____ Weight _____ Ideal body weight _____   More than body
Current therapy   requirements
   NPO _____ NG suction _____   Less than body requirements
   Tube feeding _____
   TPN _____
Labs
   Na _____ K _____ CL _____ Glucose _____

Elimination
Gastrointestinal/bowel   Bowel elimination
   Usual bowel habits _____   Constipation
   Alterations from normal _____   Diarrhea
   Abdominal examination _____   Incontinence
   _____   Gastrointestinal tissue
Renal/urinary   perfusion
   Usual urinary pattern _____   Urinary elimination
   Alteration from normal _____   Incontinence
   Urine color _____ Odor _____ Catheter _____   Retention
   External genitalia examination _____   Renal tissue perfusion
   Bladder distention _____
   Urine output: 24 hours _____ Average hourly _____
   BUN _____ Creatinine _____ Specific gravity _____
   Other urine studies _____
Genitalia
   Male: Prostate problems _____
   Female: LMP _____ Vaginal discharge _____   Menstrual patterns
     Unusual vaginal bleeding _____   Premenstrual syndrome

Fig. 5-1, cont'd   *Continued.*

CHOOSING ■ A pattern involving the selection of alternatives

Coping

Patient's usual problem-solving methods _____   Ineffective individual coping
_____   Ineffective family coping

Family's usual problem-solving methods _____
_____

Patient's method of dealing with stress _____
_____

Family's method of dealing with stress _____
_____

Patient's affect _____
Physical manifestations _____
Support systems available _____

Participation

Compliance with past/current health regimens _____   Noncompliance
_____   Ineffective participation

Willingness to comply with future health care regimen _____
_____

Judgment

Decision making ability   Judgment
   Patient's perspective _____   Indecisiveness
   Others' perspectives _____

Prioritized nursing diagnosis/problem list

1. _____
2. _____
3. _____
4. _____
5. _____
6. _____

Signature _____ Date _____

Fig. 5-1, cont'd

PULMONARY ASSESSMENT TOOL

Name _Mr. P. D._   Age _62_   Sex _MALE_
Address _111 First Street, Chicago, Ill._   Telephone _555-1111_
Significant other _Wife, Mrs. D._   Telephone _Same_
Date of admission _16 June_   Medical diagnosis _C.O.P.D._
Allergies _None_

Nursing Diagnosis
(Potential or Altered)

COMMUNICATING ▪ A pattern involving sending messages
(Read, write, understand) English (circle) _____ Communication
Other languages _None_   Verbal
Intubated _No_ Speech impaired _No_   Nonverbal
Alternate form of communication _—_

VALUING ▪ A pattern involving the assigning of relative worth
Religious preference _Lutheran_   Spiritual state
Important religious practices/concerns _None_   Distress
   Despair
Cultural orientation _Caucasian, American_
Cultural practices _Nothing Specific_

RELATING ▪ A pattern involving establishing bonds
Role
Marital status _Married_   Role performance
Age & health of significant other _Wife, 62 yrs., Good Health_   Parenting
   Sexual dysfunction
Number of children _6_ Ages _40, 38, 37, 33, 30, 24_   Work
Role in home _Major Decision Maker_   Social/leisure
Financial support _Pension, Disability_
Occupation _Recently Retired_
   Job satisfaction/concerns _While working, job was satisfactory_   Family processes
Sexual relationships ((Satisfactory)/unsatisfactory) _____ Sexuality patterns

Socialization
Quality of relationships with others _Good_   Impaired social interaction
   Patient's description _"Get along c̄ people"_
   Significant others' descriptions _(Wife) "He's a real talker"_
   Staff observations _Cooperative_
Verbalizes feelings of being alone _No_   Social isolation
Attributed to _—_   Social withdrawal

KNOWING ▪ A pattern involving the meaning associated with information
Current health problems _Emphysema, Chronic Bronchitis_   Knowledge deficit

Current medications _Aminophylline, 200 mg po q̄ 6hrs; Methylpred-_
nisolone, 6 mg po qd; Ampicillin 250 mgm po q̄ 6hr
Previous illness/hospitalizations/surgeries _Annual Hospitalizations_
for Bronchitis & Pneumonia

Fig. 5-2

Continued.

History of the following problems:

Heart __No__   Hypertension __No__   Knowledge deficit

Kidney __No__   Liver __No__

Diabetes __No__   Cancer __No__

Anemia __No__

Lung: Asthma __No__   Bronchitis __YES__   Emphysema __YES__

     Fibrocystic disease __No__   Pneumonia __YES__

     Pneumothorax __No__   Pulmonary edema/embolus __No__

     Tuberculosis __No__   Smoking __YES, 2 ppd x42 YEARS__

Exposure to environmental/chemical irritants __WORKED FOR 40 YEARS IN__
__AN INDUSTRIAL AREA OF TOWN__

Perception/knowledge of illness/tests/surgery __"I WILL GET MEDICATION__
__IV TO HELP ME BREATHE."__

Recognizes relationship between history and illness __YES, BUT HE__
__CLAIMS HE CANNOT QUIT SMOKING__

Misconceptions __NONE__

Readiness to learn __QUESTIONABLE__

     Requesting information concerning __NOT REQUESTING INFORMATION__

     Educational level __HIGH SCHOOL__

     Learning impeded by __DYSPNEA__   Thought processes

Orientation   Orientation

Level of alertness __FULLY ALERT__   Confusion

     Orientation: Person __YES__   Place __YES__   Time __YES__   Level of consciousness

     Appropriate behavior/communication __YES__

Memory

     Memory intact: (yes)/no   Recent __YES__   Remote __YES__   Memory

FEELING ▪ A pattern involving the subjective awareness of information

Comfort

     Pain/discomfort: yes/(no)   Comfort

        Onset __—__   Duration _____   Pain/chronic

        Location __—__   Pain/acute

        Quality __—__   Radiation __—__

        Aggravating factors __—__   Discomfort

        Alleviating factors __—__

Emotional Integrity/States   Anxiety

     Recent stressful life events __RETIREMENT WAS A STRESSFUL__   Fear

     __PERIOD__   Grieving

     Verbalizes feelings of __—__   Anger

        Source __—__   Shame

        Sadness

     Physical manifestations __NONE OBSERVED__   Guilt

MOVING ▪ A pattern involving activity

Activity

     History of physical disability __NO HISTORY__   Impaired physical mobility

        Use of device (cane, walker) __—__   (Activity intolerance)

     Limitations in daily activities __LIMITED BY DYSPNEA, TIRES WITH__
     __MINIMAL EXERTION__

     Verbal report of fatigue or weakness __YES, FATIGUE & WEAKNESS HAS__
     __INCREASED OVER LAST WEEK__

     Exercise habits __NONE__

     Exercise tolerance (treadmill) __NOT SCHEDULED__

Fig. 5-2, cont'd

Self-Care

Ability to perform ADLs: Independent   Dependent   Self-care

    Feeding   ✓   Feeding

    Bathing   ✓   Bathing/hygiene

    Dressing   ✓   Dressing/grooming

    Toileting   ✓   Toileting

Discharge planning needs _—_

Rest

Hours slept/night __6__ Feels rested: yes/(no)   (Sleep pattern disturbances)

Sleep aids (pillows, meds, food) _2 PILLOWS_   Hypersomnia

Difficulty falling/remaining asleep _AT TIMES WHEN DYSPNEIC_   Insomnia

    Nightmares

Recreation

Leisure/social activities _MAINLY READING_   Deficit in diversional activity

Environmental Maintenance

Home maintenance management

    Size & arrangement of home (stairs, bathroom) _4 BEDROOM, ONE_   Impaired home maintenance

STORY Safety needs _—_   management

    Home responsibilities _"MINOR REPAIRS AROUND HOUSE, PAY BILLS;_   Safety hazards

KIDS DO YARDWORK & HEAVY REPAIRS"

    Neighborhood pollutants/pets _1 DOG_   Sanitation hazards

Health Maintenance

    Health insurance _YES, FROM WORK & MEDICARE_   Health maintenance

    Regular physical checkups _YES, ABOUT EVERY 4-5 MONTHS_

PERCEIVING ▪ A pattern involving the reception of information

Self-Concept

Presenting appearance _TIRED, DRAWN LOOK, DYSPNEIC_   Self-concept

Patient's description of self _"STRONG MAN WHO DOESN'T BREATHE WELL"_

Effects of illness/surgery _"I'VE LEARNED TO LIVE WITH IT, SHORTNESS_   Body image

OF BREATH"   Self-esteem

    Personal identity

Meaningfulness   Hopelessness

Verbalizes hopelessness _No_   (Powerlessness)

Perceives/verbalizes loss of control _YES, CANNOT CONTROL OWN_   Loneliness

ABILITY TO BREATHE

Sensory/Perception   Sensory perception

History of restrictive environment _No_

Vision impaired _YES, CORRECTED_ Glasses ✓, _HAS IN POSSESSION_   Visual

Auditory impaired _No_ Hearing aid _No_   Auditory

Kinesthetic impaired _No_   Kinesthetic

Gustatory impaired _No_   Gustatory

Tactile impaired _No_   Tactile

Olfactory impaired _No_   Olfactory

Reflexes: Biceps   R _2+_ L _2+_   Triceps R _2+_ L _2+_

    Brachioradialis R _2+_ L _2+_   Knee   R _2+_ L _2+_

    Ankle   R _2+_ L _2+_   Plantar R _2+_ L _2+_

Fig. 5-2, cont'd

Continued.

EXCHANGING ▪ A pattern involving mutual giving and receiving
Circulation

Neurologic changes/symptoms *NONE NOTED*

Cerebral (circle appropriate response)   Cerebral tissue perfusion

Pupils	Eye Opening
L 2 ③ 4 5 6 mm	None (1)
R 2 ③ 4 5 6 mm	To pain (2)
Reaction: Brisk ✓	To speech (3)
Sluggish ____ Nonreactive ____	Spontaneous ④

Fluid volume
  Deficit
  Excess

Best verbal	Best Motor
No Response (1)	Flaccid (1)
Incomprehensible sounds (2)	Extensor response (2)
Inappropriate words (3)	Flexor response (3)
Confused conversation (4)	Semipurposeful (4)
Oriented ⑤	Localized to pain (5)
	Obeys commands ⑥

Glasgow Coma Scale total *15*

Cardiac

Pacemaker ___—___ Apical rate & rhythm *98, REGULAR*   Cardiopulmonary tissue
                                                                                                                                        perfusion
Heart sounds/murmurs *S_1, S_2 HEARD*
Dysrhythmias ___—___   Fluid volume
BP: Sitting   Lying
        R $^{130}/_{76}$ L $^{130}/_{76}$ R $^{126}/_{76}$ L $^{130}/_{70}$ Decreased cardiac output
IV fluids *D_5 ¼ NS AT TKO FOR IV MEDICATIONS*

Peripheral   Peripheral tissue perfusion
Jugular venous distention: yes (no)   Right ____ Left ____   Fluid volume
Pulses: *ALL PRESENT, PALPABLE, STRONG*   Deficit
Skin temp *WARM*   Color *PALE*   Excess
Capillary refill *SLOW, 4-5 SEC* Clubbing *MILD*   Decreased cardiac output
Edema *No*

Physical Integrity

Tissue integrity *INTACT SKIN* Rashes ___—___   Impaired skin integrity
  Lesions ___—___ Petechiae ___—___   Impaired tissue integrity
  Erythematous ___—___
  Surgical incision ___—___
  Other ___—___

Oxygenation

Thoracic examination: Pectus excavatum *No* Pectus carinatum *No*   (Ineffective airway clearance)
  Barrel *YES* Scoliosis *No* Other ___—___
Complaints of dyspnea *YES* Precipitated by *ACTIVITY*
Orthopnea *INTERMITTENT*
Rate *20* Rhythm *REGULAR* Depth *DEEP*
(Labored) unlabored (circle) *AT TIMES, c̄ FORCED EXPIRATION*
Use of accessory muscles *YES*   (Ineffective breathing patterns)
Pursed lips *YES* Nasal flaring *No*   (Impaired gas exchange)
Cough: (productive) nonproductive *UNABLE TO COMPLETELY CLEAR SECRETIONS*
Sputum: Color *YELLOW* Amount *MODERATE*
        Character *THICK* Odor ___—___
Breath sounds *DECREASED IN ALL LOBES, BILATERAL RHONCHI*

Arterial blood gases: pH *7.33* Po_2 *60 mm Hg* Pco_2 *56 mm Hg*
O_2 saturation *90%* Bicarbonate *34 mM* BE *−1 mEq/L*
Hemoglobin *12.4 g/dl* Hematocrit *37%*
Pulmonary function tests *FEV DECREASED, FVC DECREASED*

Fig. 5-2, cont'd

CXR _FLAT DIAPHRAGM c̄ ↑ A-P DIAMETER, NO ACUTE INFILTRATES_
Bronchoscopy _RESULTS REVEAL GRAM-NEGATIVE DIPLOCOCCI) COUNT TO FOLLOW_
Oxygen percent and device _3 LITERS PER MIN PER NASAL CANNULA_
Ventilator settings _____

Physical Regulation
Immune
    Lymph nodes enlarged _No_   Location _—_   Infection
    WBC count _14,500_
    Differential: Neutrophils _63%_   Hypothermia
      Lymphocytes _31%_ Basophils _∅_   Hyperthermia
      Monocytes _3%_ Eosinophils _1%_   Body temperature
    PT _____ PTT _____ Platelets _—_   Ineffective thermoregulation
    Temperature _99.8°F_ Route _ORAL_

Nutrition
                                          Nutrition
Eating patterns
    Number of meals per day _3, EATS VERY LITTLE_
    Special diet/supplements _No_
    Food preferences/intolerances _—_
    Food allergies _NONE_
    Fluid intake _APPROXIMATELY 1800 cc PER DAY_
    Appetite changes _DECREASED WHEN DYSPNEIC_
    Difficulty swallowing _No_   Impaired swallowing
    History of ulcers _No_ Heartburn _No_
    Anorexia/nausea/vomiting _No_
    Dyspnea while eating _USUALLY A LITTLE, LATELY A GREAT DEAL_
  Condition of mouth/throat _MOIST MUCOUS MEMBRANES, NO LESIONS,_ Oral mucous membrane
NO REDNESS, NO SWELLING
  Height _5'6"_ Weight _136 lbs_ Ideal body weight _142 lbs_ More than body
                                          requirements
  Current therapy
    NPO _—_ NG suction _—_   (Less than body requirements)
    Tube feeding _____
    TPN _____   (POTENTIAL)
  Labs
    Na _137 mEq/L_ K _3.0 mEq/L_ CL _98 mEq/L_ Glucose _116 mg/dl_

Elimination
Gastrointestinal/bowel   Bowel elimination
    Usual bowel habits _DAILY BOWEL MOVEMENT_   Constipation
    Alterations from normal _—_   Diarrhea
    Abdominal examination _SOFT ABDOMEN, NO MASSES OR TENDERNESS,_ Incontinence
BOWEL SOUNDS IN ALL FOUR QUADRANTS   Gastrointestinal tissue
                                          perfusion
Renal/urinary
    Usual urinary pattern _VOIDS WITHOUT DIFFICULTY_ Urinary elimination
    Alteration from normal _—_   Incontinence
    Urine color _YELLOW_ Odor _No_ Catheter _—_ Retention
    External genitalia examination _WITHIN NORMAL LIMITS_ Renal tissue perfusion
    Bladder distention _ABSENT_
    Urine output: 24 hours _—_ Average hourly _75 cc_
    BUN _15 mg/dl_ Creatinine _1.2 mg/dl_ Specific gravity _1.010_
    Other urine studies _—_
Genitalia
    Male: Prostate problems _NO EVIDENCE OF PROBLEMS_
    Female: LMP _N/A_ Vaginal discharge _N/A_   Menstrual patterns
      Unusual vaginal bleeding _N/A_   Premenstrual syndrome

Fig. 5-2, cont'd

Continued.

CHOOSING ▪ A pattern involving the selection of alternatives
Coping

Patient's usual problem-solving methods *"TALK TO MY WIFE OR A CLOSE FRIEND"*

Family's usual problem-solving methods *"WE SIT & DISCUSS THE PROBLEM & MAKE A DECISION"*

Patient's method of dealing with stress *"HOLD IT IN, USUALLY, SMOKE MORE"*

Family's method of dealing with stress *"WE DO NOTHING IN PARTICULAR"*

Patient's affect *FLAT BUT OTHERWISE APPROPRIATE*
Physical manifestations *NONE OBSERVED*
Support systems available *WIFE AND CHILDREN*

POTENTIAL
Ineffective individual coping
Ineffective family coping
POTENTIAL

Participation

Compliance with past/current health regimens *HAS PAST HISTORY OF COMPLIANCE WHILE IN HOSPITAL; NOT WILLING TO STOP SMOKING*

Willingness to comply with future health care regimen *YES, WHILE IN HOSPITAL*

Noncompliance
Ineffective participation

Judgment

Decision making ability
Patient's perspective *"I FEEL MY JUDGMENT IS GOOD"*
Others' perspectives *(WIFE) "I TRUST HIS JUDGMENT"*

Judgment
Indecisiveness

Prioritized nursing diagnosis/problem list
1. *IMPAIRED GAS EXCHANGE, RELATED TO RETENTION OF CO_2*
2. *INEFFECTIVE AIRWAY CLEARANCE/BREATHING PATTERN, RELATED TO INABILITY TO CONTROL SECRETIONS*
3. *ACTIVITY INTOLERANCE, RELATED TO DYSPNEA* *FATIGUE*
4. *POWERLESSNESS, RELATED TO PERCEIVED INABILITY TO CONTROL OWN BREATHING PATTERNS*
5. *POTENTIAL FOR WEIGHT LESS THAN BODY REQUIREMENTS*
6. *NONCOMPLIANCE RELATED TO SMOKING HABITS*

Signature *Shelia Bunton, Maj, AN* Date *16 JUNE, 1130 HOURS*

Fig. 5-2, cont'd

CHAPTER 6

NEUROLOGIC ASSESSMENT TOOL

ANITA P. SHERER
SUSAN FICKERTT WILSON

The Neurologic Assessment Tool was designed to assess neurologic patients who have unique biopsychosocial assessment needs. The tool incorporates specific signs and symptoms pertinent to the neurologic patient that facilitate identification of nursing diagnoses. It also incorporates the *Standards of Neurological and Neurosurgical Nursing Practice* developed by the American Nurses' Association and the American Association of Neurosurgical Nurses. This chapter includes:

- *The way the tool was developed and refined*
- *The patient population and settings to which it applies*
- *Selected neurologic emphasis areas*
- *The way to use the tool*
- *Specific neurologic focus questions and parameters to assist the nurse in eliciting appropriate data*
- *The Neurologic Assessment Tool*
- *A case study*
- *A completed version of the tool based on the case study*

DEVELOPMENT AND REFINEMENT OF THE TOOL

The Neurologic Assessment Tool was developed from the nursing data base prototype (see Chapter 2). Many cardiovascular variables originally incorporated into the prototype were deleted and replaced with more in-depth neurologic and musculoskeletal assessment variables more applicable to such an assessment. Emphasis was placed on comparing current patterns and habits to the patient's pre-hospitalization status, as well as communication and sen-

sory/perceptual deficits. The resultant tool was then modified based on recommendations of neurologic nurse experts. Further, the content of the tool was supported by the literature.

After the tool was developed and refined, it was clinically tested on 10 neurologic patients by neurologic nurse experts and clinical nurse specialists. It was tested on adult neurosurgical patients in acute care hospitals, emergency room patients, and children with neurologic problems. The testing evaluated the adequacy of the tool in terms of flow, space for recording data, and completeness of assessment variables. Based on the results, the tool was revised.

PATIENT POPULATION AND SETTINGS

The Neurologic Assessment Tool was developed for use with neurologic patients in any inpatient setting who need an admission assessment to determine their nursing care needs. Such settings might include neurologic critical care units, general neurologic or neurosurgical units, or emergency room settings. Specific hemodynamic monitoring variables could be deleted when the tool is used in general neurologic or neurosurgical units. When using the tool in the emergency room setting, sections of the tool might be reorganized to provide a screening assessment. An ongoing assessment could be provided by initiating tool completion in the emergency room and finalizing completion after transfer to the inhospital units. Assessment variables within the tool are designed for use with adults. However, the tool could easily be modified for use with pediatric patients by adding growth and development and parent–child–interaction assessment variables.

Sophisticated hemodynamic monitoring variables have been added to the tool to adequately assess the "exchanging pattern" in the critical care setting. This tool can be used with stable and unstable neurologic patients. For unstable patients, the nurse should begin assessment with the physiologic "exchanging pattern" and direct attention to the "ABCs" of basic life support. When the patient is more stable, the other assessment variables can be completed, usually within 24 hours. Depending on the patient's level of consciousness and physical condition, the family or significant other may help in providing some of the necessary data in the other patterns.

NEUROLOGIC EMPHASIS AREAS

Neurologic patients have specialized problems and needs. The Neurologic Assessment Tool includes appropriate assessment variables within each of the nine human response patterns of the Unitary Person Framework and focuses on prevalent problems in this patient population. Table 6-1 outlines these emphasis areas.

Table 6-1
Selected neurologic emphasis areas

Patterns	Emphasis areas to determine
Communicating	Speech impairment
	Aphasia
Valuing	Spiritual despair related to illness
	Religion or culture as support systems
Relating	Support systems
	Effect of illness on roles or relationships
Knowing	Neurologic history
	Orientation or memory
Feeling	Comprehensive data related to pain
	Anxiety, fear, grief, or loss
Moving	Musculoskeletal examination
	Effects of illness on home maintenance
	Self-care deficits
Perceiving	Effects of illness on self-concept
	Sensory/perceptual deficits
Exchanging	Neurologic assessment
Choosing	Patient and family's adequacy in dealing with problems or stress
	Future compliance with health care regimen

HOW TO USE THE TOOL

To use the tool effectively, nurses must first familiarize themselves with the Unitary Person Framework (see Chapter 2), which provides the underlying framework for Taxonomy I. The nine response patterns of the Unitary Person Framework serve as the major category headings for Taxonomy I and this assessment tool. The sequence of the response patterns, as it appears in Taxonomy I, has been changed to permit a logical ordering of assessment variables. Nursing diagnoses pertinent to the neurologic patient, along with the signs and symptoms necessary to identify them, are incorporated under the appropriate human response pattern.

Nurses must also realize that this tool is very different from conventional assessment tools. As a result, nurses may encounter some initial difficulty in using it. Nurses should remember however, that this tool was *not* designed to follow the organization or content of a traditional medical data base; the data collected do not solely reflect medical patterns. Rather, this tool elicits data about holistic patterns in ways not traditionally assessed by nurses. It provides a new method of collecting and synthesizing data and requires new thinking when processing data. This tool represents a nursing data base developed from a nursing model that permits a holistic nursing assessment to take place so nursing diagnoses can be identified.

Although nurses agree that a holistic nursing data base is desirable, it is realized that changing traditional assessment methods is not an easy task. For this reason, a trial usage period is recommended before any decisions about the merits of this tool are made. During this period, the nurse should assess 10 patients using the tool to become familiar and progressively more comfortable with the tool's organization and data-collection methods. With experience, nurses will become accustomed to new ways of clustering and processing information. With continued use, the time necessary to complete the tool will be reduced. Most important, nurses will recognize the unique ability of the tool to elicit appropriate signs and symptoms. They will discover that nursing diagnoses are easily identified when using this tool.

When using the Neurologic Assessment Tool, the nurse need not complete the entire tool in one session. Completion of priority sections can be designated for the initial assessment. Other designated sections or patterns can be completed later, within a time frame acceptable to the institution. To elicit appropriate data, nurses should familiarize themselves with the associated focus questions and parameters (see the next section). When assessing specific signs and symptoms that may indicate a diagnosis, the nurse circles the diagnosis in the right-hand column when deviations from normal are found. A circled diagnosis does not confirm a problem but simply alerts the nurse to

Table 6-2

Neurologic assessment tool: focus questions and parameters

Variables	Focus questions and parameters
COMMUNICATING	
Aphasia	Is aphasia present?
Expressive	If yes, what type? Can the patient name common objects? Does the patient use gestures to convey needs? Is the patient's speech halting or nonfluent? Does the patient demonstrate an awareness of a speech problem?
Receptive	Does the patient follow one- or two-step commands; repeat; require gestures to follow commands? Is the patient's speech smooth or fluent, yet lack meaning or substance?
Ability to articulate	Does the patient have difficulty articulating or expressing thoughts verbally?
RELATING	
Previous role in home	"Before this hospitalization, what was your major role in the home? Major breadwinner? Decision maker? Provider of child care?"
	Based on current status, what changes can be predicted in the patient's responsibilities or relationships after this illness?
Quality of relationship with others	Does the patient have such severe communication deficits that impaired social interaction can be predicted?
KNOWING	
Knowledge of medications	"Can you name your medications? Can you tell me the reason you are taking each medication?
	What are the side effects of your medications?
	What side effects should you report to the physician?"
Difficulties taking medications	"Have you noticed any side effects when taking your medications?
	Can you identify which medicine you think might be causing _____? Do you have problems remembering to take your medications?"
Results of diagnostic tests	What are the results of the diagnostic tests, including electroencephalography, computerized tomography, magnetic resonance imaging, or other tests?
Learning impeded by	Does the patient have aphasia, hallucinations, hyperventilation, depression, nervousness, insomnia that may impede learning?
Attention span	Is the patient's attention span unusually short?
	Is the patient easily distracted? Will the patient's attention span allow learning to take place?
MOVING	
Performs volitional movement	Is the patient able to execute a motor act on command (e.g., stick out tongue or wash face)?
Involuntary movements present	Does the patient exhibit movements (hand, arm, or facial twitching) that cannot be controlled?
	Does the patient have tremors?
Orthotic devices in use	Does the patient use a cane, walker, or splint?
Safety precautions needed	Does the patient's musculoskeletal status indicate possible safety hazards (e.g., falls)?
PERCEIVING	
Effects of illness/surgery on self-concept	"How would you describe yourself before hospitalization? How would you describe yourself now? How do you think other people would describe you at those times?"
Patient's description of own strengths/ weaknesses	"What are your strengths as a person? Your weaknesses?"

Continued.

Table 6-2—cont'd

Neurologic assessment tool: focus questions and parameters

Variables	Focus questions and parameters
EXCHANGING	
Abnormal breathing pattern	Is the patient's breathing pattern abnormal?
	Does the patient seem to hold his or her breath frequently in between breaths (Cheyne-Stokes respiration)? Does the patient breathe rapidly (hyperventilation)? Does the patient breathe rapidly and then hold his or her breath (posthyperventilation apnea)? Does the patient inhale, pause, and then exhale (apneustic breathing)? Is there some deep and some shallow breathing in an irregular pattern (ataxic breathing)? Is the breathing disorganized with some periods where the patient holds his or her breath (cluster breathing)?
Methods of control	"What do you do for diarrhea? Change your diet or take medications? What do you do
Bowel elimination	for constipation? Take medications, eat a high-fiber diet, or use enemas? How do you control incontinence? Diapers?"
Urinary elimination	"How do you control incontinence? Diapers, frequent trips to the bathroom, catheter, or fluid restriction?"

the possibility that it exists. After completing the tool, the nurse scans the circled problems, synthesizes the data to determine whether other clusters of signs and symptoms support the existence of a problem, and judges whether the actual or potential diagnosis is present.

Some diagnoses are repeated several times. These repetitions occur only within the appropriate response pattern and are convenient for identifying certain data directly with their nursing diagnosis. These diagnoses are not absolute but are intended to focus thinking and direct more detailed attention to a possible problem.

Certain signs and symptoms can indicate many diagnoses. For example, decreased blood pressure can indicate altered cerebral tissue perfusion and altered cardiopulmonary tissue perfusion, as well as other nursing diagnoses. To avoid unnecessary repetition of assessment parameters, variables were arranged with the diagnosis most likely to result from the data assessed. Thus data to support a specific diagnosis may occasionally be found in other patterns or arranged with other diagnoses. Therefore, synthesis of all data is essential.

The Neurologic Assessment Tool is not intended to be the standardized and final format for assessing neurologic patients across the country. An assessment tool must meet the needs and requirements of the individual institutions and nurses using it. The Neurologic Assessment Tool is simply a working demonstration tool that is expected to be changed and revised by nurses in clinical practice. Further evaluation and refinement are necessary before adopting

the tool for use within an institution. Nurses interested in changing, revising, and adapting the tool in a specific clinical setting should refer to Chapter 4. Nurses interested in adapting the Neurologic Assessment Tool to the pediatric setting should also refer to the Pediatric Assessment Tool (see Chapter 21).

HOW TO ELICIT APPROPRIATE DATA

Because the Unitary Person Framework and the Neurologic Assessment Tool contain some terminology that may be unfamiliar to nurses, specific neurologic focus questions and parameters were developed and refined to help the nurse to elicit appropriate information. These questions and parameters are outlined in Table 6-2, which follows the order of the content of the Neurologic Assessment Tool (Fig. 6-1). The data in bold type in the tool are described more fully in Table 6-2. For example, under the "communicating pattern," the aphasia variable is in bold type. If the nurse is unsure about which questions to ask to elicit the presence of aphasia, the questions and parameters in Table 6-2 can be used to direct the line of questioning. These questions and parameters were developed to provide clarity and guidance in eliciting data and are not all inclusive. Nurses should not feel limited by them. There are many other questions that could be used to elicit the appropriate information, based on the situation or condition and the skill of the nurse. Focus questions and parameters for most of the other data not in bold type were presented in Chapter 3.

CASE STUDY

The case study models the process a nurse uses when assessing a patient and, based on the clustering of information obtained during assessment, nursing diagnoses are formulated.

Mrs. N.A. was assessed when admitted to a neurologic stepdown unit. Mrs. N.A. has been diagnosed with amyotrophic lateral sclerosis (ALS) and has been hospitalized due to her deteriorating condition. She is 63 years old, widowed, and lives with her elderly mother. Because Mrs. N.A. was mechanically ventilated, her mother served as a source of information for parts of the nursing assessment. The Neurologic Assessment Tool (Fig. 6-2) was used to assess Mrs. N.A.

BIBLIOGRAPHY

Allmond B: Management of cervical and thoracic spine/cord injured patients, J Neurosurg Nurs 13:97, 1981.

American Nurses' Association and American Association of Neurosurgical Nurses: Standards of neurological and neurosurgical nursing practice, Kansas City, 1977, ANA, Inc.

Bates B: A guide to physical examination and history taking, ed 4, Philadelphia, 1987, JB Lippincott Co.

Hickey JV: The clinical practice of neurological and neurosurgical nursing, ed 2, Philadelphia, 1986, JB Lippincott Co.

Ricci M, editor: Core curriculum for neuroscience nursing, Chicago, 1984, American Association of Neuroscience Nurses.

Rudy EB: Advanced neurological and neurosurgical nursing, St Louis, 1984, The CV Mosby Co.

Thompson JM et al: Clinical nursing, St Louis, 1986, The CV Mosby Co.

NEUROLOGIC ASSESSMENT TOOL

Name _____ Age _____ Sex _____

Address _____ Telephone _____

Significant other _____ Telephone _____

Date of admission _____ Medical diagnosis _____

Allergies _____

Nursing Diagnosis
(Potential or Altered)

COMMUNICATING ▪ A pattern involving sending messages

Read, write, understand English (circle)

Other languages _____

Intubated _____ Speech impaired _____

Aphasia _____ **Expressive** _____ **Receptive** _____

Alternate form of communication _____

Ability to articulate _____

Communication
  Verbal
  Nonverbal

VALUING ▪ A pattern involving the assigning of relative worth

Religious preference _____

Important religious practices _____

Spiritual concerns _____

Cultural orientation _____

Cultural practices _____

Spiritual state
  Distress
  Despair

RELATING ▪ A pattern involving establishing bonds
Role

  Marital status _____

  Age & health of significant other _____

  _____

  Number of children _____ Ages _____

  Previous role in home _____

  Financial support _____

  Occupation _____

    Job satisfaction/concerns _____

    Physical/mental energy expenditures _____

  Sexual relationships (satisfactory/unsatisfactory) _____

    Physical difficulties/effects of illness related to sex _____

  _____

Role performance
  Parenting
  Sexual dysfunction
  Work
  Family
  Social/leisure
Family processes

Sexuality patterns

Socialization

  Quality of relationships with others _____

    Patient's description _____

    Significant others' descriptions _____

    Staff observations _____

  Verbalizes feelings of being alone _____

    Attributed to _____

Impaired social interaction

Social isolation
Social withdrawal

KNOWING ▪ A pattern involving the meaning associated with information

Current health problems _____

_____

Current medications _____

_____

Knowledge of medications _____

Difficulties taking medications _____

Knowledge deficit

Fig. 6-1

Previous illnesses/hospitalizations/surgeries _____

_____

History of the following:
    Head trauma _____ Meningitis _____ Encephalitis _____   Knowledge deficit
    Aneurysm _____ Seizures _____ Alzheimer's disease _____
    Viral infection _____ Venereal disease _____ Polio _____
    Otitis media _____ Mastoiditis _____ Tuberculosis _____
    Cardiac disease _____ Lung disease _____ Diabetes _____
    Liver disease _____ Renal disease _____ Other _____
    Anticoagulant usage _____ Alcohol usage _____
    Smoking _____ Oral contraceptives _____
Family history of the following:
    Migraines _____ Diabetes _____ Seizure disorder _____
    Tremors _____ Spinocerebellar degeneration _____
    Hereditary spastic paralysis _____
    Huntington's chorea _____ Parkinson's disease _____
Results of diagnostic tests _____
Perception/knowledge of illness/tests/surgery _____

_____

Expectations of therapy _____
Misconceptions _____
Readiness to learn _____
    Educational level _____
    Learning impeded by _____   Thought processes
    Attention span _____

Orientation
Level of alertness _____   Orientation
Orientation: Person _____ Place _____ Time _____   Confusion
Appropriate behavior/communication _____

Memory
Memory intact: yes/no _____ Immediate _____ Recent _____ Remote _____   Memory

FEELING ▪ A pattern involving the subjective awareness of information
Comfort   Comfort
    Pain/discomfort: yes/no _____
        Onset _____ Duration _____   Pain/chronic
        Location _____   Pain/acute
        Quality _____ Radiation _____   Discomfort
        Associated factors _____
        Aggravating factors _____
        Alleviating factors _____

Emotional Integrity/States
    Recent stressful life events _____   Anxiety
    _____   Fear
    Verbalizes feelings of _____   Grieving
        Source _____   Anger
    _____   Guilt
        Physical manifestations _____   Shame
    _____   Sadness

MOVING ▪ A pattern involving activity
Activity
    History of physical disability _____   Impaired physical mobility
    _____

Fig. 6-1, cont'd

Continued.

Previous limitations in daily activities _____

_____

Previous exercise habits _____
Strength: RUE _____ RLE _____ LUE _____ LLE _____
ROM: RUE _____ RLE _____ LUE _____ LLE _____
Tone: RUE _____ RLE _____ LUE _____ LLE _____
Coordination—finger/nose: Right _____ Left _____
Performs volitional movement _____   Activity intolerance
Involuntary movements present (describe) _____
Balance impaired _____ Sitting _____ Standing _____
Gait impaired _____ Posture _____
Orthotic devices in use _____
Safety precautions needed _____   Safety hazards

Rest
Hours slept/night _____ Feels rested: yes/no _____   Sleep pattern disturbance
Sleep aids (pillows, meds, food) _____   Hypersomnia
Difficulty falling/remaining asleep _____   Insomnia
       Nightmares

Recreation
Leisure activities _____   Deficit in diversional activity
Social activities _____

Environmental Maintenance
Home maintenance management
Size & arrangement of home (stairs, bathroom) _____

_____   Impaired home maintenance
Transportation _____ Safety needs _____   management
Previous home responsibilities _____   Safety hazards

_____

Health Maintenance
Health insurance _____   Health maintenance
Regular physical checkups _____
Access to health care _____

Self-Care   Self-care
Ability to perform ADLs: Independent _____ Dependent _____   Feeding
Specify deficits _____   Bathing/hygeine
Discharge planning needs _____   Dressing/grooming
       Toileting
_____   Impaired swallowing

PERCEIVING ▪ A pattern involving the reception of information
Self-Concept   Self-concept
Patient's description of self _____   Body image
Effects of illness/surgery on self-concept _____   Self-esteem
     Personal identity
_____
Patient's description of own strengths/weaknesses _____

_____

Meaningfulness
Verbalizes hopelessness _____   Hopelessness
Verbalizes/perceives loss of control _____   Powerlessness

Sensory/Perception   Sensory/perception
History of restricted environment _____
Vision impaired _____   Visual
_____ Glasses _____

Fig. 6-1, cont'd

Auditory impaired _____ Auditory
  Tinnitus _____ Hearing Aid _____
Kinesthetics (position sense) impaired _____ Kinesthetic
Gustatory impaired _____ Gustatory
  Gag/swallowing reflex _____ Facial weakness _____ Impaired swallowing
Tactile impaired _____ Tactile
  Paresthesia _____ Analgesia _____
Olfactory impaired _____ Olfactory
Reflexes: +4 = hyperactive   +3 = more brisk than average
      +2 = average   +1 = somewhat diminished   0 = no response
     Biceps   R _____ L _____   Triceps R _____ L _____
     Brachioradialis R _____ L _____   Knee   R _____ L _____
     Ankle   R _____ L _____   Plantar R _____ L _____
     Ankle clonus R _____ L _____ Nuchal rigidity _____
     Corneal reflex _____ Oculocephalic reflex _____

EXCHANGING ▪ A pattern involving mutual giving and receiving
Circulation
  Cerebral
    Neurologic changes/symptoms _____
    _____
    _____
    Seizure activity _____ Type _____ Cerebral tissue perfusion
    Pupils   Eye Opening
      L 2 3 4 5 6 mm   Spontaneously (4)
      R 2 3 4 5 6 mm   To speech (3)
      Direct reaction: Brisk _____ To pain (2)
      Sluggish _____ Nonreactive _____ No response (I)
      Consensual reaction: R to L _____ L to R _____
    Best Verbal   Best Motor
      Oriented (5)   Obeys commands (6)
      Confused conversation (4) Localizes pain (5)
      Inappropriate words (3)   Flexion withdrawal (4)
      Incomprehensible sound (2) Abnormal flexion (3)
      No response (1)   Abnormal extension (2)
                       No response (1)
    Glascow Coma Scale total _____
    ICP _____ Cerebral perfusion pressure _____
  Cardiac
    PMI _____ Pacemaker _____ Cardiopulmonary tissue
    Apical rate & rhythm _____   perfusion
    Heart sounds/murmurs _____
    Dysrhythmias _____ Fluid volume
    BP: Sitting   Lying   Standing   Deficit
       R _____ L _____   R _____ L _____   R _____ L _____ Excess
    A-Line reading _____
    MAP _____ Pulse pressure _____
    Cardiac index _____ Cardiac output _____ Cardiac output
    CVP _____ PAP _____ PCWP _____
  Peripheral   Peripheral tissue perfusion
    Jugular venous distension: yes/no   R _____ L _____
    Pulses _____
    Skin temp _____ Color _____ Fluid volume
    Capillary refill _____ Clubbing _____ Deficit
    Edema _____ Excess

Fig. 6-1, cont'd

Continued.

Physical Integrity

Tissue integrity _____ Rashes _____ Lesions _____   Impaired skin integrity
  Petechiae _____ Bruises _____   Impaired tissue integrity
  Abrasions _____ Surgical incision _____   Potential for injury
  Present pressure sores (site/grade) _____
_____
  Current treatment _____

Oxygenation

Complaints of dyspnea _____ Precipitated by _____
Orthopnea _____
Rate _____ Rhythm _____ Depth _____   Ineffective airway clearance
Labored/unlabored (circle) Use of accessory muscles _____   Ineffective breathing pattern
Abnormal breathing pattern _____
Chest expansion _____ Splinting _____
Cough: productive/nonproductive _____
Sputum: Color _____ Amount _____ Consistency _____
Breath sounds _____   Impaired gas exchange
Arterial blood gases _____
Oxygen percent and device _____
Ventilator _____

Physical Regulation

Immune
  Lymph nodes enlarged _____ Location _____   Infection
  RBC count _____ Hemoglobin _____ Hematocrit _____
  Platelets _____ WBC count _____ Neutrophils _____
  Lymphocytes _____ Monocytes _____ Basophils _____
  Eosinophils _____ Other _____
Body temperature   Body temperature
  Temperature _____ Route _____   Hypothermia
   Hyperthermia
   Ineffective thermoregulation

Nutrition

Eating patterns   Nutrition
  Number of meals per day _____ Where eaten _____
  Previous special diet _____
  Food preferences/intolerances/allergies _____
  Caffeine intake (coffee, tea, soft drinks)
_____
  Appetite changes _____
  Nausea/vomiting _____
Condition of mouth/throat _____   Oral mucous membrane
Height _____ Weight _____ Ideal body weight _____   More than body
  Current therapy   requirements
    Current diet _____ NPO _____ NG suction _____   Less than body requirements
    Tube feeding _____
    TPN _____
    Fluid intake _____ IV fluids _____   Fluid volume
Labs   Deficit
  Na _____ K _____ CL _____ Glucose _____ Fasting _____   Excess
  Albumin _____ Total protein _____ Other _____

Elimination

Gastrointestinal/bowel   Bowel elimination
  Usual bowel habits _____   Constipation
  Alterations from normal _____   Diarrhea
  Methods of control _____   Incontinence
  Abdominal physical examination _____

Fig. 6-1, cont'd

Renal/genitourinary
    Menstrual cycle _____ LMP _____   Menstrual patterns
    Abnormalities _____   Premenstrual syndrome
    Usual urinary pattern _____   Urinary elimination
    Alterations from normal _____   Incontinence
    Methods of control _____   Retention
    Color _____ Catheter _____   Enuresis
    Urine output: 24 hour _____ Average hourly _____   Renal tissue perfusion
    Bladder distention _____
    Serum: BUN _____ Creatinine _____ Specific gravity _____
    Urine studies _____

CHOOSING: ▪ A pattern involving the selection of alternatives
Coping
    Patient's usual problem-solving methods _____   Ineffective individual coping
    _____   Ineffective family coping
    Family's usual problem-solving methods _____
    _____
    Patient's method of dealing with stress _____
    _____
    Family's method of dealing with stress _____
    _____
    Patient's affect _____
    Physical manifestations _____
    Coping mechanisms used _____
    Support system/resources _____

Participation
    Compliance with past/current health care regimens _____   Noncompliance
    _____   Ineffective participation
    Willingness to comply with future health care regimen _____
    _____

Judgment
    Decision-making ability
        Patient's perspective _____   Judgment
        Others' perspectives _____   Indecisiveness

Prioritized nursing diagnoses/problem list
1. _____
2. _____
3. _____
4. _____
5. _____
6. _____
7. _____
8. _____
9. _____
10. _____

Signature _____   Date _____

Fig. 6-1, cont'd

NEUROLOGIC ASSESSMENT TOOL

Name _N. A._   Age _63_   Sex _F_
Address _88 NINTH STREET, BAYTOWN, TEXAS_   Telephone _243-5324_
Significant other _MOTHER — C.K._   Telephone _243-5324_
Date of admission _2/1_   Medical diagnosis _AMYOTROPHIC LATERAL SCLEROSIS_
Allergies _PENICILLIN, CODEINE_

Nursing Diagnosis
(Potential or Altered)

COMMUNICATING ■ A pattern involving sending messages
(Read) (write,) (understand) English (circle)
Other languages _NODS HEAD FOR "YES," SHAKES HEAD FOR "NO"_
Intubated _TRACH_   Speech impaired _SPEECH SLURRED_
Aphasia _NO_   Expressive _____   Receptive ——
Alternate form of communication _SIGNBOARD, WRITING_
Ability to articulate _COMPROMISED DUE TO TRACH_

(Communication)
(Verbal)
Nonverbal

VALUING ■ A pattern involving the assigning of relative worth
Religious preference _BAPTIST_
Important religious practices _LIKES TO ATTEND CHURCH_
Spiritual concerns _"THINKS A LOT ABOUT DYING" (MOTHER)_
Cultural orientation _BLACK AMERICAN_
Cultural practices _NONE VOICED_

(Spiritual state)
(Distress)
Despair

RELATING ■ A pattern involving establishing bonds
Role
  Marital status _WIDOW 12 YEARS_
  Age & health of significant other _80 y/o MOTHER IN GOOD HEALTH_

  Number of children _3_   Ages _35 y/o SON, 40 y/o DAUGHTER 45y/o_
  Previous role in home _HOMEMAKER_   _SON_
  Financial support _MEDICAID, PENSION_
  Occupation _PREVIOUSLY SECRETARY FOR SCHOOL SYSTEM_
    Job satisfaction/concerns _RETIRED ON DISABILITY_
    Physical/mental energy expenditures _JOB WAS MENTALLY STRESSFUL_
  Sexual relationships (satisfactory/unsatisfactory) _NOT SEXUALLY ACTIVE_
    Physical difficulties/effects of illness related to sex _____

Role performance
  Parenting
  Sexual dysfunction
  Work
  Family
  Social/leisure
Family processes

Sexuality patterns

Socialization
  Quality of relationships with others _GOOD IN GENERAL_
    Patient's description _DIFFICULTY COMMUNICATING_
    Significant others' descriptions _GOOD RELATIONSHIPS_
    Staff observations _SUPPORTIVE FAMILY c̄ POSITIVE INTERACTIONS_
  Verbalizes feelings of being alone _TERRIFIED OF BEING ALONE_
    Attributed to _FEARS VENTILATOR WILL BE DISCONNECTED_

Impaired social interaction

(Social isolation)
Social withdrawal

KNOWING ■ A pattern involving the meaning associated with information
Current health problems _PARALYSIS OF LOWER EXTREMITIES AND SEVERE WEAKNESS_
OF UPPER EXTREMITIES DUE TO AMYOTROPHIC LATERAL SCLEROSIS
Current medications _ALBUTEROL 2 mg TID, VITAMIN C 50 mg qd, ELAVIL_
25 mg TID, ZANTAC 150 mg BID, BACTRIM ÷ q12h, LASIX 20mg qd, KCL 20 mEq BID
Knowledge of medications _FAIR UNDERSTANDING OF PURPOSE- KNOWS SCHEDULE_
Difficulties taking medications _"HARD TO KEEP TRACK OF ALL THESE MEDICINES" (MOTHER)_

Knowledge deficit

Fig. 6-2

Previous illnesses/hospitalizations/surgeries _APPENDECTOMY @ AGE 13,_
BIRTH OF 3 CHILDREN

History of the following:

Head trauma _No_	Meningitis _No_	Encephalitis _No_	Knowledge deficit
Aneurysm _No_	Seizures _No_	Alzheimer's disease _No_	
Viral infection _No_	Venereal disease _No_	Polio _No_	
Otitis media _No_	Mastoiditis _No_	Tuberculosis _No_	
Cardiac disease _No_	Lung disease _No_	Diabetes _No_	
Liver disease _No_	Renal disease _No_	Other _No_	
Anticoagulant usage _No_	Alcohol usage _No_		
Smoking _No_	Oral contraceptives _No_		

Family history of the following:

Migraines _NO_   Diabetes _No_   Seizure disorder _No_
Tremors _NO_   Spinocerebellar degeneration _No_
Hereditary spastic paralysis _No_
Huntington's chorea _No_   Parkinson's disease _No_

Results of diagnostic tests _ELECTROMYOGRAPH → MUSCULAR WASTING, ATROPHY FASCICULATIONS_
Perception/knowledge of illness/tests/surgery _"HAS A DISEASE FOR WHICH_
THERE IS NO CURE" (MOTHER) PATIENT NODS AGREEMENT
Expectations of therapy _"TO KEEP FROM GETTING CONTRACTURES & BEDSORES" (MOTHER)_
Misconceptions _NONE_
Readiness to learn _GOOD_
   Educational level _HIGH SCHOOL & 1 YEAR COLLEGE_
   Learning impeded by _PHYSICAL DISABILITY & IMPAIRED COMMUNICATION_   Thought processes
   Attention span _½ - 1 HR_

Orientation
Level of alertness _ALERT_   Orientation
Orientation: Person _✓_   Place _✓_   Time _✓_   Confusion
Appropriate behavior/communication _UNDERSTANDS WHAT IS HAPPENING AROUND HER_

Memory
Memory intact: yes/no _YES_ Immediate _✓_ Recent _✓_ Remote _✓_   Memory

FEELING ▪ A pattern involving the subjective awareness of information
Comfort   (Comfort)
   Pain/discomfort: yes/no _YES_
      Onset _2/88_ Duration _CONSTANT_   Pain/chronic
      Location _BACK_   Pain/acute
      Quality _DULL_ Radiation _NONE_   (Discomfort)
      Associated factors _NONE_
      Aggravating factors _BAD POSITIONING_
      Alleviating factors _BACK RUB_

Emotional Integrity/States
   Recent stressful life events _BEING DIAGNOSED c̄ ALS_   Anxiety
                                     (Fear)
   Verbalizes feelings of _FEAR; SADNESS_   Grieving
      Source _BEING ALONE - FEARS VENTILATOR WILL DISCONNECT;_   Anger
   SADNESS OVER HER ILLNESS/DISABILITY   Guilt
      Physical manifestations _HOLDS ON TO FAMILY/FRIENDS' HANDS -_   Shame
   DOESN'T WANT THEM TO LEAVE; SAD FACIAL EXPRESSION   (Sadness)

MOVING ▪ A pattern involving activity
Activity
   History of physical disability _NONE_   (Impaired physical mobilitety)

Fig. 6-2, cont'd

Continued.

Previous limitations in daily activities _NONE_

Previous exercise habits _WALKED_

Strength: RUE _WEAK_ RLE _0_ LUE _WEAK_ LLE _0_

ROM: RUE _FULL_ RLE _FULL_ LUE _FULL_ LLE _FULL_

Tone: RUE _SPASTIC_ RLE _SPASTIC_ LUE _SPASTIC_ LLE _SPASTIC_

Coordination—finger/nose: Right _SLOWED_ Left _SLOWED_

Performs volitional movement _YES c̄ UPPER EXTREMITIES_   Activity intolerance

Involuntary movements present (describe) _NONE_

Balance impaired _YES_ Sitting _YES_ Standing _0_

Gait impaired _YES, PARALYSIS_ Posture _UNABLE TO STAND_

Orthotic devices in use _SPLINT, PILLOW FOR PROPER POSITIONING_

Safety precautions needed _SIDE RAILS UP_   Safety hazards

Rest

Hours slept/night _6-8 HRS_ Feels rested: yes/no _YES_   Sleep pattern disturbance

Sleep aids (pillows, meds, food) _NONE_   Hypersomnia

Difficulty falling/remaining asleep _SLEEPS 2-3 HRS @ A TIME_   Insomnia

Nightmares

Recreation

Leisure activities _WATCHES TV IN HOSPITAL, USED TO GARDEN_   Deficit in diversional activity

Social activities _VISITS c̄ FAMILY_

Environmental Maintenance

Home maintenance management

    Size & arrangement of home (stairs, bathroom) _3 BEDROOM — 1 STORY — NOT ACCESSIBLE_   (POTENTIAL)

    Transportation _CAR_ Safety needs _MAKE HOME ACCESSIBLE_   (Impaired home maintenance management)

    Previous home responsibilities _HOUSEKEEPING, COOKING, CLEANING WILL NEED HELP c̄ THESE p̄ DISCHARGE. MOTHER IS ABLE TO MAINTAIN HOUSEHOLD AT PRESENT._   Safety hazards

Health Maintenance

Health insurance _YES_   Health maintenance

Regular physical checkups _YES_

Access to health care _EASILY AVAILABLE_

Self-Care

Ability to perform ADLs: Independent _____ Dependent _✓_   (Self-care)

Specify deficits _FEEDING, BATHING, DRESSING, TOILETING_   (Feeding)

Discharge planning needs _____   (Bathing/hygeine)

WILL NEED HELP c̄ ADL's   (Dressing/grooming)

    (Toileting)

    Impaired swallowing

PERCEIVING ▪ A pattern involving the reception of information

Self-Concept

Patient's description of self _"STRONG PERSON" (MOTHER)_   (Self-concept)

Effects of illness/surgery on self-concept _"FEELS HELPLESS" (MOTHER)_   Body image

DOES MAINTAIN APPEARANCE c̄ HELP FROM MOTHER   Self-esteem

Patient's description of own strengths/weaknesses _"I ALWAYS HAVE HOPE."_   Personal identity

Meaningfulness

Verbalizes hopelessness _IS HOPEFUL OF GETTING BETTER_   Hopelessness

Verbalizes/perceives loss of control _YES, FEELS HELPLESS_   (Powerlessness)

Sensory/Perception

History of restricted environment _PREVIOUS ICU STAY_   Sensory/perception

Vision impaired _NO_   Visual

_____ Glasses _NO_

Fig. 6-2, cont'd

Auditory impaired __No__   Auditory
   Tinnitus __No__   Hearing Aid __No__
Kinesthetics (position sense) impaired __No__   Kinesthetic
Gustatory impaired __YES__   Gustatory
   Gag/swallowing reflex __No GAG REFLEX__ Facial weakness __No__   Impaired swallowing
Tactile impaired __No__   Tactile
   Paresthesia __No__   Analgesia __No__
Olfactory impaired __No__   Olfactory
Reflexes: +4 = hyperactive   +3 = more brisk than average
       +2 = average   +1 = somewhat diminished   0 = no response
       Biceps   R __2__ L __2__   Triceps R __2__ L __2__
       Brachioradialis R __2__ L __2__   Knee   R __0__ L __0__
       Ankle   R __0__ L __0__   Plantar R __0__ L __0__
       Ankle clonus   R __0__ L __0__ Nuchal rigidity __0__
       Corneal reflex __NORMAL__ Oculocephalic reflex __NORMAL__

EXCHANGING ▪ A pattern involving mutual giving and receiving

Circulation

Cerebral
   Neurologic changes/symptoms __PARALYSIS OF LOWER EXTREMITIES,__
__WEAKNESS IN UPPER EXTREMITIES, NO GAG REFLEX__

   Seizure activity __NONE__   Type __—__   Cerebral tissue perfusion
   Pupils   Eye Opening
     L (2) 3 4 5 6 mm   Spontaneously (4)
     R (2) 3 4 5 6 mm   To speech (3)
     Direct reaction: Brisk __✓__   To pain (2)
     Sluggish ____ Nonreactive ____   No response (I)
     Consensual reaction: R to L __✓__ L to R __✓__
   Best Verbal   Best Motor
     Oriented (5)   Obeys commands (6) __c̄ UPPER EXTREMITIES__
     Confused conversation (4)   Localizes pain (5)
     Inappropriate words (3)   Flexion withdrawal (4)
     Incomprehensible sound (2)   Abnormal flexion (3)
     No response (1)   Abnormal extension (2)
                         No response (1)
   Glasgow Coma Scale total __15__
   ICP __N/A__   Cerebral perfusion pressure __N/A__
Cardiac
   PMI __5TH ICS @ MCL__ Pacemaker __No__   Cardiopulmonary tissue
   Apical rate & rhythm __80 REGULAR__   perfusion
   Heart sounds/murmurs __S₁ S₂__
   Dysrhythmias __NONE — NORMAL SINUS RHYTHM s̄ ECTOPY__   Fluid volume
   BP: Sitting   Lying   Standing   Deficit
     R __130/70__ L __128/70__   R __140/70__ L __132/70__   R __—__ L __—__   Excess
   A-Line reading __N/A__
   MAP __N/A__   Pulse pressure __40__
   Cardiac index __N/A__   Cardiac output __N/A__   Cardiac output
   CVP __N/A__   PAP __N/A__   PCWP __N/A__
Peripheral   Peripheral tissue perfusion
   Jugular venous distension: yes (no)   R____ L ____
   Pulses __PALPABLE BILATERALLY__
   Skin temp __WARM__   Color __BLACK__   Fluid volume
   Capillary refill __< 2 SEC.__   Clubbing __None__   Deficit
   Edema __None__   Excess

Continued.

Fig. 6-2, cont'd

Physical Integrity

Tissue integrity _INTACT_ Rashes _No_ Lesions _No_   Impaired skin integrity
  Petechiae _No_ Bruises _No_   Impaired tissue integrity
  Abrasions _No_ Surgical incision _TRACH_   Potential for injury
  Present pressure sores (site/grade) _NONE_

  Current treatment _—_

Oxygenation

Complaints of dyspnea _No_ Precipitated by _—_
Orthopnea _No_
Rate _12_ Rhythm _REGULAR_ Depth _DEEP_   Ineffective airway clearance
Labored/(unlabored) (circle) Use of accessory muscles _No_   (Ineffective breathing pattern)
Abnormal breathing pattern _No_
Chest expansion _SYMMETRICAL_ Splinting _—_
Cough: productive/nonproductive _No_
Sputum: Color _WHITE_ Amount _SMALL_ Consistency _THIN_
Breath sounds _CLEAR BILATERALLY_   Impaired gas exchange
Arterial blood gases _pH 7.47 Pco₂ 28 mmHg, Po₂ 104 mm Hg, O₂ SAT 98% BASE EXCESS + 4.41 mEq/L_
Oxygen percent and device _21%_
Ventilator _MONAHAMS ASSIST/CONTROL TV 900 cc; RATE 12_

Physical Regulation

Immune
  Lymph nodes enlarged _No_ Location _—_   Infection
  RBC count _3.61×10⁶/μL_ Hemoglobin _11.0 g/dl_ Hematocrit _32.6 %_
  Platelets _400,000 μL_ WBC count _6.4×10³/μL_ Neutrophils _50%_
  Lymphocytes _34%_ Monocytes _3%_ Basophils _0.3%_
  Eosinophils _2%_ Other _BANDS 2%_
Body temperature   Body temperature
  Temperature _98.2°F_ Route _ORAL_   Hypothermia
    Hyperthermia
    Ineffective thermoregutlation

Nutrition

Eating patterns   Nutrition
  Number of meals per day _4 FEEDINGS_ Where eaten _PT'S HOSPITAL ROOM_
  Previous special diet _No_
  Food preferences/intolerances/allergies _NONE_
  Caffeine intake (coffee, tea, soft drinks)

  Appetite changes
  Nausea/vomiting _No_
Condition of mouth/throat _INTACT; TRACHEOSTOMY_   Oral mucous membrane
Height _5'5'_ Weight _140 lbs_ Ideal body weight _135_   More than body
  Current therapy   requirements
    Current diet _TUBE FEEDING_ NPO _YES_ NG suction _—_   Less than body requirements
    Tube feeding _GASTROSTOMY TUBE c̄ FEEDINGS q6h_
    TPN _—_
    Fluid intake _2000 cc/DAY_ IV fluids _D5¼ NS_   Fluid volume
Labs   Deficit
  Na _138 mEq/L_ K _3.8 mEq/L_ CL _103 mEq/L_ Glucose _90 mg/dl_ Fasting _YES_   Excess
  Albumin _4.5 g/dl_ Total protein _6.0 g/dl_ Other _—_

Elimination

Gastrointestinal/bowel   Bowel elimination
  Usual bowel habits _DAILY BOWEL MOVEMENTS_   Constipation
  Alterations from normal _No_   Diarrhca
  Methods of control _DULCOLAX DAILY_   Incontinence
  Abdominal physical examination _SOFT, ⊕ BS IN ALL 4 QUADS_

Fig. 6-2, cont'd

Renal/genitourinary *POST*
   Menstrual cycle *MENOPAUSAL* LMP *52 YEARS*   Menstrual patterns
   Abnormalities *No*   Premenstrual syndrome
   Usual urinary pattern *6-8 × /DAY*   Urinary elimination
   Alterations from normal *No*   Incontinence
   Methods of control *VOIDS C̄ ASSISTANCE*   Retention
   Color *CLEAR YELLOW* Catheter *No*   Enuresis
   Urine output: 24 hour *1450* Average hourly *60*   Renal tissue perfusion
   Bladder distention *No*
   Serum: BUN *9 mg/dl* Creatinine *0.6 mg/dl* Specific gravity *1,020*
   Urine studies

CHOOSING: ■ **A pattern involving the selection of alternatives**

Coping
   Patient's usual problem-solving methods *CRYS ; MAINTAINS HOPE; LOOKS*   Ineffective individual coping
@ PROS ∗ CONS ∗ CHOOSES WHAT'S BEST   Ineffective family coping
   Family's usual problem-solving methods *EVALUATES PROS ∗ CONS ∗ CHOOSES*
BEST ALTERNATIVE
   Patient's method of dealing with stress *PRAYS*

   Family's method of dealing with stress *TALK TO EACH OTHER*

   Patient's affect *APPROPRIATE — DEMONSTRATES SADNESS @ TIMES*
   Physical manifestations *CRYS FREQUENTLY*
   Coping mechanisms used *ANXIETY*
   Support system/resources *MOTHER AND CHILDREN*

Participation
   Compliance with past/current health care regimens *COMPLIANT*   Noncompliance
                                              Ineffective participation
   Willingness to comply with future health care regimen *YES, WILLING TO*
COMPLY

Judgment
   Decision-making ability
      Patient's perspective *SOUND DECISION MAKER*   Judgment
      Others' perspectives *MOTHER AGREES SHE IS SOUND DECISIONMAKER*   Indecisiveness

Prioritized nursing diagnoses/problem list
1. *ALTERED VERBAL COMMUNICATION R/T TRACHEOSTOMY*
2. *IMPAIRED PHYSICAL MOBILITY R/T PARALYSIS ∗ WEAKNESS*
3. *ALTERED SELF-CARE R/T PARALYSIS ∗ WEAKNESS*
4. *INEFFECTIVE BREATHING PATTERN R/T DISEASE PROCESS ∗ VENTILATOR DEPENDENCY*
5. *ALTERED COMFORT R/T BACK DISCOMFORT*
6. *ALTERED SELF-CONCEPT R/T DISABILITY*
7. *POWERLESSNESS R/T LIMITATIONS IMPOSED BY DISEASE PROCESS*
8. *FEAR R/T POTENTIAL ACCIDENTAL VENTILATOR DISCONNECTION*
9. *SADNESS R/T PHYSICAL LIMITATIONS*
10.

Signature *Anita P. Sherer, RN*   Date *5/3*

Fig. 6-2, cont'd

CHAPTER 7

RENAL ASSESSMENT TOOL

CHAROLD L. BAER
LINDA A. PRINKEY

The Renal Assessment Tool is designed to assess patients with renal dysfunction who have unique biopsychosocial assessment needs. The tool incorporates specific assessment variables pertinent to renal patients that facilitate identification of nursing diagnoses for this patient group. This chapter includes:

- *The way the tool was developed and refined*
- *The patient populations and settings to which it applies*
- *Selected renal emphasis areas*
- *The way to use the tool*
- *Specific renal focus questions and parameters to assist the nurse in eliciting appropriate data*
- *The Renal Assessment Tool*
- *A case study*
- *A completed version of the tool based on the case study*

DEVELOPMENT AND REFINEMENT OF THE TOOL

The Renal Assessment Tool was developed from the nursing data base prototype (see Chapter 2). Many hemodynamic and critical care variables originally incorporated into the prototype were deleted and replaced with variables applicable to renal assessment. The resultant tool was then modified based on the recommendations of renal nurse experts. Further, the content of the tool was supported by the literature.

After the tool was developed and refined it was clinically tested on 10 patients by renal nurse experts and a clinical nurse specialist. The tool was tested on adult patients in a renal dysfunction and transplant unit of a metropolitan tertiary care facility. The testing evaluated the adequacy of the tool in terms of flow, space for recording data, and completeness of assessment variables. Based on the results, the tool was revised.

PATIENT POPULATION AND SETTING

The Renal Assessment Tool was developed to assess the problems and needs of adult patients experiencing renal insufficiency, or acute or chronic renal failure. It was designed for use in the hospital, particularly for renal and medical-surgical units where patients with alterations in renal function are admitted. This tool is also appropriate for use in free-standing dialysis centers, provided that minor modifications, such as deleting assessment variables concerning arterial blood gases and oxygen delivery devices, are made. Patients with renal dysfunction who are admitted to intensive care units may be more adequately assessed using the Critical Care Assessment Tool (see Chapter 12).

RENAL EMPHASIS AREAS

Patients with renal disease have unique problems and needs. The Renal Assessment Tool provides a holistic assessment by allowing evaluation of an individual's level of functioning in each of the nine human response patterns of the Unitary Person Framework. In addition, the tool focuses on prevalent problems among renal patients. Table 7-1 outlines these renal emphasis areas.

HOW TO USE THE TOOL

To use the Renal Assessment Tool effectively, nurses must first familiarize themselves with the Unitary Person

Table 7-1
Selected renal emphasis areas

Patterns	Emphasis areas to determine
Communicating	Ability to express thoughts and feelings verbally and nonverbally
Valuing	Religious and cultural beliefs about dialysis, transplantation, and blood transfusions
Relating	Effect of renal disease on role performance, including parenting, work, and sexual relationships
Knowing	Expectations of therapy, particularly dialysis
Feeling	Response to diagnosis of renal disease
Moving	Health maintenance practices, including the ability to keep dialysis appointments
Perceiving	Effect of the disease process and treatment on self-concept and body image
Exchanging	Fluid volume status Electrolyte balance Condition of dialysis access Dialysis routine Assessment for infection
Choosing	Assessment of compliance with health care regimen

Framework (see Chapter 2), which provides the underlying framework for Taxonomy I. The nine human response patterns of the Unitary Person Framework serve as the major category headings for Taxonomy I and the Renal Assessment Tool. The sequence of the response patterns, as it appears in Taxonomy I, has been changed in the tool to permit a more logical ordering of assessment variables. Nursing diagnoses pertinent to the renal patient are incorporated under the appropriate human response patterns and are arranged with assessment variables necessary to identify these diagnoses.

Nurses must also realize that this tool is very different from conventional assessment tools. As a result, nurses may initially encounter some difficulty in using it. They should remember, however, that this tool was not designed to follow the organization or content of a traditional medical data base; the data collected do not solely reflect medical patterns. Rather, this tool elicits data about holistic patterns in ways not traditionally used by nurses. This tool represents a nursing data base developed from a nursing model. The use of this tool results in a holistic nursing assessment that facilitates identification of nursing diagnoses.

Although many nurses would agree that a holistic nursing data base is desirable, changing traditional assessment methods is not an easy task. For this reason, a trial usage period is recommended before any decisions are made about the tool's merits. During this period, nurses will become familiar and progressively more comfortable with the tool's organization and data-collection methods. With experience, nurses will become accustomed to new ways of clustering and processing information. Further, with continued use, the time necessary to complete the tool will be reduced. Most importantly, nurses will discover that nursing diagnoses are easily identified because of the tool's unique ability to elicit appropriate signs and symptoms in a readily understandable fashion.

It is not necessary to complete the entire tool in one session. Priority sections can be completed during the initial assessment. Other sections or patterns can be completed later, within a time frame acceptable to the patient, the nurse, and the institution. Further, depending on the patient's condition and degree of orientation, the family or significant other may help in providing necessary data.

When assessing for specific signs and symptoms that may indicate a particular diagnosis, the nurse circles the diagnosis in the right-hand column when deviations from normal are found. A circled diagnosis does not confirm the existence of the problem but merely alerts the nurse to a possible problem or alteration. After completing the tool, the nurse scans the circled diagnoses, synthesizes the data to determine whether other clusters of data also support the existence of a problem, and decides whether the actual or potential diagnosis is present.

Some diagnoses are repeated several times in the right-hand column. These repetitions occur only within the appropriate response pattern and are convenient for identifying data with their corresponding nursing diagnosis. These diagnoses are not absolute but are intended to focus thinking and direct attention to a possible problem.

Certain signs and symptoms can indicate any number of diagnoses. For example, disorientation and inappropriate behavior can indicate confusion, altered thought processes, altered cerebral perfusion, or impaired gas exchange. For renal patients, confusion can also result from an elevated blood urea nitrogen level, which may stem from altered renal tissue perfusion. To avoid unnecessary repetition of assessment parameters, variables are arranged with the diagnosis most likely to result from the data assessed. Thus, data to support a specific diagnosis may occasionally be found in other patterns or arranged with other diagnoses.

Table 7-2
Renal assessment tool: focus questions and parameters

Variables	Focus questions and parameters
COMMUNICATING	
Communication barriers	Does the patient demonstrate extreme fatigue or decreased level of consciousness that interferes with the ability to express needs?
VALUING	
Important religious or cultural practices	"Does your religion or culture permit you to have surgery, blood transfusions, dialysis, or organ transplantation?"
RELATING	
Financial support	Does the patient receive Social Security Disability?
Job satisfaction/concerns	Does therapy interfere with the patient's ability to work?
Sexual concerns	Does the patient experience impotency? (Determine source such as drugs or fatigue.)
	Does the patient complain of decreased libido?
KNOWING	
Expectations of therapy	Does the patient believe that renal function will return? Is this belief realistic? What are the patient's expectations of dialysis?
Learning impeded by	Is the blood urea nitrogen level so elevated that it interferes with mentation?
FEELING	
Recent stressful life events	When was renal disease first diagnosed in the patient? What was the reaction to the diagnosis?
MOVING	
Home maintenance management concerns	"Will your treatment interfere with your ability to perform housekeeping or shopping duties? Other household chores?"
Health maintenance	Does the patient express concerns about maintaining the dialysis regimen?
Discharge planning needs	Can the patient adequately care for the fistula or perform continuous ambulatory peritoneal dialysis (CAPD) appropriately?
	Can the patient take medications as prescribed?
PERCEIVING	
Effects of illness/surgery	"How do you feel about having kidney disease? Being on dialysis? Needing a kidney transplant?"
EXCHANGING	
Convulsions	Has the patient experienced convulsions? Last episode?
Tetany	Does the patient exhibit: carpopedal spasm? Chvostek's sign (twitching of facial muscles in response to tapping or stroking the cheek just below the zygomatic bone in front of the ear)? Positive Trousseau's sign (carpal spasm induced by inflating a blood pressure cuff above systolic blood pressure or creating ischemia in the extremity)?
Dialysis access: current condition of access	*General:* What is the condition of the skin around the access? Is there any drainage or signs of infection?
	Fistula: Does the patient have a bruit?
	A-V Shunt: Is the tubing clotted? Are there kinks in the tubing?
	Peritoneal dialysis catheter: Is the catheter patent?
	Central line: Is the line patent and free of kinks?
WBC Differential	See Chapter 3 and Appendix II.
	PMNs increase with infection, gout, hemolysis, and drug intoxication; Eos increase with allergic conditions; Baso decreases with corticosteroid use or production

Table 7-2—cont'd
Renal assessment tool: focus questions and parameters

Variables	Focus questions and parameters
EXCHANGING—cont'd	
Special diet	Is the patient on a sodium-, potassium-, protein-, or phosphate-restricted diet?
Dry weight	Individually determined after ideal dialysis
Labs	See Chapter 3 and Appendix II.
Frequency of dialysis	How often does the patient dialyze?
Duration	How long does the patient dialyze? How many exchanges?
CHOOSING	
Compliance with past/current health care	If on dialysis, does the patient adhere to instructions for diet, dialysis, and medications? Are there extenuating circumstances preventing the desired level of compliance (e.g., family or monetary problems, lack of transportation, or inadequate facilities such as running water, storage space for supplies, and difficulty obtaining supplies)?

Therefore, synthesis of all data is essential before formulating the nursing diagnoses.

The Renal Assessment Tool is not intended to be a standardized, final format for evaluating renal patients across the country. An assessment tool must meet the needs of the individual institutions and nurses using it. Thus, it is a working demonstration tool that is expected to be revised by nurses in clinical practice. Further, evaluation and refinement are necessary before adopting the tool for use within an institution. Nurses interested in changing and revising the tool for use in a specific clinical setting should refer to Chapter 4.

HOW TO ELICIT APPROPRIATE DATA

Because the Unitary Person Framework and the Renal Assessment Tool contain terminology that may be unfamiliar to nurses, specific renal focus questions and parameters were developed and refined to elicit appropriate information. These questions and parameters appear in Table 7-2 and correspond with the assessment variables in bold type in the tool (Fig. 7-1). For example, the learning impeded by variable found under the "knowing pattern" is in bold type. If the nurse is unsure what questions to ask to elicit this information, Table 7-2 can be used to direct the assessment. Questions and parameters for data not in bold type appear in Chapter 3.

The questions and parameters in this book provide clarity and guidance in eliciting data, but these questions are not all inclusive. Nurses should not feel limited to ask only the questions or assess only the parameters provided.

There are many other methods of eliciting appropriate information. Assessment methods should be tailored to the patient's level of understanding and the situation, as well as to the skill and comfort level of the nurse.

CASE STUDY

The case study models the process a nurse uses to assess a patient using the Renal Assessment Tool. Based on clustering of information gathered during assessment, the nurse formulates nursing diagnoses (Fig. 7-2), and at the end then lists them in order of priority.

W.H. is a 66-year-old Chinese American with end-stage renal disease and is receiving hemodialysis. The Renal Assessment Tool (Fig. 7-2) contains data obtained from W.H. Nursing diagnoses, ordered by priority, have been derived from this data.

BIBLIOGRAPHY

Brundage DJ: Nursing management of renal problems, ed 2, St Louis, 1980, The CV Mosby Co.

Carpenito LJ: Nursing diagnosis: application to clinical practice, ed 2, Philadelphia, 1987, JB Lippincott Co.

Kenner CV, Guzzetta CE, and Dossey BM: Critical care nursing: body-mind-spirit, ed 2, Boston, 1985, Little, Brown & Co, Inc.

Lancaster LE: The patient with end stage renal disease, ed 2, New York, 1984, John Wiley & Sons, Inc.

Lancaster LE: Core curriculum for nephrology nursing, Pitman, NJ, 1987, American Nephrology Nurses' Association.

RENAL ASSESSMENT TOOL

Name _____ Age _____ Sex _____
Address _____ Telephone _____
Significant other _____ Telephone _____
Date of admission _____ Medical diagnosis _____
Allergies _____

Nursing Diagnosis
(Potential or Altered)

COMMUNICATING ▪ A pattern involving sending messages
English: Read _____ Write _____ Understand _____   Communication
Other languages _____   Verbal
Communication barriers _____   Nonverbal
Alternate form of communication _____

VALUING ▪ A pattern involving the assigning of relative worth
Religious preference _____   Spiritual state
Important religious practices _____   Distress
Spiritual concerns _____   Despair
Cultural orientation _____
Cultural practices _____

RELATING ▪ A pattern involving establishing bonds
Role
  Marital status _____   Role performance
  Age & health of significant other _____   Parenting
  _____   Sexual dysfunction
  Number of children _____ Ages _____   Work
  Role in home _____   Family
  Financial support _____   Social/leisure
  Occupation _____   Family processes
    Job satisfaction/concerns _____
    _____
  Sexual concerns _____   Sexuality patterns
    _____

Socialization
  Quality of relationships with others _____   Impaired social interaction
  Patient's description _____
  Significant others' descriptions _____
  Staff observations _____
    Verbalizes feelings of being alone _____   Social isolation
      Attributed to _____   Social withdrawal

KNOWING ▪ A pattern involving the meaning associated with information
Current health problems _____
_____
_____
Previous illnesses/hospitalizations/surgeries _____
_____
_____
_____
_____

Fig. 7-1

History of the following diseases: Knowledge deficit

    Heart _____ Hypertension _____

    Peripheral vascular _____

    Cerebrovascular _____

    Lung _____

    Liver _____

    Kidney _____

    Thyroid _____

    Drug abuse _____ Alcoholism _____

Current medications _____

_____

_____

_____

_____

Risk factors for heart disease	Present	Perceptions/knowledge of
1. Hypertension	_____	_____
2. Hyperlipidemia	_____	_____
3. Smoking	_____	_____
4. Obesity	_____	_____
5. Diabetes	_____	_____
6. Sedentary living	_____	_____
7. Stress	_____	_____
8. Alcohol use	_____	_____
9. Oral contraceptives	_____	_____
10. Family history	_____	

_____

Perception/knowledge of illness/tests/surgery _____

_____

Expectations of therapy _____

Misconceptions _____

Readiness to learn _____ Learning

    Requests information concerning _____

    Educational level _____ Thought processes

    Learning impeded by _____ Impaired problem solving

Orientation

Level of alertness _____ Orientation

Orientation: Person _____ Place _____ Time _____ Confusion

Appropriate behavior/communication _____

Memory

Memory intact: Yes _____ No _____ Recent _____ Remote _____ Memory

FEELING ▪ A pattern involving the subjective awareness of information

Comfort

    Pain/discomfort: Yes _____ No_____ Comfort

        Onset _____ Duration _____

        Location _____ Quality _____ Radiation _____ Pain/chronic

        Associated factors _____ Pain/acute

        Aggravating factors _____ Discomfort

        Alleviating factors _____

Emotional Integrity/States

    Recent stressful life events _____ Grieving

_____ Anxiety

    Verbalizes feelings of _____ Fear

        Source _____ Anger

_____ Guilt

Fig. 7-1, cont'd

Continued.

Physical manifestations _____ Shame
_____ Sadness

MOVING ▪ A pattern involving activity
Activity
  History of physical disability _____ Impaired physical mobility
  _____ Activity intolerance
  Limitations in daily activities _____
  _____
  Verbal report of fatigue/weakness _____
  Exercise habits _____

Rest   Sleep pattern disturbance
  Hours slept/night _____ Feels rested: Yes ____ No ____ Hypersomnia
  Sleep aids (pillows, meds, food) _____ Insomnia
  Difficulty falling/remaining asleep _____ Nightmares

Recreation
  Leisure/social activities _____ Deficit in diversional activity
  _____

Environmental Maintenance
  Home maintenance management   Impaired home maintenance
    Concerns _____   management
    _____
    _____

Health Maintenance
  Regular physical checkups _____ Health maintenance
  Transportation to appointments _____
  Distance from home to dialysis _____

Self-care   Self-care
  Ability to perform ADLs: Independent _____ Dependent _____   Feeding
    Needs assistance ____   Bathing/hygiene
    Specify deficits _____ Dressing/grooming
  Discharge planning needs _____ Toileting
  _____

PERCEIVING ▪ A pattern involving the reception of information
Self-Concept   Self-concept
  Patient's description of self_____ Body image
  Effects of illness/surgery _____ Self-esteem
  _____ Personal identity

Meaningfulness
  Verbalizes hopelessness _____ Hopelessness
  Verbalizes/perceives loss of control _____ Powerlessness

Sensory/Perception   Sensory/perception
  Vision impaired _____ Glasses _____   Visual
  Auditory impaired _____ Hearing aid _____   Auditory
  Kinesthetics impaired _____   Kinesthetic
  Gustatory impaired _____   Gustatory
  Tactile impaired _____   Tactile
  Olfactory impaired _____   Olfactory
  Reflexes: Grossly intact ____ Alterations _____
  _____

Fig. 7-1, cont'd

EXCHANGING ▪ A pattern involving mutual giving and receiving
Circulation
Cerebral
 Neurologic changes/symptoms _____ Cerebral tissue perfusion

Pupils	Eye Opening
Size: Equal _____	None (1)
Unequal _____	To pain (2)
Reaction: Brisk _____	To speech (3)
Sluggish _____ Nonreactive _____	Spontaneous (4)

Fluid volume
 Deficit
 Excess

Best Verbal	Best Motor
No response (1)	Flaccid (1)
Incomprehensible sound (2)	Extensor response (2)
Inappropriate words (3)	Flexor response (3)
Confused conversation (4)	Semipurposeful (4)
Oriented (5)	Localized to pain (5)
	Obeys commands (6)

Cardiac output

 Glasgow Coma Scale total _____
Cardiac
 Pacemaker _____
 Apical rate & rhythm _____ Cardiopulmonary tissue
 Heart sounds/murmurs _____   perfusion
 Dysrhythmias _____ Fluid volume

BP:	Sitting	Lying	Standing	Deficit
	R _____ L _____	R _____ L _____	R _____ L _____	Excess

 IV fluids _____ Cardiac output
 _____

Peripheral   Peripheral tissue perfusion
 Jugular venous distension R _____ L _____
 Pulses: A = absent   B = bruits   D = doppler
    +3 = bounding   +2 = palpable   +1 = faintly palpable

Carotid R _____ L _____	Popliteal R _____ L _____
Brachial R _____ L _____	Posterior tibial R _____ L _____
Radial R _____ L _____	Dorsalis pedis R _____ L _____
Femoral R _____ L _____	

Fluid volume
 Deficit
 Excess

 Skin temp _____ Color _____ Turgor _____
 Capillary refill _____ Clubbing _____   Cardiac output
 Edema_____

Physical Integrity
Injury   Injury
 Convulsions _____ Tetany _____
 Dialysis access: Infection
    Fistula _____ A-V shunt _____ PD cath _____ Central line _____
    Current condition of access _____
Tissue integrity: Rashes _____ Lesions _____   Impaired skin integrity
 Petechiae _____ Bruises _____   Impaired tissue integrity
 Abrasions _____ Surgical incisions _____
 _____

Oxygenation
 Complaints of dyspnea _____ Precipitated by _____
 Orthopnea _____ Ineffective airway clearance
 Rate _____ Rhythm _____ Depth _____ Ineffective breathing patterns
 Labored/unlabored (circle) Use of accessory muscles _____ Impaired gas exchange
 Chest expansion _____ Splinting _____
 Breath sounds _____

Fig. 7-1, cont'd

Continued.

Cough: productive/nonproductive _____
Sputum: Color _____ Amount _____ Consistency_____
Arterial blood gases _____
Oxygen percent and device _____

Physical Regulation
Immune
  WBC count _____ **Differential: PMN** _____ **Mono** _____
           Eos _____ **Baso** _____ **Lymph** _____
Temperature _____ Route _____

Infection
Hypothermia
Hyperthermia
Body temperature
Ineffective thermoregulation

Nutrition
Eating patterns
  Number of meals per day _____
  Special diet _____
  Food preferences _____
  Food allergies/intolerances _____
  Appetite changes _____
  Presence of nausea/vomiting _____
Condition of mouth/throat _____
_____
Height _____ Weight _____ **Dry weight** _____
Current therapy
  NPO _____ NG suction _____
  Tube feeding _____
  TPN _____
Labs
  Na _____ **K** _____ **CL** _____ **CO₂** _____ **Glu** _____ **Ca** _____
  Phos _____ **Mg** _____ **Uric acid** _____ **Total bilirubin** _____
  Total protein _____ **Albumin** _____ Cholesterol _____
  Hct _____ Hb _____ **RBC** _____ Platelets _____
  PT _____ **PTT** _____ Other _____

Nutrition

Less than body requirements
More than body
    requirements

Oral mucous membrane

Less than body requirements
More than body
    requirements

Elimination
Gastrointestinal/bowel
  Usual bowel habits _____
  Alterations from normal _____
  Abdominal physical examination _____
    Ascites _____ Girth _____
Renal/Urinary
  Frequency of dialysis _____ **Duration** _____
  Urinary pattern _____
  Urine output: 24 hour _____ Color _____
  Specific gravity _____
  Urine studies _____
  Serum BUN _____ Serum creatinine _____

Elimination
  Bowel
    Constipation
    Diarrhea
    Incontinence
GI tissue perfusion

Renal tissue perfusion
Urinary patterns
  Incontinence
  Retention
Fluid volume
  Deficit
  Excess
Cardiac output

CHOOSING ▪ A pattern involving the selection of alternatives
Coping
Patient's usual problem-solving methods _____
_____
Family's usual problem-solving methods _____
_____

Ineffective individual coping
Ineffective family coping

Fig. 7-1, cont'd

Patient's method of dealing with stress _____

_____

Family's method of dealing with stress _____

_____

Participation
Compliance with past/current health care regimen _____ Noncompliance
_____ Ineffective participation

Willingness to comply with future health care regimen _____

_____

Decision-making ability Judgment
   Patient's perspective _____ Indecisiveness
   Others' perspectives _____

Prioritized nursing diagnosis/problem list
1. _____
2. _____
3. _____
4. _____
5. _____

Signature _____ Date _____

Fig. 7-1, cont'd

RENAL ASSESSMENT TOOL

Name _W. H._   Age _66_   Sex _M_
Address _21 PLUMTREE DRIVE, SEVERNA, GA._   Telephone _526-3330_
Significant other _WIFE, MRS. H._   Telephone _SAME_
Date of admission _2/23_   Medical diagnosis _HYPERTENSIVE NEPHROPATHY; END-_
Allergies _CODEINE_   _STAGE RENAL DISEASE_

**Nursing Diagnosis
(Potential or Altered)**

COMMUNICATING ▪ A pattern involving sending messages
English: Read _✓_   Write _✓_   Understand _✓_   Communication
Other languages _MINIMAL CHINESE_   Verbal
Communication barriers _NONE_   Nonverbal
Alternate form of communication _NONE_

VALUING ▪ A pattern involving the assigning of relative worth
Religious preference _NONE_   Spiritual state
Important religious practices _NONE_   Distress
Spiritual concerns _NONE_   Despair
Cultural orientation _CHINESE AMERICAN_
Cultural practices _NONE IN PARTICULAR_

RELATING ▪ A pattern involving establishing bonds
Role
Marital status _MARRIED_   Role performance
Age & health of significant other _WIFE 60 YEARS GOOD HEALTH_   Parenting
   Sexual dysfunction
Number of children _2_   Ages _33 AND 35_   Work
Role in home _HUSBAND, MONEY MANAGER_   Family
Financial support _SOCIAL SECURITY DISABILITY_   Social/leisure
Occupation _RETIRED CONSTRUCTION SUPERVISOR_   Family processes
   Job satisfaction/concerns _NONE_

Sexual concerns _DECREASED LIBIDO, OCCASIONAL IMPOTENCY_   (Sexuality patterns)

Socialization
Quality of relationships with others _INTERACTS WELL WITH OTHERS_   Impaired social interaction
Patient's description _"I LIKE PEOPLE — THEY LIKE ME."_
Significant others' descriptions _"HE HAS LOTS OF FRIENDS." (WIFE)_
Staff observations _INTERACTS WELL WITH FAMILY AND STAFF_
   Verbalizes feelings of being alone _No_   Social isolation
   Attributed to _N/A_   Social withdrawal

KNOWING ▪ A pattern involving the meaning associated with information
Current health problems _END STAGE RENAL DISEASE; HYPERTENSION_

Previous illnesses/hospitalizations/surgeries _HERNIA REPAIR 1975, LEFT
NEPHRECTOMY 1980, LEFT ARM FISTULA MAY 1987_

Fig. 7-2

History of the following diseases: (Knowledge deficit)
  Heart *MURMUR*_____ Hypertension *YES X.30 YEARS*
  Peripheral vascular *INTERMITTENT CLAUDICATION*
  Cerebrovascular *No*
  Lung *ASTHMA SINCE CHILD HOOD, MILD COPD*
  Liver *No*
  Kidney *LEFT NEPHRECTOMY 1980; END STAGE RENAL DISEASE*
  Thyroid *No*
  Drug abuse *No*_____ Alcoholism *No*
  Current medications *NORMODYNE 100mg PO bID; ALLOPURINOL 150mg PO q̄d; NEPHROVIT ī PO q̄d; CALCITRIOL .25mcg PO q̄d; DUCOSATE Na 100mg PO TID; FERROUS SULFATE 325mg PO TID; ALUCAPS ī PO c̄ BREAKFAST; ALUCAPS IV PO c̄ LUNCH AND DINNER*

Risk factors for heart disease   Present   Perceptions/knowledge of
  1. Hypertension   *YES* *AWARE ↑BP LEADS TO STROKE AND MI*
  2. Hyperlipidemia   *No*
  3. Smoking   *YES* *AWARE OF CANCER RISK; NOT HEART DISEASE*
  4. Obesity   *No*
  5. Diabetes   *No*
  6. Sedentary living   *YES* *NOT AWARE OF RISK FOR HEART DISEASE*
  7. Stress   *No*
  8. Alcohol use   *No*
  9. Oral contraceptives   *N/A*
  10. Family history *MOTHER DIED—80 YEARS OF STROKE; SISTER AND BROTHER HAVE HYPERTENSION*
Perception/knowledge of illness/tests/(surgery) *AWARE OF DISEASE PROGRESSION; VERBALIZES KNOWLEDGE OF POSSIBLE TRANSPLANT PROCEDURE*
Expectations of therapy *HOPES TO RECEIVE TRANSPLANT*
Misconceptions *NONE AT PRESENT*
Readiness to learn *VERBALIZES EAGERNESS TO LEARN ABOUT TRANSPLANT*   (Learning)
  Requests information concerning *LIFE AFTER TRANSPLANTATION*
  Educational level *BACHELOR'S DEGREE— ENGINEERING*   Thought processes
  Learning impeded by *NOTHING*   Impaired problem solving

Orientation
Level of alertness *VERY ALERT*   Orientation
Orientation: Person ✔ Place ✔ Time ✔   Confusion
Appropriate behavior/communication *VERY APPROPRIATE*

Memory
Memory intact: Yes ✔ No ___ Recent *YES* Remote *YES*   Memory

FEELING ▪ A pattern involving the subjective awareness of information
Comfort
  Pain/discomfort: Yes ___ No ✔   Comfort
    Onset ___ Duration ___
    Location ___ Quality ___ Radiation ___   Pain/chronic
    Associated factors ___   Pain/acute
    Aggravating factors ___   Discomfort
    Alleviating factors ___

Emotional Integrity/States
  Recent stressful life events *FAILURE OF REMAINING KIDNEY* (Grieving)
                                                              (Anxiety)
  Verbalizes feelings of *ANXIETY AND LOSS*   Fear
    Source *ANXIETY—EVALUATION FOR TRANSPLANT; LOSS—LOSS OF KIDNEY FUNCTION*   Anger
                                                              Guilt

Fig. 7-2, cont'd   *Continued.*

Physical manifestations *OCCASIONALLY WITHDRAWS — STARES OUT WINDOW, DOESN'T PAY ATTENTION TO ACTIVITY AROUND HIM*

Shame
Sadness

MOVING ▪ A pattern involving activity
Activity
History of physical disability *NONE*

Limitations in daily activities *BECOMES FATIGUED DOING YARD WORK OR HOUSEHOLD REPAIRS*
Verbal report of (fatigue)/weakness *p̄ 15 TO 20 MIN. OF ACTIVITY*
Exercise habits *No REGULAR ROUTINE*

Impaired physical mobility
(Activity intolerance)

Rest
Hours slept/night *6-8 HOURS*   Feels rested: Yes ✓ No ____
Sleep aids (pillows, meds, food) *NONE*
Difficulty falling/remaining asleep *No*

Sleep pattern disturbance
Hypersomnia
Insomnia
Nightmares

Recreation
Leisure/social activities *LIKES TO PLAY GOLF, PLAYS CARDS WITH FRIENDS 1X/MONTH, LIKES TO READ*

Deficit in diversional activity

Environmental Maintenance
Home maintenance management
 Concerns *NONE — WIFE DOES HOUSEKEEPING AND SHOPPING. SON HELPS WITH REPAIRS*

Impaired home maintenance
management

Health Maintenance
Regular physical checkups *SEEN REGULARLY IN CLINIC*
Transportation to appointments *HAS CAR; DRIVES SELF*
Distance from home to dialysis *15 MILES*

Health maintenance

Self-care
Ability to perform ADLs: Independent ___✓___ Dependent _____
 Needs assistance ____
 Specify deficits *NONE*
Discharge planning needs *NONE*

Self-care
 Feeding
 Bathing/hygiene
 Dressing/grooming
 Toileting

PERCEIVING ▪ A pattern involving the reception of information
Self-Concept
Patient's description of self *FEELS GOOD ABOUT SELF*
Effects of (illness)/surgery *FEELS LESS IN CONTROL — REQUIRING DIALYSIS AND FATIGUE*

Self-concept
Body image
(Self-esteem)
Personal identity

Meaningfulness
Verbalizes hopelessness *No*
Verbalizes/perceives loss of control *YES, AS ABOVE*

Hopelessness
Powerlessness

Sensory/Perception
Vision impaired *YES*   Glasses *CORRECTED c̄ GLASSES*
Auditory impaired *No*   Hearing aid *No*
Kinesthetics impaired *No*
Gustatory impaired *No*
Tactile impaired *No*
Olfactory impaired *No*
Reflexes: Grossly intact ✓ Alterations _____

Sensory/perception
 Visual
 Auditory
 Kinesthetic
 Gustatory
 Tactile
 Olfactory

Fig. 7-2, cont'd

EXCHANGING ▪ A pattern involving mutual giving and receiving
Circulation
Cerebral
Neurologic changes/symptoms _NONE_   Cerebral tissue perfusion
Pupils   Eye Opening
Size: Equal ✔   None (1)
Unequal ____   To pain (2)
Reaction: Brisk ✔   To speech (3)   Fluid volume
Sluggish ____ Nonreactive ____   Spontaneous (4)   Deficit
Excess

Best Verbal   Best Motor
No response (1)   Flaccid (1)
Incomprehensible sound (2)   Extensor response (2)   Cardiac output
Inappropriate words (3)   Flexor response (3)
Confused conversation (4)   Semipurposeful (4)
Oriented (5)   Localized to pain (5)
Obeys commands (6)
Glasgow Coma Scale total _15_
Cardiac
Pacemaker _No_
Apical rate & rhythm _84 REGULAR_   Cardiopulmonary tissue
Heart sounds/murmurs _II/VI SYSTOLIC CRESCENDO—DECRESCENDO-_   perfusion
Dysrhythmias _NONE_   _AORTIC_   Fluid volume
BP: Sitting   Lying   Standing   Deficit
R¹⁶⁰/₉₀ L¹⁶²/₉₀   R¹⁶²/₉₀ L¹⁶⁴/₉₂   R¹⁵⁰/₉₀ L¹⁵²/₉₀   Excess
IV fluids _NONE_   Cardiac output

Peripheral   Peripheral tissue perfusion
Jugular venous distension R _NO_ L _NO_
Pulses: A = absent   B = bruits   D = doppler
+3 = bounding   +2 = palpable   +1 = faintly palpable
Carotid R +3 L +3   Popliteal   R +2 L +2
Brachial R +2 L +2   Posterior tibial R +1 L +1   (Fluid volume)
Radial R +2 L +2   Dorsalis pedis R +1 L +1   Deficit
Femoral R +2 L +2   (Excess)
Skin temp _WARM_   Color _LIGHT YELLOW_ Turgor _NORMAL_
Capillary refill _BRISK_   Clubbing _NONE_   Cardiac output
Edema _+1 ANKLES_

Physical Integrity
Injury   Injury
Convulsions _NO HISTORY_ Tetany _NONE_
Dialysis access: (Infection) (POTENTIAL)
Fistula ✔ A-V shunt ____ PD cath ____ Central line ____
Current condition of access _GOOD_
Tissue integrity: Rashes _No_   Lesions _No_   Impaired skin integrity
Petechiae _No_   Bruises _No_   Impaired tissue integrity
Abrasions _No_   Surgical incisions _NO RECENT; OLD— RIGHT_
GROIN, LEFT LATERAL (NEPHRECTOMY) THORAX

Oxygenation
Complaints of dyspnea _OCCASIONAL_ Precipitated by _EXERTION_
Orthopnea _No_   Ineffective airway clearance
Rate _16_   Rhythm _REGULAR_   Depth _MODERATE_   Ineffective breathing patterns
Labored/unlabored (circle) Use of accessory muscles _No_   Impaired gas exchange
Chest expansion _EQUAL_   Splinting _No_
Breath sounds _CLEAR s̄ CRACKLES, RHONCHI, WHEEZING_

Fig. 7-2, cont'd

Continued.

Cough: productive/(nonproductive) _____
Sputum: Color _____ Amount ____—____ Consistency___—___
Arterial blood gases _NOT PERFORMED_ _____
Oxygen percent and device _NONE_ _____

Physical Regulation

Immune   Infection
  WBC count _7,700x10³/μl_ Differential: PMN _66%_____ Mono _5%_____   Hypothermia
                   Eos _2.5%_ Baso _1%_____ Lymph _20%_   Hyperthermia
  Temperature _98.6°F_ Route _____ _ORAL_ _____   Body temperature
                                           Ineffective thermoregulation

Nutrition

Eating patterns   Nutrition
  Number of meals per day _3 TO 4_ _____   (_POTENTIAL_)
  Special diet _2 gm Na, 2 gm K+_ _____   (Less than body requirements)
  Food preferences _LIKES STEAK_ _____   More than body
  Food allergies/(intolerances) _MILK_ _____   requirements
  Appetite changes _RECENTLY DECREASED APPETITE_ __
  Presence of nausea/vomiting _No_ _____
Condition of mouth/throat _No LESIONS_ _____   Oral mucous membrane

Height _5'4"_ Weight _135 lbs_ Dry weight _131 lbs_ ___   Less than body requirements
Current therapy   More than body
  NPO ____—____ NG suction ____—____ _____   requirements
  Tube feeding ____—_____
  TPN ____—_____
Labs
  Na _140 mEq/L_ K _5.7 mEq/L_ CL _96 mEq/L_ CO₂ _21 mM_ Glu _95 mg/dl_ Ca _9.9 mg/dl_
  Phos _8.5 mg/dl_ Mg _2.6 mEq/L_ Uric acid _9.2 mg/dl_ Total bilirubin _1.3 mg/dl_
  Total protein _7.1 g/dl_ Albumin _4.5 g/dl_ Cholesterol _222 mg/dl_
  Hct _30.6%_ Hb _9.8%_ RBC _4.02x10⁶/μL_ Platelets _337,000/μL_
  PT _12.6_ PTT _30.0_ Other _AMYLASE 225 SOMOGYI UNITS/dl_

Elimination   Elimination
Gastrointestinal/bowel   Bowel
  Usual bowel habits _1 STOOL/DAY_ _____   Constipation
  Alterations from normal _OCCASIONAL CONSTIPATION—NOT AT PRESENT_   Diarrhea
  Abdominal physical examination _ACTIVE BOWEL SOUNDS ALL QUADRANTS_   Incontinence
    Ascites _No_ Girth ____—____ _____   GI tissue perfusion
Renal/Urinary
  Frequency of dialysis _3x/wk_ Duration _3-4 HOURS_ ___   (Renal tissue perfusion)
  Urinary pattern _VOIDS 1-2 TIMES/DAY_ _____   Urinary patterns
  Urine output: 24 hour _60 cc_ Color _LIGHT YELLOW_   Incontinence
  Specific gravity _1.013_ _____   Retention
  Urine studies _pH 6; PROTEIN 100 mg; GLUCOSE .1 gm; KETONE NEGATIVE_ Fluid volume
  Serum BUN _97 mg/dl_ Serum creatinine _15.5 mg/dl_ ___   Deficit
                                           Excess
                                        Cardiac output

CHOOSING ▪ A pattern involving the selection of alternatives

Coping
  Patient's usual problem-solving methods _SEEKS INFORMATION; CONSULTS_   Ineffective individual coping
  WITH OTHERS _____   Ineffective family coping
  Family's usual problem-solving methods _SAME AS ABOVE_ ___

Fig. 7-2, cont'd

Patient's method of dealing with stress _TALKS ABOUT SOURCE OF STRESS; GOES GOLFING_

Family's method of dealing with stress _ATTEMPTS TO ELIMINATE SOURCE OF STRESS; LISTENS TO MUSIC_

Participation

Compliance with past/current health care regimen _GOOD-HAS TAKEN MEDICINES AS PRESCRIBED; KEEPS DIALYSIS APPOINTMENTS_ Noncompliance
Ineffective participation

Willingness to comply with future health care regimen _VERBALIZES WILLINGNESS TO COMPLY WITH TRANSPLANT FOLLOW-UP_

Decision-making ability Judgment
  Patient's perspective _"METHODICAL, DECISIVE"_   Indecisiveness
  Others' perspectives _"GOOD JUDGMENT" (WIFE)_

Prioritized nursing diagnosis/problem list
1. _KNOWLEDGE DEFICIT RELATED TO POSSIBLE KIDNEY TRANSPLANT_
2. _ACTIVITY INTOLERANCE RELATED TO ANEMIA_
3. _ALTERED SELF-ESTEEM RELATED TO PERCEIVED LOSS OF CONTROL_
4. _ANXIETY RELATED TO LOSS OF KIDNEY FUNCTION & POSSIBLE TRANSPLANT_
5. _POTENTIAL FOR INFECTION RELATED TO REPEATED VENIPUNCTURE OF FISTULA_

Signature _Linda A. Prinkey, RN_ Date _2/23_

Fig. 7-2, cont'd

CHAPTER 8

ENDOCRINE ASSESSMENT TOOL

LINDA A. PRINKEY
CHRISTINE A. KESSLER

The Endocrine Assessment Tool was designed to assess patients who have major endocrine disorders such as adrenal insufficiency, diabetes (all forms), and hyperthyroidism or hypothyroidism. It incorporates assessment variables pertinent to patients with endocrine dysfunction to facilitate identification of nursing diagnoses. This chapter includes:

- *The way the tool was developed and refined*
- *The patient populations and settings to which it applies*
- *Selected endocrine emphasis areas*
- *The way to use it*
- *Specific endocrine focus questions and parameters to assist the nurse in eliciting appropriate data*
- *The Endocrine Assessment Tool*
- *A case study*
- *A completed version of the tool based on the case study*

DEVELOPMENT AND REFINEMENT OF THE TOOL

The Endocrine Assessment Tool was developed from the nursing data base prototype (see Chapter 2). Many hemodynamic monitoring and critical care variables originally incorporated in the prototype were deleted and replaced with specific variables more applicable to endocrine assessment. The resultant tool was then modified, based on the recommendations of endocrine nurse experts. Further, the content of the tool was supported by the current literature.

After the tool was developed and refined, it was clinically tested on seven patients by endocrine nurse experts and a clinical specialist with expertise in caring for patients with endocrine disorders. The tool was tested on patients in acute-care settings only. The testing evaluated the adequacy of the tool in terms of flow, space for recording data, and completeness of assessment variables. Based on the results, the tool was revised.

PATIENT POPULATION AND SETTING

The Endocrine Assessment Tool assesses the problems and needs of patients with many types of endocrine disorders, particularly those hospitalized with acute exacerbations of endocrine disease. Some examples of endocrine disorders include diabetic ketoacidosis, pheochromocytoma, thyroid crisis, acute hyperparathyroidism, pituitary tumors or lesions, Addison's disease, Cushing's syndrome, and galactorrhea. Many less-common conditions can also be assessed using this tool; in these cases the knowledge and expertise of the nurse performing the assessment are crucial when eliciting pertinent and appropriate information from patients.

The Endocrine Assessment Tool is designed for use in the hospital. However, the tool can also be used in clinics. Although the tool is intended for use with stable patients, it can also be used to assess unstable patients. For more information about the use of this tool in assessing unstable individuals, nurses can refer to the section on how to use the tool.

ENDOCRINE EMPHASIS AREAS

Patients with endocrine disorders have unique and complex problems and needs. Clinical manifestations of endocrine dysfunction are expressions of the accentuation or

Table 8-1
Selected endocrine emphasis areas

Patterns	Emphasis areas to determine
Communicating	Voice changes due to hormonal or other endocrine disturbances
Valuing	No endocrine-specific emphasis areas
Relating	Male and female infertility and the effects on sexual relationships
Knowing	Medications that alter or supplement endocrine function
	Knowledge and perception of the effects of the endocrine disorder
Feeling	Pain and discomfort related to headaches and bone and joint pain
	Emotional manifestations of endocrine dysfunction
Moving	Characteristics of any complaints of weakness and fatigue
	Alterations in muscle tone and joint function
	Alterations in growth and development resulting from endocrine dysfunction
Perceiving	Effects of illness on body image and self-concept
	Changes in sensory perception
Exchanging	Changes in physical habitus and physiological function resulting from endocrine dysfunction
	Changes in patient tolerance of environmental temperature
Choosing	Patient's and family's methods of dealing with stress

absence of specific hormone activities. Because of the widespread effects of hormones on the body, patients with endocrine disorders have many signs and symptoms that can be confused with the signs and symptoms of other disorders. The subtleties of early endocrine manifestations challenge the assessment capabilities of the nurse. The Endocrine Assessment Tool provides a guide for a holistic patient assessment that focuses on several problems prevalent among this patient population. Table 8-1 outlines these endocrine assessment areas.

HOW TO USE THE TOOL

To use the Endocrine Assessment Tool effectively, nurses must first familiarize themselves with the Unitary Person Framework, which provides the underlying structure for Taxonomy I (see Chapter 2). The nine human response patterns of the Unitary Person Framework serve as the major category headings for Taxonomy I and the Endocrine Assessment Tool. The sequence of the response patterns, as it appears in Taxonomy I, has been changed in the tool to permit a more logical ordering of assessment variables. Nursing diagnoses pertinent to patients with endocrine disorders are incorporated under the appropriate human response patterns and are arranged with assessment variables necessary to identify these diagnoses.

Nurses must also realize that this tool is very different from conventional assessment tools. As a result, nurses may encounter some initial difficulty in using it. They should remember, however, that the tool was not designed to follow the organization or content of a traditional medical data base; the data collected do not solely reflect medical patterns. Rather, this tool elicits data about holistic patterns in ways not traditionally used by nurses. It represents a nursing data base developed from a nursing model. Use of this tool results in a holistic nursing assessment that facilitates the identification of nursing diagnoses.

Although many nurses would agree that a holistic nursing data base is desirable, changing traditional assessment methods is not an easy task. For this reason, a trial usage period is recommended before any decisions are made about the tool's merits. During this period, nurses will become familiar and progressively more comfortable with the tool's organization and data-collection methods. With experience, nurses will become accustomed to new ways of clustering and processing information. Further, with continued use, the time necessary to complete the tool will be reduced. Most important, nurses will discover that nursing diagnoses are more easily identified because of the tool's unique ability to elicit appropriate signs and symptoms in a readily understandable fashion.

It is not necessary to complete the tool in one session. Completion of priority sections can be designated for the initial assessment, particularly when the patient is unstable. In this case, starting the assessment with the "exchanging pattern" is recommended because this pattern contains important physiological data such as vital signs. Other designated sections or patterns can be completed later, within a time frame acceptable to the institution. Further, depending on the patient's condition and degree of orientation, the family or significant others may help in providing necessary data.

When signs and symptoms indicating a particular diagnosis are found, the nurse circles the diagnosis in the right-hand column. A circled diagnosis does not confirm a problem but simply alerts the nurse to the possibility of its existence. After completing the tool, the nurse scans the

Table 8-2
Endocrine assessment tool: focus questions and parameters

Variables	Focus questions and parameters
COMMUNICATING	
Voice changes	Has the patient's voice become hoarse or lower in pitch?
Physical barriers to communication	Does the patient's goiter displace the trachea?
VALUING	
Cultural practices	What folk remedies or treatments has the patient tried?
RELATING	
Difficulties related to sex	Has there been a decline in libido (male or female)?
Inability to conceive	"Have you experienced difficulty in becoming pregnant? Have you ever had a miscarriage?"
Male infertility	"Have you ever been told that you might have difficulty fathering a child?"
	Are there concerns about impotency?
	Is there a problem with the patient's sperm count or motility?
KNOWING	
Diabetes: type	*Diabetes mellitus:* Type I, insulin dependent; type II, noninsulin dependent; secondary, develops in association with other disorders (Cushing's syndrome, acromegaly, or pancreatic disease)
	Gestational: onset of recognition during pregnancy
Current medications:	
Insulin	Give the type of insulin and the dose and frequency.
	Does the patient mix types?
Hypoglycemic agent	Does the patient take an oral medication to control diabetes? Give the type, dose, and frequency.
Steroids	Does the patient take steroid medication such as prednisone (orally or topically) or receive intravenous corticosteroid medications? Give dose and frequency.
Thyroid preparation	Does the patient take thyroid hormone supplements? Does the patient receive medication to decrease thyroid hormone secretion (methimazole, propylthiouricil, or radioactive iodine)? Give dose and frequency.
	Has the patient stopped, decreased, or increased the dosage of the above medications recently?
FEELING	
Pain/discomfort	Is there evidence of bone pain or arthralgia?
Physical manifestations	Does the patient appear disheveled or neglectful of basic hygiene?
	Does the patient pace the room or handle objects in an nonpurposeful manner?
	Also see Chapter 3.
MOVING	
Weakness/fatigue: characteristics	Does weakness become progressively worse during activity?
	Does the patient complain of generalized or localized fatigue?
Muscle tremors	Does the patient complain of tremor (especially during periods of sustained posture)?
Muscle tone	What is the overall muscle tone? Does the patient complain of muscle spasms?
Joint enlargement	Does the patient have spinal deformities (acromegaly)?
Growth and development (refer to a pediatric text for normals)	Is the body height, weight, alignment, and symmetry of paired structures appropriate?
	Does the child or adolescent seem to have social, emotional, intellectual, or motor skill developmental delays? Has any specific testing been performed?
PERCEIVING	
Effects of altered physical characteristics	Does the patient or family report a tendency to avoid social interactions?
	Does the patient express embarrassment, disgust, or despair about changes?
Vision impaired	Is there a loss of peripheral vision?
Tactile impaired	Does the patient report any numbness, tingling, or loss of sensation of the face or extremities? Give location.

Table 8-2—cont'd

Endocrine assessment tool: focus questions and parameters

Variables	Focus questions and parameters
EXCHANGING	
Galactorrhea	Does the patient exhibit inappropriate excretion of breast milk?
Altered physical charac- teristics	Has the patient experienced a recent increase in hat, glove, ring, or shoe size?
	Has the patient experienced an increase or loss of body hair?
	Is the distribution of body hair appropriate?
	Does the patient have abnormal skin texture or pigmentation (e.g., excess dryness, sca- liness, oiliness, or perspiration; striae, or vitiligo)?
	Is there abnormal fat distribution around the face, between the scapula, or around the abdomen?
	Are the secondary sexual characteristics appropriate for gender?
Response to temperature changes	Is the patient unable to tolerate hot or cold weather?
Dysmenorrhea: type	*Congestive:* due to congestion of pelvic viscera
	Essential: no apparent cause
	Inflammatory: due to inflammation
	Membranous: discharge contains shreds of membrane
	Obstructive: due to mechanical obstruction of menstrual flow.
Amenorrhea	*Primary:* failure to begin menstration before age 16; *secondary:* cessation of menstrua- tion for more than 3 months in a previously normally menstruating woman.
	"When was your last normal menstrual period?"
Alterations in normal men- strual cycle	"Do your periods come at regular intervals or are they frequently late or early?"
	"Is your menstrual discharge unusually heavy or light?"
Hysterectomy	Give type and reason for surgery.
Menopause	Give date of onset.
	Does the patient complain of "hot flashes," fatigue, crying spells, insomnia, or other symptoms?
Labs	See Chapter 3 and Appendix II.
Serum osmo (osmolality)	See Appendix II.
CHOOSING	
Patient's/family's methods of dealing with stress	See Chapter 3.

circled diagnoses, synthesizes the data to determine whether other clusters of data also support the existence of the problem, and judges whether the actual or potential diagnosis is present.

Some diagnoses are repeated several times in the right-hand column. These repetitions occur only within the appropriate response pattern and are convenient for correlating data directly with appropriate nursing diagnosis. These diagnoses are not absolute but are intended to focus thinking and direct attention to a possible problem.

Certain signs and symptoms can indicate many diagnoses. For example, fever can indicate infection or ineffective thermoregulation. It can also indicate altered metabolic patterns such as hypermetabolism, which occurs in hyperthyroidism. To avoid unnecessary repetition of assessment parameters, variables are arranged with the diagnosis most likely to result from the data assessed. Thus, data to support a specific diagnosis may occasionally be found in other patterns or arranged with other diagnoses. Therefore, synthesis of all data is essential.

The Endocrine Assessment Tool is not intended to be the standardized and final format for evaluating patients with endocrine dysfunctions in all health institutions. An assessment tool must meet the needs of the institution and nurses using it. This tool is simply a working model that is expected to be changed and revised by nurses in clinical practice. Furthermore, evaluation and refinement are necessary before adopting the tool for use within a particular institution. Nurses interested in changing and revising the tool for use in a specific clinical setting should refer to Chapter 4.

HOW TO ELICIT APPROPRIATE DATA

Because the Unitary Person Framework and the Endocrine Assessment Tool contain some terms that may be unfamiliar to nurses, specific endocrine focus questions and parameters were developed and refined to elicit appropriate information. These questions and parameters appear in Table 8-2 and correspond with the assessment variables in bold type in the tool (Fig. 8-1). For example, the altered physical characteristics variable found in the "exchanging pattern" is in bold type; if the nurse is unsure about what to ask when assessing physical characteristics, Table 8-2 can be used to direct the assessment. Questions and parameters for data not in bold type appear in Chapter 3.

The focus questions and parameters in this book provide clarity and guidance in eliciting data and are not intended to be all inclusive. Nurses should not feel limited to asking only the questions or assessing the parameters provided. There are many other methods of eliciting appropriate information. Assessment methods should be tailored to the patient's level of understanding and the situation, as well as to the nurse's skill and comfort level.

CASE STUDY

The case study demonstrates the process a nurse uses to assess a patient with the Endocrine Assessment Tool. Based on clustering of information gathered during assessment, the nurse formulates appropriate nursing diagnoses and lists them in order of priority at the end of the tool.

M.D. is a 30-year-old man who has recently developed hypertension. He has also experienced increasing fatigue and mood swings. He is in the hospital for testing to rule out the possibility of pheochromocytoma and Cushing's syndrome. The Endocrine Assessment Tool (Fig. 8-2) was used to assess Mr. M.D.

BIBLIOGRAPHY

Block G and Nolan J: Health assessment for professional nursing: a developmental approach, ed 2, Norwalk, Conn, 1986, Appleton-Century-Crofts.

Carpenito L: Nursing diagnosis: application to clinical practice, Philadelphia, 1983, JB Lippincott Co, Inc.

Kenner C, Guzzetta C, and Dossey B: Critical care nursing: body-mind-spirit, ed 2, Boston, 1985, Little, Brown & Co, Inc.

Kessler C: Assessment of endocrine function. In Patrick M et al, editors: Medical-surgical nursing: a pathophysiologic approach, Philadelphia, 1985, JB Lippincott Co.

Malasanos L: Health assessment, ed 3, St Louis, 1986, The CV Mosby Co.

ENDOCRINE ASSESSMENT TOOL

Name _____ Age _____ Sex _____
Address _____ Telephone _____
Significant other _____ Telephone _____
Date of admission _____ Medical diagnosis _____
Allergies _____

Nursing Diagnosis
(Potential or Altered)

COMMUNICATING ▪ A pattern involving sending messages
Read, write, understand English (circle) _____ Communication
Other languages_____ Verbal
Voice changes _____ Nonverbal
Physical barriers to communication _____
Alternate form of communication _____

VALUING ▪ A pattern involving the assigning of relative worth
Religious preference _____ Spiritual state
Important religious practices _____ Distress
Spiritual concerns _____ Despair
Cultural orientation _____
Cultural practices _____

RELATING ▪ A pattern involving establishing bonds
Role
  Marital status _____ Role performance
  Age & health of significant others _____ Parenting
  _____ Sexual dysfunction
  Number of children _____ Ages _____ Work
  Role in home _____ Family
  Financial support _____ Social/leisure
  Occupation _____ Family processes
  Job satisfaction/concerns _____
  Sexual relationships (satisfactory/unsatisfactory) _____ Sexuality patterns
    Difficulties related to sex _____
    Inability to conceive _____ **Male infertility** _____

Socialization
  Quality of relationships with others _____ Impaired social interaction
    Patient's description _____

    Significant others' descriptions _____

    Staff observations _____
  Verbalizes feelings of being alone _____ Social isolation
    Attributed to _____ Social withdrawal

KNOWING: ▪ A pattern involving the meaning associated with information
Current health problems _____
_____
Previous illnesses/hospitalizations/surgeries _____
_____
_____
_____
_____

Fig. 8-1

Continued.

History of the following problems:
Heart _____
Peripheral vascular _____
Lung _____
Liver _____ Kidney _____ Adrenal _____   Knowledge deficit
Cerebrovascular _____ Rheumatic fever _____
Thyroid _____ Pituitary _____
Diabetes _____ **Type** _____
Other _____
Current medications: **Insulin** _____
   Hypoglycemic agent _____ **Steroids** _____
   Thyroid preparation _____ Other _____
   _____
   _____
   _____

Risk factors for heart disease
                         Present   Perceptions/knowledge
 1. Hypertension   _____ _____
 2. Hyperlipidemia   _____ _____
 3. Smoking   _____ _____
 4. Obesity   _____ _____
 5. Diabetes   _____ _____
 6. Sedentary living _____ _____
 7. Stress   _____ _____
 8. Alcohol/drug use _____ _____
 9. Oral contraceptives ____ _____
10. Family history _____
   _____

Perception/knowledge of illness/tests/surgery _____
   _____
Misconceptions _____
Readiness to learn _____
   Requests information concerning _____
   Educational level _____   Thought processes
   Learning impeded by _____   Impaired problem solving

Orientation
Level of alertness _____   Orientation
Orientation: Person _____ Place _____ Time _____   Confusion
Appropriate behavior/communication _____

Memory
Memory intact: Yes_____ No _____ Recent _____ Remote _____   Memory

FEELING: ▪ A pattern involving the subjective awareness of information
Comfort
   Pain/discomfort: Yes _____ No _____   Comfort
      Onset _____ Duration _____   Pain/chronic
      Location _____ Quality _____ Radiation _____   Pain/acute
      Associated factors _____
      Aggravating factors _____   Discomfort
      Alleviating factors _____
      Headaches: Yes _____ No _____ Frequency _____

Fig. 8-1, cont'd

Emotional Integrity/States
Recent stressful life events _____ Grieving
_____ Anxiety
Verbalizes feelings of: Fear _____ Anxiety _____ Depression _____ Fear
   Nervousness _____ Mood swings _____ Irritability _____ Anger
   Other _____ Guilt
   Attributed to _____ Shame
_____ Sadness

Physical manifestations _____
_____

MOVING ▪ A pattern involving activity
Activity
History of physical disability _____ Impaired physical mobility
_____
Mobility aids _____
Limitations in daily activities _____ Activity intolerance
_____
Exercise habits _____
Weakness/fatigue _____ **Characteristics** _____
Muscle tremors _____ **Muscle tone** _____
Joint enlargement _____ Location _____
Paralysis _____ Describe _____

Rest
Hours slept/night _____ Feels rested: Yes _____ No _____   Sleep pattern disturbance
Sleep aids (pillows, meds, food) _____   Hypersomnia
Difficulty falling/remaining asleep _____   Insomnia
   Nightmares

Recreation
Leisure activities _____ Deficit in diversional activity
Social activities _____

Environmental Maintenance
Home maintenance management
   Size & arrangement of home (stairs, bathroom) _____ Impaired home maintenance
   _____ Safety needs _____   management
   Home responsibilities _____ Safety hazards
_____

Self-Care
Ability to perform ADLs: Independent _____ Dependent _____ Self-care
Specify deficits _____   Feeding
   Difficulty swallowing _____   Impaired swallowing
Discharge planning needs _____   Bathing/hygiene
_____   Dressing/grooming
   Toileting

Growth and Development
Height and weight appropriate for age? _____ Growth and Development
   If no, specify alteration _____
Personal/social skills appropriate for age? _____
   If no, specify alteration _____
Motor skills appropriate for age? _____
   If no, specify alteration _____
Language/cognitive skills appropriate for age? _____
   If no, specify alteration _____
Diagnosed retardation or learning disabilities _____
_____

Fig. 8-1, cont'd

Continued.

Health Maintenance
   Health insurance _____   Health maintenance
      Regular physical checkups _____

PERCEIVING: ▪ A pattern involving the reception of information
Self-Concept
   Patient's description of self _____   Self-concept
   Effects of illness/surgery _____   Body image
   _____   Self-esteem
   Effects of altered physical characteristics _____   Personal identity
   _____   Gender
                                                                            Social

Meaningfulness
   Verbalizes hopelessness _____   Hopelessness
   Verbalizes/perceives loss of control _____   Powerlessness

Sensory/Perception
   Vision impaired _____ Glasses _____   Visual
   Auditory impaired _____ Hearing aid _____   Auditory
   Kinesthetics impaired _____   Kinesthetic
   Gustatory impaired _____   Gustatory
   Tactile impaired _____   Tactile

   _____
   Olfactory impaired _____   Olfactory
   Reflexes: Biceps   R _____ L _____   Triceps R _____ L _____
              Brachioradialis R _____ L _____   Knee   R _____ L _____
              Ankle   R _____ L _____   Plantar R _____ L _____

EXCHANGING ▪ A pattern involving mutual giving and receiving
Circulation
   Cerebral
      Neurologic changes/symptoms _____   Cerebral tissue perfusion
      Pupils   Eye Opening
         L 2 3 4 5 6 mm   None (1)
         R 2 3 4 5 6 mm   To pain (2)
         Reaction: Brisk _____   To speech (3)   Fluid volume
         Sluggish _____ Nonreactive _____   Spontaneous (4)   Deficit
                                                                            Excess

      Best Verbal   Best Motor
         No response (1)   Flaccid (1)
         Incomprehensible sound (2)   Extensor response (2)   Cardiac output
         Inappropriate words (3)   Flexor response (3)
         Confused conversation (4)   Semipurposeful (4)
         Oriented (5)   Localized to pain (5)
                                         Obeys commands (6)

      Glasgow Coma Scale total _____
   Cardiac
      PMI _____ Pacemaker _____   Cardiopulmonary tissue
      Apical rate rhythm _____   perfusion
      Heart sounds/murmurs _____
      Dysrhythmias _____   Fluid volume
      BP: Sitting   Lying   Standing   Deficit
            R _____ L _____   R _____ L _____   R _____ L _____   Excess
                                                                        Peripheral tissue perfusion

Fig. 8-1, cont'd

Peripheral
 Jugular venous distension R ＿＿＿ L ＿＿＿
 Pulses: A = absent   B = bruits   D = doppler
 Carotid   R ＿＿＿ L ＿＿＿   Popliteal   R ＿＿＿ L ＿＿＿
 Brachial R ＿＿＿ L ＿＿＿   Posterior tibial R ＿＿＿ L ＿＿＿   Peripheral tissue perfusion
 Radial   R ＿＿＿ L ＿＿＿   Dorsalis pedis R ＿＿＿ L ＿＿＿   Fluid volume
 Femoral R ＿＿＿ L ＿＿＿   Deficit
 Skin temp ＿＿＿＿＿＿ Color ＿＿＿＿＿＿ Turgor ＿＿＿＿＿＿＿＿＿＿   Excess
 Capillary refill ＿＿＿＿＿＿ Clubbing ＿＿＿＿＿＿＿＿＿＿＿＿＿
 Edema ＿＿＿＿＿＿＿＿＿＿＿＿＿＿＿＿＿＿＿＿＿＿＿＿＿

Physical Integrity
 Tissue integrity ＿＿＿＿＿＿＿＿＿＿＿＿＿＿＿＿＿＿＿＿＿＿＿＿   Impaired tissue integrity
 Skin integrity ＿＿＿＿＿＿＿＿＿＿＿＿＿＿＿＿＿＿＿＿＿＿＿＿＿   Impaired skin integrity
  Rashes ＿＿＿＿＿＿ Lesions ＿＿＿＿＿＿＿＿＿＿＿＿＿＿＿＿＿
  Petechiae ＿＿＿＿＿＿ Bruises ＿＿＿＿＿＿＿＿＿＿＿＿＿＿＿＿
  Abrasions ＿＿＿＿＿＿ Surgical incisions ＿＿＿＿＿＿＿＿＿＿＿   Infection
  Exophthalmos ＿＿＿＿＿＿ **Galactorrhea** ＿＿＿＿＿＿＿＿＿＿＿   Injury
  Poor wound healing ＿＿＿＿＿＿ Recent bone fractures ＿＿＿＿＿＿
  Altered physical characteristics ＿＿＿＿＿＿＿＿＿＿＿＿＿＿＿
  ＿＿＿＿＿＿＿＿＿＿＿＿＿＿＿＿＿＿＿＿＿＿＿＿＿＿＿＿＿

Oxygenation
 Complaints of dyspnea ＿＿＿＿＿＿ Precipitated by ＿＿＿＿＿＿＿＿
 Orthopnea ＿＿＿＿＿＿＿＿＿＿＿＿＿＿＿＿＿＿＿＿＿＿＿＿＿
 Rate ＿＿＿＿＿＿ Rhythm ＿＿＿＿＿＿ Depth ＿＿＿＿＿＿＿＿＿   Ineffective breathing patterns
 Labored/unlabored (circle) Chest expansion ＿＿＿＿＿＿＿＿＿＿
 Splinting ＿＿＿＿＿＿＿＿＿＿＿＿＿＿＿＿＿＿＿＿＿＿＿＿＿＿
 Use of accessory muscles ＿＿＿＿＿＿ Stridor ＿＿＿＿＿＿＿＿＿＿   Ineffective airway clearance
 Cough: productive/nonproductive ＿＿＿＿＿＿＿＿＿＿＿＿＿＿＿＿
 Sputum: Color ＿＿＿＿＿＿ Amount ＿＿＿＿＿＿ Consistency ＿＿＿＿＿
 Breath sounds ＿＿＿＿＿＿＿＿＿＿＿＿＿＿＿＿＿＿＿＿＿＿＿＿   Impaired gas exchange
 Arterial blood gases ＿＿＿＿＿＿＿＿＿＿＿＿＿＿＿＿＿＿＿＿＿
 Oxygen percent and device ＿＿＿＿＿＿＿＿＿＿＿＿＿＿＿＿＿＿
 Ventilator ＿＿＿＿＿＿＿＿＿＿＿＿＿＿＿＿＿＿＿＿＿＿＿＿

Physical Regulation
 Immune
  Lymph nodes enlarged ＿＿＿＿＿＿ Location ＿＿＿＿＿＿＿＿＿＿＿   Infection
  WBC count ＿＿＿＿＿＿ Differential ＿＿＿＿＿＿＿＿＿＿＿＿＿＿   Hypothermia
 Altered body temperature   Hyperthermia
  Temperature ＿＿＿＿＿＿ Route ＿＿＿＿＿＿＿＿＿＿＿＿＿＿＿＿   Ineffective thermoregulation
  Response to temperature changes ＿＿＿＿＿＿＿＿＿＿＿＿＿＿

Hormonal/Metabolic Patterns
 Altered Menstrual Patterns   Hormonal/metabolic patterns
  Dysmenorrhea ＿＿＿＿＿＿ **Type** ＿＿＿＿＿＿ Severity ＿＿＿＿＿＿＿
  Amenorrhea ＿＿＿＿＿＿＿＿＿＿＿＿＿＿＿＿＿＿＿＿＿＿＿＿
  Alterations in normal menstrual cycle ＿＿＿＿＿＿＿＿＿＿＿＿＿
  Hysterectomy ＿＿＿＿＿＿ **Menopause** ＿＿＿＿＿＿＿＿＿＿＿

Fig. 8-1, cont'd

Continued.

Nutrition

Eating patterns   Nutrition

 Number of meals per day _____

 Special diet _____   Less than body requirements

 Where eaten _____

 Food preferences/intolerances _____

 Food allergies _____   More than body

 Caffeine intake (coffee, tea, soft drinks)   requirements

 _____

 Appetite changes _____

 Excessive thirst _____   Fluid volume

 Nausea/vomiting _____   Deficit

 Condition of mouth/throat (e.g., moniliasis) _____   Excess

 _____   Oral mucous membrane

 Height _____ Weight _____ Ideal body weight _____   More than body

 Recent changes in weight/height/proportions (circle) _____   requirements

 Current therapy   Less than body requirements

 NPO _____ NG suction _____

 Tube feeding _____

 TPN _____

Labs

 Na _____ **K** _____ **CL** _____ **Glucose** _____ **(Fasting?)** _____

 Cholesterol _____ **Triglycerides** _____ **Albumin** _____

 Ca _____ **Mg** _____ **Phosphate** _____ **Other** _____

Elimination

Gastrointestinal/bowel

 Usual bowel habits _____   Bowel elimination

 Alterations from normal _____   Constipation

 Bowel regulatory aids _____   Diarrhea

 Abdominal physical examination _____   Incontinence

                                                                        GI tissue perfusion

Renal/urinary   Urinary elimination

 Usual urinary pattern _____   Incontinence

 Alteration from normal _____   Retention

 Color _____ Catheter _____

 Urine output: 24 hour _____ Average hourly _____   Renal tissue perfusion

 Bladder distention _____

 Serum BUN _____ Serum Creatinine _____ **Serum osmo** _____   Fluid volume

 Urine studies _____   Deficit

 Specific gravity _____   Excess

                                                                        Cardiac output

CHOOSING ▪ A pattern involving the selection of alternatives

Coping

 Patient's usual problem-solving methods _____   Ineffective individual coping

 _____   Ineffective family coping

 Family's usual problem-solving methods _____

 _____

 Patient's method of dealing with stress _____

 _____

 Family's method of dealing with stress _____

 _____

 Support systems available _____

 _____

Fig. 8-1, cont'd

Participation

Compliance with past/current health care regimens ＿＿＿＿＿＿＿＿＿＿＿＿＿＿＿＿   Noncompliance
＿＿＿＿＿＿＿＿＿＿＿＿＿＿＿＿＿＿＿＿＿＿＿＿＿＿＿＿＿＿＿＿＿＿＿＿＿   Ineffective participation

Willingness to comply with future health care regimen ＿＿＿＿＿＿＿＿＿＿＿＿＿
＿＿＿＿＿＿＿＿＿＿＿＿＿＿＿＿＿＿＿＿＿＿＿＿＿＿＿＿＿＿＿＿＿＿＿＿＿

Judgment

Decision-making ability   Judgment
  Patient's perspective ＿＿＿＿＿＿＿＿＿＿＿＿＿＿＿＿＿＿＿＿＿＿＿＿＿＿＿＿   Indecisiveness
  Others' perspectives ＿＿＿＿＿＿＿＿＿＿＿＿＿＿＿＿＿＿＿＿＿＿＿＿＿＿＿＿＿

Prioritized nursing diagnosis/problem list

1. ＿＿＿＿＿＿＿＿＿＿＿＿＿＿＿＿＿＿＿＿＿＿＿＿＿＿＿＿＿＿＿＿＿＿＿＿＿＿
2. ＿＿＿＿＿＿＿＿＿＿＿＿＿＿＿＿＿＿＿＿＿＿＿＿＿＿＿＿＿＿＿＿＿＿＿＿＿＿
3. ＿＿＿＿＿＿＿＿＿＿＿＿＿＿＿＿＿＿＿＿＿＿＿＿＿＿＿＿＿＿＿＿＿＿＿＿＿＿
4. ＿＿＿＿＿＿＿＿＿＿＿＿＿＿＿＿＿＿＿＿＿＿＿＿＿＿＿＿＿＿＿＿＿＿＿＿＿＿
5. ＿＿＿＿＿＿＿＿＿＿＿＿＿＿＿＿＿＿＿＿＿＿＿＿＿＿＿＿＿＿＿＿＿＿＿＿＿＿
6. ＿＿＿＿＿＿＿＿＿＿＿＿＿＿＿＿＿＿＿＿＿＿＿＿＿＿＿＿＿＿＿＿＿＿＿＿＿＿
7. ＿＿＿＿＿＿＿＿＿＿＿＿＿＿＿＿＿＿＿＿＿＿＿＿＿＿＿＿＿＿＿＿＿＿＿＿＿＿
8. ＿＿＿＿＿＿＿＿＿＿＿＿＿＿＿＿＿＿＿＿＿＿＿＿＿＿＿＿＿＿＿＿＿＿＿＿＿＿

Signature ＿＿＿＿＿＿＿＿＿＿＿＿＿＿＿＿＿＿＿＿＿＿＿＿＿＿＿＿＿   Date ＿＿＿＿＿＿＿＿＿＿＿

Fig. 8-1, cont'd

ENDOCRINE ASSESSMENT TOOL

Name __M.D.__ Age __30__ Sex __M__
Address __2115 WALTER'S COURT, BOSTON, MA__ Telephone __421-5830__
Significant other __WIFE — C.__ Telephone __SAME__
Date of admission __2/15__ Medical diagnosis __R/O PHEOCHROMOCYTOMA/CUSHING'S SYNDROME__
Allergies __NONE KNOWN__

Nursing Diagnosis
(Potential or Altered)

COMMUNICATING ▪ A pattern involving sending messages
(Read,) (write,) (understand) English (circle) __NO DIFFICULTIES__   Communication
Other languages __No__   Verbal
Voice changes __No__   Nonverbal
Physical barriers to communication __No__
Alternate form of communication __NONE__

VALUING ▪ A pattern involving the assigning of relative worth
Religious preference __BAPTIST__   Spiritual state
Important religious practices __PERIODS OF SILENT PRAYER__   Distress
Spiritual concerns __NONE AT PRESENT__   Despair
Cultural orientation __ANGLO – AMERICAN__
Cultural practices __NO SPECIFIC PRACTICES IMPORTANT__

RELATING ▪ A pattern involving establishing bonds
Role
  Marital status __MARRIED__   Role performance
  Age & health of significant others __WIFE – C. 28 YEARS, GOOD__   Parenting
  __HEALTH__   (Sexual dysfunction)
  Number of children __1__ Ages __2 YEARS (ALEX)__   (Work)
  Role in home __HUSBAND, HOME MAINTENANCE, "BREAD WINNER"__   Family
  Financial support __PRIMARILY PATIENT; WIFE WORKS PART-TIME__   Social/leisure
  Occupation __STOCK CLERK – GROCERY STORE__   Family processes
  Job satisfaction (concerns) __WORK BECOMING INCREASINGLY FATIGUING__
  Sexual relationships (satisfactory (unsatisfactory)) __PATIENT (WIFE)__   Sexuality patterns
    Difficulties related to sex __DECREASED LIBIDO ATTRIBUTED TO FATIGUE__
    Inability to conceive __N/A__ Male infertility __No__

Socialization
  Quality of relationships with others __"GOOD UNTIL RECENTLY"__   (Impaired social interaction)
    Patient's description __"LATELY I SEEM TO BE UPSET EASILY__

  Significant others' descriptions __"UNPREDICTABLE, MOODY" (WIFE)__

  Staff observations __EMOTIONAL LABILITY__
  Verbalizes feelings of being alone __No__   Social isolation
    Attributed to __N/A__   Social withdrawal

KNOWING: ▪ A pattern involving the meaning associated with information
Current health problems __"EMOTIONAL PROBLEMS", HYPERTENSION,__
__SWELLING IN FACE, HANDS, ⌄ FEET__
Previous illnesses/hospitalizations/surgeries __TONSILLECTOMY AGE 6__

Fig. 8-2

History of the following problems:
Heart _No_
Peripheral vascular _No_
Lung _No_
Liver _No_ Kidney _No_ Adrenal _"Possible"_   (Knowledge deficit)
Cerebrovascular _No_ Rheumatic fever _No_
Thyroid _No_ Pituitary _No_
Diabetes _No_ Type _—_
Other _Peptic ulcer 2 yrs. ago_
Current medications: Insulin _No_
Hypoglycemic agent _No_ Steroids _No_
Thyroid preparation _No_ Other _Xanax 0.25 mg PO Bid;_
Clonidine hydrochloride 0.3 mg PO Bid

Risk factors for heart disease

	Present	Perceptions/knowledge
1. Hypertension	✓	_Unaware of ↑ risk of heart disease_
2. Hyperlipidemia	—	
3. Smoking	✓	_"Causes lung cancer"_
4. Obesity	—	
5. Diabetes	—	
6. Sedentary living	—	
7. Stress	✓	_Unaware of ↑ risk of heart disease_
8. Alcohol/drug use	✓	_1-2 beers/day "It's okay"_
9. Oral contraceptives	_N/A_	
10. Family history		_Father-MI at age 50, hypertension_

Perception/knowledge of illness/tests/surgery _"They tell me I might have_
some kind of tumor on my adrenal gland"
Misconceptions _"I might have cancer"_
Readiness to learn _Seems receptive_
Requests information concerning _Tests to be performed_
Educational level _High school (12th grade)_   Thought processes
Learning impeded by _Anxiety_   Impaired problem solving

Orientation
Level of alertness _Very aware of surroundings_   Orientation
Orientation: Person _✓_ Place _✓_ Time _✓_   Confusion
Appropriate behavior/communication _Both appropriate_

Memory
Memory intact: Yes _✓_ No ___ Recent _✓_ Remote _✓_   Memory

FEELING: ▪ A pattern involving the subjective awareness of information
Comfort
Pain/discomfort:Yes ___ No _✓_   Comfort
Onset _—_ Duration _—_   Pain/chronic
Location _—_ Quality _—_ Radiation _—_   Pain/acute
Associated factors _—_
Aggravating factors _—_   Discomfort
Alleviating factors _—_
Headaches: Yes _✓_ No ___ Frequency _Occasional; severe_

Emotional Integrity/States

Recent stressful life events _RECENTLY PURCHASED 1ST HOUSE_   Grieving

                             (Anxiety)

Verbalizes feelings of: Fear _—_ Anxiety _✓_ Depression _✓_   Fear

     Nervousness _✓_ Mood swings _✓_ Irritability _✓_   Anger

     Other _____   Guilt

     Attributed to _DOES NOT KNOW CAUSE OF FEELINGS "THEY JUST_   Shame

COME ON ME SUDDENLY" "I FEEL LIKE I'M LOSING MY MIND"   Sadness

ANXIETY — POSSIBLE TUMOR

Physical manifestations _OCCASIONALLY TEARFUL; SLIGHT HAND_

TREMOR

MOVING ▪ A pattern involving activity

Activity

History of physical disability _No_   Impaired physical mobility

Mobility aids _No_

Limitations in daily activities _LESS STAMINA_   (Activity intolerance)

Exercise habits _MEN'S SOFTBALL TEAM_

Weakness (fatigue) _✓_ Characteristics _INCREASES THROUGHOUT DAY_

Muscle tremors _SLIGHT (HANDS)_ Muscle tone _NORMAL; GENERALIZED ATROPHY_

Joint enlargement _No_ Location _—_

Paralysis _No_ Describe _—_

Rest   (Sleep pattern disturbance)

Hours slept/night _4-8 HOURS_ Feels rested: Yes ____ No _✓_   Hypersomnia

Sleep aids (pillows, meds, food) _XANAX_   (Insomnia)

Difficulty (falling/remaining) asleep _"I HAVE TROUBLE SLEEPING"_   Nightmares

Recreation

Leisure activities _PLAYS GUITAR, "TINKERS" AROUND HOUSE_   Deficit in diversional activity

Social activities _BASEBALL TEAM; GOES OUT WITH FRIENDS OCCASIONALLY_

Environmental Maintenance

Home maintenance management

     Size & arrangement of home (stairs, bathroom) _2 STORY — BATHROOM_   Impaired home maintenance

EACH FLOOR Safety needs _—_   management

     Home responsibilities _"FIX THINGS", YARDWORK, ASSIST WITH_   Safety hazards

GROCERY SHOPPING

Self-Care

Ability to perform ADLs: Independent _✓_ Dependent _____   Self-care

Specify deficits _—_   Feeding

     Difficulty swallowing _—_   Impaired swallowing

Discharge planning needs _—_   Bathing/hygiene

                             Dressing/grooming

                             Toileting

Growth and Development

Height and weight appropriate for age? _____   Growth and Development

     If no, specify alteration _____

Personal/social skills appropriate for age? _____

     If no, specify alteration _____ _N/A_

Motor skills appropriate for age? _____ _(ADULT)_

     If no, specify alteration _____

Language/cognitive skills appropriate for age? _____

     If no, specify alteration _____

Diagnosed retardation or learning disabilities _No_

Fig. 8-2, cont'd

Health Maintenance
  Health insurance *HEALTH MAINTENANCE ORGANIZATION*   Health maintenance
  Regular physical checkups *YEARLY (FOR BASEBALL)*

PERCEIVING: ▪ A pattern involving the reception of information
Self-Concept
  Patient's description of self *"INDEPENDENT, CAPABLE*   (Self-concept)
  Effects of illness/surgery *"I'M NOT MYSELF" "I'M NOT MUCH OF A MAN*   Body image
  ANYMORE"– (DECREASED LIBIDO)   (Self-esteem)
  Effects of altered physical characteristics *NONE*   Personal identity
                                                                           Gender
                                                                           Social

Meaningfulness
  Verbalizes hopelessness *"I DON'T KNOW IF I'LL GET BETTER"*   (Hopelessness)
  Verbalizes/perceives loss of control *"I'M LOSING MY MIND*   (Powerlessness)

Sensory/Perception
  Vision impaired *No*   Glasses ———   Visual
  Auditory impaired *No*   Hearing aid ——   Auditory
  Kinesthetics impaired *No*   Kinesthetic
  Gustatory impaired *No*   Gustatory
  Tactile impaired *No*   Tactile

  Olfactory impaired *No*   Olfactory
  Reflexes:Biceps   R *+2* L *+2*   Triceps R *+2* L *+2*
           Brachioradialis R *+2* L *+2*   Knee   R *+2* L *+2*
           Ankle   R *+2* L *+2*   Plantar R *+2* L *+2*

EXCHANGING ▪ A pattern involving mutual giving and receiving
Circulation
Cerebral
  Neurologic changes/symptoms *NONE*   Cerebral tissue perfusion
  Pupils   Eye Opening
    L 2 ③ 4 5 6 mm   None (1)
    R 2 ③ 4 5 6 mm   To pain (2)
    Reaction: Brisk ✓   To speech (3)   Fluid volume
    Sluggish ——— Nonreactive ——— Spontaneous ④   Deficit
                                                                           Excess

  Best Verbal   Best Motor
    No response (1)   Flaccid (1)
    Incomprehensible sound (2) Extensor response (2)   Cardiac output
    Inappropriate words (3)   Flexor response (3)
    Confused conversation (4) Semipurposeful (4)
    Oriented ⑤   Localized to pain (5)
                              Obeys commands ⑥

  Glasgow Coma Scale total *15*
Cardiac *5TH INTERCOSTAL,*
  PMI *MIDCLAVICULAR* Pacemaker *No*   Cardiopulmonary tissue
  Apical rate rhythm *85, REGULAR*   perfusion
  Heart sounds/murmurs *S₁ & S₂, NO MURMURS, CLICKS, OR RUBS*
  Dysrhythmias *No*   Fluid volume
  BP: Sitting   Lying   Standing   Deficit
     R *¹⁹⁴/₁₁₄* L *¹⁹⁴/₁₁₄*   R *¹⁹⁸/₁₁₄* L *¹⁹⁸/₁₁₄*   R *¹⁶⁸/₁₀₀* L *¹⁶⁸/₁₀₀*   Excess
                                                                           Peripheral tissue perfusion

Fig. 8-2, cont'd

Continued.

Peripheral
  Jugular venous distension R _No_ L _No_
  Pulses: A = absent   B = bruits   D = doppler
  Carotid   R _+2_ L _+2_   Popliteal   R _+2_ L _+2_
  Brachial R _+2_ L _+2_   Posterior tibial   R _+2_ L _+2_   Peripheral tissue perfusion
  Radial   R _+2_ L _+2_   Dorsalis pedis   R _+2_ L _+2_   Fluid volume
  Femoral   R _+2_ L _+2_   Deficit
  Skin temp _WARM_ Color _LIGHT TAN_ Turgor _TAUNT_   Excess
  Capillary refill _BRISK_ Clubbing _No_
  Edema _GENERALIZED, BUT ESPECIALLY HANDS, FEET, AND FACE_

Physical Integrity
  Tissue integrity _BRUISING (SEE BELOW)_   (Impaired tissue integrity)
  Skin integrity _INTACT_   Impaired skin integrity
  Rashes _—_ Lesions _—_
  Petechiae _—_ Bruises _INCREASED FREQUENCY; LEFT FOREARM_
  Abrasions _—_ Surgical incisions _—_   (Infection) (POTENTIAL)
  Exophthalmos _—_ Galactorrhea _—_   Injury
  Poor wound healing _YES_ Recent bone fractures _—_
  Altered physical characteristics _ROUNDING OF FACIAL FEATURES,_
  EDEMA, MUSCLE WASTING OF EXTREMITIES

Oxygenation
  Complaints of dyspnea _No_ Precipitated by _—_
  Orthopnea _No_
  Rate _16_ Rhythm _REGULAR_ Depth _MODERATE_   Ineffective breathing patterns
  Labored/unlabored (circle) Chest expansion _EQUAL_
  Splinting _No_
  Use of accessory muscles _No_ Stridor _No_   Ineffective airway clearance
  Cough: productive/nonproductive _No_
  Sputum: Color _—_ Amount _—_ Consistency _—_
  Breath sounds _NORMAL VESICULAR THROUGHOUT_   Impaired gas exchange
  Arterial blood gases _NOT OBTAINED_
  Oxygen percent and device _N/A_
  Ventilator _N/A_

Physical Regulation
  Immune
    Lymph nodes enlarged _No_ Location _—_   Infection
    WBC count _8,500×10³/µL_ Differential _NORMAL_   Hypothermia
  Altered body temperature   Hyperthermia
    Temperature _37° C_ Route _ORAL_   Ineffective thermoregulation
    Response to temperature changes _SENSITIVE TO THE COLD_

Hormonal/Metabolic Patterns
  Altered Menstrual Patterns _N/A — MALE PATIENT_   Hormonal/metabolic patterns
    Dysmenorrhea _____ Type _____ Severity _____
    Amenorrhea _____
    Alterations in normal menstrual cycle _____
    Hysterectomy _____ Menopause _____

Fig. 8-2, cont'd

Nutrition

Eating patterns

Number of meals per day _2 - 3_

Special diet _No_

Where eaten _DINNER AT HOME; BREAKFAST & LUNCH AT McDONALD'S_

Food (preferences)/intolerances _FRENCH FRIES, HAMBURGERS_

Food allergies _NONE_

Caffeine intake (coffee, tea, soft drinks)
COFFEE — 2 CUPS/DAY SOFT DRINKS — 2 (12 OZ. CANS)/DAY

Appetite changes _DECREASED APPETITE X3 MONTHS_

Excessive thirst _No_

Nausea/vomiting _No_

Condition of mouth/throat (e.g., moniliasis) _No LESIONS; TEETH IN_
GOOD REPAIR; GUMS IN GOOD CONDITION

Height _5FT 11INCHES_ Weight _166 lbs_ Ideal body weight _172 lbs_

Recent changes in (weight) height (proportions) (circle) _DECREASED_

Current therapy

NPO _No_ NG suction _NONE_

Tube feeding _No_

TPN _No_

Labs

Na _130 mEq/L_ K _3.0 mEq/L_ CL _92 mEq/L_ Glucose _160 mg/dl_ (Fasting?) _YES_

Cholesterol _200 mg/dl_ Triglycerides _135 mg/dl_ Albumin _3.5 g/dl_

Ca _5.1 mEq/L_ Mg _1.8 mEq/L_ Phosphate _2.5 mg/dl_ Other _—_

Gastrointestinal Elimination

bowel

Usual bowel habits _X 2/DAY_

Alteratiojns from normal _NONE_

Bowel regulatory aids _BRAN CEREAL_

Abdominal physical examination _NORMAL SOUNDS; SOFT, NONTENDER, NO MASSES_

Renal/urinary

Usual urinary pattern _X 4–5/DAY_

Alteration from normal _NONE_

Color _AMBER_ Catheter _No_

Urine output: 24 hour _2400_ Average hourly _APPROX. 100 cc_

Bladder distention _NONE_

Serum BUN _30 mg/dl_ Serum Creatinine _1.5 mg/dl_ Serum osmo _300 mOsm/kg_

Urine studies _24 HR. URINE FOR VANILLYLMANDELIC ACID IN PROGRESS_

Specific gravity _1.035_

CHOOSING ▪ A pattern involving the selection of alternatives

Coping

Patient's usual problem-solving methods _TALKS PROBLEM OVER WITH WIFE,_
COWORKERS, OR PARENTS

Family's usual problem-solving methods _TALKS PROBLEM OVER WITH_
PATIENT; SEEKS FURTHER INFORMATION

Patient's method of dealing with stress _PLAYS GUITAR; RECENTLY_
GETS VERY ANGRY

Family's method of dealing with stress _WATCHES TV, READS A BOOK_

Support systems available _WIFE, PATIENT'S PARENTS_

Nutrition

(Less than body requirements)
(POTENTIAL)

More than body
requirements

Fluid volume
Deficit
Excess
Oral mucous membrane
More than body
requirements
(Less than body requirements)
(POTENTIAL)

Bowel elimination
Constipation
Diarrhea
Incontinence
GI tissue perfusion
Urinary elimination
Incontinence
Retention

Renal tissue perfusion

(Fluid volume)
(Deficit)
Excess
Cardiac output

(Ineffective individual coping)
Ineffective family coping

Fig. 8-2, cont'd

Continued.

Participation

Compliance with past/current health care regimens *HAS NOT HAD PREVIOUS SERIOUS ILLNESS*

Noncompliance
Ineffective participation

Willingness to comply with future health care regimen *VERBALIZES DESIRE TO COMPLY*

Judgment

Decision-making ability

Patient's perspective *"USUALLY GOOD — NOT LATELY"*

Others' perspectives *SAME AS ABOVE (WIFE)*

Judgment
Indecisiveness

Prioritized nursing diagnosis/problem list

1. *ANXIETY RELATED TO DIAGNOSIS OF POSSIBLE ADRENAL TUMOR*
2. *KNOWLEDGE DEFICIT RELATED TO DISEASE PROCESS AND NECESSARY TESTING*
3. *ALTERED SELF-ESTEEM RELATED TO DECREASED LIBIDO AND CHANGES IN PHYSICAL HABITUS*
4. *INEFFECTIVE INDIVIDUAL COPING RELATED TO EMOTIONAL LABILITY*
5. *POWERLESSNESS RELATED TO EMOTIONAL LABILITY*
6. *POTENTIAL FOR INFECTION RELATED TO POOR WOUND HEALING*
7. *SEXUAL DYSFUNCTION RELATED TO DECREASED LIBIDO*
8. *ACTIVITY INTOLERANCE RELATED TO DECREASED STAMINA AND FATIGUE*

Signature *Linda A. Prinkey, RN*   Date *2/23*

Fig. 8-2, cont'd

■ UNIT III ■
ASSESSING PATIENTS WITH MAJOR SPECIALTY DYSFUNCTIONS

CHAPTER 9

MEDICAL-SURGICAL ASSESSMENT TOOL

SHELIA D. BUNTON
CYNTHIA A. GOLDBERG

The Medical-Surgical Assessment Tool was designed to assess patients with unique biopsychosocial assessment needs. This tool incorporates signs and symptoms pertinent to medical-surgical patients and facilitates identification of nursing diagnoses. It also incorporates the American Nurses' Association's *Standards for Medical-Surgical Nursing Practice*. This chapter includes:

- *The way the tool was developed and refined*
- *The patient population and settings to which it applies*
- *Selected medical-surgical emphasis areas*
- *The way to use the tool*
- *Specific medical-surgical focus questions and parameters to assist the nurse in eliciting appropriate data*
- *The Medical-Surgical Assessment Tool*
- *A case study*
- *A completed version of the tool based on the case study*

DEVELOPMENT AND REFINEMENT OF THE TOOL

The Medical-Surgical Assessment Tool was developed from the nursing data base prototype (see Chapter 2). Many hemodynamic monitoring and critical care variables originally incorporated in the prototype were deleted and replaced with variables more applicable to assessment of unit-level medical-surgical patients. The resultant tool, supported by the American Nurses' Association's standards and current literature, was modified based on the recommendations of medical and surgical nurse experts.

Masters-prepared clinical nurse specialists and nurse experts then tested the tool on nine adult patients in a medical intensive care unit and medical-surgical, neurologic, or neurosurgical units. These patients, ranging in age from 34 to 74 years, had a variety of medical, surgical, and neurologic problems, including renal disease, hypoxia, aneurysms, and meningiomas. The testing evaluated the adequacy of the tool in terms of flow, space for recording data, and completeness of assessment variables. Based on the results, the tool was revised.

PATIENT POPULATION AND SETTING

The Medical-Surgical Assessment Tool was developed to assist the nurse in assessing the needs of adult patients with diseases and illnesses requiring treatment by medications or surgery. Originally designed for use within acute and chronic care hospital settings, the tool was difficult to use when assessing medical intensive care patients. Nurses should therefore use this particular tool for assessing general or intermediate care inpatients in multiservice medical-surgical units. Medical intensive care populations could then be assessed using the Critical Care Assessment Tool (see Chapter 12) or a form of the Medical-Surgical Assessment Tool adapted for use in a particular setting (see Chapter 4).

Although most patients can tolerate a long assessment, the nurse may complete the tool over two sessions, preferably within the first 24 hours after admission. Depending on the patient's degree of distress and the unit's laboratory and testing schedule, a family member, friend, or significant other may help in providing necessary information.

MEDICAL-SURGICAL EMPHASIS AREAS

Medical-surgical patients have specialized problems and needs. This tool, developed to include assessment variables within each of the nine human response patterns, focuses on prevalent problems in this population. Table 9-1 outlines these emphasis areas.

HOW TO USE THE TOOL

To use the Medical-Surgical Assessment Tool effectively, nurses must first familiarize themselves with the human response patterns of the Unitary Person Framework (see Chapter 2), which provides the underlying framework for Taxonomy I. The human response patterns of the Unitary Person Framework serve as the major category headings for Taxonomy I and the Medical-Surgical Assessment Tool. The sequence of the response patterns, as it appears in Taxonomy I, has been changed in this tool to permit better ordering of assessment variables. Nursing diagnoses pertinent to medical-surgical patients, along with the signs and symptoms necessary to identify them, have been added to the appropriate response patterns.

Nurses must also realize that this tool is very different from conventional medical or surgical assessment tools. As a result, nurses may encounter some initial difficulty in using it. They should remember, however, that the tool

was not designed to follow the organization or content of the traditional medical data base; the data collected do not reflect only medical patterns. Rather, the tool elicits information about holistic patterns in ways not traditionally assessed by nurses. It represents a new way of collecting and synthesizing data that further requires new thinking when processing data. This tool represents a nursing data base developed from a nursing model that permits a holistic nursing assessment to take place so nursing diagnoses can be identified.

Although nurses probably agree that a holistic nursing data base would help in practice, it is realized that changing traditional assessment methods is not an easy task. For this reason, a trial usage period is recommended before nurses judge the tool's merits. During this trial period, nurses should assess 10 patients using the tool to become familiar and progressively more comfortable with its organization and data-collection methods. With experience, nurses will become accustomed to new ways of clustering and processing information. With continued use, the time necessary to complete the tool will be reduced. Most important, nurses will recognize the unique ability of the tool to elicit appropriate signs and symptoms. Nurses will also discover that nursing diagnoses are easily identified when using this tool.

It is not necessary to complete the entire tool in one session. Priority sections can be designated for the initial assessment. Other sections or patterns can be completed within a time frame acceptable to the institution. To elicit data, nurses should familiarize themselves with the focus questions and parameters in the next section. When assessing specific signs and symptoms to affirm a diagnosis, the nurse circles the diagnosis in the right-hand column. The circled diagnosis does not confirm a problem but simply alerts the nurse to the possibility that it exists. After completing the assessment, the nurse scans the circled problems, synthesizes the data to determine whether other clusters of signs and symptoms support the existence of a problem, and judges whether the diagnosis is actually present.

Some diagnoses are repeated in more than one place. These repetitions occur only within the appropriate response pattern and are convenient for identifying data directly with their corresponding nursing diagnoses. These diagnoses are not absolute but are intended to focus thinking and direct more detailed attention to collecting data concerning a possible problem.

Some signs and symptoms can indicate many diagnoses. For example, increased secretions at the tracheostomy site may indicate ineffective breathing patterns or ineffective airway clearance. To avoid repetition of assessment parameters, variables are arranged with the diagnosis most likely to result from the data assessed. Thus, data to support one diagnosis may occasionally be found in other pat-

---

Table 9-1
Medical-surgical emphasis areas

Patterns	Emphasis areas to determine
Communicating	Tracheostomy
	The need for speech therapy consultant
Valuing	The need for ministry consultant
Relating	Role and sexual habits
Knowing	In-depth disease history of patient and family members
Moving	Rest and sleep environment
	Environmental maintenance and the need for social service consultant
	Self-care and the need for community health nurse consultant
Exchanging	Expanded examination of skin and tissue integrity
	The need for enterostomal therapy consultant
	Current therapy (expanded)
	Laboratory variables (expanded)
	Stoma or ostomy for bowel or urinary control
	Brief genitalia examination

terns or arranged with other diagnoses. Therefore, synthesis of all data is essential.

The Medical-Surgical Assessment Tool is not intended to be the standardized and final format for nationwide assessment of medical-surgical patients. An assessment tool must meet the needs of the individual institutions and nurses using it. The Medical-Surgical Assessment Tool is simply a working demonstration tool that is expected to be changed and revised by nurses in clinical practice. Further evaluation and refinement are necessary before adopting the tool for use within an institution. Nurses interested in revising the tool for a specific clinical setting should refer to Chapter 4.

HOW TO ELICIT APPROPRIATE DATA

Because the Unitary Person Framework and the Medical-Surgical Assessment Tool contain some terms that may be unfamiliar to nurses, specific medical-surgical focus questions and parameters were developed and refined to help the nurse to elicit appropriate information. These questions and parameters are outlined in Table 9-2, which is ordered to follow the content of the Medical-Surgical Assessment Tool (Fig. 9-1). The variables in bold type are described more fully in the questions and parameters in Table 9-2. For example, the sexual habits variable under the "relating pattern" is in bold type; if nurses do not know what questions to ask to elicit appropriate information about it, they can use Table 9-2 to direct the line of questioning. The questions and parameters in Table 9-2 are only suggestions to assist the nurse in focusing content when collecting data; they are not static or absolute. Nurses should not feel confined to asking only the questions or assessing only the parameters provided because there are many other ways to elicit the appropriate infor-

Table 9-2
Medical-surgical assessment tool: focus questions and parameters

Variables	Focus questions and parameters
RELATING	
Sexual habits	"How many sexual partners do you have?"
	"Would you say you have promiscuous sexual habits?"
	"Are you aware of the problems associated with sexually transmitted diseases?"
Problems verbalized	Does the patient discuss or allude to any difficulties in relationships with others?
KNOWING	
Learning impeded by	Does the patient exhibit anxiety, language barriers, educational difficulties, past experiences, lack of support systems, or physical handicaps that might impede learning?
FEELING	
Pain intensity	"On a scale of 1 to 10, with 10 being the worst level of pain, what number would you assign to your pain?"
PERCEIVING	
Nonverbal cues	Does the patient demonstrate cues such as shoulder shrugging, throwing hands into the air, constant weeping or crying, lack of eye contact, or the fetal position?
Kinesthetics impaired	Can the patient maintain a sense of balance?
	Can the patient walk across the room appropriately?
	While ambulating, does the patient sway or appear unable to remain upright?
EXCHANGING	
Cardiac pulses	On palpation, are peripheral pulses bounding, palpable, or faintly palpable?
	Is a doppler ultrasonic anemometer required to ascertain the presence of a pulse? If so, note the location.
	Are the pulses paradoxical?
Thoracic examination, other	Does the patient have pectus excavatum or carinatum?
	Does the patient have a tracheostomy?
Oxygen percent and device	If the patient receives oxygen, what percent?
	What type of device is used to deliver the oxygen (i.e., nasal cannula or mask)?
For consultant	In your opinion, does the patient's condition warrant a request for a consultant to ____?
	If so, on what date was the request sent?

mation based on the patient's situation and condition and the nurse's skill. Focus questions and parameters for most other data were presented in Chapter 3.

CASE STUDY

The case study models the process a nurse uses when assessing a patient. Based on the clustering of information obtained during assessment, the nurse formulates nursing diagnoses.

Ms. S.R., 34 years old, has been admitted to the hospital numerous times in the past year. She has undergone a cesarean section, the removal of a brain tumor, three shunt revisions, and six hospitalizations for episodes of hyperemesis. After the initial surgery for removal of the tumor, she experienced weakness and spasticity on the right side. During this assessment, she had nausea and vomiting, which she felt indicated the need for another shunt revision. The Medical-Surgical Assessment Tool (Fig. 9-2) was used to assess Ms. S.R.

BIBLIOGRAPHY

American Nurses' Association: Standards of medical-surgical nursing practice, Kansas City, Mo, 1974, ANA, Inc.

Bellack JP and Bamford PA: Nursing assessment: a multidimensional approach, Monterey, Calif, 1984, Wadsworth, Inc.

Kenner C, Guzzetta C, and Dossey B: Critical care nursing, ed 2, Boston, 1985, Little, Brown & Co, Inc.

Lewis SM and Collier IC: Medical-surgical nursing: assessment and management of clinical problems, ed 2, New York, 1987, McGraw-Hill, Inc.

Ruby EB: Advanced neurological and neurosurgical nursing, St Louis, 1984, The CV Mosby Co.

Thompson J, McFarland G, Hirsch J, Tucker S, and Bowers A: Clinical nursing, St Louis, 1986, The CV Mosby Co.

MEDICAL-SURGICAL ASSESSMENT TOOL

Name _____ Age _____ Sex _____
Address _____ Telephone _____
Significant other _____ Telephone _____
Date of admission _____ Medical diagnosis _____
Allergies _____

Nursing Diagnosis
(Potential or Altered)

COMMUNICATING ▪ A pattern involving sending messages
English (circle): read, write, understand
Other languages _____
Tracheostomy _____ Speech impaired _____
Alternate form of communication _____
Speech therapy consultant: yes/no   Date sent _____

Communication
  Verbal
  Nonverbal

VALUING ▪ A pattern involving the assigning of relative worth
Religious preference _____
Important religious practices _____
Cultural orientation _____
Cultural practices _____
Ministry consultant: yes/no   Date sent _____

Spiritual state
  Distress
  Despair

RELATING ▪ A pattern involving establishing bonds
Role
  Marital status _____
  Age & health of significant other _____
  _____
  Number of children _____ Ages _____
  Role in home _____
  Financial support _____
  Occupation _____
    Job satisfaction/concerns _____
  Sexual relationships (satisfactory/unsatisfactory)
    Physical difficulties/effects of illness on relationship _____
  _____
  Sexual habits _____
  Sexual concerns or problems _____
  _____

Role performance
  Parenting
  Sexual dysfunction
  Work
  Family
  Social/leisure

Family processes
Sexuality patterns

Socialization
  Relationships with others _____
    Patient's description _____
    Significant others' descriptions _____
    Staff observations _____
  Problems verbalized_____
  Verbalizes feelings of being alone _____
  Attributed to _____

Impaired social interaction

Social isolation
Social withdrawal

Fig. 9-1

Continued.

KNOWING ▪ A pattern involving the meaning associated with information
Current health problems _____
_____
_____

Current medications _____

Previous illnesses/hospitalizations/surgeries _____
_____

History of the following: Patient   Family Member   Knowledge deficit
  Anemia/blood dyscrasias _____
  Cancer _____
  Diabetes _____
  Heart disease _____
  Hypertension _____
  Peripheral vascular _____
  Kidney disease _____
  Stroke _____
  Tuberculosis _____
  Alcohol/substance use _____
  Smoking _____
  Other _____
Perception/knowledge of illness/tests/surgery _____
_____

Expectations of therapy _____
Misconceptions _____
Readiness to learn _____
  Requesting information concerning _____
  Educational level _____
Learning impeded by _____   Thought processes

Orientation
  Level of alertness _____   Orientation
  Orientation: Person _____ Place _____ Time _____   Confused
  Appropriate behavior/communication _____

Memory
  Memory intact: yes/no   Recent _____ Remote _____   Memory

FEELING ▪ A pattern involving the subjective awareness of information
Comfort
  Pain/discomfort: yes/no
    Onset _____ Duration _____   Comfort
    Location _____   Pain/chronic
    Intensity _____ Radiation _____   Pain/acute
    Associated factors _____   Discomfort
    Aggravating factors _____
    Alleviating factors _____

Emotional Integrity/States
  Recent stressful life events _____   Grieving
  _____   Anxiety
  Verbalizes feelings of: _____   Fear
    Source _____   Anger
  Physical manifestations _____   Guilt
  _____   Shame
       Sadness

Fig. 9-1, cont'd

MOVING ▪ A pattern involving activity

Activity History of physical disability _____   Impaired physical mobility
   Use of device (cane, walker, artificial limb) _____   Activity intolerance
   Limitations in daily activities _____
_____
   Verbal report of fatigue or weakness _____
_____
   Exercise habits _____
   Physical therapy consultant: yes/no   Date sent _____

Rest
   Sleep environment: Hours slept/night _____ Feels rested: yes/no   Sleep pattern disturbances
     Sleeps alone: yes/no _____ Temperature _____   Hypersomnia
     Position preference _____   Insomnia
     Naps during the day _____   Nightmares
     Other _____
   Sleep aids (pillows, meds, food) _____
   Difficulty falling/remaining asleep _____

Recreation
   Leisure activities _____   Deficit in diversional activity
   Social activities _____

Environmental Maintenance
   Home maintenance management   Impaired home maintenance
     Size & arrangement of home (stairs, bathroom) _____   management
_____ Safety needs _____   Safety hazards
     Housekeeping responsibilities _____
_____
   Social services consultant: yes/no   Date sent _____

Health Maintenance
     Health insurance _____
     Regular physical checkups _____

Self-Care   Self-care
   Ability to perform ADLs: Independent _____ Dependent _____   Feeding
   Specific deficits _____   Bathing/hygiene
_____   Dressing/grooming
   Discharge planning needs _____   Toileting
_____
   Community health nurse consultant: yes/no   Date sent _____

PERCEIVING ▪ A pattern involving the reception of information

Self-Concept
   Presenting appearance _____
   Patient's description of self _____   Body image
   Effects of illness/surgery _____   Self-esteem
_____   Personal identity

Meaningfulness
   Verbalizes hopelessness _____   Hopelessness
   Perceives/verbalizes loss of control _____   Powerlessness

Nonverbal cues _____

Fig. 9-1, cont'd

Continued.

Sensory/Perception

History of restrictive environment _____ Sensory perception

Vision impaired _____ Glasses _____ Visual

Auditory impaired _____ Hearing aid _____ Auditory

Kinesthetic impaired _____ Kinesthetic

Reflexes grossly intact _____

EXCHANGING ▪ A pattern involving mutual giving and receiving

Circulation

Cerebral   Cerebral tissue perfusion

  Neurologic changes/symptoms _____

  _____

  Pupils: Left 2 3 4 5 6 mm   Right 2 3 4 5 6 mm

        Reaction: Brisk _____ Sluggish _____ Nonreactive _____

  Verbal response _____

  Motor response _____

Cardiac   Cardiopulmonary tissue

  Pacemaker (brand, frequency, mode) _____   perfusion

  Heart rate rhythm _____   Fluid volume

  Heart sounds/murmurs _____   Deficit

  Blood pressure: R _____ L _____ Position _____   Excess

  Pulses _____

  Skin temp _____ Color _____

  Capillary refill _____ Clubbing _____   Cardiac output

  Edema _____

Physical Integrity

Tissue integrity/location of changes: Impaired skin integrity

  Abrasions _____ Bruises _____   Impaired tissue integrity

  Burns _____

  Lacerations _____

  Lesions _____ Petechiae _____

  Pressure sores _____

  Rashes _____

  Stoma/ostomy _____

  Surgical incision _____

  Surgical dressings _____

  Turgor _____

  Enterostomal therapy consult: yes/no   Date sent _____

Oxygenation

Thoracic examination: Barrel _____ Scoliosis _____   Ineffective airway clearance

  Other _____   Ineffective breathing patterns

Complaints of dyspnea _____ Precipitated by _____   Impaired gas exchange

Orthopnea _____

Rate _____ Rhythm _____ Depth _____

Labored/unlabored (circle)

Use of accessory muscles _____

Chest expansion _____

Pursed lips _____ Nasal flaring _____

Cough: productive/nonproductive _____

Sputum: Color _____ Amount _____ Consistencey _____

Splinting _____ Breath sounds _____

Arterial blood gases _____

Oxygen percent and device _____

Fig. 9-1, cont'd

Physical Regulation

Immune
    Lymph nodes enlarged _____ Location _____
    WBC count _____ Differential _____
    PT _____ PTT _____ Platelets _____
    Temperature _____ Route _____

Infection
Hyperthermia
Hypothermia
Body temperature
Ineffective thermoregulation

Nutrition

Eating patterns
    Number of meals per day: Usual _____ Current _____
    Special diet _____
    Where eaten _____
    Food preferences/intolerances _____
    Food allergies _____
    Fluid intake _____
    Appetite changes _____
    Difficulty swallowing _____
    History of ulcers _____ Heartburn _____
    Anorexia/nausea/vomiting _____
    Condition of mouth/throat _____
    _____
Height _____ Weight _____ Ideal body weight _____
Dietary consultant: yes/no   Date sent _____
Current therapy
    NPO _____ NG suction _____
    Enteral nutrition _____ TPN _____
    IV fluids _____
Labs (place * by abnormal values)
    Hemoglobin _____ Hematocrit _____ RBC _____
    Na _____ K _____ CL _____ Glucose _____
    Cholesterol _____ Triglycerides _____ Fasting _____
    Total protein _____ Albumin _____ Iron _____

Nutrition

Impaired swallowing

Oral mucous membrane
More/less than body
    requirements

Fluid volume
    Deficit
    Excess

Elimination

Gastrointestinal/bowel
    Usual bowel habits _____
    Alterations from normal _____ Stoma/ostomy: yes/no
    Remedies used _____
    Abdominal physical examination _____
    _____
    Liver: Enlarged _____ Ascites _____
    Occult blood test _____
Renal/urinary
    Usual urinary patterns _____
    Alteration from normal _____ Stoma/ostomy: yes/no
    Urine: Color _____ Odor _____ Catheter _____
    Urine output: 24 hour _____ Average hourly _____
    Bladder distention _____
Genitalia
    External genitalia examination _____
    Male: Prostate problems _____
    Female: LMP _____ Vaginal discharge _____
        Unusual vaginal bleeding _____

Bowel elimination
    Constipation
    Diarrhea
    Incontinence
Gastrointestinal tissue
    perfusion

Urinary elimination
    Incontinence
    Retention

Renal tissue perfusion

Menstrual patterns
Premenstrual syndrome

Fig. 9-1, cont'd

Continued.

CHOOSING ▪ A pattern involving the selection of alternatives

Coping

Patient's usual problem-solving methods _____   Ineffective individual coping

_____   Ineffective family coping

Family's usual problem-solving methods _____

_____

Patient's method of dealing with stress _____

_____

Family's method of dealing with stress _____

_____

Patient's affect _____

Physical manifestations _____

Support systems available _____

_____

Participation

Compliance with past/current health regimens _____   Noncompliance

_____

Willingness to comply with future health care regimen _____   Ineffective participation

_____

Judgment

Decision-making ability   Judgment

    Patient's perspective _____   Indecisiveness

    Others' perspectives _____

Prioritized nursing diagnosis/problem list

1. _____

2. _____

3. _____

4. _____

5. _____

Signature _____   Date _____

Fig. 9-1, cont'd

MEDICAL-SURGICAL ASSESSMENT TOOL

Name _Mrs. S.R._   Age _34_ Sex _F_
Address _444 Fourth Avenue, Seattle Washington_   Telephone _555-4444_
Significant other _Husband; Mr. R._   Telephone _Same_
Date of admission _27 August_   Medical diagnosis _R/O Inoperative shunt vs gastric ulcer_
Allergies _Erythromycin (causes nausea & vomiting)_

Nursing Diagnosis
(Potential or Altered)

COMMUNICATING ■ A pattern involving sending messages
English (circle): (read) (write) (understand)
Other languages _Nonfluent – German_
Tracheostomy _Ø_   Speech impaired _Ø_
Alternate form of communication _Ø_
Speech therapy consultant: yes (no)   Date sent _____

Communication
  Verbal
  Nonverbal

VALUING ■ A pattern involving the assigning of relative worth
Religious preference _Catholic, Byzantine_
Important religious practices _"Prayer – it's a little support"_
Cultural orientation _"Born & brought up in Tacoma, Washington_
Cultural practices _"Nothing specific"_
Ministry consultant: yes (no)   Date sent _____

Spiritual state
  Distress
  Despair

RELATING ■ A pattern involving establishing bonds
Role
Marital status _Married 5 years_
Age & health of significant other _34 yrs., excellent health_

Number of children _1_ Ages _5 months, girl (Mary)_
Role in home _"Housewife now" (medically retired army officer)_
Financial support _Husband's income & military disability pay_
Occupation _Husband – realtor, patient was finance officer_
  Job satisfaction/concerns _Prior to illness, enjoyed job_
Sexual relationships (satisfactory/unsatisfactory) _(see concerns)_
  Physical difficulties/effects of illness on relationship _Exhausted, (R) arm spasticity_
  Sexual habits _↓ intercourse, one partner_
  Sexual concerns or problems _"Has not had sexual intimacy with husband for over a year, it's not a problem or a necessity at this point"_

Role performance
  Parenting
  Sexual dysfunction
  Work
  Family
  Social/leisure

Family processes
Sexuality patterns

Socialization
Relationships with others _"Most relationships are strong"_
  Patient's description _"Fine, not a lot of friends but good ones"_
  Significant others' descriptions _____
  Staff observations _Quiet, keeps to herself, slightly introverted_
Problems verbalized _None_
Verbalizes feelings of being alone _No_
Attributed to _____

Impaired social interaction

Social isolation
Social withdrawal

Fig. 9-2   *Continued.*

KNOWING ▪ A pattern involving the meaning associated with information

Current health problems *↑ NAUSEA & VOMITING OVER LAST FEW WEEKS*

Current medications *TYLENOL #3, 1-2 TABS, PO, PRN FOR HEADACHE*

Previous illnesses/hospitalizations/surgeries *① RESECTION OF MENINGIOMA, ② SHUNT REVISION X3, ③ HOSPITALIZATION X6 FOR HYPEREMESIS ④ C-SECTION Ē DAUGHTER*

History of the following:　　　Patient　　　　　　　　　　Family Member　　　(Knowledge deficit)
Anemia/blood dyscrasias _∅_　　　　　　　　_∅_
Cancer _∅_　　　　　　　　*MOTHER- UTERINE CA*
Diabetes _∅_　　　　　　　　_∅_
Heart disease _∅_　　　　　　　　_∅_
Hypertension _∅_　　　　　　　　_∅_
Peripheral vascular _∅_　　　　　　　　_∅_
Kidney disease _∅_　　　　　　　　_∅_
Stroke _∅_　　　　　　　　_∅_
Tuberculosis _∅_　　　　　　　　_∅_
Alcohol/substance use _∅_　　　　　　　　_∅_
Smoking _∅_　　　　　　　　_∅_
Other 　　　　　*BOTH PARENTS HAVE ULCERS*

Perception/knowledge of illness/tests/surgery *KNOWLEDGABLE CONCERNING SHUNT REVISIONS, UNDERSTANDS THE NEED FOR SHUNT TO WORK CORRECTLY. QUESTIONS CAUSE OF CONTINUED NAUSEA & VOMITING*

Expectations of therapy *EVALUATE NAUSEA & VOMITING, CORRECT PROBLEM SOURCE (i.e., SHUNT)*

Misconceptions *FEELS NAUSEA & VOMITING CAN ONLY BE RELATED TO INOPERATIVE SHUNT*

Readiness to learn *ASKING APPROPRIATE QUESTIONS, APPEARS READY TO LEARN*

Requesting information concerning *NOTHING AT THIS TIME*

Educational level *COLLEGE — BS*　　　　　　　(POTENTIAL)

Learning impeded by *WHEN SHUNT WAS NOT WORKING — THOUGHT PROCESSES ARE SLOWER, MORE CONFUSED*　(Thought processes)

Orientation
Level of alertness *FULLY ALERT AT THIS TIME*　　　Orientation
Orientation: Person _YES_　Place _YES_　Time _YES_　Confused
Appropriate behavior/communication _YES_

Memory　*PARTIAL*
Memory intact:(yes)/no　　Recent _YES_　Remote _USUALLY_　Memory

FEELING ▪ A pattern involving the subjective awareness of information
Comfort
Pain/discomfort:(yes)/no
Onset *1-2 HRS. AFTER MEALS*　Duration *VARIES*　Comfort
Location *UPPER ABDOMEN MAINLY*　Pain/chronic
Intensity *BURNING/GASEOUS PRESSURE (7)*　Radiation _—_　(Pain/acute)
Associated factors *HEAD & NECK PAIN WHICH IS DULL IN NATURE*　Discomfort
Aggravating factors *MOVEMENT*
Alleviating factors *SOMETIMES FOOD OR LIQUID, TYLENOL #3 FOR HEADACHE*

Emotional Integrity/States
Recent stressful life events *"BIRTH OF BABY AT 8 MONTHS BY C-SECTION & REMOVAL OF BRAIN TUMOR SAME DAY*　Grieving / Anxiety
Verbalizes feelings of: *"FEAR & GUILT"*　(Fear)
Source *"RECURRENT TUMORS & NOT CARING FOR HER CHILD"*　Anger
Physical manifestations *PATIENT DOES NOT FEEL NAUSEA & VOMITING MAY BE RELATED TO THESE EVENTS.*　(Guilt) / Shame / Sadness

Fig. 9-2, cont'd

MOVING ▪ A pattern involving activity

Activity   History of physical disability _YES, FOLLOWING BRAIN SURGERY_   (Impaired physical mobility)
   Use of device (cane, walker, artificial limb) _4-POINT CANE_   Activity intolerance
   Limitations in daily activities _FULL RANGE OF MOTION, DECREASED_
COORDINATION, (R) ARM JERKS
   Verbal report of fatigue or (weakness) _"MY BODY IS ALWAYS WEAK."_

   Exercise habits _WALK, SWIM_
   Physical therapy consultant: (yes)/no   Date sent _27 AUGUST_

Rest
   Sleep environment: Hours slept/night _8_   Feels rested: (yes)/no   Sleep pattern disturbances
     Sleeps alone: yes/(no) _c̄ HUSBAND_ Temperature _"NORMAL ROOM"_   Hypersomnia
     Position preference _"EITHER SIDE"_   Insomnia
     Naps during the day _OCCASIONALLY_   Nightmares
     Other _—_
   Sleep aids (pillows, meds, food) _NONE_
   Difficulty falling/remaining asleep _NO_

Recreation
   Leisure activities _"READ A LOT"_   Deficit in diversional activity
   Social activities _"HAVE COMPANY OVER — OCCASIONALLY WE DINE OUT"_

Environmental Maintenance
   Home maintenance management   Impaired home maintenance
     Size & arrangement of home (stairs, bathroom) _2 FLOORS, LARGE HOME_   management
     Safety needs _STAIRS c̄ ASSISTANCE_   Safety hazards
     Housekeeping responsibilities _"I DO VERY LITTLE. WE HIRED A HOUSE-_
KEEPER & MY PARENTS HELP. MY HUSBAND CARES FOR THE BABY, COOKS, DOES IT ALL."
     Social services consultant: (yes)/no   Date sent _27 AUGUST_
(DISCHARGE NEEDS & CHILD CARE

Health Maintenance
   Health insurance _MILITARY_
   Regular physical checkups _"THEY ARE DONE WITH MY CT SCANS."_

Self-Care
   Ability to perform ADLs: Independent _____ Dependent _✓_   (Self-care)
   Specific deficits _PT. RIGHT HANDED; FINE MOTOR SKILLS, COORDINATION_   Feeding
& CONTROL DECREASED. ATAXIC   Bathing/hygiene
   Discharge planning needs _LEARNING ADAPTATIONS TO COMPENSATE_   Dressing/grooming
FOR CURRENT LOSSES & DECREASES (PT. CONSULT SENT AS ABOVE)   Toileting
   Community health nurse consultant: yes/(no)   Date sent ___

PERCEIVING ▪ A pattern involving the reception of information

Self-Concept
   Presenting appearance _NEAT, NO MAKE-UP, DOES NOT WEAR WIG OR SCARF OVER HEAD._
   Patient's description of self _"IT'S AMAZING WHAT YOU CAN DO WITH NO HAIR."_ Body image
   Effects of illness/surgery _"I'D LIKE TO SEE WHAT I LOOK LIKE MORE_   Self-esteem
OFTEN, BUT NO ONE OFFERS ME A MIRROR."   Personal identity

Meaningfulness
   Verbalizes hopelessness _"IT'S NOT HOPELESS YET"_   Hopelessness
   Perceived/verbalized loss of control _YES — "THE THOUGHT OF GOING IN_   (Powerlessness)
AGAIN MAKES ME SICK."
   Nonverbal cues _NEGATIVE (LEFT TO RIGHT) SHAKING OF HEAD_

Fig. 9-2, cont'd

Continued.

Sensory/Perception

History of restrictive environment ___No___ | Sensory perception

Vision impaired ___No___ Glasses ___No___ | Visual

Auditory impaired ___No___ Hearing aid ___No___ | Auditory

Kinesthetic impaired ___YES — ATAXIC___ | (Kinesthetic)

Reflexes grossly intact ___ℝ SIDE= HYPERREFLEXIA___

EXCHANGING ▪ A pattern involving mutual giving and receiving

Circulation

Cerebral | Cerebral tissue perfusion

Neurologic changes/symptoms ___WORD/THOUGHT SEARCH ALTERED___
___"I MUST STOP TO GROPE FOR CORRECT WORDS"___

Pupils: Left 2 3 4 ⑤ 6 mm   Right 2 3 4 ⑤ 6 mm

     Reaction: Brisk ___R/L___ Sluggish _____ Nonreactive _____

Verbal response ___APPROPRIATE___

Motor response ___ALTERED BALANCE, JERKING ℝ ARM___

Cardiac | Cardiopulmonary tissue perfusion

Pacemaker (brand, frequency, mode) ___—___

Heart rate rhythm ___78, STRONG RHYTHMIC___ | Fluid volume

Heart sounds/murmurs ___$S_1 S_2$ No MURMURS NOTED___ | Deficit

Blood pressure: R ___130/80___ L ___130/76___ Position ___SITTING___ | Excess

Pulses ___ALL PALPABLE, STRONG___

Skin temp ___WARM___ Color ___PALE___

Capillary refill ___< 2 SECONDS___ Clubbing ___—___ | Cardiac output

Edema ___—___

Physical Integrity

Tissue integrity/location of changes: | Impaired skin integrity

Abrasions ___—___ Bruises ___OLD IV SITES, BLOOD DRAWING___ | Impaired tissue integrity

Burns ___∅___

Lacerations ___∅___

Lesions ___∅___ Petechiae ___∅___

Pressure sores ___∅___

Rashes ___∅___

Stoma/ostomy ___∅___

Surgical incision ___ABDOMEN/C-SECTION; SCALP/SHUNT, TUMOR REMOVAL___

Surgical dressings ___∅___

Turgor ___FAIR, EVIDENCE OF DEHYDRATION___

Enterostomal therapy consult: yes/(no)   Date sent _____

Oxygenation

Thoracic examination: Barrel ___∅___ Scoliosis ___∅___ | Ineffective airway clearance

Other ___NONE___ | Ineffective breathing patterns

Complaints of dyspnea ___∅___ Precipitated by ___∅___ | Impaired gas exchange

Orthopnea ___∅___

Rate ___16___ Rhythm ___EVEN___ Depth ___NORMAL___

Labored/(unlabored)(circle)

Use of accessory muscles ___NO___

Chest expansion ___SYMMETRICAL___

Pursed lips ___No___ Nasal flaring ___No___

Cough: productive/nonproductive ___No___

Sputum: Color ___—___ Amount ___—___ Consistencey ___—___

Splinting ___∅___ Breath sounds ___CLEAR BILATERALLY___

Arterial blood gases ___—___

Oxygen percent and device ___—___

Fig. 9-2, cont'd

Physical Regulation

Immune   Infection

    Lymph nodes enlarged *No*   Location *—*   Hyperthermia

    WBC count *13,500*   Differential *NEUTROPHILS — 60%*   Hypothermia

    PT *—*   PTT *—*   Platelets *—*   Body temperature

    Temperature *98.8° F*   Route *ORALLY*   Ineffective thermoregulation

Nutrition   Nutrition

    Eating patterns

        Number of meals per day: Usual *3*   Current *3 SMALL*

        Special diet *No*

        Where eaten *HOME OR OCCASIONALLY OUT*

        Food preferences/~~intolerances~~ *EASTERN EUROPEAN, FRUIT, CHICKEN LIVERS*

        Food allergies *NONE*

        Fluid intake *DECREASED c̄ NAUSEA & VOMITING*

        Appetite changes *"NOT HUNGRY, USUALLY JUST NAUSEATED"*

        Difficulty swallowing *Ø*   Impaired swallowing

        History of ulcers *YES, PARENTS* Heartburn *No*

        Anorexia/nausea/vomiting *"YES — ALL THREE FOR A FEW WEEKS"*

    Condition of mouth/throat *MOIST MUCOUS MEMBRANES, NO REDNESS,*   Oral mucous membrane

    NO LESIONS; TONGUE DRY   ~~More~~/less than body

    Height *5'10"*   Weight *117#*   Ideal body weight *150# (HAS ALWAYS*   (requirements)

    Dietary consultant: yes/no   Date sent _____ *BEEN BELOW)* (*POTENTIAL*)

    Current therapy

        NPO *FOR TESTING* NG suction *—*   Fluid volume

        Enteral nutrition *—*   TPN *—*   Deficit

        IV fluids *—*   Excess

    Labs (place * by abnormal values)

        Hemoglobin *11 g/dl **   Hematocrit *35% **   RBC *—*

        Na *150 mEq/L **   K *3.2 mEq/L **   CL *90 mEq/L **   Glucose *110 mg/dl*

        Cholesterol *180 mg/dl*   Triglycerides *94 mg/dl*   Fasting *No*

        Total protein *8.8 g/dl **   Albumin *5.4 g/dl **   Iron *70 μg/dl*

Elimination

    Gastrointestinal/bowel   Bowel elimination

        Usual bowel habits *ONCE A DAY, "NO PROBLEMS IF I EXERCISE."*   (Constipation) (*POTENTIAL*)

        Alterations from normal *SLIGHTLY HARDER STOOL* Stoma/ostomy: yes/(no)   Diarrhea

        Remedies used *NONE*   Incontinence

        Abdominal physical examination *ABDOMEN SLIGHTLY TYMPANIC*   Gastrointestinal tissue

                                       perfusion

        Liver: Enlarged *Ø*   Ascites *Ø*

        Occult blood test *—*

    Renal/urinary   Urinary elimination

        Usual urinary patterns *SEVERAL TIMES A DAY*   Incontinence

        Alteration from normal *SMALLER AMOUNTS*   Stoma/ostomy: yes/(no)   Retention

        Urine: Color *DK. YELLOW* Odor *STRONG* Catheter *—*

        Urine output: 24 hour *—*   Average hourly *20 cc*   Renal tissue perfusion

        Bladder distention *ABSENT*

    Genitalia

        External genitalia examination *WITHIN NORMAL LIMITS*

        Male: Prostate problems *N/A*

        Female: LMP *LAST YEAR*   Vaginal discharge *Ø*   Menstrual patterns

             Unusual vaginal bleeding *NO MENSES SINCE ILLNESS BEGAN*   Premenstrual syndrome

Fig. 9-2, cont'd

Continued.

CHOOSING ▪ A pattern involving the selection of alternatives

Coping

Patient's usual problem-solving methods *"Think through — deal c̄ problems as they come"*

Family's usual problem-solving methods *"We talk, argue, & eventually resolve"*

Patient's method of dealing with stress *"Hold it in and do nothing"*

Family's method of dealing with stress *"Mom, Dad, & husband are patient & wait it out — they seem to handle it well."*

Patient's affect *Inappropriate*

Physical manifestations *Smiling inappropriately throughout assessment*

Support systems available *Husband, both parents in area*

(Ineffective individual coping)
Ineffective family coping

Participation

Compliance with past/current health regimens *Compliant in past, cooperative today.*

Willingness to comply with future health care regimen *Agrees to follow medical/health care regimen*

Noncompliance

Ineffective participation

Judgment

Decision-making ability

Patient's perspective *"Before surgery it was sound, not sure now."*

Others' perspectives *Appropriate, but questionable.*

Judgment
Indecisiveness

Prioritized nursing diagnosis/problem list

1. *Guilt related to physical difficulties which decrease pts. involvement in child care.*
2. *Knowledge deficit related to misconception of nausea & vomiting etiology,*
3. *Ineffective individual coping related to guilt & fear which manifest as nausea &*
4. *Altered comfort related to abdominal pain.* vomiting.
5. _____

Signature *Stelia Bunton, Maj, AN*   Date *27 August, 2000 hours*

Fig. 9-2, cont'd

CHAPTER 10

GYNECOLOGIC ASSESSMENT TOOL

SHELIA D. BUNTON
CANDICE J. SULLIVAN

The Gynecologic Assessment Tool was designed to assess female patients with unique biopsychosocial assessment needs. This tool incorporates specific signs and symptoms pertinent to the gynecologic patient and facilitates identification of nursing diagnoses. This chapter includes:

- *The way the tool was developed and refined*
- *The patient population and settings to which it applies*
- *Selected gynecologic emphasis areas*
- *The way to use the tool*
- *Specific gynecologic focus questions and parameters to assist the nurse in eliciting appropriate data*
- *The Gynecologic Assessment Tool*
- *A case study*
- *A completed version of the tool based on the case study*

DEVELOPMENT AND REFINEMENT OF THE TOOL

The Gynecologic Assessment Tool was developed from the nursing data base prototype (see Chapter 2). Many detailed hemodynamic monitoring and critical care variables incorporated into the prototype were generalized; specific variables applicable to gynecologic conditions were added. The resultant tool, supported by current gynecologic literature, was then tested by gynecologic nurse experts and a clinical nurse specialist on eight female patients. The testing evaluated the adequacy of the tool in terms of flow, space for documenting data, and completeness of assessment variables. Based on the results, the tool was revised.

PATIENT POPULATION AND SETTING

The Gynecologic Assessment Tool was developed to assess the needs and problems of female patients between 18 and 59 years with diseases or illnesses related to the reproductive system. For patients 60 years or older, the Gerontologic Assessment Tool (see Chapter 23) should be used because it incorporates detailed assessment parameters for the elderly patient.

The Gynecologic Assessment Tool is designed for use in the hospital with gynecologic or female general surgery patients and in the gynecology clinic. Female cancer patients may be assessed with this tool; however, use of the Oncologic Assessment Tool (see Chapter 17) better captures the assessment parameters for cancer patients, particularly those with end-stage and malignant disease.

For an acutely ill woman, the nurse may complete the tool in two sessions. Depending on the patient's degree of distress, a family member, friend, or significant other may help in providing necessary information.

GYNECOLOGIC EMPHASIS AREAS

Gynecology patients have specialized problems and needs. The Gynecologic Assessment Tool includes appropriate assessment variables within the nine human patterns of the Unitary Person framework. The tool focuses on prevalent problems among female patients. Table 10-1 outlines these emphasis areas.

HOW TO USE THE TOOL

To use the Gynecologic Assessment Tool effectively, nurses must first familiarize themselves with the nine human response patterns of the Unitary Person Framework (see Chapter 2), which provides the underlying framework

Table 10-1

Selected gynecologic emphasis areas

Patterns	Emphasis areas to determine
Role	Quality of relationships
	Expanded sexual relationships section to include elements of rape-trauma syndrome
Knowing	History focusing on female-related problems, including diseases, menstruation or menopause, or sexual assault
Moving	Environmental maintenance and individualized statements of home responsibilities of patient, partner, and children
Feeling	Emotional integrity and states related to rape-trauma syndrome
Perceiving	Self-concept related to feminity
Exchanging	Nutrition and diet history
	Renal/urinary examination and expanded genitalia examination

for Taxonomy I. The human response patterns serve as the major category headings for Taxonomy I and the Gynecologic Assessment Tool. The sequence of the response patterns, as it appears in Taxonomy I, has been changed in this tool to permit better ordering of assessment variables. Nursing diagnoses pertinent to female patients, along with signs and symptoms necessary to identify them, have been added to the appropriate response patterns in the tool.

Nurses must also realize that this tool is very different from conventional gynecologic assessment tools. As a result, nurses may encounter some initial difficulty in using it. They should remember, however, that the tool was not designed to follow the organization or content of a traditional medical data base; the data collected do not solely reflect medical patterns. Rather, the tool elicits information about holistic patterns in ways not traditionally assessed by nurses. It represents a new way of collecting and synthesizing data that requires new thinking when processing data. This tool represents a nursing data base developed from a nursing model that permits a holistic nursing assessment to take place so nursing diagnoses can be identified.

Although nurses probably agree that a holistic nursing data base would help in practice, it is realized that changing traditional assessment methods is not an easy task. For this reason, a trial usage period is recommended before nurses make decisions about the tool's merits. During this trial period, nurses should assess 10 patients using the tool to become familiar and progressively more comfortable

with its organization and data-collection methods. With experience, nurses will become accustomed to new ways of clustering and processing information. With continued use, the time necessary to complete the tool will be reduced. Most important, nurses will recognize the unique ability of the tool to elicit appropriate signs and symptoms. Nurses will also discover that nursing diagnoses are easily identified when using the tool.

It is not necessary to complete the tool in one session. Priority sections can be designated for initial assessment. Other sections or patterns can be completed later, within a time frame acceptable to the institution. To elicit appropriate data, nurses should familiarize themselves with the focus questions and parameters in the next section. When assessing specific signs and symptoms to affirm a diagnosis, the nurse circles the diagnosis in the right-hand column. The circled diagnosis does not confirm a problem but alerts the nurse to the possibility that it exists. After completing the assessment, the nurse scans the circled problems, synthesizes the data to determine whether other clusters of signs and symptoms support a problem, and judges whether the diagnosis is present.

Some diagnoses may be repeated in more than one place. These repetitions occur only within the appropriate response pattern and are convenient for identifying data directly with their corresponding nursing diagnosis. These diagnoses are not absolute but are intended to focus thinking and direct attention to collecting data about a possible problem.

Some signs and symptoms can indicate many diagnoses. For example, fatigue or general malaise may indicate activity intolerance or infection. To avoid repetition of assessment parameters, variables are arranged with the diagnosis most likely to result from the data assessed. Thus, data to support a specific diagnosis may occasionally be found in other patterns or arranged with other diagnoses. Therefore, synthesis of all data is essential.

The Gynecologic Assessment Tool is not intended to be the standardized and final format for nationwide assessment of female patients. An assessment tool must meet the needs of the individual institutions and nurses using it. The Gynecologic Assessment Tool is simply a working demonstration tool that is expected to be changed and revised by nurses in clinical practice. Further evaluation and refinement are necessary before adopting the tool for use within an institution. Nurses interested in changing, revising, and adapting the tool to specific clinical settings should refer to Chapter 4.

HOW TO ELICIT APPROPRIATE DATA

Because the Unitary Person Framework and the Gynecologic Assessment Tool contain some terms that may be unfamiliar to nurses, specific gynecologic focus questions and parameters were developed and refined to facilitate the

Table 10-2
Gynecologic assessment tool: focus questions and parameters

Variables	Focus questions and parameters
RELATING	
Quality of relationship with partner/children	Does the patient verbalize satisfaction in her relationship with her husband, partner, or children? "How do you get along with your _____?" "Is there anything you would change about the relationship with your _____?" "If so, what would those changes be?"
Fear of intercourse	"Do you find that you are sometimes apprehensive, worried, fearful, or too tired to have sex with your partner?" "Does the thought of intercourse frighten you?"
Mistrust of men	"Generally speaking, do you trust or distrust men?" "Can you share the reasons why or why not?"
KNOWING	
Cancer	"Do you, or any of your family members, have a history of cancer? Breast or uterine, in particular?"
Vaginal infections or vene-real disease	"Do you have a history of yeast, candida, or other vaginal infections or pelvic inflammatory disease?" "Have you, to the best of your knowledge, ever had syphilis, gonorrhea, herpes, other sexually transmitted diseases, or been diagnosed as HIV positive?" "To the best of your knowledge, has your partner ever contracted a sexually transmitted disease?"
Maternal diethylstilbestrol use	"Do you know if your mother received a drug to prevent miscarriage while she was pregnant with you?"
Type of contraception used	"What have you used as a family planning method?" "Are you or your partner currently using any type of birth control method?" "If so, what type?" "If not, have you ever considered using any birth control method?"
History of sexual assault	"Have you ever been sexually assaulted?"
Time/place/brief description of events	"Could you briefly describe this event (to include year, time, place, and sequence of events)?"
Authorities notified	"Were the authorities notified for the past sexual assault? Current sexual assault?"
FEELING	
Recent stressful life events	"Have recent stressful events led to feelings you might not otherwise have?"
Verbalizes feelings of	Does the patient verbalize guilt or shame about her reproductive system? "Do you feel your body is better than, equal to, or not as good as the bodies of other women?"
Evidence of posttrauma response	If the patient has been sexually assaulted, does she state or do you observe any of the responses listed on the tool?
PERCEIVING	
Verbalizes positive feelings about being female	Does the patient verbalize pride in her womaness? "Do you enjoy being a female?" Does the patient verbalize positive feelings about being female? "Are there times when you wish you were born male?"
Perceives/verbalizes loss of control	"Do you feel you have lost control over your body because of your illness?" "Do you feel your surgery will change the way you feel about your body?"

nurse in eliciting appropriate information. These questions and parameters are outlined in Table 10-2, which is ordered to follow the content of the Gynecologic Assessment Tool (Fig. 10-1). The variables in bold type are described more fully in Table 10-2. For example, verbalizing positive feelings about being female, found under the "perceiving pattern," is in bold type. If the nurse is unsure what questions to ask to elicit information about this variable, Table 10-2 can be used to direct the line of questioning. These questions and parameters are only suggestions intended to assist the nurse in focusing content when collecting data. They are not static or absolute; nurses should not feel confined to asking only the questions or assessing only the parameters provided because there are many other ways to elicit the information, based on the patient's situation and condition and the nurse's skill. Focus questions and parameters for other data were presented in Chapter 3.

CASE STUDY

The case study models the process a nurse uses when assessing a patient. Based on the clustering of information obtained during assessment, nursing diagnoses are formulated.

Ms. G.A., 22 years old, was initially seen in the emergency room for intermittent abdominal pain and malodorous vaginal discharge. She was partially assessed in the emergency room using the Gynecologic Assessment Tool. After Ms. G.A. was admitted to the gynecology unit, the tool (Fig. 10-2) was completed.

BIBLIOGRAPHY

Bates B: A guide to physical examination and history taking, ed 4, Philadelphia, 1987, JB Lippincott Co.

Freeman R and Heinrich J: Community health nursing practice, ed 2, Philadelphia, 1981, WB Saunders Co.

Humenick S: Analysis of current assessment strategies in the health care of young children and childbearing families, Norwalk, Conn, 1982, Appleton-Century-Crofts.

Sonstegard L, Kowalski K, and Jennings B: Women's health, vol 2, New York, 1983, Grune & Stratton, Inc.

Wright L and Leachey M: Nurses and families: a guide to family assessment and intervention, Philadelphia, 1984, FA Davis Co.

GYNECOLOGIC ASSESSMENT TOOL

Name _____ Age _____ Sex _____
Address _____ Telephone _____
Significant other _____ Telephone _____
Date of admission _____ Medical diagnosis _____
Allergies _____

Nursing Diagnosis
(Potential or Altered)

COMMUNICATING ▪ A pattern involving sending messages
Read, write, understand English (circle) _____ Communication
Other languages _____ Verbal
Intubated _____ Speech impaired _____ Nonverbal
Alternate form of communication _____

VALUING ▪ A pattern involving the assigning of relative worth
Religious preference _____ Spiritual state
Important religious practices _____ Distress
Cultural orientation _____ Despair
Cultural practices _____

RELATING ▪ A pattern involving establishing bonds
Role   Role performance
  Marital status _____
    Age & health of significant other _____
    Patient's description of marriage _____ Social leisure

  Quality of relationship with partner _____
Sexual relationships (satisfactory/unsatisfactory)   Sexuality patterns
  Physical difficulties/effects of illness on relationship _____ Sexual dysfunction

  Changes in sexual behavior _____
  Abnormal lesions/discharges in sexual partner _____
  Fear of intercourse _____ **Mistrust of men** _____ Rape-trauma syndrome
Role in home _____ Family processes
Number of children _____ Ages _____   Parenting
  Quality of relationship with children _____   Family
Occupation _____   Work
  Financial support _____
  Job satisfaction/concerns _____
  Physical/mental energy expenditures _____

Socialization
  Quality of relationships with others _____ Impaired social interaction
    Patient's description _____
    Significant others' descriptions _____
    Staff observations _____
  Verbalizes feelings of being alone _____ Social isolation
  Attributed to _____ Social withdrawal

Fig. 10-1

Continued.

KNOWING ▪ A pattern involving the meaning associated with information

Current health problems _____ Knowledge deficit

_____

Current medications _____

_____

Previous illnesses/hospitalizations/surgeries _____

_____

History of the following: Patient   Family member

Anemia/blood dyscrasias _____

   Cancer _____

   Diabetes _____

   Heart disease _____

   Hypertension _____

   Hysterectomy _____

   Sickle cell disease _____

   Smoking _____

   Stroke _____

   Thyroid disease _____

   Vaginal infection _____

   Venereal disease _____

   Maternal diethylstilbestrol use _____

   Other _____

Menstrual/menopause history   Menstrual patterns

   Age of onset _____ Length of cycle _____   Premenstrual syndrome

   Amount/type of flow _____

   Type of contraception used _____

     Complications of contraception _____

   Last menstrual period _____

     Associated symptoms _____

   Number & outcome of each pregnancy _____

_____

   Complications of pregnancy, delivery, or abortions _____

_____

History of sexual assault: yes/no

   Time/place _____

   Brief description of events _____

_____

   Authorities notified: yes/no

Perceptions/knowledge of illness/tests/surgery _____

_____

_____

Expectations of therapy _____

Misconceptions _____

Readiness to learn _____

   Request information concerning _____

   Educational level _____

   Learning impeded by _____ Thought processes

Orientation

Level of alertness _____ Orientation

   Orientation: Person _____ Place _____ Time _____ Confusion

   Appropriate behavior/communication _____

Memory

   Memory intact: yes/no   Recent _____ Remote _____ Memory

Fig. 10-1, cont'd

FEELING ▪ A pattern involving the subjective awareness of information
Comfort
Pain/discomfort: yes/no   Comfort
   Onset _____ Duration _____   Pain/chronic
   Location _____ Quality _____ Radiation _____   Pain/acute
   Associated factors _____   Discomfort
   Aggravating factors _____
   Alleviating factors _____

Emotional Integrity/States
Recent stressful life events _____
_____   Grieving
Verbalizes feelings of _____   Anxiety
   Source _____   Fear
Evidence of posttrauma response: Anger _____   Anger
   Phobias/nightmares _____ Self-blame/shame _____   Guilt
   Depression/guilt _____ Denial/emotional shock _____   Shame
   Expressions of numbness _____   Sadness
   Physical manifestations: Crying _____ Silence _____   Rape-trauma syndrome
     Trembling hands _____ Avoids interactions with others _____   Compound reaction
     Hysterical _____ Other _____   Silent reaction

MOVING ▪ A pattern involving activity
Activity
History of physical disability _____   Impaired physical mobility
   Use of device (cane, walker, artificial limb) _____   Activity intolerance
   Limitations in daily activities _____
Verbal report of fatigue or weakness _____
Exercise habits _____

Rest   Sleep pattern disturbances
   Hours slept/night _____ Feels rested: yes/no   Hypersomnia
   Sleep aids (pillows, meds, food) _____   Insomnia
   Difficulty falling/remaining asleep _____   Nightmares

Recreation
   Leisure activities _____   Deficit in diversional activity
   Social activities _____

Environmental Maintenance
   Home maintenance management
     Size arrangement of home (stairs, bathroom) _____   Impaired home maintenance
     _____ Safety needs _____   management
     Home responsibilities (patient) _____   Safety hazards
     Home responsibilities (partner and/or children) _____
_____

Health Maintenance
   Health insurance _____   Health maintenance
   Regular physical checkups _____

Self-Care   Self-care
   Ability to perform ADLs: Independent _____ Dependent _____   Feeding
   Specific deficits _____   Bathing/hygiene
   Discharge planning needs _____   Dressing/grooming
                                                     Toileting

Continued.

Fig. 10-1, cont'd

PERCEIVING ▪ A pattern involving the reception of information
Self-Concept   Self-concept
  Presenting appearance _____
  Patient's description of self _____   Body image
  Effects of illness/surgery on self-concept _____   Self-esteem
  _____   Personal identity
  Verbalizes positive feelings about being female _____
  _____

Meaningfulness
  Verbalizes hopelessness _____   Hopelessness
  Perceives/verbalizes loss of control _____   Powerlessness

Sensory/Perception   Sensory perception
  History of restrictive environment _____
  Vision impaired _____ Glasses/contacts _____   Visual
  Auditory impaired _____ Hearing aid _____   Auditory
  Kinesthetic impaired _____   Kinesthetic
  Gustatory impaired _____   Gustatory
  Tactile impaired _____   Tactile
  Olfactory impaired _____   Olfactory
  Reflexes: Biceps   R _____ L _____   Triceps R _____ L _____
            Brachioradialis R _____ L _____   Knee   R _____ L _____
            Ankle   R _____ L _____   Plantar R _____ L _____
            Ankle clonus _____ Nuchal rigidity _____
            Other _____

EXCHANGING ▪ A pattern involving mutual giving and receiving
Circulation
  Cerebral   Cerebral tissue perfusion
    Neurologic changes/symptoms _____   Fluid volume
    _____   Deficit
    Pupils: Left 2 3 4 5 6 mm   Right 2 3 4 5 6 mm   Excess
            Reaction: Brisk_____ Sluggish _____ Nonreactive _____   Cardiac output
    Verbal response _____
    Motor response _____
  Cardiac
    Apical rate & rhythm _____   Cardiopulmonary tissue
    Heart sounds/murmurs _____   perfusion
    Dysrhythmias _____
    BP: R _____ L _____ Position _____
  Peripheral   Peripheral tissue perfusion
    Jugular venous distension: yes/no   R _____ L _____
    Pulses: _____
    Skin temp _____ Color _____ Turgor _____
    Capillary refill _____ Edema _____

Physical Integrity
  Tissue integrity: Rashes _____ Lesions _____   Impaired skin integrity
    Petechiae _____ Bruises _____   Impaired tissue integrity
    Ecchymosis _____
    Abrasions _____ Lacerations _____
    Surgical incisions/dressings _____

Fig. 10-1, cont'd

Oxygenation

Complaints of dyspnea _____ Precipitated by _____ Ineffective airway clearance
Orthopnea _____ Ineffective breathing patterns
Rate _____ Rhythm _____ Depth _____ Impaired gas exchange
Labored/unlabored (circle)
Breath sounds _____
Cough: productive/nonproductive _____
Sputum: Color _____ Amount _____ Consistency _____

Physical Regulation

Immune Infection
  Lymph nodes enlarged _____ Location _____ Hyperthermia
  WBC count _____ Differential _____ Hypothermia
  PT _____ PTT _____ Platelets _____ Body temperature
Body temperature Ineffective thermoregulation
  Temperature _____ Route _____
  Intervention _____

Nutrition

Nutrition

Eating patterns
  Number of meals per day _____
  Special diet _____
  Food preferences/intolerances _____
  Food allergies _____
  Fluid intake _____
  Diet history: sample diet _____
  _____
  Appetite changes _____
  Difficult swallowing _____ Impaired swallowing
  History of ulcers _____ Heartburn _____
  Presence of anorexia/nausea/vomiting _____
Condition of mouth/throat _____ Oral mucous membrane
_____ More/less than body
Weight _____ Height _____ Ideal body weight _____   requirements
Current therapy
  NPO _____ NG suction _____ Fluid volume
  Enteral nutrition _____   Deficit
  IV fluids _____   Excess
  TPN _____
Labs
  Hemoglobin _____ Hematocrit _____ RBC _____
  Na _____ K _____ CL _____ Glucose _____
  Cholesterol _____ Triglycerides _____ Fasting _____
  Thyroid function test _____

Elimination

Gastrointestinal/bowel Bowel elimination
  Usual bowel habits _____   Constipation
  Alterations from normal _____   Diarrhea
  Remedies used _____   Incontinence
  Abdominal examination _____ Gastrointestinal tissue
    Bowel sounds _____   perfusion

Fig. 10-1, cont'd

Continued.

Renal/urinary
  Usual urine pattern _____ Urinary elimination
  Alterations from normal _____ Incontinence
  Urine: Color _____ Odor _____ Catheter _____ Retention
  Urine output: 24 hour _____ Average hourly _____
  Bladder distention _____
Genitalia
  Breast examination _____
  External genitalia examination _____
  _____
  Vaginal discharge _____ Odor _____
  Unusual vaginal discharge _____
  HCG _____ LH _____ FSH _____

CHOOSING ▪ A pattern involving the selection of alternatives
Coping
Patient's usual problem-solving methods _____ Ineffective individual coping
_____ Ineffective family coping
Family's usual problem-solving methods _____
_____
Patient's method of dealing with stress _____
_____
Family's method of dealing with stress _____
_____
Patient's affect _____
Physical manifestations _____
Support systems available _____
_____

Participation
  Compliance with past/current health regimens _____ Noncompliance
  _____ Ineffective participation
  Willingness to comply with future health care regimen _____
  _____

Judgment
  Decision-making ability   Judgment
    Patient's perspective _____   Indecisiveness
    Others' perspectives _____

Prioritized nursing diagnosis/problem list
1. _____
2. _____
3. _____
4. _____

Signature _____ Date _____

Fig. 10-1, cont'd

Gynecologic assessment tool 155

GYNECOLOGIC ASSESSMENT TOOL

Name _Ms. G.A._   Age _22_   Sex _F_
Address _222 SECOND STREET, RADCLIFF KY_   Telephone _555-2222_
Significant other _HUSBAND, MR. A._   Telephone _SAME_
Date of admission _24 JANUARY_   Medical diagnosis _PELVIC INFECTION_
Allergies _PENICILLIN (CAUSES RASH + HIVES)_

Nursing Diagnosis
(Potential or Altered)

COMMUNICATING ▪ A pattern involving sending messages
(Read, write, understand) English (circle) _____   Communication
Other languages _READS, WRITES + UNDERSTANDS KOREAN_   Verbal
Intubated ___—___ Speech impaired _No_   Nonverbal
Alternate form of communication _NONE REQUIRED_

VALUING ▪ A pattern involving the assigning of relative worth
Religious preference _BUDDIST_   Spiritual state
Important religious practices _DAILY PRAYER_
Cultural orientation _KOREAN_
Cultural practices _PREFERS KOREAN FOODS_

RELATING ▪ A pattern involving establishing bonds
Role   Role performance
Marital status _MARRIED_
  Age & health of significant other _24, GOOD HEALTH_
  Patient's description of marriage _"USUALLY THE MARRIAGE IS GOOD"_   Social leisure

  Quality of relationship with partner _"NORMAL TO GOOD"_
Sexual relationships (satisfactory / unsatisfactory)   (Sexuality patterns) (POTENTIAL)
  Physical difficulties/effects of illness on relationship _"VERY PAINFUL"_   Sexual dysfunction

  Changes in sexual behavior _"HAVE INTERCOURSE MUCH LESS"_
  Abnormal lesions/discharges in sexual partner _NONE REPORTED_
  Fear of intercourse _No_ Mistrust of men _No_   Rape-trauma syndrome
Role in home _SECOND IN CHARGE, HUSBAND IS DOMINANT_   Family processes
Number of children _1_ Ages _3 YEARS, SON_   Parenting
  Quality of relationship with children _EXCELLENT_   Family
Occupation _HOUSEWIFE; HUSBAND IS ACTIVE DUTY SUPPLY SERGEANT_   Work
  Financial support _BI-MONTHLY PAY CHECK, NO OTHER INCOME_
  Job satisfaction/concerns _"HE ENJOYS WORK, BUT HOURS ARE LONG"_
  Physical/mental energy expenditures _"VERY TAXING FOR HIM TO WORK IN SUPPLY"_

Socialization
  Quality of relationships with others _VERY GOOD, LOTS OF FRIENDS_   Impaired social interaction
  Patient's description _"I ENJOY MY FRIENDS"_
  Significant others' descriptions (HUSBAND) _"SHE'S WELL LIKED"_
  Staff observations _CHEERFUL, TALKATIVE, NUMEROUS VISITORS_
  Verbalizes feelings of being alone _No_   Social isolation
  Attributed to _—_   Social withdrawal

Fig. 10-2

Continued.

KNOWING ▪ A pattern involving the meaning associated with information

Current health problems _ONSET OF ABDOMINAL PAIN YESTERDAY, c̄_   ⬭ Knowledge deficit

VAGINAL DISCHARGE

Current medications _VITAMIN (OVER THE COUNTER) 1 DAILY PO_

Previous illnesses/hospitalizations/surgeries _CHILDBIRTH, NO OTHER_

SIGNIFICANT ILLNESS

History of the following:	Patient	Family member
Anemia/blood dyscrasias	_No_	_No_
Cancer	_No_	_FATHER — STOMACH_
Diabetes	_No_	_NO_
Heart disease	_No_	_No_
Hypertension	_No_	_No_
Hysterectomy	_No_	_No_
Sickle cell disease	_No_	_No_
Smoking	_NONE_	_FATHER & MOTHER_
Stroke	_No_	_No_
Thyroid disease	_No_	_NO_

Vaginal infection _OCCASIONAL, RECURRENT_

Venereal disease _QUESTIONABLE_

Maternal diethylstilbestrol use _NOT KNOWN BY PATIENT_

Other _—_

Menstrual/menopause history   Menstrual patterns

Age of onset _11 YEARS_ Length of cycle _3-4 DAYS_   Premenstrual syndrome

Amount/type of flow _MODERATE TO HEAVY_

Type of contraception used _NONE_

  Complications of contraception _—_

Last menstrual period _LAST WEEK_

  Associated symptoms _STOMACH CRAMPS, WORSE THAN USUAL_

Number & outcome of each pregnancy _ONE PREGNANCY, HEALTHY BOY,_

3 YEARS OLD

Complications of pregnancy, delivery, or abortions _NONE_

History of sexual assault: yes/ⓝⓞ

  Time/place _—_

  Brief description of events _—_

  Authorities notified: yes/no

Perceptions/knowledge of illness/tests/surgery _PT. UNSURE AS TO HOW SHE_

MAY HAVE CONTRACTED INFECTION, REALIZES POSSIBLE

SEVERITY OF UNTREATED ILLNESS & INABILITY TO HAVE CHILDREN IN THE FUTURE

Expectations of therapy _"TO CLEAR UP INFECTION"_

Misconceptions _"ALL PELVIC INFECTIONS ARE CAUSED BY VENEREAL DISEASE"_

Readiness to learn _ACCEPTS DISEASE, PREPARED TO LEARN_

  Request information concerning _PREVENTION OF RECURRENT DISEASE_

  Educational level _HIGH SCHOOL_

  Learning impeded by _—_   Thought processes

Orientation

Level of alertness _FULLY ALERT_   Orientation

  Orientation: Person _YES_ Place _YES_ Time _YES_   Confusion

  Appropriate behavior/communication _YES_

Memory

  Memory intact: ⓨⓔⓢ/no   Recent _YES_   Remote _YES_   Memory

Fig. 10-2, cont'd

FEELING ▪ A pattern involving the subjective awareness of information

Comfort

Pain/discomfort: (yes)/no   Comfort
  Onset _YESTERDAY_ Duration _COMES & GOES, LASTS 10-60 MINUTES_   Pain/chronic
  Location _ABDOMEN_ Quality _MODERATELY STRONG_ Radiation _NONE_   (Pain/acute)
  Associated factors _NONE RECOGNIZED_   Discomfort
  Aggravating factors _MOVING AROUND, WALKING_
  Alleviating factors _"NOTHING — IT JUST GOES AWAY"_

Emotional Integrity/States

Recent stressful life events _"VISITING FAMILY IN KOREA, THEN HAD TO RETURN HERE WITHOUT THEM"_   Grieving
Verbalizes feelings of _SHAME, "I'M SO ASHAMED."_   Anxiety
  Source _"I'VE GOTTEN AN UNEXPLAINED DISEASE."_   Fear
Evidence of posttrauma response: Anger ___—___   Anger
  Phobias/nightmares ___—___ Self-blame/shame ___—___   Guilt
  Depression/guilt ___—___ Denial/emotional shock ___—___   (Shame)
  Expressions of numbness ___—___   Sadness
Physical manifestations: Crying ___—___ Silence ___✓___   Rape-trauma syndrome
  Trembling hands _____ Avoids interactions with others ___—___   Compound reaction
  Hysterical ___—___ Other _____   Silent reaction

MOVING ▪ A pattern involving activity

Activity

History of physical disability _NONE_   Impaired physical mobility
  Use of device (cane, walker, artificial limb) _No_   Activity intolerance
  Limitations in daily activities _No_
Verbal report of fatigue or weakness _"A LITTLE TIRED TODAY"_
Exercise habits _WORKS 30 MINUTES EACH DAY_

Rest

Hours slept/night _6-7 HOURS_ Feels rested: (yes)/no _USUALLY_   Sleep pattern disturbances
Sleep aids (pillows, meds, food) _NONE, 1 PILLOW_   Hypersomnia
Difficulty falling/remaining asleep _No_   Insomnia
           Nightmares

Recreation

Leisure activities _NEEDLEPOINT_   Deficit in diversional activity
Social activities _OCCASIONAL PARTY OR DINING OUT_

Environmental Maintenance

Home maintenance management
  Size arrangement of home (stairs, bathroom) _SMALL HOUSE, TWO STORY, 2 BEDROOM_ Safety needs _____   Impaired home maintenance management
  Home responsibilities (patient) _SHOPPING, CLEANING, COOKING, CHILD CARE_   Safety hazards
  Home responsibilities ((partner) and/or children) _PAYS BILLS, DOES WORK AROUND YARD, HELPS WITH CARE OF SON_

Health Maintenance

Health insurance _MILITARY BENEFITS_   Health maintenance
Regular physical checkups _YEARLY_

Self-Care

Ability to perform ADLs: Independent ___✓___ Dependent _____   Self-care
Specific deficits _NONE_   Feeding
Discharge planning needs _NONE_   Bathing/hygiene
           Dressing/grooming
           Toileting

Fig. 10-2, cont'd

Continued.

PERCEIVING ▪ A pattern involving the reception of information
Self-Concept

Presenting appearance _NEAT, WELL GROOMED_

Patient's description of self _"I LIKE MYSELF"_

Effects of illness/surgery on self-concept _"I FEEL BAD ABOUT THIS DISEASE_
BECAUSE I MIGHT NOT BE ABLE TO HAVE MORE CHILDREN"

Verbalizes positive feelings about being female _YES_

(Self-concept)

Body image
Self-esteem
Personal identity

Meaningfulness

Verbalizes hopelessness _No_

Perceives/verbalizes loss of control _No_

Hopelessness
Powerlessness

Sensory/Perception

History of restrictive environment _No_

Vision impaired _NO IMPAIRMENT_ Glasses/contacts _NONE_

Auditory impaired _NO IMPAIRMENT_ Hearing aid _NONE_

Kinesthetic impaired _No_

Gustatory impaired _No_

Tactile impaired _No_

Olfactory impaired _No_

Sensory perception

Visual
Auditory
Kinesthetic
Gustatory
Tactile
Olfactory

Reflexes: Biceps   R _2+_ L _2+_   Triceps R _2+_ L _2+_
Brachioradialis R _2+_ L _2+_   Knee   R _2+_ L _2+_
Ankle   R _2+_ L _2+_   Plantar R _2+_ L _2+_
Ankle clonus _No_   Nuchal rigidity _No_
Other _—_

EXCHANGING ▪ A pattern involving mutual giving and receiving
Circulation

Cerebral

Neurologic changes/symptoms _NONE_

Pupils: Left 2 3 ④ 5 6 mm   Right 2 3 ④ 5 6 mm
Reaction: Brisk_____ Sluggish _____ Nonreactive _____
Verbal response _APPROPRIATE_
Motor response _APPROPRIATE IN ALL EXTREMITIES & MODES_

Cardiac

Apical rate & rhythm _78, REGULAR_

Heart sounds/murmurs _NORMAL, NO MURMURS_

Dysrhythmias _—_

BP: R _90/64_   L _92/60_   Position _SITTING_

Peripheral

Jugular venous distension: yes (no)   R _____ L _____

Pulses: _ALL PRESENT, FULL & STRONG_

Skin temp _WARM_   Color _PINK → RED_ Turgor _GOOD_

Capillary refill _LESS THAN_ Edema _NONE_
2 SEC.

Physical Integrity

Tissue integrity: Rashes _NONE_   Lesions _NONE_

Petechiae _NONE_   Bruises _NONE_

Ecchymosis _NONE_

Abrasions _NONE_   Lacerations _____

Surgical incisions/dressings _NONE_

Cerebral tissue perfusion
Fluid volume
  Deficit
  Excess
Cardiac output

Cardiopulmonary tissue
  perfusion

Peripheral tissue perfusion

Impaired skin integrity
Impaired tissue integrity

Fig. 10-2, cont'd

Oxygenation

Complaints of dyspnea __*No*__ Precipitated by __—__
Orthopnea __*No*__
Rate __*20*__ Rhythm __*REGULAR*__ Depth __*NORMAL*__
Labored/(unlabored)(circle)
Breath sounds __*CLEAR IN ALL BASES*__
Cough: productive/(nonproductive)
Sputum: Color __—__ Amount __—__ Consistency __—__

Ineffective airway clearance
Ineffective breathing patterns
Impaired gas exchange

Physical Regulation

Immune
  Lymph nodes enlarged __*No*__ Location __—__
  WBC count __*18,000*__ Differential __*ELEVATED NEUTROPHILS – 65%*__
  PT __—__ PTT __—__ Platelets __—__
Body temperature
  Temperature __*101.0°F*__ Route __*ORAL*__
  Intervention __*NOTHING AT THIS TIME*__

(Infection)
Hyperthermia
Hypothermia
Body temperature
Ineffective thermoregulation

Nutrition

Eating patterns
  Number of meals per day __*USUALLY 3*__
  Special diet __*No, FREQUENTLY EATS KOREAN FOODS*__
  Food preferences/intolerances __—__
  Food allergies __*NONE*__
  Fluid intake __*"DRINK A LOT OF FLUIDS, ABOUT 4 LITERS A DAY"*__
  Diet history: sample diet __*BREAKFAST = NOODLES OR EGGS*__
__*LUNCH = SANDWICH, COFFEE, FRUIT DINNER = MEAT, VEGETABLES, DESSERT*__
  Appetite changes __*NOT HUNGRY LATELY*__
  Difficult swallowing __*No*__
  History of ulcers __*No*__ Heartburn __*No*__
  Presence of anorexia/nausea/vomiting __*YES, OVER THE LAST COUPLE DAYS*__
Condition of mouth/throat __*No REDNESS, LESIONS, OR SWELLING*__
__*TEETH & GUMS IN EXCELLENT CONDITION*__
Weight __*87.5#*__ Height __*4'10"*__ Ideal body weight __*90#*__
Current therapy
  NPO __—__ NG suction __—__
  Enteral nutrition __—__
  IV fluids __*IV TO BE PLACED FOR MEDICATIONS*__
  TPN __—__
Labs
  Hemoglobin __*12 g/dl*__ Hematocrit __*36%*__ RBC __*4.2 × 10⁶/μL*__
  Na __*PENDING*__ K __*PENDING*__ CL __*PENDING*__ Glucose __*PENDING*__
  Cholesterol __—__ Triglycerides __—__ Fasting __—__
  Thyroid function test __—__

(Nutrition) (POTENTIAL)

Impaired swallowing

Oral mucous membrane
More/less than body
  requirements

Fluid volume
  Deficit
  Excess

Elimination

Gastrointestinal/bowel
  Usual bowel habits __*ONCE A DAY*__
  Alterations from normal __*SLIGHTLY HARDER STOOLS*__
  Remedies used __*NONE*__
  Abdominal examination __*TENDER TO TOUCH, NO GROSS MASSES*__
    Bowel sounds __*SLIGHTLY DECREASED IN LOWER QUADRANTS*__

Bowel elimination
(Constipation) (POTENTIAL)
Diarrhea
Incontinence
Gastrointestinal tissue
  perfusion

Fig. 10-2, cont'd

Continued.

Renal/urinary
    Usual urine pattern *SEVERAL TIMES A DAY, NO LARGE AMOUNTS*   Urinary elimination
    Alterations from normal *No*   Incontinence
    Urine: Color *YELLOW-CLEAR* Odor *No*   Catheter *No*   Retention
    Urine output: 24 hour ———— Average hourly *80- 90 cc*
    Bladder distention *NONE*
Genitalia
    Breast examination *WITHIN NORMAL LIMITS, NO TENDERNESS OR MASSES*
    External genitalia examination *No EVIDENCE OF LESIONS, REDNESS,*
    OR ABNORMALITIES
    Vaginal discharge *YES*   Odor *YES—MALODOROUS*
    Unusual vaginal discharge *PURULENT*
    HCG ———— LH ———— FSH ————

CHOOSING ▪ A pattern involving the selection of alternatives
Coping
    Patient's usual problem-solving methods *"THINK IT OUT, SELECT WHAT*   Ineffective individual coping
    I THINK IS THE BEST SOLUTION."   Ineffective family coping
    Family's usual problem-solving methods *"WE TALK THINGS OUT; MY*
    HUSBAND IS VERY GOOD AT THIS."
    Patient's method of dealing with stress *"CRY, TALK TO HUSBAND"*

    Family's method of dealing with stress *"DISCUSSION, EXERCISE"*

    Patient's affect *APPROPRIATE*
    Physical manifestations *NERVOUS, ANXIOUS, WRINGING HANDS*
    Support systems available *HUSBAND PRESENT, HAS FRIENDS IN*
    THE AREA CARING FOR CHILD

Participation
    Compliance with past/current health regimens *HAS READ & UNDERSTANDS*   Noncompliance
    UNIT RULES, STATES SHE WILL COMPLY   Ineffective participation
    Willingness to comply with future health care regimen *YES*

Judgment
    Decision-making ability   Judgment
        Patient's perspective *"MY DECISIONS ARE USUALLY GOOD."*   Indecisiveness
        Others' perspectives *(HUSBAND) "SHE USUALLY MAKES SOUND, TIMELY*
                                    DECISIONS."

Prioritized nursing diagnosis/problem list
1. *INFECTION RELATED TO DISEASE PROCESS.*
2. *ALTERED SELF-CONCEPT AND SHAME RELATED TO DISEASE & POTENTIAL LOSS OF CHILDBEARING*
3. *KNOWLEDGE DEFICIT RELATED TO DISEASE ETIOLOGY & MISCONCEPTIONS.*   *FUNCTION.*
4. *ALTERED COMFORT RELATED TO ABDOMINAL PAIN.*

Signature *Stelia Buxton, Maj. AN*   Date *24 JANUARY/1100*
                                                                HOURS

Fig. 10-2, cont'd

CHAPTER 11

PSYCHIATRIC ASSESSMENT TOOL

PATRICIA C. SEIFERT
CORNELIA BECK

The Psychiatric Assessment Tool is designed to assess adult psychiatric patients with unique biopsychosocial assessment needs. The tool incorporates specific signs and symptoms to facilitate identification of nursing diagnoses. It also incorporates the American Nurses' Association's *Standards for Psychiatric and Mental Health Nursing Practice,* and the *Standards of Child and Adolescent Psychiatric and Mental Health Nursing Practice.* This chapter includes:

- *The way the tool was developed and refined*
- *The patient populations and settings to which it applies*
- *Selected psychiatric emphasis areas*
- *The way to use the tool*
- *Specific psychiatric focus questions and parameters to assist the nurse in eliciting appropriate data*
- *The Psychiatric Assessment Tool*
- *A case study*
- *A completed version of the tool based on the case study*

DEVELOPMENT AND REFINEMENT OF THE TOOL

The Psychiatric Assessment Tool was developed from the nursing data base prototype (see Chapter 2). Many hemodynamic monitoring and critical care variables originally incorporated in the prototype were deleted and replaced with specific variables more applicable to psychiatric assessment. The resultant tool was then modified based on the recommendations of psychiatric nurse experts. Further, the content of this tool is supported by the literature from this field of nursing.

After the tool was developed and refined, it was clinically tested by psychiatric nurse experts and clinical nurse specialists. All 10 patients had been diagnosed with psychiatric problems. Many patients were chronically ill with acute exacerbations of previous problems or the development of new problems. The testing evaluated the adequacy of the tool in terms of flow, space for recording data, and completeness of assessment variables. Based on the results, the tool was revised.

PATIENT POPULATION AND SETTING

The Psychiatric Assessment Tool was developed to assess the needs and problems of psychiatric patients in the hospital; home care, long-term care, or adult day-care settings; or psychiatric clinics. It is intended for use in nonemergency situations. It may be necessary to complete the assessment tool in two sessions, preferably within 24 hours. Depending on the patient's degree of orientation, the family or significant other may help in providing necessary data.

PSYCHIATRIC EMPHASIS AREAS

Psychiatric patients have specialized problems and needs. The Psychiatric Assessment Tool includes appropriate assessment variables within each of the nine human response patterns of the Unitary Person Framework. Table 11-1 outlines these emphasis areas.

HOW TO USE THE TOOL

To use the Psychiatric Assessment Tool effectively, nurses must first be familiar with the Unitary Person Framework (see Chapter 2), which provides the underlying framework for Taxonomy I. The nine human response patterns of the Unitary Person Framework serve as the major

Table 11-1

Selected psychiatric emphasis areas

Patterns	Emphasis areas to determine
Communicating	Verbal communication
	Nonverbal communication
	Grooming and appearance
Knowing	Orientation
	Perception or knowledge of planned therapy
	Readiness to learn
Exchanging	Physical integrity
	Toxicology screen
Moving	Leisure or social activities
	Access to firearms and weapons
	Self-care
Perceiving	Sensory perception
	Self-concept
	Meaningfulness
Relating	Role (home or occupation)
	Quality of relationships with others
Feeling	Emotional or integrity states
	Recent stressful life events
	Cognitive manifestations
	Coping with anxiety, fear, anger, guilt, envy, shame, and sadness
Choosing	Patient and family coping methods
	Patient's usual defense methods
	Compliance with health care regimen
	Judgment or decision-making ability
Valuing	Important religious practices
	Important life values

category headings for Taxonomy I and the Psychiatric Assessment Tool. The sequence of the response patterns, as it appears in Taxonomy I, has been changed in the tool to permit a logical ordering of assessment variables. Nursing diagnoses pertinent to the psychiatric patient, along with the signs and symptoms necessary to identify them are incorporated under the appropriate human response patterns.

Nurses must also realize that this tool is very different from conventional assessment tools. As a result, nurses may encounter some initial difficulty in using it. They should remember, however, that the tool was not designed to follow the organization or content of a traditional medical data base; the data collected do not solely reflect medical patterns. Rather, the tool elicits data about holistic patterns in ways not traditionally assessed by nurses. It provides a new method of collecting and synthesizing data and requires new thinking in processing data. This tool represents a nursing data base developed from a nursing model that permits a holistic nursing assessment to take place so that nursing diagnoses can be identified.

Although nurses probably agree that a holistic nursing data base is desirable, it is realized that changing traditional assessment methods is not an easy task. For this reason, a trial usage period is recommended before any decisions about the tool's merits are made. During the trial period, nurses should assess 10 psychiatric patients using the tool to become familiar and progressively more comfortable with its organization and data-collection methods. With experience, nurses will become accustomed to new ways of clustering and processing information. With continued use, the time necessary to complete the tool will be reduced. Most important, nurses will recognize the unique ability of the tool to elicit appropriate signs and symptoms. Nurses will also discover that nursing diagnoses are easily identified when using the tool.

It is not necessary to complete the tool in one session. Priority sections can be completed during the initial assessment. Other sections or patterns can be completed later, within a time frame acceptable to the institution and patient. To elicit appropriate data, nurses should familiarize themselves with the focus questions and parameters in the next section. When assessing specific signs and symptoms to indicate a particular diagnosis, the nurse circles the diagnosis in the right-hand column when deviations from normal are found. A circled diagnosis does not confirm a problem but simply alerts the nurse to the possibility that it exists. After completing the tool, the nurse scans the circled problems, synthesizes the data to determine whether other clusters of signs and symptoms support the existence of a problem, and judges whether the diagnosis is present.

Some diagnoses are repeated several times in the right-hand column. These repetitions occur only within the appropriate response pattern and are convenient for identifying data directly with their corresponding nursing diagnosis. These diagnoses are not absolute and are intended to focus thinking and direct more detailed attention to a problem.

Some signs and symptoms can indicate many diagnoses. For example, a patient's inability to follow directions can indicate inattention or a disturbance in thought processes. To avoid unnecessary repetition of assessment parameters, variables are arranged with the diagnosis most likely to result from the data assessed. Thus, data to support one di-

Table 11-2

Psychiatric assessment tool: focus questions and parameters

Variables	Focus questions and parameters
COMMUNICATING	
Verbal communication	Does the patient demonstrate disturbances in thought (blocking or flight of ideas)?
Nonverbal communication	Describe the patient's posture, facial expression, gestures, and eye contact.
Grooming and dress appearance	What is the patient's general appearance?
KNOWING	
Orientation	"Do you experience a sense of loss of time or place?"
	"Do you ever find it difficult to think clearly?"
	"Do you have disorganized thoughts?"
Perception/knowledge of planned therapy	"What is your biggest problem?"
	"What does this illness mean to you?"
	"What has been planned to help you?"
	"What do you think would help you?"
Readiness to learn	Does the patient deny that a problem exists?
	Does the patient's emotional or psychologic status permit or prohibit learning?
EXCHANGING	
Physical integrity	Assess for history of head injury, trauma, substance abuse, bruises on skin, and cuts.
Toxicology screen	Is there evidence of drug abuse?
MOVING	
Leisure and social activities	"What do you do that is fun or relaxing? How often? With whom?"
Access to firearms/weapons	Does the family describe availability of weapons or firearms?
Self-care	"Can you bathe and groom yourself?"
PERCEIVING	
Sensory perception	Is there altered sensation related to substance abuse?
	Does the patient demonstrate delusions, hallucinations, phobias, or obsessions?
Self-concept	"If you had to describe what kind of person you are, what would you say?"
	"Are you comfortable about how you look, feel, and function?"
	"How would others describe you?"
Meaningfulness	"Do you believe there is a solution to your problem?"
	Does the patient verbalize hopelessness or violent or homicidal intentions?
RELATING	
Occupation/job concerns	"Do you have a job? Tell me about it."
	"Do you worry about any major job-related problems?"
Quality of relationships with others	"How do you like others to treat you?"
	"How do you and _____ get along?"
FEELING	
Recent stressful life events	"Has anything bad or stressful happened this year?"
	"Do you feel anxious, angry, sad, etc.?"
Cognitive manifestations	Does the patient demonstrate blocking of words, inattention, difficulty concentrating, defensiveness, anger, or withdrawal?
Usual method for coping	What is the patient's usual method of coping with anxiety, fear, anger, guilt, envy, shame, or sadness?

Continued

Table 11-2—cont'd

Psychiatric assessment tool: focus questions and parameters

Variables	Focus questions and parameters
CHOOSING	
Patient's and family's coping methods	"Describe a problem you have had. How did you solve it?"
	"Who helps you to solve problems?"
	"When you have a problem, do you smoke, drink, or take drugs? Ask someone for help? Call your family? Try to put it out of your mind?"
Patient's usual defense mechanisms	Does the patient demonstrate conversion, rationalization, sublimation, regression, introjection, projection, or denial or repression?
Compliance with past/current health care regimens	"In the future, do you think you will have problems following the therapy recommended for you?"
	What is the family's opinion of the patient's ability to comply?
Judgment	"Why are you in the hospital?"
VALUING	
Important religious practices	"What is meaningful in your life?"
Important life values	"Tell me about the things that are important to you?"
	"Are there any medical or nursing treatments that you cannot or will not accept?"
	"Are family members or significant others usually with you during special times or during periods of illness?"

agnosis may occasionally be found in other patterns or arranged with other diagnoses. Therefore, synthesis of all data is essential.

The Psychiatric Assessment Tool is not intended to be the standardized and final format for assessment of patients across the country. An assessment tool must meet the needs of the individual institutions and nurses using it. The Psychiatric Assessment Tool is simply a working demonstration tool that is expected to be changed and revised by nurses in clinical practice. Further evaluation and refinement are necessary before adopting it for use in an institution. Nurses interested in changing, revising, and adapting the tool to a specific clinical setting should refer to Chapter 4.

HOW TO ELICIT APPROPRIATE DATA

Because the Unitary Person Framework and the Psychiatric Assessment Tool contain some terms that may be unfamiliar to nurses, specific psychiatric focus questions and parameters were developed and refined to elicit appropriate information. These questions and parameters are in Table 11-2, which follows the order of the Psychiatric Assessment Tool (Fig. 11-1). The variables in bold type are described more fully in Table 11-2. For example, the self-concept variable under the "perceiving pattern" is in bold type. If the nurse does not know what questions to ask about self-concept, Table 11-2 can be used to direct the line of questioning. The questions and parameters provide clarity and guidance in eliciting data. They are not intended to be all inclusive, and nurses should not feel limited by them. There are many other ways, based on the pa-

tient's situation and condition and the nurse's skill, to elicit the appropriate information. Focus questions and parameters for other data were presented in Chapter 3.

CASE STUDY

The case study models the process a nurse uses when assessing a patient. Based on the clustering of information obtained during assessment, the nurse formulates nursing diagnoses.

Mr. H.R. was assessed after his wife left him. He is 63 years old and lives alone. The Psychiatric Assessment Tool (Fig. 11-2) was used to assess Mr. H.R.

BIBLIOGRAPHY

American Nurses' Association: Standards of psychiatric and mental health nursing practice, Kansas City, Mo, 1982, ANA, Inc.

American Nurses' Association: Standards of child and adolescent psychiatric and mental health nursing practice, Kansas City, Mo, 1985, ANA, Inc.

Barry PD: Psychosocial nursing assessment and intervention, Philadelphia, 1984, JB Lippincott Co.

Beck C, Rawlins R, and Williams S: Mental health psychiatric nursing: a holistic life-cycle approach, St Louis, 1988, The CV Mosby Co.

McFarland G and Wasli E: Nursing diagnosis and process in psychiatric mental health nursing, Philadelphia, 1986, JB Lippincott Co.

Rawlins R and Heacock P: Clinical manual of psychiatric nursing, St Louis, 1988, The CV Mosby Co.

Stockwell F: The nursing process in psychiatric nursing, London, 1985, Croom Helm Ltd.

PSYCHIATRIC ASSESSMENT TOOL

Name _____ Age _____ Sex _____
Address _____ Telephone _____
Significant other _____ Telephone _____
Date of admission _____ Medical diagnosis: _____
Allergies _____ Detention: Yes _____ No _____
Legal proceedings pending: Yes _____ No _____

Nursing Diagnosis
(Potential or Altered)

COMMUNICATING ▪ A pattern involving sending messages
Verbal: Presence of: (circle) thought blocking, flight of ideas, perseveration,
circumstantiality, punning, rhyming, tangential blocking, loose
association

Speech impaired _____
Verbal coherence _____ Aphasia _____
Mutism _____ Echopraxia _____
   Rate: _____ Volume _____ Intonation _____
Nonverbal: Posture _____ Facial expression _____
   Gesture _____ Eye contact _____
Read, write, understand English (circle) _____   Communication
Other languages _____   Verbal
Physical impairment affecting communication _____   Nonverbal
Alternate form of communication _____
Grooming and dress _____
General appearance _____
Other observations _____

KNOWING ▪ A pattern involving the meaning associated with information
Orientation
   Level of alertness _____   Orientation
   Orientation: Person _____ Place _____ Time _____   Confusion
   Appropriate behavior/communication _____

Memory
   Memory intact: yes/no Immediate _____ Recent _____   Memory
   Remote _____
   Level/fund of knowledge _____
   Ability to abstract _____
Current physical health problems _____   Knowledge deficit
Previous illnesses/hospitalizations/surgeries _____
_____

History of the following problems:
   Heart _____
   Peripheral vascular _____
   Lung _____
   Liver _____ Kidney _____
   Cerebrovascular _____
   Thyroid _____
   Diabetes _____ Medication _____
   Substance abuse _____
   Alcohol use _____
   Other _____
Current medications _____
_____

Fig. 11-1

Continued.

Perception/knowledge of planned therapy _____

_____

Expectations of therapy _____

_____

Misconceptions _____

Readiness to learn _____

   Request information concerning _____   Thought processes

   Educational level _____   Impaired problem solving

   Learning impeded by _____

EXCHANGING ▪ A pattern involving mutual giving and receiving

Hormonal/Metabolic Patterns

   Hematocrit _____ Hemoglobin _____ Platelets _____   Menstrual patterns

   NA _____ K _____ CL _____ Glucose _____   Premenstrual syndrome

   Medications which potentiate blood dyscrasias _____

   Other labs _____

   Menstrual patterns _____

   BCP _____ Other methods _____

Physical Integrity

   Tissue integrity _____ Rashes _____ Lesions _____   Impaired skin integrity

      Petechiae _____ Bruises _____   Impaired tissue integrity

      Abrasions _____ Lacerations _____   Violence

      Surgical incisions _____ Scars _____   Injury

                                          Trauma

Circulation

Neurologic changes/symptoms _____   Cerebral tissue perfusion

Glascow Coma Scale total _____

CT scan _____ MRI _____

ECG reading _____ Heart rate _____

Nutrition   Nutrition

Eating patterns

   Number of meals per day _____

   Special diet _____

   Where eaten _____

   Food preferences/intolerances _____

   Food allergies _____

   Caffeine intake (coffee, tea, soft drinks, chocolate)

   _____

   Appetite changes _____

   Nausea/vomiting _____

   Anorexia _____ Bulimia _____

   Other observations: _____

Condition of mouth/throat _____   Oral mucous membranes

   Height _____ Weight _____   More/less than body

   Weight loss/gain _____   requirements

Physical Regulation

   Immune

      Lymph nodes enlarged _____ Location _____   Infection

      WBC count _____   Hypothermia

   Body temperature   Hyperthermia

      Temperature _____ Route _____   Ineffective thermoregulation

Medications with anticholinergic action _____

History of malignant neurolepsis syndrome _____

History of EPS _____

Fig. 11-1, cont'd

Oxygenation

Smoker _____ Number per day _____ How long _____

Color of nail beds _____ Nicotine stain _____

Complaints of dyspnea _____ Precipitated by _____

Rate _____ Rhythm _____ Depth _____

Labored/unlabored (circle) Chest expansion _____

Cough: productive/nonproductive _____

Sputum: Color _____ Amount _____ Consistency _____

Breath sounds _____

Ineffective airway clearance
Ineffective breathing patterns
Impaired gas exchange

Elimination

Gastrointestinal/bowel

  Usual bowel habit _____

  Alterations from normal _____

  Laxative use _____

    Incontinence _____

  Abdominal physical examination _____

Renal/urinary

  Usual urinary pattern _____

  Alteration from normal _____

  Color _____ Appearance _____

  Urine output: 24 hour _____

  Intake _____

  Bladder distention _____

_____

Bowel elimination
  Constipation
  Diarrhea
  Incontinence

GI tissue perfusion

Urinary elimination
  Incontinence
  Retention
  Enuresis

Renal tissue perfusion

Toxicology screen _____

BUN _____

Lithium/other medications _____

MOVING ▪ A pattern involving activity

Activity

History of physical disability _____

_____

Verbal report of fatigue or weakness _____

_____

Motor activity: Tics _____ Tremors _____

  Gait disturbances _____ Agitation _____

  Compulsive behavior _____ Lethargy _____

  Retardation _____

  Hyperactivity _____

  History of medications related to involuntary movements _____

_____

  Other observations _____

Impaired physical mobility

Activity intolerances

Rest

Hours slept/night _____ Feels rested: yes/no

Sleep aids (pillows, meds, food) _____

Difficulty falling/remaining asleep _____

Changes from usual sleep patterns _____

Other observations _____

Sleep pattern disturbance
  Hypersomnia
  Insomnia
  Nightmares

Recreation

Leisure activities _____

Increase/decrease from usual _____

Social activities _____

Other observations _____

(Deficit in) diversional activity

Fig. 11-1, cont'd

Continued.

Environmental Maintenance

Home maintenance management

Size & arrangement of home (stairs, bathroom) _____
_____ Safety needs _____
Access to firearms/weapons _____   Violence
Limitations in daily activities _____   Injury
Exercise habits _____
Home responsibilities _____   Impaired home maintenance
_____   management
Other observations _____   Safety hazards

Health Maintenance

Health insurance _____   Health maintenance
Regular physical checkups _____
Other observations _____

Self-Care

Ability to perform ADLs: Independent _____ Dependent _____   Self-care
Specify deficits _____   Feeding
Discharge planning needs _____   Bathing/hygiene
          Dressing/grooming
          Toileting

PERCEIVING ▪ A pattern involving the reception of information

Sensory Perception   Sensory/perception

Vision _____ Last examination _____ Glasses/contacts _____   Visual
Auditory _____ Last examination _____ Hearing aid _____   Auditory
Prostheses _____   Kinesthetic
Gustatory _____ Changes in taste _____   Gustatory
Tactile examination _____ Numbness _____   Tactile
Olfactory examination _____ Changes in smell _____   Olfactory
Reflexes: Grossly intact _____
Content of thought: Intact memory _____ Obsessions _____
  Hallucinations _____ Phobias _____
  Delusions _____ Other _____

Attention

Patient's ability to follow directions _____   Unilateral neglect
_____   (Distractibility)
Responds to verbal cues _____   (Hyperalertness)
Responds to visual cues _____   (Inattention)
          (Selective attention)

Self-Concept   Self-concept

Patient's description of self _____   Body image
Negative self-concept _____   Self-esteem
Poor self-esteem _____   Personal identity
Perceived strengths _____   Growth & development
Perceived weaknesses _____   Socialization

Meaningfulness

Verbalizes hopelessness/powerlessness _____   Hopelessness
Perceives/verbalizes loss of control _____   Powerlessness
Verbalizes suicidal ideations _____

Fig. 11-1, cont'd

Verbalizes violent intentions _____   Violence
Verbalizes homicidal intentions _____   Injury
Engages in self destructive acts _____
Awareness of values _____
Awareness of conflicts _____
Desired/stated goals of hospitalization/treatment _____
_____

RELATING ▪ A pattern involving establishing bonds
Role

Marital status _____   Role performance
Age & health of significant other _____   Parenting
_____   Work
Number of children _____ Ages _____   Family
Role in home _____   Social/leisure
Multiple roles _____
Role-related problems _____
Financial support _____   Family processes
Occupation _____
   Job satisfaction/**concerns** _____
Sexual relationships (satisfactory/unsatisfactory)_____   Sexual dysfunction
   Physical difficulties related to sex _____   Sexuality patterns
_____

Socialization

Patient's identification of additional significant others
_____
Quality of relationships with others _____   Impaired social interaction
   Patient's description _____
   Significant others' descriptions _____
   Staff observations _____
   Verbalizes feelings of being alone _____   Social isolation
   Loneliness attributed to _____   Social withdrawal
   Level of trust in relationships _____
   Level of dependence/independence _____
_____

FEELING ▪ A pattern involving the subjective awareness of information
Comfort

Pain/discomfort: yes/no   Comfort
Onset _____ Duration _____   Pain/chronic
Location _____ Quality _____ Radiation _____   Pain/acute
Associated factors _____   Discomfort
Aggravating factors _____
Alleviating factors _____

Altered Emotional Integrity States
Recent stressful life events _____
Verbalizes feelings of anxiety _____   Anxiety
Source of anxiety _____   Fear
Object of fear _____
Usual method(s) for coping with anxiety/fear _____
Physical manifestations: Muscle tension _____
   Dry mouth _____ Skin pallor _____ Nausea/vomiting _____
   Difficulty sleeping _____ Unsteady voice _____
   Increased pulse rate _____ Increased respiratory rate _____
Other observations _____

Fig. 11-1, cont'd

Continued.

Cognitive manifestations: Narrowed sensory perception _____   Anxiety
    Selective inattention _____ Blocking of words _____   Fear
    Difficulty concentrating _____ Defensiveness _____
Social manifestations: withdrawal _____
Demanding or aggressive behavior _____
Other observations _____

Event that precipitated anger _____   Anger
Usual method for coping with anger _____   Violence
Manifestations: Flushed face _____   Aggression
    Shallow breathing _____ Sweating _____
    Use of sarcasm _____ Argumentative _____   Disorganized behavior
    Fault finding _____ Dominating _____   Compulsive behavior
    Use of violence _____
Other observations _____

Event that precipitated guilt/envy/shame _____   Guilt/envy/shame
Usual method of coping with guilt/envy/shame _____
Manifestations: Embarrassment _____ Regret _____
    Inappropriate affect _____ Self-punishing thoughts
    Preoccupation with what "should" have been _____
    Isolation _____
    Lack of self-forgiveness _____
Other observations _____

Event that precipitated sadness _____   Sadness
Usual method of coping with sadness _____
    Manifestations: Emptiness _____ Unworthiness _____
    Helplessness _____ Powerlessness _____
    Hopelessness _____ Withdrawal _____
    Suicidal ideas _____
Other observations _____

CHOOSING ■ A pattern involving the selection of alternatives
Coping
    Patient's usual coping methods _____   Ineffective individual coping
    _____   Ineffective family coping
    Family's usual coping methods _____   Impaired adjustment
    _____   Impaired problem solving
    Patient's usual defense mechanisms: Rationalization _____
    Conversion _____ Sublimation _____ Regression _____
    Introjection _____ Projection _____ Denial/repression _____

Participation
    Compliance with past/current health care regimens _____   Noncompliance
    Conflicts/obstacles _____
    Noncompliance _____
    _____   Ineffective participation
    Willingness to comply with future health care regimen _____
    _____
    Family's ability to support patient _____   Family processes
Judgment
    Decision-making ability: Judgment
    Patient's perspective _____   Indecisiveness
    Others' perspectives _____

Fig. 11-1, cont'd

VALUING ▪ A pattern involving the assigning of relative worth

Religious preference _____ Spiritual distress

Important religious practices _____

   Does religion/spirituality offer comfort/hope? _____

   Or guilt and fear? _____

Changes in religious practices _____

Cultural practices _____ Despair

Important life values _____

Influence of illness on values _____

Creativity _____

Aesthetic sense _____

Prioritized nursing diagnosis/problem list

1. _____

2. _____

3. _____

4. _____

5. _____

Signature _____ Date _____

Fig. 11-1, cont'd

PSYCHIATRIC ASSESSMENT TOOL

Name _H.R._   Age _63_   Sex _M_
Address _120 LEWIS ST., LEWISVILLE, VA._   Telephone _222-3131_
Significant other _WIFE (SEPARATED), SISTER, CHILDREN_   Telephone _543-1234 (SISTER)_
Date of admission _5/1_   Medical diagnosis: _POSTTRAUMATIC STRESS, CHRONIC DEPRESSION_
Allergies _NKA_   Detention: Yes ___ No _✔_
Legal proceedings pending: Yes ___ No _✔_

Nursing Diagnosis
(Potential or Altered)

COMMUNICATING ■ A pattern involving sending messages
Verbal: Presence of: (circle) thought blocking, flight of ideas, (perseveration,) circumstantiality, punning, rhyming, tangential blocking, loose association
Speech impaired _No_
Verbal coherence _YES_   Aphasia _No_
Mutism _No_   Echopraxia _No_
  Rate: _NORMAL_   Volume _NORMAL_   Intonation _LOW VOICE (SADNESS)_
Nonverbal: Posture _SLUMPS_   Facial expression _OCCASIONAL DRAWN SMILES_
  Gesture _WRINGS HANDS_ Eye contact _USUALLY DIRECT_
(Read) (write,) (understand) English (circle) _✔_   Communication
Other languages _No_   Verbal
Physical impairment affecting communication _↓SIGHT, ↓HEARING, DENTURES_   Nonverbal
Alternate form of communication _N/A_
Grooming and dress _CLEAN, PRESSED SHIRT; TENNIS SHOES; SLACKS_
General appearance _DRESSED APPROPRIATELY_
Other observations _FIDGETS_

KNOWING ■ A pattern involving the meaning associated with information
Orientation
  Level of alertness _ALERT_   Orientation
  Orientation: Person _✔_   Place _✔_   Time _✔_   Confusion
  Appropriate behavior/communication _YES_

Memory
  Memory intact: (yes) no Immediate _✔_   Recent _✔_   Memory
  Remote _✔_
  Level/fund of knowledge _NARROW_
  Ability to abstract _LIMITED_
Current physical health problems _CHEST PAIN, HEARING, SEEING_   Knowledge deficit
Previous illnesses/hospitalizations/surgeries _1984-85 X1-2 MOS. FOR DEPRESSION; 1950 APPENDECTOMY_
History of the following problems:
  Heart _OCCASIONAL C/O CHEST PAIN_
  Peripheral vascular _No_
  Lung _No_
  Liver _No_   Kidney _No_
  Cerebrovascular _No_
  Thyroid _No_
  Diabetes _No_   Medication _⊖_
  Substance abuse _No_
  Alcohol use _↑ BEER PER DAY_
  Other _SHRAPNEL Ⓛ ARM_
Current medications _SINEQUAN (DEPRESSION, ANXIETY) 40 mg qd PO, NITRO 1/150 gr. PRN. SL_

Fig. 11-2

Perception/knowledge of planned therapy *PT. BELIEVES PLAN INVOLVES MEDS; MDs HAVE NOT COMMUNICATED PLAN*
Expectations of therapy *MEDS WILL MAKE HIM "FEEL BETTER"*

Misconceptions *ABILITY OF MEDS TO SOLVE PROBLEMS*
Readiness to learn *YES, NEED TO INVOLVE FAMILY*
   Request information concerning *MEDS*
   Educational level *10TH GRADE*
   Learning impeded by *DEPRESSION, SEPARATION FROM WIFE 3 MOS. AGO, WITHDRAWAL*

Thought processes
(Impaired problem solving (?))

EXCHANGING ▪ A pattern involving mutual giving and receiving
Hormonal/Metabolic Patterns
Hematocrit *45.2 %* Hemoglobin *15.3 g/dl* Platelets *300,000/µL*
NA *138 mEq/L* K *4.5 mEq/L* CL *103 mEq/L* Glucose *100 mg/dl*
Medications which potentiate blood dyscrasias *Ø*
Other labs *URINE, TOXICOLOGY (BELOW)*
Menstrual patterns *N/A*
BCP *N/A* Other methods *—*

Menstrual patterns
Premenstrual syndrome

Physical Integrity
Tissue integrity *INTACT* Rashes *NO* Lesions *NO*
   Petechiae *NO* Bruises *NO*
   Abrasions *NO* Lacerations *NO*
   Surgical incisions *RLQ* Scars *RLQ, (L) ARM*
     (APPENDECTOMY)

Impaired skin integrity
Impaired tissue integrity
Violence
Injury
Trauma

Circulation
Neurologic changes/symptoms *NONE APPARENT*
Glasgow Coma Scale total *—*
CT scan *No* MRI *No*
ECG reading *NSR* Heart rate *85*
   NO SOB OR DYSPNEA, NO GALLOPS OR MURMURS

Cerebral tissue perfusion

Nutrition
Eating patterns
   Number of meals per day *UP TO 6 PER DAY (SMALL)*
   Special diet *SEE BELOW*
   Where eaten *HOME, DINER (3 X PER WEEK)*
   Food preferences/intolerances *NO CAFFIENE, CHEESE, OR CHOCOLATE (DUE TO TRICYCLIC INTERACTION)*
   Food allergies *NKA*
Caffeine intake (coffee, tea, soft drinks, chocolate)
   NO CAFFEINE (COFFEE, SOFT DRINKS, OR CHOCOLATE)
Appetite changes *REPORTS EATING LESS*
Nausea/vomiting *YES, DOESN'T REPORT HOW OFTEN (NOT OBSERVED)*
Anorexia *No* Bulimia *No*
Other observations: *EFFECTS OF STRESS ON EATING*
Condition of mouth/throat *GOOD; PARTIAL PLATE (UPPER)*
Height *5'10"* Weight *150*
Weight (loss)/gain *1-2 lbs.*

Nutrition

Oral mucous membranes
More/less than body
   requirements

Physical Regulation
Immune
   Lymph nodes enlarged *No* Location *—*
   WBC count *10.4 X 10³/µL*
Body temperature
   Temperature *98.4°F* Route *ORAL*
Medications with anticholinergic action *(SINEQUAN)*
History of malignant neurolepsis syndrome *No*
History of EPS *No*

Infection
Hypothermia
Hyperthermia
Ineffective thermoregulation

Fig. 11-2, cont'd

Continued.

Oxygenation

Smoker __*No*__ Number per day __—__ How long __—__   Ineffective airway clearance
Color of nail beds __*PINK*__ Nicotine stain __—__   Ineffective breathing patterns
Complaints of dyspnea __*No*__ Precipitated by __—__   Impaired gas exchange
Rate __*16*__ Rhythm __*REGULAR*__ Depth __*NORMAL—ABDOMINAL*__
Labored (unlabored) (circle) Chest expansion __*ABDOMINAL*__
Cough: productive/nonproductive __*NONE*__
Sputum: Color __—__ Amount __—__ Consistency __—__
Breath sounds __*CLEAR*__

Elimination

Gastrointestinal/bowel   Bowel elimination
  Usual bowel habit __*1 X 9 1–2 DAYS*__   (Constipation?)
  Alterations from normal __*CONSTIPATION*__   Diarrhea
  Laxative use __*ENEMA 1 X WEEK*__   Incontinence
    Incontinence __*No*__
  Abdominal physical examination __*SOFT NON-TENDER*__   GI tissue perfusion
Renal/urinary
  Usual urinary pattern __*AM, 2–3 X DAY*__   Urinary elimination
  Alteration from normal __*No*__   Incontinence
  Color __*YELLOW*__ Appearance __*CLEAR*__   Retention
  Urine output: 24 hour __*WNL (LOW NORMAL)*__   Enuresis
  Intake __*ENCOURAGED TO DRINK MORE WATER/FLUIDS*__
  Bladder distention __*No*__   Renal tissue perfusion

Toxicology screen __*NEGATIVE*__
BUN __*19 mg/dl*__
Lithium/other medications __*No*__

MOVING ▪ A pattern involving activity

Activity

History of physical disability __*No*__   Impaired physical mobility

Verbal report of (fatigue) or weakness __*? DEPRESSION, DIFFICULTY*__
__*SLEEPING*__
Motor activity: Tics __*No*__ Tremors __*No*__
  Gait disturbances __*No*__ Agitation __*YES*__   Activity intolerances
  Compulsive behavior __*No*__ Lethargy __*OCCASIONAL*__
  Retardation __*No*__
  Hyperactivity __*No*__
  History of medications related to involuntary movements __*No*__

Other observations __(L) *ARM FUNCTIONAL (WAR INJURY)*__

Rest

Hours slept/night __*4–5 HR.*__ Feels rested: yes (no)   (Sleep pattern disturbance)
Sleep aids (pillows, meds, food) __*MEDS (?) "OVER-THE-COUNTER"*__   Hypersomnia
Difficulty falling/remaining asleep __*YES*__   (Insomnia)
Changes from usual sleep patterns __*No*__   Nightmares
Other observations __*CIRCLES UNDER EYES*__

Recreation

Leisure activities __*FEW, TV*__
Increase/decrease from usual __*No*__   (Deficit in) diversional activity
Social activities __*SEES GRANDCHILDREN ≤1 X PER MO.*__
Other observations __*"I HAVE NO HOBBIES"*__

Fig. 11-2, cont'd

Environmental Maintenance

Home maintenance management

Size & arrangement of home (stairs, bathroom) *3 BEDROOMS, 2 BATHS,*
SPLITLEVEL Safety needs *OK*

Access to firearms/weapons *DOES NOT OWN ANY* — Violence

Limitations in daily activities *No* — Injury

Exercise habits *NONE (BESIDES ADL)*

Home responsibilities *LIVES ON FARM, HAS A HOUSEKEEPER* — Impaired home maintenance
4 HRS M-F — management

Other observations *RAISES PIGS AND CHICKENS (IN PARTNERSHIP)* — Safety hazards

(POTENTIAL)

Health Maintenance

Health insurance *70% SERVICE CONNECTED (VETERAN)* — (Health maintenance)

Regular physical checkups *No*

Other observations *DOESN'T SEE "NEED" FOR REGULAR CHECKUPS*

Self-Care — Self-care

Ability to perform ADLs: Independent ✓ Dependent _____ — Feeding

Specify deficits *NONE* — Bathing/hygiene

Discharge planning needs *SOCIALIZATION NEEDS; TEACH SIDE EFFECTS OF* — Dressing/grooming
SINEQUAN (ESPECIALLY AVOIDING HAZARDOUS — Toileting
ACTIVITIES: DRIVING, USING FARM EQUIPMENT)

PERCEIVING ▪ A pattern involving the reception of information

Sensory Perception — Sensory/perception

Vision *GLASSES* Last examination *NOT KNOWN* (Glasses) contacts ✓ — Visual

Auditory *H. AID* Last examination *NOT KNOWN* Hearing aid ✓ — Auditory

Prostheses *No* — Kinesthetic

Gustatory *INTACT* Changes in taste *No* — Gustatory

Tactile examination *NORMAL* Numbness *No* — Tactile

Olfactory examination *NORMAL* Changes in smell *No* — Olfactory

Reflexes: Grossly intact *YES*

Content of thought: Intact memory ✓ Obsessions *WIFE, WAR*

Hallucinations *No* Phobias *No*

Delusions *No* Other *No*

Attention

Patient's ability to follow directions *INTACT ABILITY, BUT DOES NOT BECOME* — Unilateral neglect
ACTIVELY INVOLVED c̄ THERAPY — (Distractibility)

Responds to verbal cues *YES, WHEN PT. WISHES TO* — (Hyperalertness)

Responds to visual cues *YES, WHEN PT. WISHES TO* — (Inattention)

(Selective attention)

Self-Concept — Self-concept

Patient's description of self *INADEQUATE, HASN'T "DONE ENOUGH FOR FAMILY"* — Body image

Negative self-concept *YES, DESPAIR* — Self-esteem

Poor self-esteem *YES* — Personal identity

Perceived strengths *RUNS OWN BUSINESS* — Growth & development

Perceived weaknesses *WIFE LEFT HIM, DOESN'T SOCIALIZE* — (Socialization)

Meaningfulness

Verbalizes (hopelessness/powerlessness) ✓ — Hopelessness

Perceives/verbalizes loss of control *YES* — Powerlessness

Verbalizes suicidal ideations *No (ON SUICIDE PRECAUTIONS)*

Fig. 11-2, cont'd

Continued.

Verbalizes violent intentions __*No*__ — Violence
Verbalizes homicidal intentions __*No*__ — Injury
Engages in self destructive acts __*No*__
Awareness of values __*POOR AWARENESS*__
Awareness of conflicts __*YES, WITH WIFE AND CHILDREN*__
Desired/stated goals of hospitalization/treatment __*HAS NO GOALS AT THIS TIME*__

RELATING ▪ A pattern involving establishing bonds
Role
Marital status __*SEPARATED X 3 MOS*__ — Role performance
Age & health of significant other __*WIFE, 61 YO, IN GOOD HEALTH, LIVES IN ANOTHER STATE*__ — Parenting / Work *(?)*
Number of children __*3*__ Ages __*32 ♂ 28 ♂ 23 ♀*__ — Family
Role in home __*INDEPENDENT (HAS A PART-TIME HOUSEKEEPER)*__ — Social/leisure
Multiple roles __*GRANDFATHER, FATHER*__
Role-related problems __*STRESS OF SEPARATION*__
Financial support __*BUSINESS INCOME, VETERAN'S BENEFITS*__ — Family processes
Occupation __*FARMER (PIGS AND CHICKENS)*__
Job satisfaction/concerns __*WORKING LESS, ↓ INTEREST*__
Sexual relationships (satisfactory/~~unsatisfactory~~) — Sexual dysfunction
Physical difficulties related to sex __*No*__ — Sexuality patterns

Socialization
Patient's identification of additional significant others
__*DOES NOT SOCIALIZE c̄ PEERS OF EITHER SEX*__
Quality of relationships with others __*POOR*__ — (Impaired social interaction)
Patient's description __*"DON'T SOCIALIZE"*__
Significant others' descriptions __*CONFIRMED BY SISTER*__
Staff observations __*CRIES EASILY*__
Verbalizes feelings of being alone __*YES*__ — Social isolation
Loneliness attributed to __*MARITAL SEPARATION*__ — (Social withdrawal)
Level of trust in relationships __*POOR*__
Level of dependence/independence __*LIVES ALONE, DENIES NEED FOR SIGNIFICANT RELATIONSHIPS; LITTLE INTERACTION c̄ HOUSEKEEPER, SISTER, OR CHILDREN*__

FEELING ▪ A pattern involving the subjective awareness of information
Comfort
Pain/discomfort: yes/(no) __*AT PRESENT*__ — Comfort
Onset __*N/A*__ Duration __*N/A*__ — Pain/chronic
Location __*N/A*__ Quality __*N/A*__ Radiation __*N/A*__ — Pain/acute
Associated factors __*No*__ ⎱ __*OCCASIONAL CHEST PAIN,*__ — Discomfort
Aggravating factors __*EXERTION*__ ⎰ __*RELIEVED WITHIN*__
Alleviating factors __*NITRO, REST*__ / __*MINUTES*__

Altered Emotional Integrity States
Recent stressful life events __*WIFE LEFT 3 MOS AGO*__
Verbalizes feelings of anxiety __*YES, ↑FREQUENCY, AGITATED s̄ MEDS*__ — (Anxiety)
Source of anxiety __*WIFE, WAR*__ — Fear
Object of fear __*N/A*__
Usual method(s) for coping with anxiety/fear __*MEDS TO SLEEP (OVER-THE-COUNTER)*__
Physical manifestations: Muscle tension __*WRINGS HANDS*__
Dry mouth __*YES*__ Skin pallor __*YES*__ Nausea/vomiting __*YES, REPORTED*__
Difficulty sleeping __*YES*__ Unsteady voice __*YES*__
Increased pulse rate __*No*__ Increased respiratory rate __*OCCASIONALLY*__
Other observations __*RESISTS INCLUDING FAMILY IN THERAPY*__

Fig. 11-2, cont'd

Cognitive manifestations: Narrowed sensory perception __No__   Anxiety
   Selective inattention __No__ Blocking of words __No__   Fear
   Difficulty concentrating __No__ Defensiveness __No__
Social manifestations: withdrawal __Yes__
Demanding or aggressive behavior __No__
Other observations __Occasional Anger__

Event that precipitated anger __Wife's Leaving__   (Anger)
Usual method for coping with anger __Withdrawal, Sleep__   Violence
Manifestations: Flushed face __No__   Aggression
   Shallow breathing __No__ Sweating __No__
   Use of sarcasm __No__ Argumentative __Occasional__   Disorganized behavior
   Fault finding __c̄ MDs, RNs__ Dominating __No__   Compulsive behavior
   Use of violence __None Noted__
Other observations __Verbalizes Anger Toward Wife__

Event that precipitated (guilt)/envy/shame __Wife's Departure__   (Guilt)/envy/shame
Usual method of coping with (guilt)/envy/shame __Withdrawal__
Manifestations: Embarrassment __Yes__ Regret __Yes__
   Inappropriate affect __Yes__ Self-punishing thoughts __"I didn't do enough."__
   Preoccupation with what "should" have been __Yes__
   Isolation __Yes__
   Lack of self-forgiveness __Yes__
Other observations __Often c/o Fatigue__

Event that precipitated sadness __Wife's Departure__   (Sadness)
Usual method of coping with sadness __Withdrawal, Sleep__
Manifestations: Emptiness __Yes__ Unworthiness __Yes__
   Helplessness __Yes__ Powerlessness __Yes__
   Hopelessness __Yes__ Withdrawal __Yes__
   Suicidal ideas __Pt. reports "no", doesn't understand why on__
Other observations __Suicide Precautions__

CHOOSING ▪ A pattern involving the selection of alternatives
Coping
   Patient's usual coping methods __Is not coping well, stays home__   (Ineffective individual coping)
__and doesn't work, withdrawn from family__   (Ineffective family coping)
   Family's usual coping methods __Sons cover bills, but family__   (Impaired adjustment)
__unable to help (? blame father for separation)__   (Impaired problem solving)
   Patient's usual defense mechanisms: Rationalization __Yes__
   Conversion __No__ Sublimation __No__ Regression __Yes__
   Introjection _____ Projection __No__ (Denial)/repression __✓__

Participation
   Compliance with past/current health care regimens __Usually complies__   Noncompliance
   Conflicts/obstacles __Would like to go home__
   Noncompliance __Does not report all meds taken, or amount__
__of vomiting (not observed)__   Ineffective participation
   Willingness to comply with future health care regimen __Expresses willing-__
__ness to comply__
   Family's ability to support patient __Offer by children, sister, business__   Family processes
__partner__
Judgment
   Decision-making ability: Judgment
      Patient's perspective __Thinks he should be able to go home__   Indecisiveness
      Others' perspectives __Can't make decision, depressed, suicidal (sister)__

Fig. 11-2, cont'd

Continued.

VALUING ▪ A pattern involving the assigning of relative worth

Religious preference *BAPTIST (NONPRACTICING)*   ⟨Spiritual distress(?)⟩

Important religious practices *NONE AT PRESENT*

   Does religion/spirituality offer comfort/hope? *SOME HOPE*

   Or ⟨guilt⟩ and fear? *GUILT*

Changes in religious practices *STOPPED ATTENDING SERVICES*

Cultural practices *INDEPENDENCE, SELF-SUFFICIENCY*   ⟨Despair⟩

Important life values *BELIEVES PEOPLE SHOULD BE SELF-SUFFICIENT*

Influence of illness on values *UNABLE "TO SUCCEED"*

Creativity *LITTLE EVIDENCE; "NO TIME FOR DAYDREAMING"*

Aesthetic sense *"NOT MUCH BEAUTY IN LIFE"*

Prioritized nursing diagnosis/problem list

1. *DISTURBANCE IN SELF-ESTEEM RELATED TO SEPARATION FROM WIFE.*
2. *INEFFECTIVE INDIVIDUAL COPING RELATED TO DEPRESSION.*
3. *IMPAIRED PROBLEM SOLVING RELATED TO WITHDRAWAL, DEPRESSION.*
4. *IMPAIRED SOCIAL INTERACTION RELATED TO FEW FRIENDS.*
5. *SLEEP PATTERN DISTURBANCE RELATED TO DEPRESSION.*

Signature *Patricia C. Seifert, RN*   Date *5/1 11 AM*

Fig. 11-2, cont'd

CHAPTER 12

CRITICAL CARE ASSESSMENT TOOL

LINDA A. PRINKEY
SHELIA D. BUNTON

The Critical Care Assessment Tool was designed to assess critically ill individuals with multiple and complex assessment needs. This tool incorporates assessment variables pertinent to the critically ill patient to facilitate identification of nursing diagnoses. The tool also incorporates the American Association of Critical-Care Nurses' *Standards for the Nursing Care of the Critically Ill*. This chapter includes:

- *The way the tool was developed and refined*
- *The patient populations and settings to which it applies*
- *Selected critical care emphasis areas*
- *The way to use the tool*
- *Specific critical care focus questions and parameters to assist the nurse in eliciting appropriate data*
- *The Critical Care Assessment Tool*
- *A case study*
- *A completed version of the tool based on the case study*

DEVELOPMENT AND REFINEMENT OF THE TOOL

The Critical Care Assessment Tool was developed from the nursing data base prototype (see Chapter 2). Because nurses in critical care units throughout the country care for medical and surgical patients with complex needs, the assessment variables of this tool address these needs. Further, because many critical care units serve as combined intensive and coronary care units, the detailed cardiovascular assessment parameters in the prototype were retained. Other assessment parameters dealing with trauma, burns, and dialysis have also been included.

The Critical Care Assessment Tool is based on current critical care literature. In addition, the tool was modified based on the recommendations of critical care nurse experts who tested it in clinical practice.

The tool was tested on 10 patients admitted to critical care units. The testing evaluated the tool's adequacy in terms of flow, space for recording data, and completeness of assessment variables. Based on the results, revisions were made.

PATIENT POPULATION AND SETTING

The Critical Care Assessment Tool was developed to assess the needs and problems of patients admitted to critical care units for specialized treatment. Because of the length of the tool and the extensive nature of the assessment variables, this tool is not recommended for emergency or recovery room settings. However, the tool could be adapted for use in these areas (see Chapter 4).

The Critical Care Assessment Tool was developed specifically for use in medical, surgical, and combined medical and surgical intensive care units. Assessment variables of the tool address a variety of patient groups such as those with complex postoperative needs, trauma or burns, or complex neurologic, pulmonary, gastrointestinal or renal, or metabolic problems. Nurses dealing with patients with these problems should also refer to the assessment tools specifically developed for these patients (see Chapters 13, 15, 6, 5, 7, and 8). These tools contain detailed assessments pertaining to the problems peculiar to these patients. Nurses caring solely for cardiovascular patients should refer to the Cardiovascular Assessment Tool (see Chapter 2), which served as the prototype for this book.

The assessment parameters of the Critical Care Assessment Tool were designed for use with critically ill adult patients. The tool can be used to assess stable and unstable patients. For more detailed information about clinical applications of the tool, nurses should refer to the section on how to use the tool.

CRITICAL CARE EMPHASIS AREAS

Critically ill patients have complex and unique problems and needs. The Critical Care Assessment Tool focuses on these problems and includes appropriate assessment variables for them within each of the nine human response patterns of Unitary Person Framework. When assessing the critically ill patient, nurses should pay particular attention to sections of the tool that address the problems and needs unique to these patients. Table 12-1 outlines emphasis areas for assessment of the critically ill patient.

HOW TO USE THE TOOL

To use the Critical Care Assessment Tool effectively, nurses must first be familiar with the nine human response

Table 12-1
Selected critical care emphasis areas

Patterns	Emphasis areas to determine
Communicating	Physical barriers to communication (i.e., intubation, laryngectomy, or paralysis)
Valuing	Cultural and religious values related to surgery, blood transfusion, or transplantation
Relating	Risk assessment for acquired immunodeficiency syndrome (AIDS)
Knowing	Risk assessment for acute renal failure
	Cardiac risk factors
Feeling	Comprehensive pain assessment
	Emotional impact of illness or injury
Moving	Effects of fractures, burns, paralysis, and amputation on mobility
Perceiving	Effects of illness, injury, or surgery on self-concept and body image
Exchanging	Current nutritional status, including nutritional support
	Skin and tissue integrity in relation to wounds, incisions, burns, and dialysis access sites
	Hemodynamic monitoring values
Choosing	Ability of the patient and significant others to cope with crisis

patterns of the Unitary Person Framework (see Chapter 2) and Taxonomy I. The sequence of the response patterns, as it appears in Taxonomy I, has been changed to permit better ordering of assessment variables. Questions, designed to elicit assessment of signs and symptoms related to specific nursing diagnoses in Taxonomy I, have been arranged according to their appropriate response patterns in this tool.

Nurses must also realize that this tool is very different from conventional assessment tools. As a result, nurses may encounter some initial difficulty in using it. They should remember, however, that the tool was not designed to follow the organization or content of a traditional medical data base; the data collected do not solely reflect medical patterns. Rather, the tool elicits data about holistic patterns in ways not traditionally assessed by nurses and provides a new method of collecting and synthesizing data. The Critical Care Assessment Tool is a nursing data base developed from a nursing model. Use of this tool results in a holistic assessment that allows nursing diagnoses to be identified.

Although many nurses probably agree that a holistic nursing data base is desirable, it is realized that changing traditional assessment methods is not an easy task. For this reason, a trial usage period is recommended before any decisions are made about the tool's merits. During the trial period, nurses will become familiar and progressively more comfortable with the tool's organization and data-collection methods. With experience, they will become accustomed to new ways of clustering and processing information. Further, with continued use, the time necessary to complete the tool will be reduced. Most important, nurses will discover that nursing diagnoses are easily identified because of the tool's unique ability to elicit appropriate signs and symptoms in a readily understandable fashion.

It is not necessary to complete the entire tool in one session. Priority sections can be completed during the initial assessment. Other sections can be completed later, within a time frame acceptable to the institution.

When assessing unstable patients, nurses should begin by collecting data within the "exchanging pattern." This pattern contains basic physiologic assessment variables (such as breathing patterns, arterial blood gases, blood pressure and other hemodynamic measurements, dysrhythmias, and level of consciousness) that relate to the "ABCs" of basic life support. When the patient becomes more stable, other assessment data can be collected, usually within 24 hours. Depending on the patient's level of consciousness and physical condition, the family or significant other may provide some of the data necessary to complete the tool.

To elicit appropriate data, nurses should familiarize themselves with the focus questions and parameters in the next section. These questions and parameters are not all

Table 12-2
Critical care assessment tool: focus questions and parameters

Variables	Focus questions and parameters
COMMUNICATING	
Physical barriers to communication	Does the patient have facial paralysis? Does the patient have a mandibular fracture? Does the patient have lacerations or burns of the face or mouth that affect the ability to speak? Is the patient intubated? Has the patient had a tracheostomy or laryngectomy?
VALUING	
Important religious practices	"Does your religion or culture permit you to have surgery, blood transfusions, and organ transplants?"
RELATING	
Sexual partner(s)	Is the patient a known homosexual, prostitute, or intravenous drug user? "Do you have more than one sexual partner? If so, how many?" Has the patient had sexual contact with a person who has a positive HIV test?
KNOWING	
Recent history of the following (NOTE: this section assesses for the *risk* of acute renal failure)	"Have you ever had a reaction to a blood transfusion?" Has the patient sustained a traumatic injury (crushing injury or car accident)? Has the patient had prolonged exposure to smoke or car exhaust? Is the patient being treated for heat stroke? Has the patient been treated recently for a severe infection? Has the patient performed any prolonged strenuous activity? Has the patient recently received anesthesia? Does the patient receive the following: neomycin, gentamicin, tobramycin, amikacin, or cyclosporine?
FEELING	
Pain/discomfort	See Chapter 3
Recent stressful life events	Was the patient involved in an accident in which other people were killed or injured?
MOVING	
Limitations in daily activities	Does the injury, condition, or surgery prevent the patient from living alone; feeding, bathing, or dressing self; combing hair, or brushing teeth?
PERCEIVING	
Verbalizes hopelessness	Has the patient attempted suicide?
Tactile impaired	Does the patient exhibit numbness, decreased sensation, or hypersensitivity?
EXCHANGING	
Intracranial pressure	Normal: 0-15 mm Hg.
Bleeding	Is the patient actively bleeding externally? If so, estimate the amount. Note the presence and extent of hematomas.
Extravasation from burns	Is there serosanguinous or serous fluid draining from the burned area?
Burns	
Degree	First degree, redness; second degree, blistering; or third degree, eschar (white, black, or cherry-red tissue and thrombosed blood vessels).
Type	Ask the patient or family how the patient was injured: Chemical injury—cleaners or battery acid; electrical injury—electrical wiring or lightening; or thermal injury—fire or stove.
___% surface area	Rule of Nines—arms, 4½% each; legs, 9% each; front, 18%; back, 18%; face and anterior portion of neck, 4½%; back of head and neck, 4½%.

Continued

Table 12-2—cont'd

Critical care assessment tool: focus questions and parameters

Variables	Focus questions and parameters
EXCHANGING—cont'd	
Dialysis access	What type of access does the patient have? Hemodialysis: fistula, arteriovenous shunt, or central lines; peritoneal dialysis: trochar catheter.
Current condition of access	What is the condition of the access (skin erosion, or clots or kinks in catheters)?
Esophageal tube	Does the patient have any type of nasogastric tube to control bleeding from esophageal varacies?
Possible kidney contusion/ other injury	Did the patient receive a forceable blow near the kidneys? Did the patient sustain a stab wound or gun shot wound near the kidneys?
CHOOSING	
Patient's and family's methods of dealing with stress	Does the patient or family appear tearful, nervous, or angry?

inclusive but rather provide clarity and guidance in eliciting data.

When assessing for specific signs and symptoms to indicate a particular nursing diagnosis, the nurse circles the appropriate diagnosis in the right-hand column when deviations from normal findings are found. A circled diagnosis does not confirm a problem but alerts the nurse to the possibility that it exists. After completing the tool, the nurse scans the circled problems and looks for other recorded data to support or refute the existence of the problems. Based on analysis of the data, the nurse then confirms the presence of an actual or potential nursing diagnosis.

Some diagnoses are repeated several times in the right-hand column. These repetitions occur only within the appropriate response pattern and are convenient for identifying data directly with corresponding nursing diagnoses.

Some signs and symptoms can indicate many diagnoses. For example, mental confusion can indicate decreased cerebral tissue perfusion, altered oxygenation, altered thought processes, altered level of consciousness, altered sensory/perception, and other nursing diagnoses. To avoid unnecessary repetition of assessment parameters, variables are arranged with the diagnosis most likely to result from the data assessed. Thus, data to support one diagnosis may occasionally be found in other patterns or arranged with other diagnoses. Therefore, synthesis of all data is essential.

HOW TO ELICIT APPROPRIATE DATA

Because the Unitary Person Framework and the Critical Care Assessment Tool contain some terms that may be unfamiliar to many nurses, specific critical care focus questions and parameters were developed to facilitate the collection of information. These questions and parameters are in Table 12-2 and correspond with the variables in bold type in the tool (Fig. 12-1). For example, many nurses may not be familiar with the methods of estimating the percentage of body-surface area affected by burns so the Rule of Nines appears in Table 12-2 as an assessment parameter for the "exchanging pattern." Further clarification of other assessment variables was presented in Chapter 3.

The focus questions and parameters are not all inclusive. Nurses should not feel they must ask only the questions or assess only the parameters provided. There are many other methods of eliciting appropriate information. Assessment methods should be tailored to the patient's level of understanding and the situation, as well as to the nurse's skill and comfort level.

CASE STUDY

The case study models the process a nurse uses when assessing a patient using the Critical Care Assessment Tool. Based on the clustering of information gathered during assessment, the nurse formulates appropriate nursing diagnoses.

Mr. B.J. was admitted to the hospital after receiving extensive burns when attempting to light the family charcoal grill. Because of Mr. B.J.'s painful facial burns, Mrs. J. provided much of the interview information. The completed tool (Fig. 12-2) contains the data obtained from Mr. and Mrs. J. and a prioritized list of nursing diagnoses derived from it.

BIBLIOGRAPHY

American Association of Critical-Care Nurses: Standards for the nursing care of the critically ill, Reston, Va, 1981, Reston Publishing Co.

Bates B: A guide to physical examination and history taking, ed 4, Philadelphia, 1987, JB Lippincott Co.

Carpenito L: Nursing diagnosis: application to clinical practice, Philadelphia, 1983, JB Lippincott Co.

Guzzetta C and Dossey B: Cardiovascular nursing: bodymind tapestry, St Louis, 1984, The CV Mosby Co.

Johanson B et al: Standards for critical care, ed 3, St Louis, 1988, The CV Mosby Co.

Kenner C, Guzzetta C, and Dossey B: Critical care nursing: body-mind-spirit, Boston, 1985, Little, Brown & Co.

Kim M, McFarland G, and McLane A: Pocket guide to nursing diagnoses, ed 2, St Louis, 1987, The CV Mosby Co.

Williams S and McVan B: Giving emergency care competently, ed 2, Springhouse, Pa, 1983, Springhouse Corp.

CRITICAL CARE ASSESSMENT TOOL

Name _____ Age _____ Sex _____
Address _____ Telephone _____
Significant other _____ Telephone _____
Date of admission _____ Medical diagnosis _____
Allergies _____

Nursing Diagnosis
(Potential or Altered)

COMMUNICATING ▪ A pattern involving sending messages
Read, write, understand English (circle) _____ Communication
Other languages _____ Verbal
Physical barriers to communication _____ Nonverbal
Alternate form of communication _____

VALUING ▪ A pattern involving the assigning of relative worth
Religious preference _____ Spiritual state
Important religious practices _____ Distress
Spiritual concerns _____ Despair
Cultural orientation _____
Cultural practices _____

RELATING ▪ A pattern involving establishing bonds
Role
  Marital status _____ Role performance
  Age & health of significant other _____ Parenting
  _____ Sexual dysfunction
  Number of children _____ Ages _____ Work
  Responsibilities in home _____ Family
  Financial support _____ Social/leisure
  Occupation _____ Family processes
    Job satisfaction/concerns _____
    Physical/mental energy expenditures _____
  Sexual relationships (satisfactory/unsatisfactory) _____ Sexuality patterns
    Sexual partner(s) _____
    Physical difficulties/effects of illness related to sex _____
  _____

Socialization   Socialization
  Quality of relationships with others _____ Impaired social interaction
    Patient's description _____
    Significant others' descriptions _____
    Staff observations _____
  Verbalizes feelings of being alone _____ Social isolation
  Attributed to _____ Social withdrawal

KNOWING ▪ A pattern involving the meaning associated with information
Current health problems _____
_____
Previous hospitalization/surgeries _____
_____

Fig. 12-1

History of the following diseases: Knowledge deficit

   Heart _____

   Peripheral vascular diseases _____ Thyroid _____

   Lung _____

   Liver _____ Kidney _____

   Cerebrovascular _____ Rheumatic fever _____

   Drug abuse _____ Alcoholism _____

Recent history of the following:

   Blood transfusion _____ **Trauma** _____ **CO poisoning** _____

   Heat stroke _____ **Sepsis** _____ **Muscle injury** _____

   Nephrotoxic medications _____

Current medications _____

_____

Risk factors for heart disease   Present   Perceptions/knowledge of

  1. Hypertension   _____ _____

  2. Hyperlipidemia   _____ _____

  3. Smoking   _____ _____

  4. Obesity   _____ _____

  5. Diabetes   _____ _____

  6. Sedentary living   _____ _____

  7. Stress   _____ _____

  8. Alcohol use   _____ _____

  9. Oral contraceptives   _____ _____

10. Family history _____

_____

Perception/knowledge of illness/tests/surgery _____

_____

Expectations of therapy _____

Misconceptions _____

Readiness to learn _____ Learning

   Requests information concerning _____

   Educational level _____ Thought processes

   Learning impeded by _____

Orientation

Level of alertness _____ Orientation

Orientation: Person _____ Place _____ Time _____ Confusion

Appropriate behavior/communication _____

Memory

Memory intact: Yes _____ No _____ Recent _____ Remote _____ Memory

FEELING ▪ A pattern involving the subjective awareness of information

Comfort

   Pain/discomfort: Yes _____ No _____   Comfort

     Onset _____ Duration _____

     Location _____ Quality _____ Radiation _____ Pain/Chronic

     Associated factors _____ Pain/Acute

     Aggravating factors _____ Discomfort

     Alleviating factors _____

Fig. 12-1, cont'd

Continued.

Emotional Integrity/States
Recent stressful life events _____ Anxiety
_____ Fear
Verbalizes feelings of _____ Grieving
  Source _____ Anger
_____ Guilt
Physical manifestations _____ Shame
_____ Sadness

MOVING ▪ A pattern involving activity
Activity
History of physical disability _____ Impaired physical mobility
_____ Activity intolerance
Limitations in daily activities _____
_____
Verbal report of fatigue/weakness _____
Exercise habits _____
Braces/casts/splints/traction (circle) _____
Fracture(s) _____ Extensive burns _____
Paralysis _____ Amputation(s) _____

Rest
Hours slept/night _____ Feels rested: Yes _____ No _____ Sleep pattern disturbances
Sleep aids (pillows, meds, food) _____   Hypersomnia
Difficulty falling/remaining asleep _____   Insomnia
  Nightmares

Recreation
Leisure activities _____ Deficit in diversional activity
Social activities _____

Environmental Maintenance
Home maintenance management
  Size & arrangement of home (stairs, bathroom) _____ Impaired home maintenance
  _____ Safety needs _____   management
  Home responsibilities_____ Safety hazards
_____

Health Maintenance
  Health insurance _____ Health maintenance
  Regular physical checkups _____

Self-Care
Ability to perform ADLs: Independent _____ Dependent _____ Self-care
Specify deficits _____   Feeding
Discharge planning needs _____   Bathing/hygiene
_____   Dressing/grooming
  Toileting

PERCEIVING ▪ A pattern involving the reception of information
Self-Concept
Patient's description of self _____ Self-concept
Effects of illness/surgery _____ Body image
_____ Self-esteem
  Personal identity

Meaningfulness
Verbalizes hopelessness _____ Hopelessness
Verbalizes/perceives powerlessness _____ Powerlessness

Sensory/Perception
History of restricted environment _____ Sensory/perception
Vision impaired _____ Glasses _____ Visual

Fig. 12-1, cont'd

Auditory impaired _____ Hearing aid _____ Auditory
Kinesthetics impaired _____ Kinesthetic
Gustatory impaired _____ Gustatory
Tactile impaired _____ Tactile
Olfactory impaired _____ Olfactory
Reflexes: Grossly intact _____

      Biceps   R _____ L _____   Triceps R _____ L _____
      Brachioradialis R _____ L _____   Knee   R _____ L _____
      Ankle   R _____ L _____   Plantar R _____ L _____

EXCHANGING ▪ A pattern involving mutual giving and receiving
Circulation
Cerebral
  Neurologic changes/symptoms _____ Cerebral tissue perfusion
  Seizure activity: Yes _____ No _____ Type _____ Aura _____
  Pupils   Eye Opening
    L 2 3 4 5 6 mm   None (1)
    R 2 3 4 5 6 mm   To pain (2)
    Reaction: Brisk _____   To speech (3)   Fluid volume
    Sluggish _____ Nonreactive _____   Spontaneous (4)   Deficit
                                                                 Excess

  Best Verbal   Best Motor
    No response (1)   Flaccid (1)   Cardiac output
    Incomprehensible sound (2)   Extensor response (2)
    Inappropriate words (3)   Flexor response (3)
    Confused conversation (4)   Semipurposeful (4)
    Oriented (5)   Localized to pain (5)
                            Obeys commands (6)

  Glascow Coma Scale total _____ Cerebral tissue perfusion
  Intracranial pressure _____
Cardiac
  PMI _____ Pacemaker _____ Cardiopulmonary tissue
  Apical rate & rhythm _____ perfusion
  Heart sounds/murmurs _____
  Dysrhythmias _____
  Bleeding: massive/moderate/minimal (circle)   Fluid volume
  Extravasation from burns _____ Deficit
  BP: Sitting   Lying   Standing   Excess
      R _____ L _____   R _____ L _____   R _____ L _____
  A-line reading _____
  Cardiac index _____ Cardiac output _____ Cardiac output
  CVP _____ PAP _____ PCWP _____
  IV fluids _____
  IV vasoactive medications _____

  Serum enzymes _____

Fig. 12-1, cont'd

Continued.

Peripheral   Peripheral tissue perfusion
  Jugular venous distension R _____ L _____
  Pulses: A = absent   B = bruits   D = doppler
      +3 = bounding   +2 = palpable   +1 = faintly palpable
  Carotid   R _____ L _____   Popliteal   R _____ L _____
  Brachial R _____ L _____   Posterior tibial   R _____ L _____   Fluid volume
  Radial   R _____ L _____   Dorsalis pedis   R _____ L _____   Deficit
  Femoral R _____ L _____   Excess
  Skin temp _____ Color _____
  Capillary refill _____ Clubbing _____ Cardiac output
  Edema _____

Physical Integrity
  Tissue integrity _____ Rashes _____ Lesions _____   Impaired skin integrity
    Petechiae _____ Surgical incision _____   Impaired tissue integrity
    Bruising _____ Abrasions _____   Infection
    Leakage of spinal fluid from ears/nose/other (circle) _____
    Burns: Degree _____ **Type** _____ **Location** _____
           Degree _____ **Type** _____ **Location** _____
           Degree _____ **Type** _____ **Location** _____
           Percentage of body surface area _____
    Dialysis access: Yes _____ **No** _____
      Fistula _____ **A-V Shunt** _____ **PD catheter** _____
      Central line _____
      Current condition of access _____

Oxygenation
  Complaints of dyspnea _____ Precipitated by _____
  Orthopnea _____
  Rate _____ Rhythm _____ Depth _____   Ineffective airway clearance
  Labored/unlabored (circle) Use of accessory muscles _____   Ineffective breathing patterns
  Chest expansion _____ Splinting _____   Impaired gas exchange
  Cough: productive/nonproductive _____
  Sputum: Color _____ Amount _____ Consistency _____
  Breath sounds _____
  Arterial blood gases _____
  Oxygen percent and device _____
  Ventilator _____

Physical Regulation   Infection
Immune   Hypothermia
  Lymph nodes enlarged _____ Location _____   Hyperthermia
  WBC count _____ Differential _____   Body temperature
  HIV testing results _____   Ineffective thermoregulation
  Temperature _____ Route _____

Nutrition   Nutrition
  Eating patterns
    Number of meals per day _____
    Special diet _____   Less than body requirements
    Where eaten _____   More than body
    Food preferences/intolerances _____   requirements
    Food allergies _____
    Caffeine intake (coffee, tea, soft drinks)

    Appetite changes _____
    Nausea/vomiting _____
  Condition of mouth/throat _____   Oral mucous membrane

Fig. 12-1, cont'd

Height _____ Weight _____ Ideal body wt _____

Current therapy

  NPO _____ NG suction _____

  Tube feeding _____

  TPN _____

Labs

  Na _____ K _____ CL _____

  CO_2 _____ Glucose _____

  Cholesterol _____ Triglycerides _____ Fasting _____

  Albumin _____ Total protein _____ Total lymphocyte count _____

  PT _____ PTT _____ Platelets _____ Hct _____ Hb _____

More than body requirements

Less than body requirements

Elimination

Gastrointestinal/bowel

  Usual bowel habits _____

  Alterations from normal _____

  Colostomy _____ Ileostomy _____

  Abdominal physical examination _____

  Liver: Enlarged _____ Ascites _____

  Bleeding: Gastric _____ frank _____ occult _____

           Intestinal_____ frank _____ occult _____

      Esophageal tube _____

Renal/Urinary

  Possible kidney contusion/other injury _____

  Usual urinary pattern _____

  Alterations from normal _____

  Urostomy _____ Dialysis _____

  Bladder distention _____

  Color _____ Catheter _____

  Urine output: 24 hour _____ Average hourly _____

  BUN _____ Creatinine _____ Specific gravity _____

  Urine studies _____

Bowel elimination

  Constipation

  Diarrhea

  Incontinence

GI tissue perfusion

Urinary elimination

  Incontinence

  Retention

Renal tissue perfusion

Fluid volume

  Deficit

  Excess

Cardiac output

CHOOSING ▪ A pattern involving the selection of alternatives

Coping

  Patient's usual problem-solving methods _____

  _____

  Family's usual problem-solving methods _____

  _____

  Patient's method of dealing with stress _____

  _____

  Family's method of dealing with stress _____

  _____

  Patient's affect _____

  Physical manifestations _____

  Support system available _____

Coping

Ineffective individual coping

Ineffective family coping

Participation

  Compliance with past/current health care regimens _____

  _____

  Willingness to comply with future health care regimen _____

  _____

Noncompliance

Ineffective participation

Fig. 12-1, cont'd

Continued.

Judgment

Decision-making ability   Judgment
 Patient's perspective _____ Indecisiveness
 Others' perspectives _____

Prioritized nursing diagnosis/problem list
1. _____
2. _____
3. _____
4. _____
5. _____

Signature _____ Date _____

Fig. 12-1, cont'd

CRITICAL CARE ASSESSMENT TOOL

Name *Mr. B.J.* _____ Age *40* __ Sex *MALE* _____
Address *2800 Anystreet Road   Anytown, Wa* ____ Telephone *333-8181*
Significant other *Mrs. B.J. (wife)* _____ Telephone *333-8181*
Date of admission *5/2* _____ Medical diagnosis *1st and 2nd degree burns to face, chest,*
Allergies *Penicillin* _____ *arms*

Nursing Diagnosis
(Potential or Altered)

COMMUNICATING ■ A pattern involving sending messages
(Read) (write) (understand) English (circle) _____ Communication
Other languages   *None* _____ (Verbal)
Physical barriers to communication *Facial Burns — Painful* ____ Nonverbal
Alternate form of communication *Nods yes & no* _____

VALUING ■ A pattern involving the assigning of relative worth
Religious preference *Protestant* _____ Spiritual state
Important religious practices *None* _____ Distress
Spiritual concerns *Would like to receive communion* ____ Despair
Cultural orientation *No special cultural identification* ____
Cultural practices *None* _____

RELATING ■ A pattern involving establishing bonds
Role
  Marital status *Married* _____ Role performance
  Age & health of significant other *Wife 38yrs in good health* ____ Parenting
  _____ Sexual dysfunction
  Number of children *2* __ Ages *10, 8 (John, Laura)* ____ (Work) (Potential)
  Responsibilities in home *Home repair, help discipline children* Family
  Financial support *Patient is main support; wife — parttime* __ Social/leisure
  Occupation *Computer operator* _____ Family processes
    Job satisfaction/concerns *Likes job; concerned about off time*
    Physical/mental energy expenditures *Mentally demanding job*
  Sexual relationships ((satisfactory)/unsatisfactory) _____ Sexuality patterns
    Sexual partner(s) *Wife* _____
    Physical difficulties/effects of illness related to sex *None* ____

Socialization
  Quality of relationships with others *Seem good* _____ Socialization
    Patient's description *"I get along with everybody"* ____ Impaired social interaction
    Significant others' descriptions *"Gets along well with others" (wife)*
    Staff observations *Relates well to wife and staff* ____
    Verbalizes feelings of being alone *"It's a little lonely here."* ____ (Social isolation)
    Attributed to *Restricted visiting hours* _____ Social withdrawal

KNOWING ■ A pattern involving the meaning associated with information
Current health problems *Burns to face, chest, arms* _____

Previous hospitalization/surgeries *Inguinal hernia repair 2 yrs ago* ____

Fig. 12-2

Continued.

History of the following diseases: Knowledge deficit
   Heart _No_
   Peripheral vascular diseases _No_   Thyroid _No_
   Lung _No_
   Liver _No_   Kidney _No_
   Cerebrovascular _No_   Rheumatic fever _No_
   Drug abuse _No_   Alcoholism _No_
Recent history of the following:
   Blood transfusion _No_   Trauma _No_   CO poisoning _No_
   Heat stroke _No_   Sepsis _No_   Muscle injury _No_
   Nephrotoxic medications _No_
Current medications _NONE BEFORE ADMISSION_

Risk factors for heart disease	Present	Perceptions/knowledge of
1. Hypertension		
2. Hyperlipidemia		
3. Smoking	✓	_AWARE THAT IT CAUSES LUNG CANCER_
4. Obesity		
5. Diabetes		
6. Sedentary living	✓	
7. Stress		
8. Alcohol use		
9. Oral contraceptives		
10. Family history	_FATHER DIED OF HEART ATTACK AT AGE 55_	

Perception/knowledge of illness/tests/surgery _"I HAVE BURNS ON MY FACE, ARMS AND CHEST."_
Expectations of therapy _THAT BURNS WILL HEAL_
Misconceptions _DOES NOT EXPECT TO HAVE SCARRING_
Readiness to learn _WANTS TO KNOW ABOUT TREATMENT BUT DISTRACTED_ (Learning)
   Requests information concerning _TREATMENT FOR BURNS_   _BY PAIN_
   Educational level _2 YEARS COLLEGE_   Thought processes
   Learning impeded by _CURRENT AMOUNT OF PAIN_

Orientation
Level of alertness _AWAKE, AWARE OF SURROUNDINGS, ALERT_   Orientation
Orientation: Person _YES_   Place _YES_   Time _YES_   Confusion
Appropriate behavior/communication _APPROPRIATE_

Memory
Memory intact: Yes ✓ No ____ Recent _YES_ Remote _YES_   Memory

FEELING ▪ A pattern involving the subjective awareness of information
Comfort
   Pain/discomfort: Yes ✓ No ____   Comfort
      Onset _AT TIME OF ACCIDENT_ Duration _3 HOURS_
      Location _FACE, ARMS, CHEST_ Quality _BURNING_ Radiation _No_   Pain/Chronic
      Associated factors _NONE_   (Pain/Acute)
      Aggravating factors _MOVEMENT OF INVOLVED AREAS; TALKING_   Discomfort
      Alleviating factors _DEMEROL_

Fig. 12-2, cont'd

Emotional Integrity/States
Recent stressful life events _MOVED INTO 1ST HOUSE 2 MONTHS AGO_ (Anxiety)
Fear
Verbalizes feelings of _ANXIETY_ Grieving
    Source _FINANCES — MISSING WORK BECAUSE OF INJURY,_ Anger
HOSPITAL BILLS, HOUSE PAYMENT Guilt
Physical manifestations _NONE_ Shame
Sadness

MOVING ▪ A pattern involving activity
Activity
    History of physical disability _NONE_ (Impaired physical mobility)
Activity intolerance

    Limitations in daily activities _NONE BEFORE ADMISSION_

    Verbal report of fatigue/weakness _NONE_
    Exercise habits _DOES NOT EXERCISE REGULARLY_
    Braces/casts/splints/traction (circle) _NONE_
    Fracture(s) _NONE_ Extensive burns _FACE, ARMS, CHEST_
    Paralysis _NO_ Amputation(s) _NONE_

Rest
    Hours slept/night _7 HOURS_ Feels rested: Yes _✓_ No _____ Sleep pattern disturbances
    Sleep aids (pillows, meds, food) _NONE_ Hypersomnia
    Difficulty falling/remaining asleep _NONE_ Insomnia
Nightmares

Recreation
    Leisure activities _BOWLING, WORKING IN YARD, READING PAPER_ Deficit in diversional activity
    Social activities _BOWLING LEAGUE_

Environmental Maintenance
    Home maintenance management
        Size & arrangement of home (stairs, bathroom) _3 BEDROOMS AND BATH_ (Impaired home maintenance
ON 2ND FLOOR Safety needs _NONE_ management)
        Home responsibilities _HOME REPAIR, YARD WORK, PAY BILLS_ Safety hazards

Health Maintenance
    Health insurance _BLUE CROSS BLUE SHIELD_ Health maintenance
    Regular physical checkups _NO_

Self-Care
    Ability to perform ADLs: Independent _____   Dependent _✓_ (Self-care)
    Specify deficits _CANNOT HOLD UTENSELS TO EAT, CANNOT BATHE SELF_ (Feeding)
    Discharge planning needs _LEARN BURN CARE_ (Bathing/hygiene)
Dressing/grooming
Toileting

PERCEIVING ▪ A pattern involving the reception of information
Self-Concept
    Patient's description of self _"SUCCESSFUL" "GOOD HUSBAND"_ Self-concept
    Effects of illness/surgery _CONCERNED ABOUT APPEARANCE; DOESN'T_ (Body image)
LIKE TO BE DEPENDENT ON OTHERS (Self-esteem)
Personal identity

Meaningfulness
    Verbalizes hopelessness _NO_ Hopelessness
    Verbalizes/perceives powerlessness _NO_ Powerlessness

Sensory/Perception
    History of restricted environment _CURRENTLY IN ICU_ Sensory/perception
    Vision impaired _YES_ Glasses _FOR READING ONLY_ Visual

Fig. 12-2, cont'd

Continued.

Auditory impaired _No_   Hearing aid _No_   Auditory
Kinesthetics impaired _No_   Kinesthetic
Gustatory impaired _No_   Gustatory
Tactile impaired _INCREASED SENSATION IN FACE, ARMS, CHEST_   (Tactile)
Olfactory impaired _YES "EVERYTHING SMELLS BURNED"_   (Olfactory)
Reflexes: Grossly intact _✓_

Biceps	R ____	L ____	Triceps	R ____	L ____
Brachioradialis	R ____	L ____	Knee	R ____	L ____
Ankle	R ____	L ____	Plantar	R ____	L ____

EXCHANGING ▪ A pattern involving mutual giving and receiving
Circulation
Cerebral

Neurologic changes/symptoms _NONE_   Cerebral tissue perfusion
Seizure activity: Yes ____ No _✓_ Type _____ Aura _____

Pupils   Eye Opening
L (2) 3 4 5 6 mm   None (1)
R (2) 3 4 5 6 mm   To pain (2)
Reaction: Brisk _✓_   To speech (3)   Fluid volume
Sluggish ____ Nonreactive ____   Spontaneous (4)   Deficit
    Excess

Best Verbal   Best Motor
No response (1)   Flaccid (1)   Cardiac output
Incomprehensible sound (2)   Extensor response (2)
Inappropriate words (3)   Flexor response (3)
Confused conversation (4)   Semipurposeful (4)
Oriented (5)   Localized to pain (5)
    Obeys commands (6)

Glasgow Coma Scale total _15_   Cerebral tissue perfusion
Intracranial pressure _N/A_

Cardiac
PMI _5TH INTERCOSTAL MIDCLAVICU-LAR_ Pacemaker _No_   Cardiopulmonary tissue
Apical rate & rhythm _85; NORMAL SINUS RHYTHM_   perfusion
Heart sounds/murmurs _S_1 & S_2_
Dysrhythmias _NONE_
Bleeding: massive/moderate/minimal (circle)   (Fluid volume
Extravasation from burns _MODERATE AMT. SEROSANG. FROM ARMS & CHEST_   Deficit)
    Excess

BP: Sitting   Lying   Standing
   R _100/80_ _100/80_   R _120/80_ L _120/80_   R _N/A_ L _N/A_
A-line reading _105/80 SITTING_
Cardiac index _4.0_   Cardiac output _8.8_   Cardiac output
CVP _2 mmHg_ PAP _12/4 mmHg_ PCWP _4 mmHg_
IV fluids _RINGER'S LACTATE @ 662 cc/HR_
IV vasoactive medications _NONE_

Serum enzymes _N/A_

Fig. 12-2, cont'd

Peripheral   Peripheral tissue perfusion

Jugular venous distension R _NO_ L _No_

Pulses: A = absent   B = bruits   D = doppler

+3 = bounding   +2 = palpable   +1 = faintly palpable

Carotid R _+2_ L _+2_   Popliteal   R _+2_ L _+2_

Brachial R _+2_ L _+2_   Posterior tibial   R _+2_ L _+2_   Fluid volume

Radial R _+2_ L _+2_   Dorsalis pedis   R _+2_ L _+2_   Deficit

Femoral R _+2_ L _+2_   Excess

Skin temp _WARM_   Color _LIGHTLY TANNED_

Capillary refill _INSTANTANEOUS_ Clubbing _No_   Cardiac output

Edema _SMALL AMOUNT IN HANDS AND FACE; NOT PITTING_

Physical Integrity

Tissue integrity _BURNS_   Rashes _NONE_   Lesions _NONE_   (Impaired skin integrity)

Petechiae _NONE_   Surgical incision _NONE_   (Impaired tissue integrity)

Bruising _NONE_   Abrasions _NONE_   Infection   (POTENTIAL)

Leakage of spinal fluid from ears/nose/other (circle) _No_   (POTENTIAL)

Burns: Degree _1 ST_   Type _THERMAL_   Location _FACE, UPPER ARMS_

Degree _2 ND_   Type _THERMAL_   Location _FACE, UPPER ARMS_

Degree _2 ND_   Type _THERMAL_   Location _CHEST_

Percentage of body surface area _31.5 %_

Dialysis access: Yes _____ No ✓

Fistula _____ A-V Shunt _____ PD catheter _____

Central line _____

Current condition of access _N/A_

Oxygenation

Complaints of dyspnea _NONE_   Precipitated by _____

Orthopnea _No_

Rate _16_   Rhythm _REGULAR_   Depth _MODERATE_   Ineffective airway clearance

Labored (unlabored) (circle) Use of accessory muscles _No_   Ineffective breathing patterns

Chest expansion _EQUAL_   Splinting _MINIMAL_   Impaired gas exchange

Cough: (productive) nonproductive _CLEAR SPUTUM_

Sputum: Color _SAME AS ABOVE_ Amount _SMALL_   Consistency _THIN_

Breath sounds _CLEAR THROUGHOUT VESICULAR_

Arterial blood gases _pH 7.42, Pco$_2$ 38mm Hg, Po$_2$ 95mm Hg, HCO$_3$ 22mM, O SAT 99%_

Oxygen percent and device _ROOM AIR FOR ABG's_

Ventilator _No_

Physical Regulation   (Infection) (POTENTIAL)

Immune   Hypothermia

Lymph nodes enlarged _No_   Location _____   Hyperthermia

WBC count _15 x 10^3/μL_ Differential _NEUTROPHILS 85%, LYMPHOCYTES 10%_   Body temperature

HIV testing results _NOT DONE_   Ineffective thermoregulation

Temperature _37.5 °C_   Route _RECTAL_

Nutrition   Nutrition

Eating patterns

Number of meals per day _3_

Special diet _NONE_   Less than body requirements

Where eaten _BREAKFAST AND DINNER AT HOME_   More than body requirements

Food preferences/intolerances _NONE_

Food allergies _NONE_

Caffeine intake (coffee, tea, soft drinks)

2 CUPS CAFFEINATED COFFEE IN AM, COLA AT LUNCH

Appetite changes _NONE BEFORE ADMISSION; DECREASED AT PRESENT_

Nausea/vomiting _No_

Fig. 12-2, cont'd

Condition of mouth/throat *LIPS HAVE MANY BLISTERS FROM BURNS,*   Oral mucous membrane
INSIDE OF MOUTH GOOD CONDITION, TEETH IN GOOD REPAIR

Height *5'11"*   Weight *185 lbs*   Ideal body wt *172 lbs*   More than body
                                                   requirements
Current therapy

  NPO *N/A*   NG suction *N/A*   (Less than body requirements)

  Tube feeding *N/A*   (POTENTIAL)

  TPN *N/A*

Labs

  Na *140 mEq/L*   K *4.5 mEq/L*   CL *105 mEq/L*

  CO_2 *22 mM*   Glucose *105 mg/dl*

  Cholesterol *200 mg/dl*   Triglycerides *185 mg/dl*   Fasting *YES*

  Albumin *40 g/dl*   Total protein *8.0 g/dl*   Total lymphocyte count *NOT DONE*

  PT *12 SEC*   PTT *60 SEC*   Platelets *300,000/*   Hct *45%*   Hb *16 g/dl*
                                        μL

Elimination

Gastrointestinal/bowel   Bowel elimination

  Usual bowel habits *1 TIME/DAY*   Constipation

  Alterations from normal *NONE AT PRESENT*   Diarrhea

  Colostomy *No*   Ileostomy *No*   Incontinence

  Abdominal physical examination *ACTIVE BOWEL SOUNDS, Abd. SOFT, NONTENDER*

  Liver: Enlarged *No*   Ascites *No*   GI tissue perfusion

  Bleeding: Gastric *No*   frank ___ occult _____

              Intestinal *No*   frank ___ occult _____

              Esophageal tube *No*

Renal/Urinary

  Possible kidney contusion/other injury *No*

  Usual urinary pattern *5-6 TIMES/DAY*   Urinary elimination

  Alterations from normal *NONE*   Incontinence

  Urostomy *No*   Dialysis *No*

  Bladder distention *No*   Retention

  Color *CLEAR AMBER* Catheter *FOLEY #16 FRENCH 5cc BALLOON*

  Urine output: 24 hour *UNKNOWN*   Average hourly *50cc/HR*   Renal tissue perfusion

  BUN *25 mg/dl*   Creatinine *N/A*   Specific gravity *1.038*   (Fluid volume)

  Urine studies *GLUCOSE & ACETONE - NEGATIVE, BLOOD - NEGATIVE*   (Deficit)
                                                             Excess
                                                             Cardiac output

CHOOSING ▪ A pattern involving the selection of alternatives

Coping

                                                            Coping

  Patient's usual problem-solving methods *TALK WITH FAMILY (WIFE,*   Ineffective individual coping

  PARENTS)   Ineffective family coping

  Family's usual problem-solving methods *TALK IT OVER*

  Patient's method of dealing with stress *TRY TO SOLVE THE PROBLEM;*

  TRY TO RELAX BY WATCHING TV

  Family's method of dealing with stress *PATIENT & WIFE TALK ABOUT*

  PROBLEMS. NO SPECIFIC STRESS RELIEVING MEASURES

  Patient's affect *ANXIOUS*

  Physical manifestations *—*

  Support system available *WIFE, PATIENT'S PARENTS*

Participation

  Compliance with past/current health care regimens *COOPERATIVE AT*   Noncompliance

  PRESENT; NO PAST SERIOUS ILLNESS   Ineffective participation

  Willingness to comply with future health care regimen *SEEMS WILLING*

Fig. 12-2, cont'd

Judgment

   Decision-making ability   Judgment

      Patient's perspective *THINKS HE HAS GOOD JUDGMENT*   Judgment

      Others' perspectives *WIFE HAS CONFIDENCE IN PATIENT'S JUDGMENT*   Indecisiveness

Prioritized nursing diagnosis/problem list

1. *ACUTE PAIN RELATED TO BURNS*
2. *FLUID VOLUME DEFICIT RELATED TO BURNS*
3. *IMPAIRED SKIN INTEGRITY RELATED TO SECOND-DEGREE BURNS*
4. *POTENTIAL FOR INFECTION RELATED TO LOSS OF SKIN INTEGRITY (BURNS)*
5. *ANXIETY RELATED TO FINANCIAL CONCERNS (LOSS OF WORK, HOSPITAL COST)*

Signature *Linda A. Prinkey, RN*   Date *5/2*

Fig. 12-2, cont'd

CHAPTER 13

PERIOPERATIVE ASSESSMENT TOOL

PATRICIA C. SEIFERT
JANE C. ROTHROCK

The Perioperative Assessment Tool is designed to assess adult surgical patients with unique biopsychosocial assessment needs. It is divided into three sections and incorporates signs and symptoms pertinent to the perioperative patient to facilitate identification of nursing diagnoses during the preoperative, intraoperative, and postoperative periods. It also incorporates the American Nurses' Association and Association of Operating Room Nurses' *Standards of Perioperative Nursing Practice*. This chapter includes:

- *The way the tool was developed and refined*
- *The patient populations and settings to which it applies*
- *Selected perioperative emphasis areas*
- *The way to use the tool*
- *Specific perioperative focus questions and parameters to assist the nurse in eliciting appropriate data*
- *The Perioperative Assessment Tool*
- *A case study*
- *A completed version of the tool based on the case study*

DEVELOPMENT AND REFINEMENT OF THE TOOL

The Perioperative Assessment Tool demonstrates that assessment and nursing diagnosis are essential elements of perioperative nursing practice. It follows the standards for patient assessment, including level of consciousness, emotional status, and baseline physical data. The tool makes it clear that perioperative nurses are interested in and need knowledge about many patient parameters in planning and giving care.

The tool was developed from the nursing data base prototype (see Chapter 2). Some hemodynamic monitoring and critical care variables originally incorporated into the prototype were deleted and replaced with variables more applicable to perioperative assessment. In addition, the tool was divided into three parts, a preoperative phase, an intraoperative phase, and a postoperative phase. The preoperative phase incorporates all nine human response patterns (see Chapter 2) and enables the perioperative nurse to anticipate or confirm patient problems. Information collected preoperatively can be used to plan intraoperative and postoperative care. The variable, perioperative implications, follows each pattern to help the nurse focus on specific concerns. The intraoperative and postoperative sections build on data collected preoperatively and include patterns and variables for assessing patients during these periods. The resultant tool was modified based on the recommendations of perioperative nurse experts. The tool's content is supported by the current literature from this field of nursing.

After being developed and refined, the tool was clinically tested on 10 patients by perioperative nurse experts and clinical nurse specialists. The tool was tested on inpatients and outpatients, many of whom were chronically ill with acute exacerbations of previous problems or development of new problems. The testing evaluated the tool's adequacy in terms of flow, space for recording data, and completeness of assessment variables. Based on the results, the tool was revised.

PATIENT POPULATION AND SETTING

The Perioperative Assessment Tool was developed to assess the needs and problems of patients undergoing surgery who may have multisystem problems, but it can also be used for patients undergoing relatively minor surgical procedures and who are otherwise healthy.

The tool is versatile and can be used in the hospital or the ambulatory care setting. Information about chronic problems to be referred to primary nurses on the hospital unit or home health nurses for follow-up care during discharge planning may be elicited. For example, inpatients may have special neurologic or cardiac problems, whereas outpatients may benefit from assistance to help them comply with prescribed regimens. If the patient is disoriented, the family or significant other may provide necessary data.

PERIOPERATIVE EMPHASIS AREAS

Perioperative patients have specialized problems and needs. The Perioperative Assessment Tool includes appropriate assessment variables within each of the nine human response patterns of the Unitary Person Framework. Table 13-1 outlines these emphasis areas for each phase of the perioperative experience.

HOW TO USE THE TOOL

To use the Perioperative Assessment Tool effectively, nurses must first familiarize themselves with the Unitary Person Framework (see Chapter 2), which provides the underlying framework for Taxonomy I. The nine human response patterns of the Unitary Person Framework serve as the major category headings for Taxonomy I and the assessment tool. The sequence of the response patterns, as it appears in Taxonomy I, has been changed in the tool to permit a logical ordering of assessment variables. Nursing diagnoses pertinent to the perioperative patient, along with the signs and symptoms necessary to identify them, are incorporated under the appropriate human response patterns. The tool is divided into three phases. Diagnoses may be elicited in each phase and recorded at the end of each section.

Nurses must also realize that this tool is very different from conventional assessment tools. As a result, nurses may encounter some initial difficulty in using it. They should remember, however, that the tool was not designed to follow the organization or content of a traditional medical data base; the data collected do not solely reflect medical patterns. Rather, the tool elicits data about holistic patterns in ways not traditionally assessed by nurses. It provides a new method of collecting and synthesizing data and requires new thinking when processing data. This tool represents a nursing data base developed from a nursing model that permits a holistic nursing assessment to take place so nursing diagnoses can be identified.

Although nurses probably agree that a holistic nursing data base is desirable, it is realized that changing tradi-

tional assessment methods is not an easy task. For this reason, a trial usage period is recommended before any decisions about the tool's merits are made. During this trial period, the nurse should assess 10 surgical patients using the tool to become familiar and progressively more comfortable with its organization and data-collection methods. With experience, nurses will become accustomed to new ways of clustering and processing information. With continued use, the time necessary to complete the tool will be reduced. Most important, nurses will recognize the unique ability of the tool to elicit appropriate signs and symptoms. Nurses will discover that nursing diagnoses are easily identified when using this tool.

It is not necessary to complete the tool in one session. Priority sections can be completed during the initial assessment. Other sections or patterns can be completed later, within a time frame acceptable to the institution. To elicit appropriate data, nurses should be familiar with the focus questions and parameters in the next section. When assessing specific signs and symptoms that indicate a diagnosis, the nurse circles the diagnosis in the right-hand column when deviations from normal are found. A circled diagnosis does not confirm a problem but simply alerts the nurse to the possibility that it exists. After completing the tool, the nurse scans the circled problems, synthesizes the data to determine whether other clusters of signs and symptoms support a problem, and judges whether the actual or potential diagnosis is present.

Some diagnoses are repeated several times in the right-hand column. These repetitions occur only within the appropriate response pattern and are convenient for identifying data directly with their corresponding nursing diagnoses. These diagnoses are not absolute but are intended to focus thinking and direct detailed attention to a possible problem.

Some signs and symptoms can indicate several diagnoses. For example, fever can indicate infection and ineffective thermoregulation. To avoid unnecessary repetition of assessment parameters, variables are arranged with the diagnosis most likely to result from the data assessed. Thus, data to support one diagnosis may occasionally be found in other patterns or arranged with other diagnoses. Therefore, synthesis of all data is essential.

The Perioperative Assessment Tool is not intended to be the standardized and final format for assessment of patients across the country. An assessment tool must meet the needs of the institutions and nurses using it. The tool is simply a working demonstration tool that is expected to be changed and revised by nurses in clinical practice. Further evaluation and refinement are necessary before adapting the tool for use within an institution. Nurses interested in changing, revising, and adapting the tool to a specific clinical setting should refer to Chapter 4.

Text continued on p. 204.

Table 13-1
Selected perioperative emphasis areas

Patterns	Emphasis areas to determine
PREOPERATIVE	
Communicating	Ability to read, write, and understand English
	Physical deformities
Valuing	Religious or cultural preferences
Relating	Preference for being alone or with family or with friends
Knowing	Current health problems
	Transfusion and transfusion reaction
	History of bleeding problems, hepatitis, or HIV
	Risk factors
	Surgical consent
	Blood ordered
	Level of alertness
Feeling	Pain or discomfort
	Verbalized feelings such as anxiety, fear, or shame
Moving	Arthritis, back pain, prosthetic devices, or muscle weakness
Perceiving	Sensory/perceptual status
Exchanging	Neurologic and cardiac status
	Skin integrity
	Proposed incision site
	Immune system: WBC, Hct, Hgb, and steroid therapy
	Nausea or vomiting
	Condition of mouth and teeth, dentures, bridges, or plates
	Laboratory information: electrolyte levels and coagulation studies
	Renal perfusion, bladder distension, or hemodialysis
Choosing	Patient's affect
	Compliance with health care regimen
INTRAOPERATIVE	
(General information)	Wound classification
Knowing	Preoperative and postoperative diagnosis
	Procedure
Feeling	Comfort
Moving	Positioning
Exchanging	Circulation
	Physical integrity
	Implants
	Counts: sponges, needles, and instruments
	Oxygenation
	Medications
	Patient status
POSTOPERATIVE	
Knowing	Knowledge of incisional care, complications, and symptoms to report
	Need for referral
Feeling	Pain or discomfort
Moving	Discharge planning needs
Perceiving	Effects of surgery on self-concept
Exchanging	Skin integrity
	Deep breathing and coughing
	Physical regulation
Choosing	Coping
	Participation and compliance

Table 13-2
Perioperative assessment tool: focus questions and parameters

Variables	Focus questions and parameters
Preoperative	
COMMUNICATING	
Read, write, understand English	Assess the patient's ability to communicate. If needed, is a translator available (before and after surgery)?
Physical deformity	Does the patient have a physical deformity that impairs communication?
VALUING	
Religious preference and cultural practices	Has a specific spiritual leader been requested? Has the patient requested to keep certain religious items (rosary)?
	Is it a cultural practice to have family and friends nearby?
	Are important cultural meanings attached to limbs or to the disposition of body parts?
RELATING	
Prefers to be alone/with family/with friends	Does the patient prefer to be alone, or with a family member or friend?
	Where will the family and significant other be during surgery?
KNOWING	
Current health problems	"Tell me why you are having surgery. Where?"
Previous transfusion/transfusion reaction	"Have you ever had a blood transfusion? Any reactions?"
History of the following problems	Do you have a history of HIV, hepatitis, malignant hyperthermia, anesthetic reaction, or prolonged recovery time?
Risk factors	Is the patient obese or diabetic or have a coagulapathic condition?
Surgical consent signed	"What has your surgeon told you about your surgery? Do you have any questions?"
Blood/blood products ordered	Determine the blood or blood products available.
Level of alertness	Is the patient alert, lethargic, or comatose?
FEELING	
Pain/discomfort	"Are you in pain? Where?"
	Are there nonverbal indicators of pain such as shallow breathing, guarding, or grimacing?
Verbalizes feelings of anxiety/fear	Does the patient demonstrate muscle tension, pallor, or increased pulse or respiration?
	Does the patient verbalize anxiety or fear regarding the surgery or outcome?
MOVING	
Limitations in daily activities	Does the patient have arthritis, back pain, prosthetic devices, or muscle weakness that will affect positioning or transferring to the OR bed?
PERCEIVING	
Sensory/perception	Are any of the patient's senses impaired?
	Have eye glasses, hearing aids, or other items been placed in a safe location?
EXCHANGING	
Neurologic and cardiac changes/symptoms	Are there any neurologic deficits that may affect positioning, or increase the potential for nerve or pressure injury?
	Does the patient have cardiovascular disease that might pose a risk under anesthesia?
Skin integrity	Assess the skin for scars, cuts, bruises, cysts, pimples, and abrasions; note color and warmth.
	What is the condition of the skin at the pressure sites of the planned surgical position? At the site of the electrocautery grounding pad?
	What invasive lines have been or will be inserted?
	"Are you allergic to any cleansing agents?"

Continued

Table 13-2—cont'd

Perioperative assessment tool: focus questions and parameters

Variables	Focus questions and parameters
EXCHANGING—cont'd	
Proposed incision site	Assess the condition of the proposed incision site.
Immune status	Is the patient at risk for infection?
	Does the patient have a cold or symptoms of a cold?
Nausea/vomiting	Does the patient complain of nausea or indicate that nausea or vomiting occurred after a previous surgery?
Condition of mouth/throat and teeth	Does the patient wear dentures? Have they been placed in a safe location? Missing teeth? Loose or chipped teeth?
Labs	Are the patient's electrolyte levels within normal limits? Are coagulation studies normal?
Renal/urinary	Has the patient voided recently? Is a urinary catheter ordered?
	Is the patient on renal dialysis? Where is the shunt or fistula?
CHOOSING	
Patient's affect	What is the patient's affect? Is it appropriate or inappropriate (i.e., extreme anger or euphoria) to the situation?
Compliance with past/current health care regimens	Will the surgery impose physical or emotional limits on the patient's ability to comply with the anticipated therapeutic regimen?
	Will the patient or family require referral to a home health agency?
	Will the patient under local anesthesia be able to comply with intraoperative instructions? (Assess patient's need to retain glasses or hearing aid.)
Intraoperative **(GENERAL INFORMATION)**	
Wound class	Does the wound class predispose the patient to a postoperative infection?
KNOWING	
Preoperative and postoperative diagnoses	What is the patient's understanding of the problem? Is it confirmed by the diagnosis and informed consent?
Procedure	Does the patient confirm the procedure posted?
FEELING	
Comfort	Is the patient uncomfortable before induction?
	For cases using local anesthetic: Is the patient in pain? What comfort measures (pillows, warm blankets, imagery techniques, or religious items) can be provided?
	Is more local anesthetic indicated? Does the patient verbalize pain at the incision site?
MOVING	
Positioning	Is the position appropriate for the procedure?
	Is adequate padding provided to prevent nerve injury? Are pressure areas protected?
EXCHANGING	
Circulation	Assess the patient's circulatory status, including BP, intraarterial pressure, capillary refill, skin color, temperature, ECG, and heart rate.
	Assess blood loss in suction cannisters, on sponges, and in drapes. What was the preoperative hematocrit?
Physical integrity	Assess skin integrity at site of the grounding pad, ECG leads, invasive lines, tourniquet site, and incision site.
	"Do you have any allergies to medications or (irrigating or cleansing) solutions?"
Implants/prostheses	Note the manufacturer, model, lot, serial number, size, and implant site. Is appropriate paperwork completed to ensure follow up?
Counts	Account for all surgical items to avoid the possibility of a retained foreign object or infection.

Table 13-2—cont'd

Perioperative assessment tool: focus questions and parameters

Variables	Focus questions and parameters
EXCHANGING—cont'd	
Oxygenation	Is the patient's airway patent? Are laboratory results within normal limits? Does positioning allow for optimum oxygenation?
Medications	Are there any allergies to medications used during surgery?
Patient status	Is the patient's status stable or unstable on entering and leaving the OR? Are there special concerns such as history of nausea and vomiting, laryngospasm, or malignant hyperthermia related to recovery?

Postoperative
KNOWING

Knowledge of	
Care of incision site	Assess patient's knowledge and understanding of incision care.
Potential complications	Assess patient's knowledge and understanding of complications.
	"Can you tell me what you should look for to be sure you're healing properly?"
Symptoms to report	"Can you describe what changes (in your incision and in how you feel) that you should report?"
Need for referral	Is there a need for follow-up wound care or dressing change?

FEELING

Pain/discomfort	Does pain interfere with deep breathing and coughing, ambulation, or exercises?
	Does the patient know how to splint the incision site?

MOVING

Discharge planning needs	"Is there someone to help you at home?"
	Assess the need for transportation, special devices, and home health referrals.

PERCEIVING

Effects of surgery on self-concept	"How do you feel about yourself now that your surgery is over? How do you think you'll feel 6 months from now?"

EXCHANGING

Skin integrity	Is there evidence of tenderness, redness, swelling, or drainage at the incision site?
	What is the appearance of the skin at the site of grounding pad, ECG leads, and pressure areas?
	Is there evidence of nerve injury?
Ability to deep breathe and cough	Is the patient able to deep breathe and cough?
	Are breath sounds clear?
	What are the results of pulmonary function studies?
Physical regulation	Is the patient's temperature elevated? WBC elevated?
	Is there evidence of infection?

CHOOSING

Coping	What is the patient's affect?
	Do family members and significant others verbalize or demonstrate concern or anxiety over their ability to care for the patient? What assistance is available?
Participation	Does the patient verbalize a willingness to comply with the prescribed regimen?
	Does the patient understand the discharge instructions?
	Does the patient have telephone numbers for health care professionals?

HOW TO ELICIT APPROPRIATE DATA

Because the Unitary Person Framework and the Perioperative Assessment Tool contain some terms that may be unfamiliar to nurses, specific perioperative focus questions and parameters were developed and refined to elicit appropriate information. These questions and parameters are in Table 13-2, which follows the content of the tool (Fig. 13-1). The variables in bold type in the tool are described more fully in Table 13-2. For example, in the preoperative section the skin integrity variable under the "exchanging pattern" is in bold type; if the nurse does not know what parameters to assess for skin integrity, Table 13-2 can be used to focus the assessment. The questions and parameters provide clarity and guidance in eliciting data and are not all inclusive. Nurses should not feel limited by them because there are many other ways, based on the patient's situation and condition and the nurse's skill, to elicit the information. Questions and parameters for other data were presented in Chapter 3.

CASE STUDY

The case study models the process a nurse uses when assessing a patient. Based on the clustering of information obtained during assessment, the nurse formulates nursing diagnoses.

Mrs. B.J. was admitted to the hospital the afternoon before her scheduled cholangiogram, cholecystectomy, and possible common bile duct exploratory surgery. She is 47 years old and lives with her husband. The Perioperative Assessment Tool (Fig. 13-2) was used to assess Mrs. B.J.

BIBLIOGRAPHY

American Nurses' Association and Association of Operating Room Nurses: Standards of perioperative nursing practice, Kansas City, Mo, 1981, ANA, Inc.

AORN: AORN standards and recommended practices for perioperative nursing, Denver, 1987, AORN.

Atkinson LJ and Kohn ML: Introduction to operating room technique, New York, 1986, McGraw-Hill Inc.

Corbett JV: Laboratory tests and diagnostic procedures with nursing diagnoses, East Norwalk, Conn, 1987, Appleton & Lange.

Fox V and Blue MR: Job analysis: National Certification Board: Perioperative Nursing, Inc., document, AORN 47(5):1256, 1988.

Gruendemann BJ and Meeker MH: Care of the patient in surgery, St Louis, 1987, The CV Mosby Co.

Kneedler JA and Dodge GH: Perioperative patient care, Boston, 1987, Blackwell Scientific Publications, Inc.

Rothrock JC: The RN first assistant: an expanded perioperative nursing role, Philadelphia, 1987, JB Lippincott Co.

Taylor CML and Cress SS: Nursing diagnosis cards, Springhouse, Pa, 1986, Springhouse Corp.

PERIOPERATIVE ASSESSMENT TOOL

Name _____ Age _____ Sex _____
Address _____ Telephone _____
Significant other _____ Telephone _____
Date of admission _____ Medical diagnosis _____
Allergies _____
Planned surgical intervention _____
Anticipated length of surgery _____
Wound classification _____
Informed consent _____

Preoperative Phase

Nursing Diagnosis
(Potential or Altered)

COMMUNICATING ▪ A pattern involving sending messages
Read, write, understand English (circle) _____ Communication
Other languages _____ Verbal
Intubated _____ Speech impaired _____ Nonverbal
Physical deformities (jaws wired, cleft palate) _____
Alternate form of communication _____
Perioperative implications _____

VALUING ▪ A pattern involving the assigning of relative worth
Religious preference _____ Spiritual state
Name of minister, priest, rabbi _____ Distress
Cultural practices _____ Dispair
Perioperative implications _____

RELATING ▪ A pattern involving establishing bonds
Role
  Marital status _____ Role performance
  Age & health of significant other _____ Parenting
  _____ Sexual dysfunction
  Number of children _____ Ages _____
  Role in home _____
  Financial support _____
  Occupation _____ Family processes
    Job satisfaction/concerns _____

Socialization
  Social relationships: functional/dysfunctional (circle) Impaired social interaction
  Perfers to be alone/with family/with friends (circle)
  Perioperative implications _____

KNOWING ▪ A pattern involving the meaning associated with information
Current health problems _____
_____
Are you or could you be pregnant? _____
Current medications _____
_____
Previous illnesses/hospitalizations/surgeries (list dates) _____
_____
Previous transfusion/transfusion reaction: _____

Fig. 13-1

Continued.

History of the following problems (specify self or family):　　　　　Knowledge deficit

Heart _____ Rheumatic fever _____

Peripheral vascular _____ Cerebrovascular _____

Lung _____ Kidney _____

Liver _____ Hepatitis _____

Thyroid _____ Cancer _____

Human immunodeficiency virus _____

Other _____

Risk factors	Present	Perceptions/knowledge of
1. Hypertension	_____	_____
2. Hyperlipidemia	_____	_____
3. Smoking	_____	_____
4. Obesity	_____	_____
5. Diabetes	_____	_____
6. Sedentary living	_____	_____
7. Stress	_____	_____
8. Alcohol use	_____	_____
9. Oral contraceptives	_____	_____
10. Bleeding	_____	_____
11. Family history		_____

_____

Perceptions/expectations of surgery _____

_____

_____

Misconceptions _____

Readiness to learn _____

　　Educational level _____　　Thought processes

　　Learning impeded by _____

Surgical consent signed: Yes _____ No _____

Blood/blood products ordered: Yes _____ No _____ Number of units _____

Orientation

Level of alertness _____　　Orientation

Orientation: Person _____ Place _____ Time _____　　Confusion

Appropriate behavior/communication _____

Memory

Memory intact: Yes _____ No _____ Recent _____ Remote _____　　Memory

Perioperative implications _____

FEELING ▪ A pattern involving the subjective awareness of information

Comfort

Pain/discomfort: Yes _____ No _____

　　Onset _____ Duration _____　　Comfort

　　Location _____ Quality _____ Radiation _____　　Pain/chronic

　　Associated factors _____　　Pain/acute

　　Aggravating factors _____　　Discomfort

　　Alleviating factors _____

Emotional Integrity/States

　　Recent stressful life events _____　　Grieving

　　_____　　Anxiety

　　Verbalizes feelings of _____　　Fear

　　　　Source _____　　Anger

　　　　_____　　Guilt

　　Physical manifestations _____　　Shame

　　Perioperative implications _____　　Sadness

Fig. 13-1, cont'd

MOVING ▪ A pattern involving activity
Activity
  Limitations in daily activities _____
    Related to: Arthritis _____ Back pain _____
      Prosthetic devices _____ Muscle weakness _____
      Fatigue _____ Other _____
    Exercise habits _____

Activity intolerance
Impaired physical mobility

Self-Care
  Ability to perform ADLs independently: Yes _____ No _____
  Specify deficits _____
  Discharge planning needs _____

Self-care
  Feeding
  Bathing/hygiene
  Dressing/grooming
  Toileting

Rest
  Hours slept/night _____ Feels rested: yes/no
  Difficulty falling/remaining asleep _____
  Sleep aids (pillows, meds, food) _____

Sleep pattern disturbance
Insomnia
Hypersomnia
Nightmares

Recreation
  Leisure activities _____
  Social activities _____

Deficit in diversional activity

Health Maintenance
  Health insurance _____
  Regular physical checkups _____

Health maintenance

Environmental Maintenance
  Home maintenance management
    Size & arrangement of home (stairs, bathroom) _____
    _____ Safety needs _____
    Housekeeping responsibilities _____
    _____
    Perioperative implications _____

Impaired home maintenance
  management
Safety hazards

PERCEIVING ▪ A pattern involving the reception of information
Self-Concept
  Verbalizes change in feeling about self due to: Diagnosis _____
    Illness _____ Surgery _____ Other _____
    _____

Body image
Self-esteem
Personal identity

Sensory/Perception
  Vision impaired _____ Glasses _____
  Auditory impaired _____ Hearing aid _____
  Kinesthetics impaired _____
  Gustatory impaired _____
  Tactile impaired _____
  Olfactory impaired _____
  Reflexes: grossly intact _____

Visual
Auditory
Kinesthetic
Gustatory
Tactile
Olfactory

Meaningfulness
Verbalizes hopelessness/powerlessness (circle)
_____

Hopelessness
Powerlessness

Perioperative implications _____

EXCHANGING ▪ A pattern involving mutual giving and receiving
Circulation
  Cerebral (circle appropriate response)
    Neurologic changes/symptoms (headaches/seizures/convulsions/blackouts)
    _____

Cerebral tissue perfusion

Fig. 13-1, cont'd

Continued.

Pupils
    Reaction: Brisk _____
    Sluggish _____ Nonreactive _____

Eye Opening
    No response (1)
    To pain (2)
    To speech (3)
    Spontaneous (4)

Cerebral tissue perfusion

Best Verbal
    No response (1)
    Incomprehensible sound (2)
    Inappropriate words (3)
    Confused conversation (4)
    Oriented (5)

Best Motor
    Flaccid (1)
    Extensor response (2)
    Flexor response (3)
    Semipurposeful (4)
    Localized to pain (5)
    Obeys commands (6)

Glasgow Coma Scale total _____

Cardiac
    Apical rate & rhythm _____
    Heart sounds/murmurs _____
    Pacemaker: Yes _____ No _____ Type _____
    BP: Reading _____ Location _____
    IV fluids/medications _____ Location _____
    Invasive monitoring: CVP _____ Swan-Ganz _____
        A-line _____ Other _____

Cardiopulmonary tissue
  perfusion
Fluid volume
  Deficit
  Excess

Peripheral
    Pulses: A = absent   B = bruits   D = doppler
        +3 = bounding   +2 = palpable   +1 = faintly palpable
        Location _____ Side _____
    Skin temp _____ Color _____
    Edema _____ Capillary refill _____

Peripheral tissue perfusion
Fluid volume
  Deficit
  Excess
Cardiac output

Physical Integrity
Skin integrity _____ Rashes _____ Lesions _____
    Petechiae _____ Bruises _____
    Abrasions _____ Scars _____
    Proposed incision site _____

Impaired skin integrity
Impaired tissue integrity
Injury
Infection

Oxygenation
    Complaints of dyspnea _____ Precipitated by _____
    Respiratory rate _____ Rhythm _____ Depth _____
    Labored/unlabored (circle)
    Use of accessory muscles _____
    Cough: productive/nonproductive _____
    Breath sounds _____
    Pulmonary function studies _____
    Last chest x-ray study _____
    Tracheostomy/endotracheal tube _____
    Ventilator _____

Impaired gas exchange
Ineffective airway clearance
Ineffective breathing patterns

Physical Regulation
Immune Status
    Lymph nodes enlarged _____ Location _____
    Compromised immune system _____
    WBC count _____ Differential _____
    HCT _____ Hb _____
    Consent for HIV testing _____ Results _____
    Chemotherapy _____ Steroid therapy _____
    Prophylactic antibiotic therapy _____
    Temperature _____ Route _____

Infection

Hypothermia
Hyperthermia

Body temperature
Ineffective thermoregulation

Nutrition
    Eating patterns: Changed _____ Unchanged _____
    Number of meals per day _____

Nutrition

Fig. 13-1, cont'd

Special diet _____

Caffeine intake (coffee, tea, soft drinks, chocolate)

_____

Nausea/vomiting _____   Oral mucous membrane

Condition of mouth/throat _____   More than body

Teeth (chipped, loose) _____   requirements

Dentures (upper, lower, full mouth) _____   Less than body requirements

Disposition of dentures _____

Height _____ Weight _____

Current therapy

NPO _____ NG suction _____ TPN _____

Labs (indicate abnormal values with *)

Na _____ K _____ CL _____ Glucose _____

Serum albumin _____ PT _____ PTT _____ BUN _____

Other _____

Elimination

Gastrointestinal/bowel   Bowel elimination

  Usual bowel habits _____   Constipation

  Alterations from normal _____   Diarrhea

                                                                                      Incontinence

Renal/urinary

  Usual urinary pattern _____ Output q.d. _____   Urinary elimination

  Alteration from normal _____   Incontinence

  Urinary catheter _____ **Bladder distention** _____   Retention

  Hemodialysis _____   Renal tissue perfusion

  Perioperative implications _____

CHOOSING ▪ A pattern involving the selection of alternatives

Coping

  Patient's usual problem-solving/coping methods _____   Ineffective individual coping

_____   Ineffective family coping

  Family's usual problem-solving/coping methods _____

_____

  Patient's affect _____

  Physical manifestations _____

Participation

  Compliance with past/current health care regimens _____   Noncompliance

_____   Ineffective participation

  Willingness to comply with future health care regimen ____

_____

Judgment

  Decision-making ability   Judgment

    Patient's perspective _____   Indecisiveness

    Others' perspectives _____

  Perioperative implications _____

Prioritized nursing diagnosis/problem list: PREOPERATIVE

1. _____

2. _____

3. _____

4. _____

5. _____

Signature _____   Date & time _____

Fig. 13-1, cont'd

Continued.

Intraoperative Phase

GENERAL INFORMATION

Name _____ Room _____ Age _____ Sex _____

Allergies _____

Patient in _____ Patient out _____

OR # _____ Anesthesia start _____ Anesthesia stop _____

Surgery start _____ Surgery stop _____

Surgeon _____ Assistant(s) _____

Circulator _____ Relief _____

Scrub _____ Relief _____

Anesthesiologist _____ CRNA _____

Other/students _____

Type of procedure: Scheduled _____ Emergency _____ Urgent _____

Wound class: Clean _____ Clean-contaminated _____ Contaminated _____ Dirty/infected _____

Informed consent _____

Nursing Diagnosis
(Potential or Altered)

KNOWING ▪ A pattern involving meaning associated with information

Preoperative diagnosis _____

Procedure _____

Postoperative diagnosis _____

Orientation

Level of alertness _____   Orientation
                                                                        Confusion

FEELING ▪ A pattern involving the subjective awareness of information

Comfort

    Anesthesia: General _____ Mask _____ Intubated _____

                Regional _____

                Local _____ Local/monitor _____

    Pain/discomfort: Yes _____ No _____   Comfort

    Location _____   Pain/acute

    Aggravating factors _____   Discomfort

    Alleviating factors _____

    Comfort measures offered (warm blanket, pillow)_____

Emotional Integrity/States   Anxiety

    Verbalizes feelings of _____   Fear
                                                                        Shame

MOVING ▪ A pattern involving activity

Positioning: Supine _____ Prone _____ Lithotomy _____   Impaired physical mobility

    Right side up _____ Left side up _____ Jack-knife _____

    Other _____

Padding/supports/restraints _____

_____

Transfer to OR bed: Self _____ Assisted _____

Presence/disposition of prosthesis _____

PERCEIVING ▪ A pattern involving the reception of information   Sensory/perception

Sensory/Perception   Visual

    Disposition of sensory aids (glasses, hearing aid) _____   Auditory

_____

Fig. 13-1, cont'd

EXCHANGING ▪ A pattern involving mutual giving and receiving

Circulation

Blood/blood products administered _____   Tissue persusion

Estimated blood loss _____   Fluid volume

Pulse checks performed: Time _____ Location _____   Deficit

     Rate _____   Excess

Monitoring: ECG _____ Rhythm _____   Cardiac output

    BP: _____ Time _____   BP: _____ Time _____

      _____   _____   _____   _____

      _____   _____   _____   _____

Physical Integrity

Invasive lines: Peripheral _____ A-line _____   Impaired skin integrity

    CVP _____ Swan-Ganz _____   Impaired tissue integrity

Skin Integrity: electrosurgery unit # _____

    Settings _____ Ground pad site _____

    Skin condition _____   Injury

Skin Prep: Iodophor _____ Hibiclens _____ Other _____   Infection

Tourniquet #: _____ Location _____ Pressure _____

    Padding _____ Time up: _____ Time down _____

Implants/Prostheses: Mfr. _____ Model _____

    Lot _____ Serial # _____ Size _____

    Site _____

Counts:	Initial	1st	2nd	3rd
Sponge	_____	_____	_____	_____
Needle	_____	_____	_____	_____
Instrument	_____	_____	_____	_____
Other	_____	_____	_____	_____
			Initials: _____	

Drains/Catheters: Type _____ Size _____ Location _____

Packing: Type _____ Location _____

Dressings: type _____

Oxygenation   Impaired gas exchange

O_2 administered by RN: Yes _____ No _____ Rate _____ Route _____   Ineffective airway clearance

                                              Ineffective breathing patterns

Physical Regulation

Temperature _____ Route _____ Time _____   Body temperature

Specimens: Pathology _____ Bacteriology _____   Hypothermia

    Cytology _____ Other _____   Hyperthermia

                                              Infection

Nutrition

Disposition of dentures _____

Elimination

Urinary catheter _____ Inserted by _____   Renal tissue perfusion

    Size _____ Output _____   Urinary elimination

Medications

Drug	Route	Time	Prepared by	Administered by	
					Fluid volume
_____	_____	_____	_____	_____	Deficit
_____	_____	_____	_____	_____	Excess
_____	_____	_____	_____	_____	Injury

Fig. 13-1, cont'd

Continued.

Discharged to _____ Via _____

  By _____ Report given: Yes _____ No _____

Patient status _____

Prioritized nursing diagnosis/problem list: INTRAOPERATIVE

1. _____

2. _____

3. _____

4. _____

5. _____

Signature _____ Date & Time _____

Postoperative Phase

Nursing Diagnosis
(Potential or Altered)

KNOWING ▪ A pattern involving the meaning associated with information

Orientation

  Level of alertness _____ | Orientation

  Orientation: Person _____ Place _____ Time _____ | Confusion

   | Memory

Perception/expectation of surgery performed _____ | Thought processes

Misconceptions _____ | Knowledge deficit

Knowledge of:

  Care of incision site _____

  Potential complications _____

  Symptoms to report _____

Need for referral to home health agency: Yes _____ No _____

FEELING ▪ A pattern involving the subjective awareness of information

Comfort

  Pain/discomfort: Yes _____ No _____ | Comfort

    Onset _____ Location _____ Duration _____ | Pain/acute

    Quality _____ Radiation _____

    Associated factors _____

    Aggravating factors _____

    Alleviating factors _____

MOVING ▪ A pattern involving activity

Ability to perform ADLs independently: Yes _____ No _____ | Impaired physical mobility

  Specify deficits _____ | Self-care

  Discharge planning needs _____

PERCEIVING ▪ A pattern involving the reception of information

Self-Concept

Effects of surgery on self-concept _____ | Body image
| Self-esteem
| Personal identity

EXCHANGING ▪ A pattern involving mutual giving and receiving

Circulation

  Neurologic changes _____ | Tissue perfusion

  Cardiovascular changes _____ | Cerbral
| Cardiopulmonary
| Peripheral

Fig. 13-1, cont'd

Physical Integrity

    Skin integrity: Incision site _____ Color _____   Infection

        Temperature _____ Drainage _____   Injury

    Electrosurgery grounding site _____   Impaired tissue integrity

    Other _____   Impaired skin integrity

Oxygenation

    Ability to deep breathe and cough _____   Impaired gas exchange

    Mechanical ventilation: Yes _____ No _____   Ineffective airway clearance

                                                                                Ineffective breathing patterns

Physical Regulation

    Temperature _____ Route _____   Hypothermia

    WBC count _____ Other labs _____   Hyperthermia

                                                                                         Infection

Nutrition

    Current therapy: NPO _____ NG suction _____   Nutrition

    TPN _____ Diet: Fluid _____ Solid _____

Elimination

    Bowel function _____   Bowel elimination

    Urinary function _____   Urinary elimination

CHOOSING ▪ A pattern involving the selection of alternatives

Coping

    Patient's affect _____   Ineffective individual coping

    Patient's coping mechanisms _____   Ineffective family coping

    Family's coping mechanisms _____

Participation

    Willingness to comply with health care regimen _____   Noncompliance

    _____   Ineffective participation

Prioritized nursing diagnosis/problem list: POSTOPERATIVE

1. _____

2. _____

3. _____

4. _____

5. _____

Inpatient: Discussed with primary nurse   Yes _____ No _____

Outpatient: Discharged to: _____ Via _____

    Accompanied by _____

Signature _____   Date & Time _____

Fig. 13-1, cont'd

PERIOPERATIVE ASSESSMENT TOOL

Name _B.J._   Age _47_   Sex _F_
Address _75 STRONG ST., SPRINGFIELD_   Telephone _543-1122_
Significant other _M.J. (HUSBAND)_   Telephone _(SAME)_
Date of admission _1/15_   Medical diagnosis _CHOLELITHIASIS, CHOLECYSTITIS_
Allergies _NONE KNOWN_
Planned surgical intervention _CHOLANGIOGRAM, CHOLECYSTECTOMY, POSSIBLE COMMON BILE DUCT EX-_
Anticipated length of surgery _2-3 HRS_   _PLORATION_
Wound classification _CLEAN-CONTAMINATED_
Informed consent _ON CHART_

Preoperative Phase

Nursing Diagnosis
(Potential or Altered)

COMMUNICATING ▪ A pattern involving sending messages
(Read), (write), (understand) English (circle) _____   Communication
Other languages _Ø_   Verbal
Intubated _Ø_   Speech impaired _Ø_   Nonverbal
Physical deformities (jaws wired, cleft palate) _Ø_
Alternate form of communication _N/A_
Perioperative implications _ABLE TO ASK/ANSWER QUESTIONS_

VALUING ▪ A pattern involving the assigning of relative worth
Religious preference _METHODIST_   Spiritual state
Name of minister, priest, rabbi _MINISTER B. SMITH (780-1331)_   Distress
Cultural practices _WHITE, MIDDLE CLASS_   Dispair
Perioperative implications _No FEAR OF DEATH, LITTLE SPIRITUAL DISTRESS_

RELATING ▪ A pattern involving establishing bonds
Role
Marital status _MARRIED_   Role performance
Age & health of significant other _50 y.o. HUSBAND, IN GOOD HEALTH_   Parenting
    Sexual dysfunction
Number of children _3_ Ages _30 y.o. ♀, 25 y.o. ♂, 23 y.o. ♂_
Role in home _HOMEMAKER, WIFE, MOTHER_
Financial support _HUSBAND'S JOB_
Occupation _HOUSEWIFE_   Family processes
   Job satisfaction/concerns _Ø_

Socialization
   Social relationships: (functional) dysfunctional (circle)   Impaired social interaction
   Prefers to be alone (with family) with friends (circle)
   Perioperative implications _FAMILY SUPPORT AVAILABLE_

KNOWING ▪ A pattern involving the meaning associated with information
Current health problems _RUQ PAIN p̄ EATING, INFLAMED GALLBLADDER_
c̄ STONES, "STOMACH ACHE"
Are you or could you be pregnant? _No_
Current medications _OCCASIONAL TYLENOL FOR HEADACHE_

Previous illnesses/hospitalizations/surgeries (list dates) _TONSILLECTOMY_
40 YRS. AGO; APPENDECTOMY 25 YRS. AGO
Previous transfusion/transfusion reaction: _Ø_

Fig. 13-2

History of the following problems (specify self or family):   Knowledge deficit

Heart ____⊖____   Rheumatic fever ____⊖____

Peripheral vascular ___⊖___   Cerebrovascular ___⊖___

Lung ___⊖___   Kidney ___⊖___

Liver ___⊖___   Hepatitis ___⊖___

Thyroid ___⊖___   Cancer ___⊖___

Human immunodeficiency virus *NOT TESTED*

Other *OCCASIONAL HEADACHES RELIEVED BY TYLENOL*

Risk factors	Present	Perceptions/knowledge of
1. Hypertension	⊖	✓
2. Hyperlipidemia	✓	✓
3. Smoking	⊖	✓
4. Obesity	✓	✓ *WANTS TO LOSE WEIGHT*
5. Diabetes	⊖	✓
6. Sedentary living	✓	✓
7. Stress	⊖	✓
8. Alcohol use	✓	*1 GLASS WINE PER WEEK*
9. Oral contraceptives	⊖	✓
10. Bleeding	⊖	
11. Family history	*NO SIGNIFICANT FAMILY HISTORY*	

Perceptions/expectations of surgery *TO BE ABLE TO EAT s̄ PAIN,*
ABDOMINAL DISCOMFORT WILL CEASE

Misconceptions *WORRIED WON'T BE ABLE TO EAT CERTAIN FOODS*

Readiness to learn *YES, REFER FOR WEIGHT LOSS*

Educational level *4 YRS. HIGH SCHOOL*   Thought processes

Learning impeded by ___⊖___

Surgical consent signed: Yes __✓__ No _____

Blood/blood products ordered: Yes __✓__ No _____ Number of units _____

Orientation   *(TYPE, SCREEN, HOLD)*

Level of alertness *ALERT*   Orientation

Orientation: Person __✓__ Place __✓__ Time __✓__   Confusion

Appropriate behavior/communication *OBESITY: POSITIONING, LONG INSTRUMENTS*
NEEDED; TEACH DEEP BREATHING & COUGHING

Memory

Memory intact: Yes __✓__ No _____ Recent __✓__ Remote __✓__   Memory

Perioperative implications __*YES*__

FEELING ▪ A pattern involving the subjective awareness of information

Comfort

Pain/discomfort: Yes __✓__ No _____ *OCCASIONAL, p̄ MEALS*

Onset *p̄ MEALS* Duration *1-2 HRS.*

Location *EPIGASTRIC* Quality *"ACHES"* Radiation *No*

Associated factors *CONSTIPATION*

Aggravating factors *FATTY FOOD, HEAVY MEAL*

Alleviating factors *LESS FAT, REST*

> Comfort
> Pain/chronic
> Pain/acute
> Discomfort

Emotional Integrity/States

Recent stressful life events *"CHRISTMAS BILLS"*   Grieving

Verbalizes feelings of *FEAR, ANXIETY*   (Anxiety)
   (Fear)

Source *SURGERY, "GETTING STUCK c̄ NEEDLES" (IV, IM)*   (Anger)
   Guilt

Physical manifestations *BECAME ANGRY c̄ IV NURSE*   Shame

Perioperative implications *SUGGEST LOCAL ANESTHETIC BEFORE PRE-OP*   Sadness
IV, CHECK PRE-OP MED, DISCUSS SURGERY, FEELINGS

Fig. 13-2, cont'd

Continued.

MOVING ▪ A pattern involving activity
Activity
Limitations in daily activities ↓ *EXERCISE*
Related to: Arthritis —⊖—   Back pain —⊖—
    Prosthetic devices —⊖—   Muscle weakness —⊖—
    Fatigue *YES*   Other *EPIGASTRIC PAIN*
Exercise habits *ADL's ONLY*

    Activity intolerance
    Impaired physical mobility

Self-Care
Ability to perform ADLs independently: Yes ✔   No
Specify deficits —⊖—
Discharge planning needs ⊖ *(FAMILY CAN HELP c̄ CHORES)*

    Self-care
      Feeding
      Bathing/hygiene
      Dressing/grooming
      Toileting

Rest
Hours slept/night *7 HRS.*   Feels rested: (yes) no
Difficulty falling/remaining asleep *WHEN IN PAIN*
Sleep aids (pillows, meds, food) *WARM BATH, EXRA PILLOW*

    Sleep pattern disturbance
      Insomnia
      Hypersomnia
      Nightmares

Recreation
Leisure activities *SEWING, HANDICRAFTS*
Social activities *CHURCH ACTIVITIES*

    Deficit in diversional activity

Health Maintenance
Health insurance *YES, HMO.*
Regular physical checkups *YES, 1 TIME/YR.*

    Health maintenance

Environmental Maintenance
Home maintenance management
    Size & arrangement of home (stairs, bathroom) *3 BEDROOMS, 2 BATHS*
      Safety needs *NONE APPARENT*
    Housekeeping responsibilities *CLEANING, COOKING, LAUNDRY,*
SHOPPING, ETC.
    Perioperative implications *NO MUSCULOSKELETAL PROBLEMS*

    Impaired home maintenance
      management
    Safety hazards

PERCEIVING ▪ A pattern involving the reception of information
Self-Concept
Verbalizes change in feeling about self due to: Diagnosis
    Illness _____ Surgery ✔ Other
    ("HOW BIG IS SCAR?")

    (Body image)
    Self-esteem
    Personal identity

Sensory/Perception
Vision impaired *YES*   Glasses *GLASSES*
Auditory impaired —⊖—   Hearing aid *N/A*
Kinesthetics impaired —⊖—
Gustatory impaired —⊖—
Tactile impaired —⊖—
Olfactory impaired —⊖—
Reflexes: grossly intact *YES*

    Visual
    Auditory
    Kinesthetic
    Gustatory
    Tactile
    Olfactory

Meaningfulness
Verbalizes hopelessness/powerlessness (circle)
    No
Perioperative implications *VISION IMPAIRED; CAUTION*

    Hopelessness
    Powerlessness

EXCHANGING ▪ A pattern involving mutual giving and receiving
Circulation
Cerebral (circle appropriate response)
    Neurologic changes/symptoms (headaches/seizures/convulsions/blackouts)
    No

    Cerebral tissue perfusion

Fig. 13-2, cont'd

Pupils
    Reaction: Brisk ✓
    Sluggish _____ Nonreactive _____

Eye Opening
    No response (1)
    To pain (2)
    To speech (3)
    Spontaneous (4) ⟵circled

Cerebral tissue perfusion

Best Verbal
    No response (1)
    Incomprehensible sound (2)
    Inappropriate words (3)
    Confused conversation (4)
    Oriented (5) ⟵circled

Best Motor
    Flaccid (1)
    Extensor response (2)
    Flexor response (3)
    Semipurposeful (4)
    Localized to pain (5)
    Obeys commands (6) ⟵circled

Glascow Coma Scale total _*15*_

Cardiac
    Apical rate & rhythm _*85 NSR*_
    Heart sounds/murmurs _*NO GALLOPS OR MURMURS*_
    Pacemaker: Yes _____ (No) _____ Type _*N/A*_
    BP: Reading _*120/85*_ Location _Ⓛ *ARM*_
    IV fluids/medications _⊖_ Location _*N/A*_
    Invasive monitoring: CVP _⊖_ Swan-Ganz _⊖_
    A-line _⊖_ Other _____

Cardiopulmonary tissue
  perfusion
Fluid volume
  Deficit
  Excess

Peripheral
    Pulses: A = absent   B = bruits   D = doppler
        +3 = bounding   (+2) = palpable   +1 = faintly palpable
        Location Ⓡ *RADIAL* Side _*R*_
    Skin temp _*WARM*_ Color _*PINK*_
    Edema _*No*_ Capillary refill _*< 2 SEC.*_

Peripheral tissue perfusion
Fluid volume
  Deficit
  Excess
Cardiac output

Physical Integrity
    Skin integrity _*INTACT*_ Rashes _⊖_ Lesions _⊖_
    Petechiae _⊖_ Bruises _⊖_
    Abrasions _⊖_ Scars _*RLQ — OLD SCAR*_
    Proposed incision site _Ⓡ *SUBCOSTAL*_

Impaired skin integrity
Impaired tissue integrity
Injury
(Infection) *POTENTIAL*

Oxygenation
    Complaints of dyspnea _*OCCASIONAL*_ Precipitated by _*? OBESITY*_
    Respiratory rate _*20*_ Rhythm _*REGULAR*_ Depth _*THORACIC*_
    Labored (unlabored) (circle)
    Use of accessory muscles _⊖_
    Cough: productive/nonproductive _⊖_
    Breath sounds _*CLEAR*_
    Pulmonary function studies _*(NOT ORDERED)*_
    Last chest x-ray study _*ON ADMISSION 1/15 — LUNGS CLEAR*_
    Tracheostomy/endotracheal tube _⊖_
    Ventilator _⊖_

Impaired gas exchange
Ineffective airway clearance
Ineffective breathing patterns
POTENTIAL

Physical Regulation
  Immune Status
    Lymph nodes enlarged _*No*_ Location _*N/A*_
    Compromised immune system _*No*_
    WBC count _*7×10³/μL*_ Differential _*WNL*_
    HCT _*45.8%*_ Hb _*12.5 g/dl*_
    Consent for HIV testing _*No*_ Results _*N/A*_
    Chemotherapy _⊖_ Steroid therapy _⊖_
    Prophylactic antibiotic therapy _*ORDERED PRE-OP: ANCEF 1 gm IV*_
    Temperature _*98.4°F*_ Route _*ORAL*_

Infection

Hypothermia
Hyperthermia

Body temperature
Ineffective thermoregulation

Nutrition
    Eating patterns: (Changed) _↓ *APPETITE*_ Unchanged _____
    Number of meals per day _*3*_

Nutrition

Fig. 13-2, cont'd

Continued.

Special diet _LESS FAT, SMALLER MEALS_
Caffeine intake (coffee, (tea,) soft drinks, chocolate)
IN A.M. AND AFTERNOON
(Nausea)/vomiting _DURING ADMISSION_
Condition of mouth/throat _WNL_   Oral mucous membrane
Teeth (chipped, loose) _INTACT_   (More than body requirements)
Dentures (upper, lower, full mouth) _No_
  Disposition of dentures _N/A_   Less than body requirements
Height _5'3"_ Weight _150 lbs_
Current therapy
  NPO _YES_   NG suction _-0-_   TPN _-0-_
Labs (indicate abnormal values with *)
  Na _141mEq/L_ K _4.0mEq/L_ CL _104mEq/L_ Glucose _86 mg/dl_
  Serum albumin _4.5 g/dl_ PT _10 SEC_ PTT _75 SEC_ BUN _15 mg/dl_
  Other _CHOLESTEROL ↑ 275mg/dl*; PLATELETS 300,000/µL_
  ** NPO p̄ MIDNIGHT

Elimination
Gastrointestinal/bowel
  Usual bowel habits _1 PER DAY_   Bowel elimination
  Alterations from normal _OCCASIONAL CONSTIPATION_   Constipation
     Diarrhea
     Incontinence

Renal/urinary
  Usual urinary pattern _3-4 x/DAY_ Output q.d. _>750cc_   Urinary elimination
  Alteration from normal _No_   Incontinence
  Urinary catheter _No_ Bladder distention _No_   Retention
  Hemodialysis _-0-_   Renal tissue perfusion
  Perioperative implications _OBESITY: (1) INCREASED RISK OF INFECTION,_
(2) DIFFICULTY c̄ POST-OP DEEP BREATHING & COUGHING. No ALLERGIES TO RENOGRAFIN;
PROTECT GROIN DURING X-RAY

CHOOSING ■ A pattern involving the selection of alternatives
Coping
Patient's usual problem-solving/coping methods _TALKS TO HUSBAND_   Ineffective individual coping
AND CHILDREN, PRAYS   Ineffective family coping
Family's usual problem-solving/coping methods _MUTUALLY DISCUSS_
PROBLEMS
Patient's affect _MILDY ANXIOUS BUT CONTROLLED_
Physical manifestations _FIDGETY, FINGERING SHEETS_

Participation
Compliance with past/current health care regimens _HAS FOLLOWED_   Noncompliance
MD's ORDERS IN PAST   Ineffective participation
Willingness to comply with future health care regimen _EXPRESSES_
WILLINGNESS TO COMPLY

Judgment
Decision-making ability
  Patient's perspective _ABLE TO MAKE DECISIONS_   Judgment
  Others' perspectives _"MY WIFE HAS A GOOD HEAD ON HER SHOULDERS"_   Indecisiveness
  Perioperative implications _POSITIVE ATTITUDE TOWARD SURGERY/(HUSBAND)_

Prioritized nursing diagnosis/problem list: PREOPERATIVE
1. _ANXIETY RELATED TO SURGERY, PAIN OF INITIATING IV_
2. _POTENTIAL FOR INFECTION RELATED TO INCISION, OBESITY_
3. _POTENTIAL FOR POSTOPERATIVE IMPAIRED GAS EXCHANGE_
4. _RELATED TO GENERAL ANESTHETIC, OBESITY_
4 5. _NUTRITION MORE THAN BODY REQUIREMENTS RELATED TO (? UNKNOWN)_

Signature _Patricia C. Seifert, R.N._   Date & time _1/15 1600_

Fig. 13-2, cont'd

Intraoperative Phase

GENERAL INFORMATION

Name *B. J.*   Room *305*   Age *47*   Sex *F*

Allergies *NKA*

Patient in *0815*   Patient out *1045*

OR # *8*   Anesthesia start *0825*   Anesthesia stop *1037*

Surgery start *0835*   Surgery stop *1032*

Surgeon *T.M., MD*   Assistant(s) *R. B, MD*

Circulator *P.C.S., RN*   Relief *M.C.R., RN*

Scrub *J.C.R., RN*   Relief *∅*

Anesthesiologist *L.M., MD*   CRNA *S.N., CRNA*

Other/students *∅*

Type of procedure: Scheduled *✔*   Emergency ____   Urgent ____

Wound class: Clean ____ Clean-contaminated *✔* Contaminated ____ Dirty/infected ____

Informed consent *"IN CHART"*

Nursing Diagnosis
(Potential or Altered)

KNOWING ▪ A pattern involving meaning associated with information

Preoperative diagnosis *CHOLELITHIASIS, CHOLECYSTITIS*

Procedure *CHOLANGIOGRAM, CHOLECYSTECTOMY*

Postoperative diagnosis *SAME*

Orientation

Level of alertness *ANESTHETIZED*   Orientation

Confusion

FEELING ▪ A pattern involving the subjective awareness of information

Comfort

Anesthesia: General *✔*   Mask *—*   Intubated *✔*

Regional *—*

Local *—*   Local/monitor ____

Pain/discomfort: Yes ____ (No)   Comfort

Location *—*   Pain/acute

Aggravating factors *—*   Discomfort

Alleviating factors *—*

Comfort measures offered (warm blanket, pillow) *(WARM BLANKET APPLIED BEFORE INTUBATION)*

Emotional Integrity/States

Verbalizes feelings of *SLIGHT ANXIETY BEFORE INTUBATION*   (Anxiety)

Fear

Shame

MOVING ▪ A pattern involving activity

Positioning: Supine *✔*   Prone ____   Lithotomy ____   Impaired physical mobility

Right side up ____ Left side up ____ Jack-knife ____

Other *SMALL ROLL UNDER ℝ SIDE*

Padding/supports/restraints *KNEE STRAP APPLIED, ℝ AND Ⓛ ARMS ON ARMBOARDS, ARMS/HANDS PADDED*

Transfer to OR bed: Self *✔*   Assisted ____

Presence/disposition of prosthesis *N/A*

PERCEIVING ▪ A pattern involving the reception of information

Sensory/perception

Sensory/Perception

(Visual)

Disposition of sensory aids ((glasses,) hearing aid) *GLASSES GIVEN TO HUSBAND*   Auditory

Continued.

Fig. 13-2, cont'd

EXCHANGING ▪ A pattern involving mutual giving and receiving

Circulation

Blood/blood products administered __No__
Estimated blood loss __150cc__
Pulse checks performed: Time _____ Location _____
　Rate __SEE ANESTHESIA RECORD__
Monitoring: ECG __YES__ Rhythm __NSR__
　BP: ___ Time ___　　　　BP: ___ Time ___

Tissue persusion
Fluid volume
　Deficit
　Excess
Cardiac output

Physical Integrity

Invasive lines: Peripheral ⓇCEPHALIC A-line __0__
　CVP __0__ Swan-Ganz __0__
Skin Integrity: electrosurgery unit # __155 11__
　Settings __30 CUT, 40 COAG__ Ground pad site Ⓛ THIGH
　Skin condition __INTACT; GROIN AREA SHIELDED DURING X-RAY__
Skin Prep: Iodophor __✓__ Hibiclens _____ Other _____
Tourniquet #: __N/A__ Location __N/A__ Pressure __N/A__
　Padding __N/A__ Time up: __N/A__ Time down __N/A__
Implants/Prostheses: Mfr. __N/A__ Model __N/A__
　Lot __N/A__ Serial # __N/A__ Size __N/A__
　Site __N/A__

(POTENTIAL)
Impaired skin integrity
Impaired tissue integrity

Injury (POTENTIAL)
Infection (POTENTIAL)

Counts:	Initial	1st	2nd	3rd
Sponge	10+10,5+5+5+5	✓	✓	✓
Needle	6+1⑦	✓	✓	✓
Instrument	70+5 ⑦⑤	✓	✓	✓
Other	BOVIE TIP 1	✓	✓	✓
	BLADES 3	✓	Initials: P.C.S/J.C.R.	✓

Drains/Catheters: Type __PENROSE__ Size __½"__ Location __RUQ__
Packing: Type __0__ Location __0__
Dressings: type __4X4, PAPER TAPE__

(POTENTIAL)
Impaired gas exchange
Ineffective airway clearance
Ineffective breathing patterns

Oxygenation

O₂ administered by RN: Yes ___ No __✓__ Rate __N/A__ Route __N/A__

Physical Regulation

Temperature __98.6°F__ Route __SKIN(FOREHEAD)__ Time __INTRA OP__
Specimens: Pathology __G.B. c̄ STONES__ Bacteriology __x1 (GALL)__
　Cytology __0__ Other __0__

Body temperature
Hypothermia
Hyperthermia
Infection (POTENTIAL)

Nutrition

Disposition of dentures __N/A__

Elimination

Urinary catheter __NO__ Inserted by __N/A__
Size __N/A__ Output __N/A__

Renal tissue perfusion
Urinary elimination

Medications

Drug	Route	Time	Prepared by	Administered by	
RENOGRAFIN	INTRADUCTAL	INTRAOP	P.C.S./J.C.R.	DR. T.M.	Fluid volume
50 cc c̄					Deficit
50 cc NS					Excess
					Injury

Fig. 13-2, cont'd

Discharged to *POST. ANES. CARE* Via *STRETCHER*
  By *P.C.S., RN* *UNIT*   Report given: Yes ✓ No ____
Patient status *STABLE, EXTUBATED*

Prioritized nursing diagnosis/problem list: INTRAOPERATIVE
  1. *IMPAIRED SKIN INTEGRITY RELATED TO INCISION.*
  2. *POTENTIAL FOR POST-OP IMPAIRED GAS EXCHANGE RELATED TO*
  2. *ANESTHESIA, OBESITY.*
  3 4. *POTENTIAL FOR INFECTION RELATED TO IMPAIRED SKIN INTEGRITY.*
  5. _____
      Signature *Patricia C. Seifert R.N.*   Date & Time *1/16 10 46*

Postoperative Phase

Nursing Diagnosis
(Potential or Altered)

KNOWING ▪ A pattern involving the meaning associated with information
Orientation
  Level of alertness *ALERT AND ORIENTED ×3*   Orientation
  Orientation: Person ✓ Place ✓ Time ✓   Confusion
Perception/expectation of surgery performed *"WON'T HAVE STOMACH ACHE*   Memory
  ANYMORE "   Thought processes
Misconceptions *DOES NOT REALIZE SHE NEEDS TO REST/RECUPERATE BEFORE*   Knowledge deficit
Knowledge of: *RETURNING TO HOUSEHOLD CHORES.*
  Care of incision site *YES*
  Potential complications *✓ (INFECTION)*
  Symptoms to report *✓ (REDNESS, TENDERNESS, SWELLING, ↑TEMP)*
Need for referral to home health agency: Yes ____ No ✓

FEELING ▪ A pattern involving the subjective awareness of information
Comfort
  Pain/discomfort: (Yes) ____ No ____   Comfort
    Onset *c̄ MOVEMENT* Location *RUQ* Duration *1-2 HRS*   Pain/acute
    Quality *DULL/SHARP* Radiation *θ*
    Associated factors *INCISIONAL PAIN*
    Aggravating factors *MOVEMENT, COUGHING + DEEP BREATHING*
    Alleviating factors *REST, PAIN MED: TYLENOL II q 4HR, PRN*

MOVING ▪ A pattern involving activity
Ability to perform ADLs independently: Yes ✓ No ____   Impaired physical mobility
  ~~Specify deficits~~ *c̄ ASSIST; NO EVIDENCE OF NERVE INJURY TO ARMS*   Self-care
  Discharge planning needs *HUSBAND/CHILDREN TO HELP c̄ HOUSE WORK*
                           DURING RECUPERATION

PERCEIVING ▪ A pattern involving the reception of information
Self-Concept
Effects of surgery on self-concept *INTERESTED IN LOSING WEIGHT; WONDERS*   Body image
IF WILL BE ABLE TO RESUME HOUSEHOLD RESPONSIBILITIES   Self-esteem
                                                                           Personal identity

EXCHANGING ▪ A pattern involving mutual giving and receiving
Circulation   Tissue perfusion
  Neurologic changes *θ*   Cerbral
  Cardiovascular changes *θ*   Cardiopulmonary
                                                                             Peripheral

Continued.

Fig. 13-2, cont'd

Physical Integrity
Skin integrity: Incision site *RUQ, INTACT* Color *PINK*
  Temperature *WARM* Drainage *(PENROSE) SEROUS DRAINAGE*
Electrosurgery grounding site *Ⓛ THIGH INTACT*
Other ____

Infection (POTENTIAL)
Injury
Impaired tissue integrity
(Impaired skin integrity)

Oxygenation
Ability to deep breathe and cough *YES, PRODUCTIVE COUGH, NO DYSPNEA*
Mechanical ventilation: Yes ____ No ✓

Impaired gas exchange
Ineffective airway clearance
Ineffective breathing patterns

Physical Regulation
Temperature *99°F* Route *ORAL*
WBC count *8×10³/µL* Other labs *Hct 45.0%, Hgb 12.0 g/dl*

Hypothermia
Hyperthermia
Infection

Nutrition
Current therapy: NPO ⊖ NG suction ⊖
TPN ⊖ Diet: Fluid ✓ Solid ____

Nutrition

Elimination
Bowel function *BOWEL SOUNDS AUSCULTATED*
Urinary function *> 30 cc/HR*

Bowel elimination
Urinary elimination

CHOOSING ▪ A pattern involving the selection of alternatives
Coping
Patient's affect *MILDLY CONCERNED ABOUT DISCHARGE, DOING HOUSEWORK*
Patient's coping mechanisms *TALK TO FAMILY & FRIENDS*
Family's coping mechanisms *VISITS, DISCUSSES CONCERNS*

Ineffective individual coping
Ineffective family coping

Participation
Willingness to comply with health care regimen *YES, UNDERSTANDS DISCHARGE INSTRUCTIONS*

Noncompliance
Ineffective participation

Prioritized nursing diagnosis/problem list: POSTOPERATIVE
1. *PAIN RELATED TO SURGERY.*
2. *IMPAIRED MOBILITY RELATED TO STRESS OF SURGERY/FATIGUE/ PAIN.*
3 4. *IMPAIRED SKIN INTEGRITY RELATED TO INCISION AND DRAINAGE SITE.*
4 5. *POTENTIAL FOR INFECTION RELATED TO INCISIONS, DRAIN.*

(Inpatient:) Discussed with primary nurse Yes ✓ No ____

Outpatient: Discharged to: *N/A* Via ____
Accompanied by *N/A*

Signature *Patricia C. Seifert, R.N.* Date & Time *1/17 1000*

Fig. 13-2, cont'd

CHAPTER 14

TRANSPLANT ASSESSMENT TOOL

CHAROLD L. BAER
JULIE A. SHINN
LINDA A. PRINKEY

The Transplant Assessment Tool is designed to assess patients who will receive or have received organ transplants. These patients have unique biopsychosocial assessment needs. The tool incorporates specific assessment variables pertinent to transplant patients to facilitate identification of nursing diagnoses. This chapter includes:

- *The way the tool was developed and refined*
- *The patient populations and settings for which it applies*
- *Selected transplant emphasis areas*
- *The way to use the tool*
- *Specific transplant focus questions and parameters to assist the nurse in eliciting appropriate data*
- *The Transplant Assessment Tool*
- *A case study*
- *A completed version of the tool based on the case study*

DEVELOPMENT AND REFINEMENT OF THE TOOL

The Transplant Assessment Tool was developed from the nursing data base prototype (see Chapter 2). Many hemodynamic and critical care variables originally incorporated in the prototype were deleted and replaced with variables more applicable to transplant patient assessment. The resultant tool was then modified based on the recommendations of transplant nurse experts. Further, the content of the tool is supported by the literature from this field of nursing.

After the tool was developed and refined, it was clini-cally tested by nurse experts and clinical nurse specialists on 10 renal transplant and 8 heart or heart and lung transplant patients in tertiary care facilities. The testing evaluated the tool's adequacy in terms of flow, space for recording data, and completeness of assessment variables. Based on the results, the tool was revised.

PATIENT POPULATION AND SETTING

The Transplant Assessment Tool was developed to assess the needs and problems of adult solid organ transplant patients in hospitals. It is most appropriate for stable postoperative transplant patients receiving care in step-down units. With some minor modifications, it could be used for pretransplant or immediate postoperative assessment. In these cases the patient may be too unstable or weak to provide all the requested information. This problem can be resolved by obtaining some of the data from family members and significant others.

TRANSPLANT EMPHASIS AREAS

Transplant patients have unique problems and needs. The Transplant Assessment Tool provides a holistic assessment by evaluating the individual's level of functioning within each of the nine human response patterns of the Unitary Person Framework. In addition, the tool focuses on prevalent problems among transplant patients. Table 14-1 outlines these emphasis areas.

HOW TO USE THE TOOL

To use the Transplant Assessment Tool effectively, nurses must first be familiar with the Unitary Person Framework (see Chapter 2), which provides the underlying

Table 14-1

Selected transplant emphasis areas

Patterns	Emphasis areas to determine
Communicating	Patient's ability to express thoughts and feelings verbally and nonverbally
Valuing	Religious and cultural beliefs about transplant
	Importance of religion to the patient
Relating	Effect of patient's hospitalization on family and sexual relationships, as well as work
Knowing	Readiness to learn about the transplant procedure and health-maintenance regimens after transplant
Feeling	Verbal and physical manifestations of fear, anxiety, anger, guilt, and other emotions
Moving	Preoperative limitations in daily activities due to the deconditioning effects of severe illness
	Ability of patient to meet follow-up care obligations such as checkups
Perceiving	Effect of transplant on self-concept, self-esteem, and body image
Exchanging	Function of the transplanted organ
	Assessment for infection
	Nutritional status
Choosing	Patient's and family's abilities to cope with life-style changes related to transplant follow-up care
	Willingness to comply with transplant follow-up care

framework for Taxonomy I. The human response patterns of the Unitary Person Framework serve as the major category headings for Taxonomy I and the Transplant Assessment Tool. The sequence of the response patterns, as it appears in Taxonomy I, has been changed in the tool to permit a more logical ordering of assessment variables. Nursing diagnoses pertinent to transplant patients are incorporated under the appropriate human response patterns and are arranged with the associated assessment variables.

Nurses must also realize that this tool is very different from conventional assessment tools. As a result, nurses may encounter some initial difficulty in using it. They should remember, however, that the tool was not designed to follow the organization or content of a traditional medical data base; the data collected do not solely reflect medical patterns. Rather, this tool elicits data about holistic patterns in ways not traditionally used by nurses. It repre-

sents a nursing data base developed from a nursing model. The use of this tool results in a holistic nursing assessment that facilitates identification of nursing diagnoses.

Although many nurses probably agree that a holistic nursing data base is desirable, it is realized that changing traditional assessment methods is not an easy task. For this reason, a trial usage period is recommended before any decisions about the tool's merits are made. During the trial period, nurses will become familiar and progressively more comfortable with the tool's organization and data-collection methods. With experience, nurses will become accustomed to new ways of clustering and processing information. Further, with continued use, the time necessary to complete the tool will be reduced. Most important, nurses will discover that nursing diagnoses are easily identified because of the tool's unique ability to elicit appropriate signs and symptoms in a readily understandable fashion.

It is not necessary to complete the tool in one session. Priority sections can be completed during the initial assessment. Other sections or patterns can be completed later, within a time frame acceptable to the nurse, patient, and institution. Further, depending on the patient's condition and degree of orientation, the family or significant others may help in providing data.

When assessing for specific signs and symptoms to indicate a particular diagnosis, the nurse circles the diagnosis in the right-hand column when deviations from normal are found. A circled diagnosis does not confirm a problem but simply alerts the nurse to the possibility that it exists. After completing the tool, the nurse scans the circled diagnoses, synthesizes the data to determine whether other clusters of data support a problem, and judges whether the actual or potential diagnosis is present.

Some diagnoses are repeated several times in the right-hand column. These repetitions occur only within the appropriate response pattern and are convenient for identifying certain data directly with their corresponding nursing diagnosis. These diagnoses are not absolute but are intended to focus thinking and direct detailed attention to a possible problem.

Some signs and symptoms can indicate several diagnoses. For example, disorientation and inappropriate behavior can indicate confusion, altered thought processes, altered cerebral perfusion, and impaired gas exchange. For transplant patients, confusion can also result from changes in blood chemistry values (e.g., blood urea nitrogen). To avoid unnecessary repetition of assessment parameters, variables are arranged with the diagnosis most likely to result from the data assessed. Thus, data to support a specific diagnosis may occasionally be found in other patterns or arranged with other diagnoses. Therefore, synthesis of all data is essential before formulating nursing diagnoses.

The Transplant Assessment Tool is not intended to be

Table 14-2

Transplant assessment tool: focus questions and parameters

Variables	Focus questions and parameters
COMMUNICATING	
Communication barriers	Does the patient demonstrate extreme fatigue or a decreased level of consciousness that interferes with the ability to express needs? Also see Chapter 3.
VALUING	
Important religious and cultural practices	"How important is religion or your culture to you? To your family?" "Does your religion or culture permit you to receive blood transfusions? A transplant?"
RELATING	
Family relationships	"Can you describe how the members of your family get along?"
Permanent/temporary relocation of family	Did the family move to be closer to the transplant center? Is this move only temporary?
Verbalizes feelings of being alone	How will the transplant affect the patient's ability to interact with others?
KNOWING	
Nephrotoxic medications	Is the patient receiving aminoglycoside antibiotics or cyclosporine?
Perception/knowledge of illness/tests/surgery	Does the patient verbalize an understanding of the transplant surgery, postoperative care, medical follow-up, and drug therapy and side effects? Does the patient understand the implications of rejection? Does the patient know any transplant recipients?
Expectations of therapy	What does the patient expect from the transplant?
FEELING	
Verbalizes feelings of	Does the patient seem to focus excessively on the organ donor (especially the heart donor)?
MOVING	
Limitations in daily activities	Is the patient deconditioned due to the severity of pretransplant illness? Does the patient have muscle atrophy?
Exercise habits	What were the patient's exercise habits before the illness?
Home maintenance management concerns	"Will your treatment interfere with your ability to perform housekeeping or shopping duties? Other household chores?"
Health care regimen concerns	Does the patient voice concerns about the ability to take or obtain prescribed medications? Keep appointments?
Discharge planning needs	Does the patient need a referral to a social worker or any agencies for assistance in caring for self or family?
PERCEIVING	
Effects of illness/surgery	"How do you feel about having a transplant? Relying on others for assistance during recovery?"
EXCHANGING	
Dialysis access: current condition of access (NOTE: Applies only to renal transplants)	Does the patient have a bruit at the fistula site? Are all tubings or catheters patent and free of clots? What is the condition of the skin around the access site?
WBC Differential	See Chapter 3 and Appendix II.
Temperature	A temperature higher than 37° C or 98.6° F should be investigated as a symptom of infection
Condition of mouth/throat	Does the patient have any herpetic lesions, *Candida*, or gingival hyperplasia?
Ideal (dry) body weight	See Chapter 3. Dry weight: weight after ideal dialysis.
Labs	See Chapter 3 and Appendix II.
CHOOSING	
Compliance with past/current health care regimens	If on dialysis, did the patient attend or perform dialysis as prescribed? Take medication as ordered? Does the patient generally follow health care instructions well?

the standardized final format for evaluating transplant patients across the country because an assessment tool must meet the needs of the institutions and nurses using it. This tool is simply a working model that is expected to be revised by nurses in clinical practice. In addition, evaluation and refinement are necessary before adopting the tool for use within an institution. Nurses interested in changing and revising the tool for use in a specific clinical setting should refer to Chapter 4.

HOW TO ELICIT APPROPRIATE DATA

Because the Unitary Person Framework and the Transplant Assessment Tool contain some terms that may be unfamiliar to nurses, specific transplant focus questions and parameters were developed and refined to elicit appropriate information. These questions and parameters appear in Table 14-2 and correspond with the variables in bold type in the tool (Fig. 14-1). For example, the effects of illness/surgery on self concept variable found in the "perceiving pattern" is in bold type. If the nurse does not know what questions to ask about this variable, Table 14-2 can be used to direct the assessment. Questions and parameters for other assessment variables were presented in Chapter 3.

The focus questions and parameters provide clarity and guidance in eliciting data and are not all inclusive. Nurses should not feel limited to asking only the questions or assessing the parameters provided. There are many other methods of eliciting information. Assessment methods should be tailored to the patient's level of understanding, the situation, and the skill and comfort level of the nurse.

CASE STUDY

The case study models the process a nurse uses when assessing a patient using the Transplant Assessment Tool. Based on the clustering of information gathered during assessment, the nurse formulates appropriate nursing diagnoses (Fig. 14-2) and lists them in order of priority at the end of the tool.

Mrs. K.L. is a 25-year-old heart transplant patient in the cardiac transplant step-down unit. Mrs. K.L.'s pretransplant cardiac dysfunction was caused by postpartum cardiomyopathy. The Transplant Assessment Tool (Fig. 14-2) contains the data obtained from Mrs. K.L. A list of nursing diagnoses has been derived from this data.

BIBLIOGRAPHY

Brundage DJ: Nursing management of renal problems, ed 2, St Louis, 1980, The CV Mosby Co.

Carpenito LJ: Nursing diagnosis: application to clinical practice, ed 2, Philadelphia, 1987, JB Lippincott Co.

Dressler D: Current trends in heart transplantation. In Kern LS, editor: Cardiac critical care nursing, Rockville, Md, 1988, Aspen Publishers, Inc.

Funk M: Heart transplantation: postoperative care during the acute period, Crit Care Nurse 6:27, 1986.

Kenner CV, Guzzetta CE, and Dossey BM: Critical care nursing: body-mind-spirit, ed 2, Boston, 1985, Little, Brown & Co, Inc.

Lancaster LE: The patient with end stage renal disease, ed 2, New York, 1984, John Wiley & Sons, Inc.

Lancaster LE: Core curriculum for nephrology nursing, Pitman, NJ, 1987, American Nephrology Nurses' Association.

Lough ME: Quality of life issues following heart transplantation, Prog Cardiovasc Nurs 1:17, 1986.

McAleer MJ: Psychological aspect of heart transplantation, Heart Transplantation 4:232, 1985.

McKelvey SA: Effects of dennervation in the cardiac transplant patient. In Douglas MK and Shinn JA, editors: Advances in cardiovascular nursing, Rockville, Md, 1985, Aspen Publishers, Inc.

Shinn JA: Cardiac transplantation. In Underhill SL et al, editors: Cardiac nursing, ed 2, Philadelphia, 1988, JB Lippincott Co.

TRANSPLANT ASSESSMENT TOOL

Name _____ Age _____ Sex _____
Address _____ Telephone _____
Significant other _____ Telephone _____
Date of admission _____ Medical diagnosis _____
Allergies _____

Nursing Diagnosis
(Potential or Altered)

COMMUNICATING ▪ A pattern involving sending messages

English: Read _____ Write _____ Understand _____
Other languages _____
Communication barriers _____
Alternate form of communication _____

Communication
  Verbal
  Nonverbal

VALUING ▪ A pattern involving the assigning of relative worth
Religious preference _____
Important religious practices _____
Spiritual concerns _____
Cultural orientation _____
Cultural practices _____

Spiritual state
  Distress
  Despair

RELATING ▪ A pattern involving establishing bonds
Role
  Marital status _____
  Age & health of significant other _____
  _____
  Number of children _____ Ages _____
  Role in home _____
  Family relationships _____
  Distance from home to hospital _____
  Family transportation arrangements _____
  Permanent/temporary (circle) relocation of family _____
  Financial support _____
  Occupation _____
    Job satisfaction/concerns _____
    _____
    Physical/mental energy expenditures _____
  Sexual concerns _____

Role performance
  Parenting
  Sexual dysfunction
  Work
  Family
  Social/leisure
Family processes

Sexuality patterns

Socialization
  Quality of relationships with others _____
    Patient's description _____
    Significant others' descriptions _____
    Staff observations _____
  Verbalizes feelings of being alone _____
    Attributed to _____

Impaired social interaction

Social isolation
Social withdrawal

KNOWING ▪ A pattern involving the meaning associated with information
Current health problems _____
_____
_____
Previous illnesses/hospitalizations/surgeries _____
_____
_____

Fig. 14-1

Continued.

History of the following problems: Knowledge deficit
  Heart _____ Hypertension _____
  Peripheral vascular disease _____
  Cerebrovascular _____ Rheumatic fever _____
  Lung _____
  Liver _____ (hepatitis?) Kidney _____
  Thyroid _____
  Rejection of transplant _____
  Drug abuse _____ Alcoholism _____
Current medications _____
_____
_____
_____
_____

Nephrotoxic medications _____
Risk factors for heart disease:
                          Present   Perceptions/knowledge of
  1. Hypertension   _____   _____
  2. Hyperlipidemia   _____   _____
  3. Smoking   _____   _____
  4. Obesity   _____   _____
  5. Diabetes   _____   _____
  6. Sedentary living   _____   _____
  7. Stress   _____   _____
  8. Alcohol use   _____   _____
  9. Oral contraceptives _____   _____
  10. Family history _____
_____

Perception/knowledge of illness/tests/surgery _____
_____

Expectations of therapy _____
Misconceptions _____
Readiness to learn _____
  Requests information concerning _____
  Educational level _____   Thought processes
  Learning impeded by _____   Impaired problem
                                                                         solving

Orientation
Level of alertness _____   Orientation
Orientation: Person _____ Place _____ Time _____   Confusion
Appropriate behavior/communication _____

Memory
Memory intact: Yes _____ No _____ Recent _____ Remote _____   Memory

FEELING ▪ A pattern involving the subjective awareness of information
Comfort
  Pain/discomfort: Yes _____ No _____   Comfort
    Onset _____ Duration _____   Pain/chronic
    Location _____ Quality _____ Radiation _____   Pain/acute
    Associated factors _____   Discomfort
    Aggravating factors _____
    Alleviating factors _____

Emotional Integrity/States
Recent stressful life events _____   Grieving
_____   Anxiety

Fig. 14-1, cont'd

Verbalizes feelings of _____   Anxiety
_____   Fear
Source _____   Anger
_____   Guilt
Physical manifestations _____   Shame
_____   Sadness

MOVING ▪ A pattern involving activity
Activity
History of physical disability _____   Impaired physical mobility
_____   Activity intolerance
Limitations in daily activities _____
_____
Verbal report of fatigue/weakness _____
Exercise habits _____

Rest   Sleep pattern disturbance
Hours slept/night _____ Feels rested: Yes ____ No ____   Hypersomnia
Sleep aids (pillows, meds, food) _____   Insomnia
Difficulty falling/remaining asleep _____   Nightmares

Recreation
Social/leisure activities _____   Deficits in diversional activity
_____

Environmental Maintenance
Home maintenance management
Home responsibilities _____   Impaired home maintenance
Home maintenance management concerns _____   management
_____   Safety hazards
_____

Health Maintenance
Health insurance _____   Health maintenance
Regular physical checkups _____
Transportation to appointments _____
Health care regimen concerns _____
_____

Self-Care   Self-care
Ability to perform ADLs: Independent _____ Dependent _____   Feeding
Needs assistance _____   Bathing/hygiene
Specify deficits _____   Dressing/grooming
Discharge planning needs _____   Toileting
_____

PERCEIVING ▪ A pattern involving the reception of information
Self-Concept
Patient's description of self _____   Body image
Effects of illness/surgery _____   Self-esteem
_____   Personal identity

Meaningfulness
Verbalizes hopelessness _____   Hopelessness
Verbalizes/perceives loss of control _____   Powerlessness
_____

Fig. 14-1, cont'd

Continued.

Sensory/Perception

Vision impaired _____ Glasses _____

Auditory impaired _____ Hearing aid _____

Kinesthetics impaired _____

Gustatory impaired _____

Tactile impaired _____

Olfactory impaired _____

Reflexes: Grossly intact _____ Altered _____

       Biceps   R _____ L _____   Knee R _____ L _____

       Ankle   R _____ L _____   Plantar R _____ L _____

Sensory/perception

  Visual

  Auditory

  Kinesthetic

  Gustatory

  Tactile

  Olfactory

EXCHANGING ▪ A pattern involving mutual giving and receiving

Circulation

Cerebral

  Neurologic changes/symptoms _____

  Cerebral tissue perfusion

Pupils	Eye Opening
L 2 3 4 5 6 mm	None (1)
R 2 3 4 5 6 mm	To pain (2)
Reaction: Brisk _____	To speech (3)
Sluggish _____ Nonreactive _____	Spontaneous (4)

Fluid volume

  Deficit

  Excess

Best Verbal	Best Motor
No response (1)	Flaccid (1)
Incomprehensible sound (2)	Extensor response (2)
Inappropriate words (3)	Flexor response (3)
Confused conversation (4)	Semipurposeful (4)
Oriented (5)	Localized to pain (5)
	Obeys commands (6)

Cardiac output

  Glasgow Coma Scale total _____

Cardiac

  Pacemaker _____

  Apical rate & rhythm _____ PMI _____

  Heart sounds/murmurs _____

  Dysrhythmias _____

  BP: Sitting   Lying   Standing

     R _____ L _____   R _____ L _____   R _____ L _____

  A-line reading _____

  CVP _____

  IV fluids _____

  IV cardiac medications _____

  _____

Cardiopulmonary tissue

  perfusion

Fluid volume

  Deficit

  Excess

Cardiac output

Peripheral

  Jugular venous distension R _____ L _____

  Pulses: A = absent   B = bruits   D = doppler

     + 3 = bounding   +2 = palpable   +1 = faintly palpable

Carotid	R _____ L _____	Popliteal	R _____ L _____
Brachial	R _____ L _____	Posterior tibial	R _____ L _____
Radial	R _____ L _____	Dorsalis pedis	R _____ L _____
Femoral	R _____ L _____		

  Skin temp _____ Color _____ Turgor _____

  Capillary refill _____ Clubbing _____

Peripheral tissue perfusion

Fluid volume

  Deficit

  Excess

Cardiac output

Physical Integrity

Injury

  Convulsions _____ Tetany _____

Injury

Fig. 14-1, cont'd

Dialysis access: Yes _____ No _____   Infection
   Fistula _____ **A-V Shunt** _____ **PD cath** _____
   Central line _____ **Current condition of access** _____
Tissue integrity: Rashes _____ Lesions _____   Impaired skin integrity
   Petechiae _____ Bruises _____   Impaired tissue integrity
   Abrasions _____ Surgical incisions _____
_____

Oxygenation
Complaints of dyspnea _____ Precipitated by _____
Orthopnea _____
Rate _____ Rhythm _____ Depth _____   Ineffective breathing patterns
Labored/unlabored (circle) Use of accessory muscles _____
Chest expansion _____ Splinting _____
Cough: productive/nonproductive _____   Ineffective airway clearance
Sputum: Color _____ Amount _____ Consistency _____
Breath sounds _____
Arterial blood gases _____   Impaired gas exchange
Oxygen percent and device _____
Ventilator _____

Physical Regulation
Immune
   Lymph nodes enlarged _____ Location _____   Infection
   WBC count _____ **Differential: PMN** _____ **Mono** _____
              Eos _____ **Baso** _____ **Lymph** _____
   Cytomegalovirus titer _____
   Cultures _____   Hypothermia
Body temperature   Hyperthermia
   Temperature _____ Route _____   Ineffective thermoregulation

Nutrition   Nutrition
Eating patterns
   Number of meals per day _____
   Special diet _____   Less than body requirements
   Food preferences/intolerances _____
   Food allergies _____
   Caffeine intake (coffee, tea, soft drinks) _____   More than body
_____   requirements
   Appetite changes _____
   Nausea/vomiting _____
Condition of mouth/throat _____   Oral mucous membrane
Height _____ Weight _____ **Ideal (dry) body weight** _____
Current therapy   Less than body requirements
   NPO _____ NG suction _____
   Tube feeding _____
   TPN _____   More than body
   IV fluids _____   requirements
Labs
   Na _____ K _____ CL _____ CO_2 _____   Fluid volume
   Glucose _____ Ca _____   Deficit
   Phos _____ Mg _____ Uric acid _____ Total bilirubin _____   Excess
   Total protein _____ Albumin _____ Cholesterol _____
   Liver enzymes _____ Amylase _____
   Hct _____ Hb _____ RBC _____ Platelets _____
   PT _____ PTT _____ Other _____

Fig. 14-1, cont'd

Continued.

Elimination
  Gastrointestinal/bowel   Bowel elimination
    Usual bowel habits _____   Constipation
    Alterations from normal _____   Diarrhea
    Abdominal physical examination _____   Incontinence
      Liver: Enlarged _____ Ascites _____   GI tissue perfusion
  Renal/urinary   Urinary elimination
    Usual urinary pattern _____   Incontinence
    Alteration from normal _____   Retention
    Currently dialyzing _____
    Color _____ Catheter _____
    Urine output: 24 hour _____ Average hourly _____   Renal tissue perfusion
    Bladder distention _____
    Specific gravity _____   Fluid volume
    Urine studies _____   Deficit
    Serum BUN _____ Serum creatinine _____   Excess
     Cardiac output

CHOOSING ▪ A pattern involving the selection of alternatives
Coping
  Patient's usual problem-solving methods _____   Ineffective individual coping
  _____   Ineffective family coping
  Family's usual problem-solving methods _____

  Patient's method of dealing with stress _____

  Family's method of dealing with stress _____

Participation
  Compliance with past/current health care regimens _____   Noncompliance
  _____   Ineffective participation
  Willingness to comply with future health care regimen _____

  Decision-making ability   Judgment
    Patient's perspective _____   Indecisiveness
    Others' perspectives _____

Prioritized nursing diagnosis/problem list
1. _____
2. _____
3. _____
4. _____
5. _____

Signature _____ Date _____

Fig. 14-1, cont'd

TRANSPLANT ASSESSMENT TOOL

Name _K.L._   Age _25_   Sex _FEMALE_
Address _2418 RIVERDRIVE CHARLOTTSVILLE, N.C._   Telephone _(704) 246-8323_
Significant other _HUSBAND — B._   Telephone _LOCAL 467-5119_
Date of admission _4/5_   Medical diagnosis _S/P HEART TRANSPLANT_
Allergies _PENICILLIN_

Nursing Diagnosis
(Potential or Altered)

COMMUNICATING ▪ A pattern involving sending messages
English: Read ___✔___ Write ___✔___ Understand ___✔___   Communication
Other languages _No_   Verbal
Communication barriers _NONE_   Nonverbal
Alternate form of communication _NONE_

VALUING ▪ A pattern involving the assigning of relative worth
Religious preference _METHODIST_   Spiritual state
Important religious practices _NONE_   Distress
Spiritual concerns _WANTS TO BE "CLOSER TO GOD"_   Despair
Cultural orientation _AMERICAN_
Cultural practices _NONE_

RELATING ▪ A pattern involving establishing bonds
Role
  Marital status _MARRIED_   Role performance
  Age & health of significant other _HUSBAND 26 YRS GOOD HEALTH_   (Parenting)
       (Sexual dysfunction)
  Number of children _2_ Ages _1½ MO., 2 YRS_   (Work)
  Role in home _CHILD CARE, HOUSEKEEPING, WIFE_   Family
  Family relationships _DESCRIBES RELATIONSHIPS AS GOOD_   Social/leisure
  Distance from home to hospital _300 MILES_   (Family processes)
  Family transportation arrangements _HUSBAND HAS CAR & DRIVES_
  Permanent (temporary) (circle) relocation of family _WITH RELATIVES_
  Financial support _PRIMARILY HUSBAND_
  Occupation _SECRETARY (BEFORE BIRTH OF SECOND CHILD) PARTTIME_
    Job satisfaction/concerns _LIKES WORKING; HOPES TO RETURN TO WORK_
    Physical/mental energy expenditures _MINIMAL_
  Sexual concerns _BEFORE TRANSPLANT SEXUAL ACTIVITY CAUSED_   Sexuality patterns
EXTREME SHORTNESS OF BREATH & FATIGUE

Socialization
  Quality of relationships with others _TENSE AT TIMES_   (Impaired social interaction)
    Patient's description _"B. DOESN'T PAY ENOUGH ATTENTION TO ME"_
    Significant others' descriptions _"I CAN'T SEEM TO PLEASE HER" (HUSBAND)_
    Staff observations _PATIENT VERY DEMANDING_
  Verbalizes feelings of being alone _YES_   (Social isolation)
    Attributed to _MISSES CHILDREN, WANTS TO SEE MORE OF HUSBAND_   Social withdrawal

KNOWING ▪ A pattern involving the meaning associated with information
Current health problems _S/P HEART TRANSPLANT_

Previous illnesses/hospitalizations/surgeries _EMERGENCY CESAREAN SECTION_
1½ MONTHS BEFORE ADMISSION _PRETRANSPLANT— CARDIO-_
GENIC SHOCK ON LEFT VENTRICULAR ASSIST DEVICE

Fig. 14-2

Continued.

History of the following problems: ⟨Knowledge deficit⟩

Heart **POSTPARTUM CARDIOMYOPATHY** Hypertension _No_____

Peripheral vascular disease ___ *No* _____

Cerebrovascular ___ *No* ____ Rheumatic fever ___ *No* _____

Lung ___ *No* _____

Liver ___ *No* ____ (hepatitis?) Kidney ___ *No* _____

Thyroid _*No*_____

R ejection of transplant ___ *No* _____

Drug abuse ___ *No* _____ Alcoholism ___ *No* _____

Current medications *CYCLOSPORINE 260 mg PO qd, AZATHIOPRINE*
105 mg PO qid, PREDNISONE 10 mg PO qd, MYCOSTATIN 5 cc SWISH
AND SWALLOW qid

Nephrotoxic medications *CYCLOSPORINE*_____

Risk factors for heart disease:

	Present	Perceptions/knowledge of
1. Hypertension	*No*	
2. Hyperlipidemia	*No*	
3. Smoking	*No*	
4. Obesity	*No*	*VERBALIZES KNOWLEDGE OF HOW*
5. Diabetes	*No*	*RISK FACTORS RELATE TO DEVELOP-*
6. Sedentary living	*YES*	*MENT OF HEART DISEASE*
7. Stress	*YES*	
8. Alcohol use	*No*	
9. Oral contraceptives	*YES*	
10. Family history	*No FAMILY HISTORY OF HEART DISEASE*	

Perception/knowledge of illness/⟨tests⟩/surgery *VERBALIZES KNOWLEDGE*
OF POST TRANSPLANT TREATMENT AND FOLLOW UP

Expectations of therapy *TO RETURN TO FAMILY RESPONSIBILITIES & WORK*

Misconceptions *RECIPIENT TAKING ON CHARACTERISTICS OF DONOR*

Readiness to learn *SEEMS EAGER*_____

Requests information concerning *MEDICATIONS ON DISCHARGE*

Educational level *1½ YRS. COLLEGE*_____   **Thought processes**
                                                                        Impaired problem
Learning impeded by ___ — _____   solving

Orientation

Level of alertness *ALERT*_____   Orientation

Orientation: Person ___✓___ Place ___✓___ Time ___✓___   Confusion

Appropriate behavior/communication *BOTH APPROPRIATE*_____

Memory

Memory intact: Yes ✓ No ____ Recent ✓ Remote ___✓___   Memory

FEELING ▪ A pattern involving the subjective awareness of information

Comfort

Pain/discomfort: Yes ✓ No ____   Comfort

Onset *WITH MOVEMENT* ____ Duration *DURING MOVEMENT*   Pain/chronic

Location *CHEST* ___ Quality *SHARP* ___ Radiation ___ *No* ___   ⟨Pain/acute⟩

Associated factors *NONE*_____   Discomfort

Aggravating factors *MOVEMENT*_____

Alleviating factors *PROPPING UP ON PILLOWS, CODEINE 60 mg PO*

Emotional Integrity/States

Recent stressful life events *BIRTH OF BABY; CARDIOGENIC SHOCK*   Grieving
*AFTER DELIVERY*_____   Anxiety

Fig. 14-2, cont'd

Verbalizes feelings of *SADNESS, ANGER AT TIMES* _____

Source *MISSES CHILDREN; SAD ABOUT NOT HAVING THE OPPORTUNITY TO BE WITH BABY; ANGRY ABOUT BEING ILL*

Physical manifestations *TEARFUL AT TIMES* _____

Anxiety
Fear
(Anger)
Guilt
Shame
(Sadness)

MOVING ▪ A pattern involving activity

Activity

History of physical disability *CARDIOGENIC SHOCK — 10 DAYS ON LEFT VENTRICULAR ASSIST DEVICE*

Limitations in daily activities *PRETRANSPLANT — UNABLE TO PERFORM ANY ACTIVITY; CURRENTLY IS EASILY FATIGUED*

Verbal report of (fatigue)/weakness *AFTER WASHING IN A.M.*

Exercise habits *PREILLNESS: RUNNING, HORSEBACK RIDING*

Impaired physical mobility
(Activity intolerance)

Rest

Hours slept/night *7-8 HOURS* _____ Feels rested: Yes ✓ No _____

Sleep aids (pillows, meds, food) *PILLOWS*

Difficulty falling/remaining asleep *NO*

Sleep pattern disturbance
Hypersomnia
Insomnia
Nightmares

Recreation

Social/leisure activities *RIDING, RUNNING, DANCING, LISTENING TO MUSIC, VISITING FRIENDS*

Deficits in diversional activity

Environmental Maintenance

Home maintenance management

Home responsibilities *CARING FOR CHILDREN, SHOPPING, CLEANING*

Home maintenance management concerns *REGARDING ALL OF ABOVE ACTIVITIES DUE TO FATIGUE AND ACTIVITY RESTRICTIONS ON DISCHARGE (LIFTING)*

Impaired home maintenance management
Safety hazards

Health Maintenance

Health insurance *CHAMPUS*

Regular physical checkups *MAINLY OB-GYN*

Transportation to appointments *YES, HUSBAND OR MOTHER*

Health care regimen concerns *NONE AT PRESENT*

Health maintenance

Self-Care

Ability to perform ADLs: Independent ✓ Dependent _____

Needs assistance _____

Specify deficits *NEEDS TO SPACE ACTIVITIES TO AVOID FATIGUE*

Discharge planning needs _____

Self-care
Feeding
Bathing/hygiene
Dressing/grooming
Toileting

PERCEIVING ▪ A pattern involving the reception of information

Self-Concept

Patient's description of self *"VERY DETERMINED"*

Effects of illness/surgery *CONCERNED ABOUT APPEARANCE — HAIR GROWTH (FACIAL) ACNE, WEIGHT LOSS*

Body image
Self-esteem
Personal identity

Meaningfulness

Verbalizes hopelessness *NO*

Verbalizes/perceives loss of control *NO*

Hopelessness
Powerlessness

Fig. 14-2, cont'd

Continued.

Sensory/Perception
Vision impaired ___No___   Glasses ___—___

Auditory impaired ___No___   Hearing aid ___—___

Kinesthetics impaired ___No___

Gustatory impaired ___No___

Tactile impaired ___No___

Olfactory impaired ___No___

Reflexes: Grossly intact ___✓___ Altered _____

Biceps	R _____	L _____		Knee	R _____	L _____
Ankle	R _____	L _____		Plantar R _____	L _____	

Sensory/perception
Visual
Auditory
Kinesthetic
Gustatory
Tactile
Olfactory

EXCHANGING ▪ A pattern involving mutual giving and receiving
Circulation
Cerebral
Neurologic changes/symptoms ___NONE___

Cerebral tissue perfusion

Pupils
L 2 ③ 4 5 6 mm
R 2 ③ 4 5 6 mm
Reaction: Brisk ___✓___
Sluggish _____ Nonreactive _____

Eye Opening
None (1)
To pain (2)
To speech (3)
Spontaneous (④)

Fluid volume
Deficit
Excess

Best Verbal
No response (1)
Incomprehensible sound (2)
Inappropriate words (3)
Confused conversation (4)
Oriented (⑤)

Best Motor
Flaccid (1)
Extensor response (2)
Flexor response (3)
Semipurposeful (4)
Localized to pain (5)
Obeys commands (⑥)

Cardiac output

Glasgow Coma Scale total ___15___

Cardiac
Pacemaker ___NOT AT PRESENT; EPICARDIAL WIRES IN PLACE___
Apical rate & rhythm ___100___ PMI ___5TH INTERCOSTAL 2 cm___
Heart sounds/murmurs ___S₁ & S₂___
Dysrhythmias ___No___

Cardiopulmonary tissue
perfusion
(Fluid volume)
(Deficit)
Excess

BP: Sitting   Lying   Standing
R ¹³²/₈₀ L ¹³⁰/₈₀   R ¹³⁰/₈₀ L ¹³⁰/₇₈   R ¹²⁰/₇₀ L ¹²⁰/₇₀

A-line reading ___N/A___
CVP ___N/A___
IV fluids ___NONE___
IV cardiac medications ___NONE___

Cardiac output

Peripheral
Jugular venous distension R ___No___ L ___No___
Pulses: A = absent   B = bruits   D = doppler
   + 3 = bounding   +2 = palpable   +1 = faintly palpable

Peripheral tissue perfusion

(Fluid volume)
(Deficit)
Excess

Carotid R +2 L +2		Popliteal	R +2 L +2
Brachial R +2 L +2		Posterior tibial	R +2 L +2
Radial R +2 L +2		Dorsalis pedis	R +2 L +2
Femoral R +2 L +2			

Skin temp ___WARM___ Color ___PALE___ Turgor ___LOOSE___
Capillary refill ___< 2 SEC___ Clubbing ___No___

Cardiac output

Physical Integrity
Injury
Convulsions ___No___ Tetany ___No___

Injury

Fig. 14-2, cont'd

Dialysis access: Yes _____ No ✓_____ (Infection) (POTENTIAL)

   Fistula _____ A-V Shunt _____ PD cath _____

   Central line _____ Current condition of access _____

Tissue integrity: Rashes *No*_____ Lesions *ACNE—FACE + CHEST*__ (Impaired skin integrity)

Petechiae *No*_____ Bruises *No*_____ Impaired tissue integrity

Abrasions *No*_____ Surgical incisions *MEDIAN STERNOTOMY*____

*CHEST TUBE INCISIONS — CLOSED*_____

Oxygenation

Complaints of dyspnea *No*_____ Precipitated by __—_____

Orthopnea *No*_____

Rate *12*_____ Rhythm *REGULAR* Depth *SHALLOW*_____ (Ineffective breathing patterns)

Labored (unlabored) (circle) Use of accessory muscles *No*_____

Chest expansion *EQUAL*_____ Splinting *YES*_____

Cough: productive (nonproductive)_____ Ineffective airway clearance

Sputum: Color ____—_____ Amount ____—_____ Consistency __—___

Breath sounds *CRACKLES IN BASES BILATERALLY*_____

Arterial blood gases *No RECENT RESULTS*_____ Impaired gas exchange

Oxygen percent and device ___—_____

Ventilator ___—_____

Physical Regulation

Immune

   Lymph nodes enlarged *No*_____ Location __—_____ Infection

   WBC count *8.1×10³/μL* Differential: PMN *56%*_____ Mono *4%*____

               Eos *2.7%* Baso *0.3%* Lymph *34%*

   Cytomegalovirus titer *NEGATIVE*_____ Hypothermia

   Cultures *SPUTUM, BLOOD AND URINE CULTURES NEGATIVE*__ Hyperthermia

Body temperature Ineffective thermoregulation

   Temperature *36.1°C*_____ Route *ORAL*_____

Nutrition Nutrition

Eating patterns

   Number of meals per day *3*_____

   Special diet *LOW SODIUM*_____ (Less than body requirements)

   Food (preferences) intolerances *LIKES "JUNK FOOD"*_____

   Food allergies *NONE*_____

   Caffeine intake (coffee, tea, soft drinks) More than body

COFFEE — 2 CUPS/DAY SOFT DRINKS — COKE 16 oz 2/DAY   requirements

   Appetite changes *UNABLE TO EAT BEFORE SURGERY (SHOCK) APPETITE GOOD NOW*

   Nausea/vomiting *No*_____

Condition of mouth/throat *CANDIDA ON TONGUE, HARD PALATE* Oral mucous membrane

Height *5'5"*_____ Weight *115 lb*_____ Ideal (dry) body weight *125 lb*__

Current therapy Less than body requirements

   NPO *No*_____ NG suction *No*_____

   Tube feeding *No*_____

   TPN *No*_____ More than body

   IV fluids *No*_____   requirements

Labs

   Na *142 mEq/L* K *4.5 mEq/L* CL *102 mEq/L* CO₂ *2.3 mM*___ Fluid volume

   Glucose *105 mg/dl* Ca *5.0 mEq/L*_____   Deficit

   Phos *2.4 mg/dl* Mg *2.5 mEq/L* Uric acid *7.0 mg/dl* Total bilirubin *0.7 mg/dl* Excess

   Total protein *5.5 g/dl* Albumin *3.0 g/dl* Cholesterol *200 mg/dl*

   Liver enzymes *SGOT 20 U/ml, SGPT 25 U/ml, LDH 180 U* Amylase __—__

   Hct *36.0%* Hb *9.8 g/dl* RBC *4.0×10⁶/μL* Platelets *300,000/μL*

   PT *12 SEC* PTT *60 SEC* Other __—_____

Fig. 14-2, cont'd

Continued.

Elimination

Gastrointestinal/bowel
 Usual bowel habits *1 X /DAY*
 Alterations from normal *NONE*
 Abdominal physical examination *SOFT, NONTENDER, ACTIVE BOWEL SOUNDS*
  Liver: Enlarged *No* Ascites *No*

Bowel elimination
 Constipation
 Diarrhea
 Incontinence
GI tissue perfusion

Renal/urinary
 Usual urinary pattern *4-5x/DAY*
 Alteration from normal *No*
 Currently dialyzing *N/A*
 Color *DARK AMBER* Catheter *No*
 Urine output: 24 hour *2,000 cc* Average hourly *80 - 90cc/HR*
 Bladder distention *NONE*
 Specific gravity *1.025*
 Urine studies *pH 6 GLUCOSE-NEGATIVE; KETONES-NEGATIVE*
 Serum BUN *10 mg/dl* Serum creatinine *0.5 mg/dl*

Urinary elimination
 Incontinence
 Retention

Renal tissue perfusion

(Fluid volume
 Deficit)
 Excess
Cardiac output

CHOOSING ▪ A pattern involving the selection of alternatives
Coping

Patient's usual problem-solving methods *EXPLORES ALL ALTERNATIVES*
BEFORE MAKING A DECISION
Family's usual problem-solving methods *HUSBAND SOMETIMES HAS*
TROUBLE CHOOSING PROPER METHOD OF ACTION
Patient's method of dealing with stress *GOES RUNNING, LISTENS*
TO MUSIC
Family's method of dealing with stress *HUSBAND-GETS ANGRY*

Ineffective individual coping
Ineffective family coping

Participation

Compliance with past/current health care regimens *CURRENTLY GIVING*
OWN MEDICATION; FOLLOWS INSTRUCTIONS
Willingness to comply with future health care regimen *VERBALIZES*
WILLINGNESS
Decision-making ability
 Patient's perspective *GOOD*
 Others' perspectives *(HUSBAND) "GOOD JUDGMENT"*

Noncompliance
Ineffective participation

Judgment
 Indecisiveness

Prioritized nursing diagnosis/problem list
1. *ALTERED COMFORT — PAIN (ACUTE) RELATED TO RECENT SURGERY*
2. *SOCIAL ISOLATION RELATED TO HOSPITALIZATION AND SEPARATION FROM CHILDREN*
3. *POTENTIAL FOR INFECTION RELATED TO IMMUNOSUPPRESSION AND ALTERED SKIN INTEGRITY*
4. *ACTIVITY INTOLERANCE RELATED TO DECONDITIONING PRETRANSPLANT*
5. *ALTERED BODY IMAGE/SELF-ESTEEM RELATED TO DRUG SIDE EFFECTS, WEIGHT LOSS*

Signature *Linda A. Prinkey, RN*   Date *4/5*

Fig. 14-2, cont'd

CHAPTER 15

TRAUMA ASSESSMENT TOOL

LINDA A. PRINKEY
LYNELLE N. BABA

The Trauma Assessment Tool is designed to assess traumatically injured patients with complex nursing care needs. This tool has assessment variables pertinent to trauma patients to facilitate identification of nursing diagnoses. The tool also incorporates the American Association of Critical-Care Nurses' *Standards for the Nursing Care of the Critically Ill*. This chapter includes:

- *The way the tool was developed and refined*
- *The patient populations and settings for which it applies*
- *Selected trauma emphasis areas*
- *The way to use the tool*
- *Specific trauma focus questions and parameters to assist the nurse in eliciting appropriate data*
- *The Trauma Assessment Tool*
- *A case study*
- *A completed version of the tool based on the case study*

DEVELOPMENT AND REFINEMENT OF THE TOOL

The Trauma Assessment Tool was developed from the nursing data base prototype (see Chapter 2). Because of the complex and severe physiological alterations experienced by trauma patients, the sequence of the human response patterns in the Trauma Assessment Tool differs from that of the prototype and all other tools. This reordering allows the nurse to assess for life-threatening physiological alterations first. Therefore, unlike the other tools, the Trauma Assessment Tool begins with the "exchanging pattern." Further, the lower-level categories within the "exchanging pattern" have been rearranged to reflect the ABCs of basic life support. The order of the remaining response patterns was also changed to reflect the needs and concerns of trauma patients. Finally, the Glasgow Coma Scale has been moved from the cerebral perfusion section of the "exchanging pattern" to the orientation section under the "knowing pattern." This change was made because nurses in trauma settings have more direct methods of measuring cerebral perfusion (e.g., intracranial pressure and cerebral perfusion pressure). Further, the Glasgow Coma Scale assesses consciousness and orientation, which are in the "knowing pattern." These changes represent several ways in which the tools can be altered to meet the unique needs of a particular nursing unit or patient population. For further information about adapting tools to a particular practice setting, nurses should see Chapter 4.

The Trauma Assessment Tool is based on the literature and was modified according to recommendations from a trauma clinical specialist and trauma nurse experts, who tested the tool in clinical practice. The Truama Assessment Tool was tested on 10 traumatically injured patients who had been admitted to surgical intensive care and trauma units. The testing evaluated the adequacy of the tool's content such as completeness, clarity, and usefulness of assessment variables, adequacy of space for recording data, and logical ordering of variables. Based on the results, the tool was revised.

PATIENT POPULATION AND SETTING

The Trauma Assessment Tool was developed to assess the needs and problems of adult patients who have experienced multiple- or single-system trauma and have been admitted to intensive care units specializing in trauma. This tool is also useful in trauma step-down units; in that setting, inclusion of additional assessment variables related to rehabilitation needs and concerns may be desirable (see Chapter 26). Because of the length of the tool and the extensive nature of assessment variables, this tool is not recommended for use in trauma admitting areas. However, it is possible to adapt the tool to these areas (see Chapter 4).

The Trauma Assessment Tool is intended for use with both stable and unstable patients. For more detailed information about the assessment of unstable patients, nurses should refer to the section on how to use the tool.

TRAUMA EMPHASIS AREAS

Trauma victims have multiple, complex, and unique problems and needs. The Trauma Assessment Tool provides a holistic assessment of all these problems and needs but focuses on problems prevalent among the trauma patient population. Table 15-1 outlines these emphasis areas.

HOW TO USE THE TOOL

To use the Trauma Assessment Tool effectively, nurses must first be familiar with the nine human response patterns of the Unitary Person Framework and with Taxonomy I (see Chapter 2). The sequence of the response patterns, as it appears in Taxonomy I, has been changed in the Trauma Assessment Tool to permit a more logical ordering of assessment variables. Questions designed to elicit assessment of signs and symptoms related to a nursing diagnosis are arranged according to their corresponding response pattern in the tool.

Nurses must also realize that this tool is very different from conventional assessment tools because it was not designed to follow the organization or content of a traditional medical data base. The data collected do not solely reflect medical patterns. Rather, this tool elicits data about holistic patterns in ways not traditionally used by nurses. Therefore, nurses may initially encounter some difficulty in using the tool. They should remember, however that the tool provides a new method of collecting and synthesizing data. It is a nursing data base developed from a nursing model. The use of this tool results in a holistic nursing assessment in which defining characteristics are clustered to facilitate the formulation of appropriate nursing diagnoses.

Although many nurses probably agree that a holistic nursing data base is desirable, it is realized that changing traditional assessment methods is not an easy task. For this reason, a trial usage period is recommended before any decisions about the tool's merits are made. During the trial period, nurses will become familiar and progressively more comfortable with the tool's organization and data-collection methods. With experience, nurses will become skilled in new ways of clustering and processing information. Further, with continued use, the time necessary to complete the tool will be reduced. Most important, nurses will discover that nursing diagnoses are easily identified because of the tool's unique ability to elicit signs and symptoms in a readily understandable fashion.

Table 15-1
Selected trauma emphasis areas

Patterns	Emphasis areas to determine
Exchanging	Chest injuries affecting breathing and oxygenation
	Head trauma affecting cerebral tissue perfusion
	Hemodynamic monitoring values to evaluate the adequacy of resuscitation and hemodynamic stability
	Bleeding and the potential for disseminated intravascular coagulation
	Wounds, crushing injuries, and incisions affecting skin and tissue integrity
	Gastrointestinal or genitourinary trauma affecting nutrition and elimination
Feeling	Comprehensive pain assessment
	Emotional impact of injuries
Communicating	Physical barriers to communication (i.e., intubation, facial injuries, or paralysis)
Knowing	Perceptions of injuries and expectations of therapy
	A thorough assessment of level of consciousness
Perceiving	Sensory losses related to nerve or spinal cord injury
	Effects of injury on self-concept and body image
Moving	Effects of fractures, amputations, and paralysis on mobility, activity tolerance, and self-care
	Necessary changes in the home environment, including safety needs
Valuing	Cultural and religious values concerning surgery, blood transfusions, treatments, and visitors
Relating	Role concerns related to current injuries
	Concerns about altered sexual function resulting from injuries
Choosing	Ability of patient and significant others to cope with crisis

It is not necessary to complete the tool in one session. When dealing with unstable trauma patients in the intensive care unit, nurses should complete the physiological assessment variables under the "exchanging pattern" within a few hours after admission. Other patterns can be completed within a time frame acceptable to the nurses and institution. When assessing unstable patients and neurologic trauma victims, it may be necessary to obtain information from family members or significant others, at least until the patient is able to confirm or refute the data.

To elicit appropriate data, nurses should be familiar with the focus questions and parameters in the next section. These questions and parameters are not all inclusive but provide clarity and guidance when eliciting data.

When assessing for specific signs and symptoms to indicate a nursing diagnosis, the nurse circles the diagnosis in the right-hand column of the tool when deviations from normal are found. A circled diagnosis does not positively confirm a problem but alerts the nurse to the possibility that it exists. After completing the tool, the nurse scans the circled problems and looks for other data to support or refute the problem. Based on this analysis, the nurse confirms an actual or potential nursing diagnosis then lists the diagnoses in order of priority for care planning.

Some of the nursing diagnoses are repeated several times in the right-hand column. These repetitions occur only within the appropriate response pattern and are convenient for identifying certain data directly with their corresponding nursing diagnosis.

Certain signs and symptoms can indicate several diagnoses. For example, mental confusion can indicate decreased cerebral tissue perfusion, altered oxygenation, altered thought processes, altered level of consciousness, and altered sensory/perception. To avoid unnecessary repetition of assessment parameters, variables are arranged with the diagnosis most likely to result from the data assessed. Thus, data to support a particular nursing diagnosis may occasionally be found in other patterns or arranged with other diagnoses. Therefore, synthesis of all data is essential.

The Trauma Assessment Tool is not intended to be the standardized or final format for assessing trauma patients across the country. An assessment tool must meet the needs of the institutions and nurses using it. This tool is merely a working demonstration tool that is expected to be changed and revised by nurses in clinical practice. Further evaluation and refinement are necessary before adopting the tool for use within a particular institution. Nurses interested in changing and revising the tool for use in a specific clinical setting should refer to Chapter 4.

HOW TO ELICIT APPROPRIATE DATA

Because the Unitary Person Framework and the Trauma Assessment Tool contain some terms that may be unfamil-

---

Table 15-2

Trauma assessment tool: focus questions and parameters

Variables	Focus questions and parameters
EXCHANGING	
Inhalation of smoke or noxious gas	Was the patient trapped in a burning building or a car that was still running?
Intracranial pressure (ICP)	ICP normal is 0 to 15 mm Hg.
Cerebral perfusion pressure (CPP)	CPP = mean arterial pressure − ICP (Adequate if ≥ 60 mm Hg).
Cardiac index/cardiac output	See Chapter 3.
Bleeding	Estimate cumulative blood loss in cubic centimeters (cc). Indicate active blood loss and location.
	Is internal bleeding suspected?
Compartment tension	Has the compartmental pressure been measured? (Abnormal is ≥ 30 mm Hg.)
Soft tissue injury	Has the patient suffered a crushing or tearing injury?
Current therapy meeting body requirements W = weight in kg H = height in cm A = age in years	Basal metabolic rate: for men, Kcal = 66 + 13.7W + 5H + 6.8A; for women, Kcal = 655 + 9.6W + 1.8H + 4.7A. Severe trauma increases energy needs 10 to 30%. Protein: Nitrogen balance = nitrogen intake − urine urea nitrogen (should not be negative). Nitrogen intake in grams = Protein (g) × 6.25. Vitamins and minerals as needed
Evisceration/injury of abdominal organs	Is there obvious evisceration of abdominal organs? Did the patient sustain blunt or penetrating trauma to the abdomen?

Continued

Table 15-2—cont'd

Trauma assessment tool: focus questions and parameters

Variables	Focus questions and parameters
EXCHANGING—cont'd	
Diagnostic peritoneal lavage (DPL)	Positive DPL: WBCs > 500/mm^3; RBCs > 1000,000/mm^3; amylase, vegetable fibers, or feces.
Possible kidney contusion/ other injury	Is there bruising over the lower posterior portion of the ribs or flank? Did the mechanism of injury indicate possible blunt or penetrating trauma to the kidney? What were the results of the intravenous pyelogram or cystogram (if performed)? Is hematuria present?
FEELING	
Pain/discomfort	See Chapter 3
Recent stressful life events	Was the patient involved in an accident in which other people were killed or injured? Is it possible that a recent event precipitated the injury (i.e., divorce, separation, death, or financial difficulties)?
COMMUNICATING	
Alternate form of communication	Is the use of the patient's writing hand impaired due to injury or therapeutic devices? Can a paralyzed patient answer yes and no questions by blinking?
KNOWING	
Neurologic changes/ symptoms	Has the patient experienced seizures? Type? Duration? Has the patient experienced a change in personality?
PERCEIVING	
Level of sensory loss	Assess heat, pain, and touch perception from neck down. List dermatome where impaired sensation begins bilaterally.
Self-inflicted injury	Was this injury an obvious suicide attempt (i.e., was there a note, plan, or expression of intent to harm self)?
MOVING	
Level of paralysis	C1 to C6 (complete quadriplegia): loss of all function below shoulders and upper arms, no hand control, innervation of diaphragm lost if lesion is at C4 and above (complete respiratory paralysis). C6 to C7 (incomplete quadriplegia): loss of motor control to parts of arm and hand, some hand control. T1 to T6 (paraplegia): loss of motor control below midchest, varying impairment of intercostal muscles. T6 to L3 (paraplegia): functional loss dependent on specific level of injury. L3 to L4 (incomplete paraplegia): loss of control of part of lower legs, ankles, and feet.
VALUING	
Important religious or cultural practices	Does the patient's religion or culture permit surgery or blood transfusions?
RELATING	
Role satisfaction/concerns	Was the patient satisfied with the position or responsibilities in the home before the injury? Does the patient voice any concerns about the ability to fulfill roles in future? Does the family have any concerns about the patient's future roles?
Physical difficulties related to sex	Will the patient have any physical sexual disability as a result of this injury?
CHOOSING	
Suspected or known substance abuse	Was a serum toxicology screen performed? Give results. Is the patient known to use alcohol, marijuana, cocaine, heroin, or other drugs regularly or occasionally?

iar to many nurses, focus questions and parameters were developed to facilitate the collection of appropriate information. These questions and parameters (Table 15-2) correspond with assessment variables in bold type in the tool (Fig. 15-1). For example, current therapy meeting body requirements is a variable under the "exchanging pattern." If the nurse does not know how to evaluate the adequacy of the patient's nutritional source, the information in Table 15-2 can be used as a guide. Questions and parameters for other assessment variables were presented in Chapter 3.

These questions and parameters are not all inclusive, so nurses should not feel confined to asking only the questions or assessing the parameters provided. There are many other methods of eliciting the information. Assessment methods should be tailored to the patient's level of understanding, the situation, and the skill and comfort level of the nurse. The questions and parameters serve only as a guide to data collection.

CASE STUDY

The case study models the process a nurse uses when assessing a patient using the Trauma Assessment Tool. Based on the clustering of information gathered during assessment, the nurse formulates nursing diagnoses (Fig. 15-2). The problem list at the end of the completed tool then serves as a guide for developing a nursing care plan.

Mr. C.P. is a 20-year-old male admitted to the trauma unit via helicopter after receiving a gunshot wound to the back. The circumstances of his injury were unknown but were suspected to be related to drugs. The Trauma Assessment Tool (Fig. 15-2) contains the data obtained from Mr. C.P., his girlfriend, and his father. A list of nursing diagnoses has also been derived from this data.

BIBLIOGRAPHY

American Association of Critical-Care Nurses: Standards for the nursing care of the critically ill, Reston, Va, 1981, Reston Publishing Co.

Cardona VD, editor: Trauma nursing, Oradell, NJ, 1985, Medical Economics Books.

Cardona VD, editor: Trauma reference manual, Maryland Institute for Emergency Medical Services Systems, Bowie, Md, 1985, Brady Communications Company, Inc.

Dunham CM: Initial evaluation and management of the trauma patient. In Cowley RA and Dunham CM, editors: Shock trauma/critical care manual, Baltimore, Md, 1982, University of Maryland Press.

Elwyn DH, Kinney JM, and Askanazi J: Energy expenditure in surgical patients, Surg Clin North Am 61:545, 1981.

Forlaw L: The critically ill patient: nutritional implications, Nurs Clin North Am 18:111, 1983.

Johanson BC, et al: Standards for critical care, ed 3, St Louis, 1988, The CV Mosby Co.

Knezevich BA: Trauma nursing: principles and practice, East Norwalk, Conn, 1986, Appleton-Century-Crofts.

Larson M, Leigh J, and Wilson LR: Detecting compartmental syndrome using continuous pressure monitoring, Focus Crit Care 13:51, 1986.

Roberts SL: Nursing diagnosis and the critically ill patient, East Norwalk, Conn, 1987, Appleton & Lange.

TRAUMA ASSESSMENT TOOL

Name _____ Age _____ Sex _____
Address _____ Telephone _____
Significant other _____ Telephone _____
Date of admission _____ Type of Injury _____
Allergies _____
Acute interventions performed _____
_____

Nursing Diagnosis
(Potential or Altered)

EXCHANGING ▪ A pattern involving mutual giving and receiving
Oxygenation

Rate _____ Rhythm _____ Depth _____
Labored/unlabored (circle) Chest expansion _____
Use of accessory muscles _____
Complaints of dyspnea _____ Splinting _____
Breath sounds _____   Ineffective breathing patterns
Flail chest _____ Bony thorax fractures _____
Chest x-ray findings _____
History of smoking _____
Inhalation of smoke or noxious gas _____
Cough: productive/nonproductive _____   Ineffective airway clearance
Sputum: Color _____ Amount _____ Consistency _____
Arterial blood gases _____
Oxygen percent and device _____   Impaired gas exchange
Ventilator settings _____
Type of airway _____

Circulation
Cerebral   Cerebral tissue perfusion
  Intracranial pathology/trauma _____
  Intracranial pressure _____ **Cerebral Perfusion Pressure** _____
  Pupils   Reaction: Brisk _____
    L 2 3 4 5 6 mm   Sluggish _____ Nonreactive _____
    R 2 3 4 5 6 mm
Cardiac
  Pacemaker _____   Cardiopulmonary tissue
  Apical rate & rhythm _____   perfusion
  Dysrhythmias _____
  Heart sounds/murmurs _____
  BP: Cuff R _____ L _____ Arterial Line _____
  Cardiac index _____ **Cardiac output** _____   Cardiac output
  CVP _____ PAP _____ PCWP _____   Fluid volume
  IV fluids _____   Deficit
  IV vasoactive medications _____   Excess
  _____

  Bleeding: Yes _____ No _____ Estimated blood loss _____
    Sites of active bleeding _____
  Labs
    Na _____ K _____ CL _____ CO_2 _____ Glucose _____
    Hct _____ Hb _____ PT _____ PTT _____ Platelets _____
    Fibrin split products _____ Cardiac enzymes _____   Cardiac output
                                                             Peripheral tissue perfusion
Peripheral   Fluid volume
  Jugular venous distention R _____ L _____   Deficit
  Skin Temp _____ Color _____ Turgor _____   Excess
  Edema _____ Capillary refill _____

Fig. 15-1

Pulses: A = absent   B = bruits   D = doppler   Peripheral tissue perfusion
+ 3 = bounding   +2 = palpable   +1 = faintly palpable   Fluid volume

Carotid R _____ L _____		Popliteal R _____ L _____	Deficit
Brachial R _____ L _____		Posterior tibial R _____ L _____	Excess
Radial R _____ L _____		Dorsalis pedis R _____ L _____	
Femoral R _____ L _____			

Compartment tension _____ **Location** _____

Physical Integrity

Tissue integrity: Rashes _____ Lesions _____   Impaired skin integrity
    Lacerations _____ Abrasions _____
    Bruises _____
    Petechiae _____   Impaired tissue integrity
    Soft tissue injury _____
    Surgical incisions/drains/tubes (type and location) _____   Infection
    _____
Leakage of spinal fluid from ears/nose/other (circle) _____

Physical Regulation

Immune
    WBC count _____ Cultures _____   Infection
    _____   Hypothermia
Body temperature   Hyperthermia
    Temperature _____ Route _____   Ineffective thermoregulation

Nutrition

Usual eating patterns   More than body
    Number of meals per day _____   requirements
    Special diet _____
    Food preferences/intolerances _____   Less than body requirements
    Food allergies _____
    Appetite changes _____
Facial injury _____
Condition of mouth/throat _____   Oral mucous membrane
Height _____ Weight _____ Ideal body weight _____
Current therapy
    NPO _____ NG suction _____ Diet _____   Fluid volume
    Tube feeding _____   Deficit
    TPN _____   Excess
    Additional insulin needs _____
    Current therapy meeting body requirements: Yes _____ No _____

Elimination

Gastrointestinal/bowel   Bowel patterns
    Alterations from normal _____   Constipation
    Colostomy _____ Ileostomy _____   Diarrhea
    Evisceration/injury of abdominal organs _____   Incontinence
    _____
    Bleeding: Gastric _____ frank _____ occult _____   GI tissue perfusion
               Intestinal _____ frank _____ occult _____
Abdominal physical examination _____
Anal sphincter tone _____
Diagnostic peritoneal lavage: Positive _____ **Negative** _____

Fig. 15-1, cont'd

Continued.

Renal/urinary
  Possible kidney contusion/other injury _____
  Alteration from normal _____
  Urine color _____ Catheter _____
  Urine output: 24 hour _____ Average hourly _____
  Bladder distention _____ Genitourinary injury _____
  BUN _____ Creatinine _____ Specific gravity _____
  Urine myoglobin _____ Other urine studies _____
  _____

Renal tissue perfusion
Urinary patterns
  Incontinence
  Retention
Cardiac output

Fluid volume
  Deficit
  Excess

FEELING ▪ A pattern involving the subjective awareness of information
Comfort
  Pain/discomfort: Yes _____ No _____
    Onset _____ Duration _____
    Location _____ Quality _____
    Aggravating factors _____
    Alleviating factors _____

Comfort

  Pain/chronic
  Pain/acute
  Discomfort

Emotional Integrity/States
  Recent stressful life events _____
  _____
  Verbalizes feelings of _____
  _____
    Source _____
  _____
  _____
  Physical manifestations _____
  _____

Grieving
Anxiety
Fear
Anger
Guilt
Shame
Sadness

COMMUNICATING ▪ A pattern involving sending messages
  Read, write, understand English (circle) _____
  Other languages _____
  Intubated _____ Speech impaired _____
  Alternate form of communication _____
  _____

Communication
  Verbal
  Nonverbal

KNOWING ▪ A pattern involving the meaning associated with information
  Current health problems _____
  _____
  Previous hospitalizations/surgeries/illnesses _____
  _____
  _____
  Current medications _____
  _____
  _____
  Last tetanus immunization _____
  Perception/knowledge of illness/planned tests/surgery _____
  _____
  _____
  Expectations of therapy _____
  Misconceptions _____
  Readiness to learn _____
    Requests information concerning _____
    Educational level _____
    Learning impeded by _____

Knowledge deficit

Learning

Thought processes
  Impaired problem solving

Fig. 15-1, cont'd

Orientation

Level of alertness _____ Orientation
Orientation: Person _____ Place _____ Time_____ Confusion
Appropriate behavior/communication _____ Thought processes
Neurologic changes/symptoms _____

_____

Eye Opening
  None (1)
  To pain (2)
  To speech (3)
  Spontaneous (4)

Best Verbal   Best Motor   Orientation
  No response (1)   Flaccid (1)   Confusion
  Incomprehensible sound (2)   Extensor response (2)   LOC
  Inappropriate words (3)   Flexor response (3)
  Confused conversation (4)   Semipurposeful (4)
  Oriented (5)   Localized to pain (5)
                         Obeys commands (6)

Glascow Coma Scale total _____

Memory

Memory intact: Yes _____ No _____ Recent _____ Remote _____ Memory

PERCEIVING ▪ A pattern involving the reception of information

Sensory/Perception

History of restricted environment _____ Sensory/perception
Vision impaired _____ Glasses _____ Visual
Auditory impaired _____ Hearing aid _____ Auditory
Kinesthetics impaired _____ Kinesthetic
Gustatory impaired _____ Gustatory
Tactile impaired _____ Tactile
Olfactory impaired _____ Olfactory
Spinal cord injury: Yes _____ No _____
Level of sensory loss: R _____ L _____

Self-Concept

Patient's description of self _____ Self-concept
Effects of injury/surgery on self-concept _____ Body image
_____ Self-esteem
                                    Personal identity

Meaningfulness

Verbalizes hopelessness _____ Hopelessness
Verbalizes/perceives loss of control _____ Powerlessness
Self-inflicted injury: Yes _____ No _____ Type _____

MOVING ▪ A pattern involving activity

Activity

History of previous/current/anticipated physical disabilities _____ Impaired physical mobility

_____

_____

Fig. 15-1, cont'd

Continued.

Verbal report of fatigue/weakness _____   Activity intolerance
Braces/casts/splints/traction (circle) _____   Impaired physical mobility

_____

Fractures _____
Amputations _____
Paralysis: Yes _____ No _____ **Level of paralysis: R** _____ **L** _____

Self-Care   Self-care
Ability to perform ADLs: Independent _____ Dependent _____   Feeding
Specify deficits _____   Bathing/hygiene

_____   Dressing/grooming
Discharge planning needs _____   Toileting

_____

Environmental Maintenance
Home maintenance management
    Limitations related to returning to previous home environment and/or   Impaired home maintenance
    responsibilities _____   management

_____

_____
    Safety needs _____   Safety hazards

Health Maintenance
    Regular physical checkups _____
    Health insurance _____   Health maintenance

Rest   Sleep pattern disturbance
    Hours slept/night _____ Feels rested: Yes _____ No _____   Hypersomnia
    Difficulty falling/remaining asleep _____   Insomnia
    Sleep aids (pillows, meds, food) _____   Nightmares

Recreation
    Leisure/diversional activities _____   Deficit in diversional activity
    Social activities _____

VALUING ▪ A pattern involving the assigning of relative worth
    Religious preference _____   Spiritual state
    Important religious practices _____   Distress
    Spiritual concerns _____   Despair
    Cultural orientation _____
    Cultural practices _____

RELATING ▪ A pattern involving establishing bonds
Role
    Marital status _____   Role performance
    Age & health of significant other _____   Parenting

_____   Sexual dysfunction
    Number of children _____ Ages _____   Work
    Role in home _____   Family
    Role satisfaction/concerns_____   Social/leisure
    Financial support _____
    Occupation _____   Family processes
        Job satisfaction/concerns _____
        Physical/mental energy expenditures _____
    Sexual relationships (satisfactory/unsatisfactory) _____   Sexuality patterns
        Physical difficulties related to sex _____

_____
        Concerns regarding sexual function as a result of injury _____

_____

Fig. 15-1, cont'd

Socialization

Quality of relationships with others _____ Impaired social interaction
  Patient's description _____
  Significant others' descriptions _____
  Staff observations _____
  Verbalizes feelings of being alone _____ Social isolation
    Attributed to _____ Social withdrawal

CHOOSING ■ A pattern involving the selection of alternatives

Coping

Patient's usual problem-solving methods _____ Ineffective individual coping
_____ Ineffective family coping

Family's usual problem-solving methods _____
_____

Patient's method of dealing with stress _____
_____

Family's method of dealing with stress _____
_____

Suspected/known (circle) substance abuse: Yes _____ No _____
  Type of substance _____
Verbalizes inability to cope _____
Patient's affect _____
  Physical manifestations _____
Support systems available _____
_____

Participation

Compliance with past/current health care regimens _____ Noncompliance
_____ Ineffective participation

Willingness to comply with future health care regimen _____
_____

Decision-making ability Judgment
  Patient's perspective _____   Indecisiveness
  Others' perspectives _____

Prioritized nursing diagnosis/problem list
1. _____
2. _____
3. _____
4. _____
5. _____

Signature _____ Date _____

Fig. 15-1, cont'd

TRAUMA ASSESSMENT TOOL

Name *C.P.* _____ Age *20* Sex *MALE*
Address *4852 BENTWOOD AVE., WASHINGTON, D.C.* _____ Telephone *523-3168*
Significant other *JANE (GIRLFRIEND)* _____ Telephone *SAME*
Date of admission *7/1* _____ Type of Injury *GUNSHOT WOUND TO LEFT POSTERIOR CHEST*
Allergies *PENICILLIN*
Acute interventions performed *LEFT CHEST TUBE FOR PNEUMOTHORAX; LEFT NEPHRECTOMY;*
EXPLORATORY LAPAROTOMY; REPAIR OF SEROSAL TEARS x2; REMOVE BULLET

Nursing Diagnosis
(Potential or Altered)

EXCHANGING ▪ A pattern involving mutual giving and receiving
Oxygenation

Rate *24* _____ Rhythm *REGULAR* Depth *SHALLOW*
Labored/(unlabored) (circle) Chest expansion *EQUAL*
Use of accessory muscles *No*
Complaints of dyspnea *No* _____ Splinting *YES*
Breath sounds *VESICULAR BILATERALLY; VERY DIMINISHED LEFT BASE* (Ineffective breathing patterns)
Flail chest *No* _____ Bony thorax fractures *No*
Chest x-ray findings *LEFT LOWER LOBE ATELECTASIS*
History of smoking *YES; 2 PACKS PER DAY*
Inhalation of smoke or noxious gas *No*
Cough: (productive)/nonproductive *STRONG COUGH EFFORT* ___ Ineffective airway clearance
Sputum: Color *BROWN* Amount *MODERATE* Consistency *THICK*
Arterial blood gases *pH 7.40, $PaCO_2$ 45mmHg, PaO_2 80mmHg, HCO_3 23mM, O_2 SAT 96%*
Oxygen percent and device *40% HIGH HUMIDITY MASK* ___ Impaired gas exchange
Ventilator settings *NONE*
Type of airway *NATURAL*

Circulation

Cerebral _____ Cerebral tissue perfusion
Intracranial pathology/trauma *NONE*
Intracranial pressure *—* Cerebral Perfusion Pressure *—*
Pupils   Reaction: Brisk *✓*
  L 2 3 (4) 5 6 mm   Sluggish ____ Nonreactive ____
  R 2 3 (4) 5 6 mm
Cardiac
Pacemaker *NONE* _____ Cardiopulmonary tissue
Apical rate & rhythm *110; SINUS TACHYCARDIA*   perfusion
Dysrhythmias *NONE*
Heart sounds/murmurs *S_1 & S_2 3 RUBS OR MURMURS*
BP: Cuff R *126/54* L *126/54* Arterial Line *123/52*
Cardiac index *4.6* _____ Cardiac output *8.56* ___ Cardiac output
CVP *14mmHg* PAP *40/20 mmHg* PCWP *16 mmHg*   Fluid volume
IV fluids *D5.45 NSE 40mEg KCl/L @ 50cc/HR; TPN@ 75cc/HR*   Deficit
IV vasoactive medications *NONE*   Excess

Bleeding: Yes *✓* No ____ Estimated blood loss *2,600 cc*
Sites of active bleeding *GUNSHOT ENTRY WOUND — LEFT POST. CHEST*
Labs
Na *145mEg/L* K *4.0mEg/L* CL *108mEg/L* CO_2 *23mM* Glucose *140 mg/dl*
Hct *32.5%* Hb *11.3g/dl* PT *12.35sec* PTT *60 sec* Platelets *200,000/µL*
Fibrin split products *—* Cardiac enzymes *—*   Cardiac output
                                      Peripheral tissue perfusion
Peripheral   Fluid volume
Jugular venous distention R *4cm* L *4cm*   Deficit
Skin Temp *WARM* Color *PINK* Turgor *GOOD*   Excess
Edema *FACE, EXTREMITIES* _____ Capillary refill *BRISK*

Fig. 15-2

Pulses: A = absent   B = bruits   D = doppler   Peripheral tissue perfusion
    + 3 = bounding   +2 = palpable   +1 = faintly palpable   Fluid volume
    Carotid   R _+2_ L _+2_   Popliteal   R _+2_ L _+2_   Deficit
    Brachial R _+2_ L _+2_   Posterior tibial R _+2_ L _+2_   Excess
    Radial   R _+2_ L _+2_   Dorsalis pedis R _+2_ L _+2_
    Femoral R _+2_ L _+2_
    Compartment tension _____ Location _MEASUREMENT NOT INDICATED_

Physical Integrity
Tissue integrity: Rashes _NONE_   Lesions _NONE_   (Impaired skin integrity)
    Lacerations _RIGHT ELBOW_ Abrasions _RIGHT KNEE_
    Bruises _RIGHT KNEE AND ELBOW; LEFT FLANK_
    Petechiae _NONE_   Impaired tissue integrity
    Soft tissue injury _BULLET ENTRY WOUND LEFT POSTERIOR CHEST WALL_
    Surgical incisions/drains/tubes (type and location) _ABDOMINAL MIDLINE;_
ABDOMINAL CHAFFIN TO LOW SUCTION; LEFT PLEURAL CHEST Infection
Leakage of spinal fluid from ears/nose/other (circle) _NONE_   _TUBE_

Physical Regulation
Immune
    WBC count _13.5x10^3/μL_ Cultures _SPUTUM, URINE, & BLOOD CULTURES_ (Infection)
PENDING; BULLET ENTRY SITE CULTURE PENDING   Hypothermia
Body temperature   Hyperthermia
    Temperature _102.2°F_ Route _RECTAL_   Ineffective thermoregulation

Nutrition
Usual eating patterns   More than body
    Number of meals per day _3_   requirements
    Special diet _No_
    Food preferences/intolerances _LIKES HAMBURGERS & TACOS_ (Less than body requirements)
    Food allergies _No_
    Appetite changes _NONE PRIOR TO ADMISSION_
Facial injury _NONE_
Condition of mouth/throat _TEETH IN GOOD CONDITION; MOUTH & THROAT LESIONS_ Oral mucous membrane
Height _5'7"_   Weight _171.6 lbs_ Ideal body weight _148 lbs_
Current therapy
    NPO _✓_   NG suction _Low_   Diet _—_   Fluid volume
    Tube feeding _No_   Deficit
    TPN _20% DEXTROSE 500cc; TRAVASOL 500cc; AMP MVI qd @ 75cc_ Excess
    Additional insulin needs _10 U REGULAR PER LITER OF TPN_   _HR; INTRALIPID @ 210cc/HR_
    Current therapy meeting body requirements: Yes ____ No _✓_

Elimination
Gastrointestinal/bowel   (Bowel patterns)
    Alterations from normal _WILL NEED BOWEL TRAINING_   Constipation
    Colostomy _No_   Ileostomy _No_   Diarrhea
    Evisceration/injury of abdominal organs _SEROSAL TEARS x 2 — DUODENUM_ (Incontinence) (POTENTIAL)
AND TRANSVERSE COLON
    Bleeding: Gastric _YES_ frank _—_ occult _✓_   (GI tissue perfusion)
      Intestinal _No_ frank _—_ occult _No STOOLS_
    Abdominal physical examination _No BOWEL SOUNDS; ABD. SLIGHTLY DISTENDED_
    Anal sphincter tone _NONE_
    Diagnostic peritoneal lavage: Positive _✓_   Negative _____

Fig. 15-2, cont'd

Continued.

Renal/urinary — **Renal tissue perfusion**
Possible kidney contusion/(other injury) *LEFT KIDNEY RUPTURE* — **Urinary patterns** (POTENTIAL)
Alteration from normal *WILL NEED BLADDER TRAINING* — (Incontinence) (POTENTIAL)
Urine color *TEA COLORED* Catheter *# 16 FRENCH FOLEY* — (Retention) (POTENTIAL)
Urine output: 24 hour *3245cc* Average hourly *135cc* — Cardiac output
Bladder distention *No* Genitourinary injury *No*
BUN *15 mg/dl* Creatinine *1.1 mg/dl* Specific gravity *1.030* — Fluid volume
Urine myoglobin *NEGATIVE* Other urine studies *GLUCOSE & ACETONE-* — Deficit
TRACE/NEGATIVE; pH 8.0; OCCULT BLOOD — LARGE — Excess

FEELING ▪ A pattern involving the subjective awareness of information
Comfort — Comfort
Pain/discomfort: Yes ✔ No _____
Onset *WITH MOVEMENT* Duration *THROUGHOUT ACTIVITY* — Pain/chronic
Location *ABDOMEN* Quality *SHARP* — (Pain/acute)
Aggravating factors *MOVEMENT; COUGHING* — Discomfort
Alleviating factors *REST, PAIN MEDICATION (DEMEROL 75 mg &*
VISTARIL 25mg IM)

Emotional Integrity/States
Recent stressful life events *RECENTLY ENTERED DRUG REHABIL-* — Grieving
ITATION — (Anxiety)
Verbalizes feelings of *FEAR AND ANXIETY* — (Fear)
— Anger
Source *CONCERNED ABOUT EXTENT OF PARALYSIS AND ITS* — Guilt
EFFECT ON HIS JOB AND SOCIAL LIFE — Shame
— Sadness
Physical manifestations *OCCASIONALLY TEARFUL*

COMMUNICATING ▪ A pattern involving sending messages
(Read) (write) (understand) English (circle) _____ — Communication
Other languages *No* — Verbal
Intubated *No* Speech impaired *No* — Nonverbal
Alternate form of communication *No*

KNOWING ▪ A pattern involving the meaning associated with information
Current health problems *PARALYSIS, POSSIBLE INFECTION, COCAINE*
ADDICTION
Previous hospitalizations/surgeries/illnesses *TONSILLECTOMY 1974*

— (Knowledge deficit)
Current medications *DEMEROL 75mg c̄ VISTARIL 25mg IM q 8h*

Last tetanus immunization *MED STAR (HELICOPTER) 7/1*
Perception/knowledge of illness/planned tests/surgery *VERBALIZES*
KNOWLEDGE OF PROCEDURE AND PURPOSE OF CAT SCAN OF
THE ABDOMEN
Expectations of therapy *HELP HIM DEAL WITH HIS PARALYSIS*
Misconceptions *NONE AT THIS TIME*
Readiness to learn *TOO ANXIOUS AT PRESENT* — Learning
Requests information concerning *PERMANENCE AND EXTENT OF PARALYSIS*
Educational level *8TH GRADE*
— Thought processes
Learning impeded by *PAIN; ANXIETY* — (Impaired problem solving)

Fig. 15-2, cont'd

Orientation

Level of alertness *VERY ALERT; EASILY AROUSED*   Orientation

Orientation: Person *YES*   Place *YES*   Time *YES*   Confusion

Appropriate behavior/communication *BOTH APPROPRIATE*   Thought processes

Neurologic changes/symptoms *LOSS OF MOVEMENT AND SENSATION:*
LEFT T12 RIGHT T11

Eye Opening
    None (1)
    To pain (2)
    To speech (3)
    Spontaneous (4)⃝

Best Verbal	Best Motor	
No response (1)	Flaccid (1)	Orientation
Incomprehensible sound (2)	Extensor response (2)	Confusion
Inappropriate words (3)	Flexor response (3)	LOC
Confused conversation (4)	Semipurposeful (4)	
Oriented (5)⃝	Localized to pain (5)	
	Obeys commands (6)⃝	

Glascow Coma Scale total *15*

Memory

Memory intact: Yes ✓ No ____ Recent *YES* Remote *YES*   Memory

PERCEIVING ▪ A pattern involving the reception of information

Sensory/Perception   ⟨Sensory/perception⟩

History of restricted environment *CURRENTLY IN ICU*

Vision impaired *No*   Glasses *No*   Visual

Auditory impaired *No*   Hearing aid *No*   Auditory

Kinesthetics impaired *YES — NO POSITION SENSE IN LEGS*   ⟨Kinesthetic⟩

Gustatory impaired *No*   Gustatory

Tactile impaired *YES; SECONDARY TO SPINAL CORD INJURY*   ⟨Tactile⟩

Olfactory impaired *No*   Olfactory

Spinal cord injury: Yes ✓ No ____

    Level of sensory loss: R *T11*   L *T12*

Self-Concept   ⟨Self-concept⟩

Patient's description of self *INDEPENDENT*   ⟨Body image⟩

Effects of injury/surgery on self-concept *CONCERNED ABOUT LEVEL*   ⟨Self-esteem⟩
OF DEPENDENCE ON OTHERS; INABILITY TO WORK   Personal identity

Meaningfulness

Verbalizes hopelessness *No*   Hopelessness

Verbalizes/perceives loss of control *RELATED TO MOVING IN BED*   ⟨Powerlessness⟩

Self-inflicted injury: Yes ____ No ✓ Type —

MOVING ▪ A pattern involving activity

Activity

History of previous/current/anticipated physical disabilities *PARALYSIS —*   ⟨Impaired physical mobility⟩
PARAPLEGIA

Fig. 15-2, cont'd

Continued.

Verbal report of fatigue/weakness *TIRES EASILY*   Activity intolerance

Braces/casts/(splints)/traction (circle) *SPLINTS ON BOTH FEET*   Impaired physical mobility

Fractures *T 12 VERTEBRAE SHATTERED*

Amputations *No*

Paralysis: Yes ✓ No _____ Level of paralysis: R *T11* L *T12*

Self-Care

Ability to perform ADLs: Independent _____ Dependent ✓   (Self-care)

Feeding

Specify deficits *CURRENTLY BATHING, DRESSING, TURNING*   (Bathing/hygiene)

(Dressing/grooming)

Discharge planning needs *BOWEL & BLADDER TRAINING; WHEEL-*   (Toileting)
CHAIR TRANSFERS; SEXUAL FUNCTIONING WITH PARAPLEGIA;
                                     DRESSING

Environmental Maintenance

Home maintenance management

   Limitations related to returning to previous home environment and/or   (Impaired home maintenance
   responsibilities *LIVES IN 2ND FLOOR APARTMENT — NO ELAVATOR;*   management)
GIRLFRIEND DOES SHOPPING; USUALLY SHARE HOUSEKEEP-
ING DUTIES (GIRLFRIEND)

Safety needs *GRIP RAILS — TUB & TOILET*   Safety hazards

Health Maintenance

   Regular physical checkups *No*

   Health insurance *CHAMPUS*   Health maintenance

Rest   Sleep pattern disturbance

   Hours slept/night *8* Feels rested: Yes ✓ No _____   Hypersomnia

   Difficulty falling/remaining asleep *No*   Insomnia

   Sleep aids (pillows, meds, food) *No*   Nightmares

Recreation

   Leisure/diversional activities *SINGS, BOXES, WATCHES MOVIES*   Deficit in diversional activity

   Social activities *GOES OUT WITH THE "GUYS" AT LEAST TWICE A WEEK*

VALUING ▪ A pattern involving the assigning of relative worth

Religious preference *PROTESTANT*   Spiritual state

Important religious practices *NONE*   Distress

Spiritual concerns *NONE*   Despair

Cultural orientation *No SPECIFIC*

Cultural practices *NONE*

RELATING ▪ A pattern involving establishing bonds

Role

Marital status *SINGLE*   (Role performance)

Age & health of significant other *GIRLFRIEND 20 YRS, GOOD HEALTH;*   Parenting
FATHER — 55 YRS, GOOD HEALTH   (Sexual dysfunction)

Number of children *1* Ages *1 YR*   (Work)

Role in home *WAGE EARNER*   (Family)

Role satisfaction/(concerns) *REGARDING FINANCES*   Social/leisure

Financial support *PATIENT*

Occupation *CONSTRUCTION WORKER*   Family processes

   Job satisfaction/concerns *LIKES JOB; WORRIED ABOUT RETURNING*

   Physical/mental energy expenditures *HEAVY LIFTING; CLIMBING*

Sexual relationships ((satisfactory)/unsatisfactory) *(GIRLFRIEND)*   Sexuality patterns

   Physical difficulties related to sex *NONE IN PAST*

Concerns regarding sexual function as a result of injury *HOW PARALYSIS*
WILL AFFECT SEXUAL FUNCTION (GIRLFRIEND)

Fig. 15-2, cont'd

Socialization

Quality of relationships with others *GOOD (FATHER)*   Impaired social interaction

 Patient's description *"I GET ALONG OK WITH PEOPLE — IF THEY DON'T CROSS ME "*

 Significant others' descriptions *"HE'S FAIRLY EASY GOING " (GIRLFRIEND)*

 Staff observations *RELATES WELL WITH FAMILY; OCCASIONALLY DEMANDING*

Verbalizes feelings of being alone *No*   Social isolation

 Attributed to   Social withdrawal

CHOOSING ▪ A pattern involving the selection of alternatives

Coping

Patient's usual problem-solving methods *KEEPS PROBLEMS TO HIMSELF;* Ineffective individual coping

"IMPULSIVE " (FATHER & GIRLFRIEND)   Ineffective family coping

Family's usual problem-solving methods *TALKING WITH EACH OTHER ;*

SEEKING FATHER'S ADVICE (GIRLFRIEND)

Patient's method of dealing with stress *"SNORT COKE" — IN THE PAST ;*

GO TO THE GYM (GIRLFRIEND)

Family's method of dealing with stress *WATCH TV ; GO FOR A WALK*

Suspected/known (circle) substance abuse: Yes ✓ No

 Type of substance *COCAINE*

Verbalizes inability to cope *No*

Patient's affect *WITHDRAWN, OCCASIONALLY DEMANDING OR ANGRY*

 Physical manifestations *SPEAKS ONLY WHEN SPOKEN TO; LITTLE EYE CONTACT*

Support systems available *GIRLFRIEND; FATHER*

Participation

Compliance with past/current health care regimens *ATTENDING DRUG* Noncompliance

REHABILITATION PROGRAM AS REQUIRED   Ineffective participation

Willingness to comply with future health care regimen *UNKNOWN AT*

PRESENT

Decision-making ability   Judgment

 Patient's perspective *NOT ASSESSED AT PRESENT*   Indecisiveness

 Others' perspectives *"FAIR " (GIRLFRIEND)*

Prioritized nursing diagnosis/problem list

1. *ALTERED COMFORT ; PAIN (ACUTE) RELATED TO SURGICAL INCISIONS*
2. *IMPAIRED PHYSICAL MOBILITY RELATED TO PARAPLEGIA*
3. *ALTERED NUTRITION : LESS THAN BODY REQUIREMENTS*

A. *RELATED TO HYPERMETABOLIC STATE CAUSED BY INJURY AND FEVER*

4/5. *POTENTIAL FOR INFECTION RELATED TO IMPAIRED SKIN AND TISSUE INTEGRITY*

5. *ALTERED SELF-CONCEPT RELATED TO DEPENDENCE ON OTHERS*

Signature *Linda A. Prinkey*   Date *7/2*

Fig. 15-2, cont'd

CHAPTER 16

ORTHOPEDIC ASSESSMENT TOOL

PATRICIA C. SEIFERT
ANN MARIE JANEK

The Orthopedic Assessment Tool is designed to assess orthopedic patients with unique biopsychosocial assessment needs. The tool incorporates specific signs and symptoms pertinent to orthopedic patients to facilitate identification of nursing diagnoses. It also incorporates the American Nurses' Association and National Association of Orthopaedic Nurses' *Standards of Orthopaedic Nursing Practice*. This chapter includes:

- *The way the tool was developed and refined*
- *The patient populations and settings to which it applies*
- *Selected orthopedic emphasis areas*
- *The way to use the tool*
- *Specific orthopedic focus questions and parameters to assist the nurse in eliciting appropriate data*
- *The Orthopedic Assessment Tool*
- *A case study*
- *A completed version of the tool based on the case study*

DEVELOPMENT AND REFINEMENT OF THE TOOL

The Orthopedic Assessment Tool was developed from the nursing data base prototype (see Chapter 2). Some hemodynamic monitoring and critical care variables originally incorporated in the prototype were deleted and replaced with variables more applicable to orthopedic assessment. The resultant tool was then modified based on the recommendations of orthopedic nurse experts. Further, the content of the tool is supported by the literature from this field of nursing.

After the tool was developed and refined, it was clinically tested by orthopedic nurse experts and clinical nurse specialists on 10 patients in acute care medical and surgical units. All patients had several problems or medical diagnoses. Many were chronically ill with acute exacerbations of previous problems or the development of new problems. The testing evaluated the adequacy of the tool in terms of flow, space for recording data, and completeness of assessment variables. Based on the results, the tool was revised.

PATIENT POPULATION AND SETTING

The Orthopedic Assessment Tool was developed to assess the needs and problems of orthopedic patients who may have multisystem problems. It is designed for use with stable patients in hospitals or home or long-term care settings. To avoid fatiguing some patients, it may be necessary to complete the assessment tool in two sessions, preferably within 24 hours.

ORTHOPEDIC EMPHASIS AREAS

Orthopedic patients have specialized problems and needs. The Orthopedic Assessment Tool includes appropriate assessment variables within each of the nine human response patterns of the Unitary Person Framework. The tool focuses on prevalent problems among these patients. Table 16-1 outlines these emphasis areas.

HOW TO USE THE TOOL

To use the Orthopedic Assessment Tool effectively, nurses must first be familiar with the Unitary Person Framework (see Chapter 2), which provides the underlying framework for Taxonomy I. The nine human response pat-

Table 16-1
Selected orthopedic emphasis areas

Patterns	Emphasis areas to determine
Communicating	Physical impairment affecting communication
Knowing	Perception and knowledge of illness, tests, surgery, or therapy
	Expectations of therapy
Valuing	Religious or cultural practices
Relating	Role and responsibilities in home
	Feelings of being alone
Feeling	Nonverbal indicators of pain
	Alleviating factors such as position, medication, or external supports
Moving	Limitations in daily activities such as casts, traction, or bed rest
	Fatigue or activity tolerance: factors increasing fatigue and energy demands
	Range of motion
	Environmental maintenance
	Altered self-care
Perceiving	Effects of illness and surgery on self-concept
Exchanging	Tissue integrity or skin breakdown (increased risk)
	Elimination: impact of impaired mobility on body systems
Choosing	Coping and problem-solving strategies, and strategies to deal with stress
	Compliance with health care regimen

terns of the Unitary Person Framework serve as the major category headings for Taxonomy I and the tool. The sequence of the response patterns, as it appears in Taxonomy I, has been changed in the tool to permit a logical ordering of assessment variables. Nursing diagnoses pertinent to the orthopedic patient, along with the signs and symptoms necessary to identify them, are under the appropriate human response patterns.

Nurses must also realize that this tool is very different from conventional assessment tools. As a result, nurses may encounter some initial difficulty in using it. They should remember, however, that this tool was not designed to follow the organization or content of a traditional medical data base; the data collected does not solely reflect medical patterns. Rather, this tool elicits data about holistic patterns in ways not traditionally assessed by nurses and provides a new method of collecting and synthesizing data. It requires new thinking when processing data. This tool represents a nursing data base developed from a nursing model to permit a holistic nursing assessment to take place so nursing diagnoses can be identified.

Although nurses probably agree that a holistic nursing data base is desirable, it is realized that changing traditional assessment methods is not an easy task. For this reason, a trial usage period is recommended before decisions about the tool's merits are made. During this trial period, nurses should assess 10 orthopedic patients using the tool to become familiar and progressively more comfortable with its organization and data-collection methods. With experience, nurses will become accustomed to new ways of clustering and processing information. With continued use, the time necessary to complete the tool will be reduced. Most important, nurses will recognize the unique ability of the tool to elicit appropriate signs and symptoms. Nurses will also discover that nursing diagnoses are easily identified when using this tool.

It is not necessary to complete the tool in one session. Priority sections can be completed during the initial assessment. Other sections or patterns can be completed later, within a time frame acceptable to the institution. To elicit appropriate data, nurses should be familiar with the focus questions and parameters in the next section. When assessing for specific signs and symptoms, the nurse circles the diagnosis in the right-hand column when deviations from normal are found. A circled diagnosis does not confirm a problem but simply alerts the nurse to the possibility that it exists. After completing the tool, the nurse scans the circled problems, synthesizes the data to determine whether other clusters of signs and symptoms support a problem, and judges whether the actual or potential diagnosis is present.

Some diagnoses are repeated several times in the right-hand column. These repetitions occur only within the appropriate response pattern and are convenient for identifying data directly with their corresponding nursing diagnosis. These diagnoses are not absolute but focus thinking and direct more attention to a possible problem.

Certain signs and symptoms can indicate several diagnoses. For example, fever can indicate infection and ineffective thermoregulation. To avoid repetition of assessment parameters, variables are arranged with the diagnosis most likely to result from the data assessed. Thus, data to support one diagnosis may occasionally be found in other

Table 16-2
Orthopedic assessment tool: focus questions and parameters

Variables	Focus questions and parameters
COMMUNICATING	
Physical impairment affecting communication	What written communication methods are available to the patient who has a fractured writing hand or who is unable to sit up?
KNOWING	
Perception/knowledge of illness/tests/surgery/ therapy and expectations of therapy	"What do you think causes your pain?" "Tell me about your illness, tests, surgery, or therapy."
VALUING	
Religious and cultural practices	"Are there special mementos or religious articles that you would like to have here with you?"
RELATING	
Role/responsibilities in home	"Is there someone at home to help you while you're in a cast or in bed?"
Verbalizes feelings of being alone	"Do you feel isolated while you're confined to a bed or in a cast?"
FEELING	
Nonverbal indications	What nonverbal indications of pain such as massaging, wincing, guarding, and reluctance to move are demonstrated?
Alleviating factors	What factors (rest, massage, relaxation techniques, exercise, specific position, heat or cold) alleviate the pain?
MOVING	
Limitations in daily activities activities	Is the patient's activity restricted by a cast, brace, traction, or bed rest? What techniques are safe and effective for bed mobility, transfer, and ambulation?
Fatigue/activity tolerance	Do these restrictions increase the patient's fatigue and energy demands? Do any factors (inefficient walking, recent surgery, or other health problems) increase energy demands?
Range of motion	What is the patient's ability to perform flexion, extension, abduction, adduction, and rotation?
Environmental maintenance	Are there special sleeping, toileting, or eating arrangements in the home for the patient with a total hip replacement or fracture?
Self-care	"Do you have any difficulty feeding, bathing, dressing, or toileting?"
PERCEIVING	
Effects of illness/surgery on self-concept	"Will your illness, surgery, or therapy affect how you think about yourself? How?"
EXCHANGING	
Tissue integrity	Are there bruises or edema?
Skin	Assess the patient's skin color, moisture, turgor, temperature, and general condition. Is there increased potential for skin pressure, friction, shearing, or moisture due to an impaired ability to change positions, orthopedic devices, or impaired sensation?
Elimination	Is there increased potential for constipation related to reduced activity or medications? Are there other effects of immobility (venous stasis or renal calculi)?
CHOOSING	
Coping	How does the musculoskeletal disruption affect coping ability and stress level? What are the patient's and family's methods of dealing with stress?
Compliance with past/ current health care regimens	"Are there physical limitations making compliance with the prescribed regimen difficult?"

patterns or arranged with other diagnoses. Therefore, synthesis of all data is essential.

The Orthopedic Assessment Tool is not intended to be the standardized and final format for assessing orthopedic patients across the country. An assessment tool must meet the needs of the institutions and nurses using it. The Orthopedic Assessment Tool is simply a working demonstration tool that is expected to be changed and revised by nurses in clinical practice. Further evaluation and refinement are necessary before adopting the tool for use in an institution. Nurses interested in changing, revising, and adapting the tool to a specific clinical setting should refer to Chapter 4.

HOW TO ELICIT APPROPRIATE DATA

Because the Unitary Person Framework and the Orthopedic Assessment Tool contain some terms that may be unfamiliar to nurses, focus questions and parameters were developed and refined to elicit appropriate information. These questions and parameters are outlined in Table 16-2, which follows the content of the assessment tool (Fig. 16-1). The variables in bold type in the tool are described in Table 16-2. For example, the variable about range of motion under the "moving pattern" is in bold type. If the nurse is unsure what to ask about range of motion, the information in Table 16-2 can guide questioning. The questions and parameters provide clarity and guidance in eliciting data. They are not all inclusive so nurses should not feel limited by them. There are many other ways based on the patient's situation and condition and the skill of the nurse to elicit the information. Focus questions and parameters for other data were presented in Chapter 3.

CASE STUDY

The case study models the process a nurse uses when assessing a patient. Based on the clustering of information obtained during assessment, the nurse formulates nursing diagnoses.

Mrs. R.L. is a 49-year-old housewife admitted to the hospital after fracturing her right ankle. The Orthopedic Assessment Tool (Fig. 16-2) was used to assess Mrs. R.L.

BIBLIOGRAPHY

American Nurses' Association and National Association of Orthopaedic Nurses: Orthopaedic nursing practice, Kansas City, Mo, 1986, ANA, Inc.

American Nurses' Association and National Association of Orthopaedic Nurses: Orthopaedic nursing practice: process and outcome criteria for selected diagnoses, Orthop Nurs 6:11, 1987.

Baird SE: Development of a nursing assessment tool to diagnose altered body image in immobilized patients, Orthop Nurs 4:47, 1985.

Pastorino CA: Using standards of care in the practice setting, Orthop Nurs 6:20, 1987.

Phipps WJ, Long BC, and Woods N, editors: Medical-surgical nursing: concepts and clinical practice, ed 2, St Louis, 1987, The CV Mosby Co.

Taylor SL: Low back pain assessment. I. History-taking, Orthop Nurs 2:11, 1983.

Vanderbeck KA: Getting the facts: a guide to orthopaedic assessment, Orthop Nurs 3:31, 1984.

ORTHOPEDIC ASSESSMENT TOOL

Name _____ Age _____ Sex _____
Address _____ Telephone _____
Significant other _____ Telephone _____
Date of admission _____ Medical diagnosis _____
Allergies _____

Nursing Diagnosis
(Potential or Altered)

COMMUNICATING ▪ A pattern involving sending messages

Read, write, understand English (circle) _____ Communication
Other languages _____ Verbal
Intubated _____ Speech impaired _____ Nonverbal
Alternate form of communication _____
Physical impairment affecting communication _____

KNOWING ▪ A pattern involving the meaning associated with information

Current health problems _____
_____
Current medications (steroids, ASA) _____
_____
Previous hospitalizations/surgeries _____
_____

History of the following problems: Knowledge deficit
   Heart _____
   Lung _____
   Gastric/duodenal ulcer _____
   Liver _____ Gallbladder _____
   Kidney _____ Urinary tract _____
   Cerebrovascular _____ Rheumatic fever _____
   Thyroid _____
   Diabetes _____ Medication _____

Risk factors   Present   Perceptions/knowledge of
  1. Hypertension   _____ _____
  2. Hyperlipidemia   _____ _____
  3. Smoking   _____ _____
  4. Obesity   _____ _____
  5. Diabetes   _____ _____
  6. Sedentary living _____ _____
  7. Stress   _____ _____
  8. Alcohol use   _____ _____
  9. Oral contraceptives _____ _____
 10. Family history   _____ _____

Perception/knowledge of illness/tests/surgery/therapy _____
_____

Expectations of therapy _____
Misconceptions _____
Readiness to learn _____
   Request information concerning _____
   Educational level _____ Thought processes
   Learning impeded by _____

Orientation

   Level of alertness _____ Orientation
   Orientation: Person _____ Place _____ Time _____ Confusion
   Appropriate behavior/communication _____

Fig. 16-1

Memory

Memory intact: Yes _____ No _____ Recent _____ Remote _____   Memory

VALUING ▪ A pattern involving the assigning of relative worth

Religious preference _____   Spiritual state

Important religious practices _____   Distress

Spiritual concerns _____   Despair

Cultural orientation/practices _____

RELATING ▪ A pattern involving establishing bonds

Role

  Marital status _____   Role performance

  Age & health of significant other _____   Parenting

_____   Sexual dysfunction

  Number of children _____ Ages _____   Work

  Role/responsibilities in home _____   Family

  Financial support _____   Social/leisure

  Occupation _____   Family processes

    Job satisfaction/concerns _____

    Physical/mental energy expenditures _____

  Sexual relationships (satisfactory/unsatisfactory) _____   Sexuality patterns

    Physical difficulties/effects of illness related to sex _____

_____

Socialization

  Quality of relationships with others _____   Impaired social interaction

    Patient's description _____

    Significant others' descriptions _____

    Staff observations _____

  Verbalizes feelings of being alone _____   Social isolation

    Attributed to _____   Social withdrawal

FEELING ▪ A pattern involving the subjective awareness of information

Comfort

  Pain/discomfort: Yes _____ No _____

    Onset _____ Duration _____   Comfort

    Location _____ Quality _____ Radiation _____   Pain/chronic

    Nonverbal indications: _____ Wincing _____   Pain/acute

      Guarding _____ Massaging _____ Reluctance to move _____   Discomfort

    Associated factors _____

    Aggravating factors _____

    Alleviating factors: position _____

      Medications _____

      External supports _____

Emotional Integrity/States

  Recent stressful life events _____   Grieving

_____   Anxiety

  Verbalizes feelings of _____   Fear

    Source _____   Anger

_____   Guilt

  Physical manifestations _____   Shame

_____   Sadness

Fig. 16-1, cont'd

Continued.

MOVING ▪ A pattern involving activity
Activity
History of physical disability _____   Impaired physical mobility
_____
Presence of: Cast _____ Braces _____
Traction _____ Crutches _____
Limitations in daily activities _____   Activity intolerance
Fatigue/activity tolerance _____
Exercise habits _____
Range of motion: Flexion _____ Extension _____
Abduction _____ Adduction _____
Rotation _____ Sensation _____
Skeleton: Posture _____ Symmetry _____
Gait _____ Appearance _____
Muscles: Strength _____ Shape _____
Movement _____
Diagnostic findings: x-ray studies _____
CT scan _____ MRI _____
Myelogram _____ Fluid aspiration _____

Rest   Sleep pattern disturbance
Hours slept/night _____   Hypersomnia
Sleep aids (pillows, meds, food) _____   Insomnia
Difficulty falling/remaining asleep _____   Nightmares

Recreation
Leisure activities _____   Deficit in diversional activity
Social activities _____

Environmental Maintenance
Home maintenance management
Size & arrangement of home (stairs, bathroom) _____   Impaired home maintenance
_____ Safety needs _____   management
Housekeeping responsibilities _____   Safety hazards
Shopping responsibilities _____

Health Maintenance
Health insurance _____   Health maintenance
Regular physical checkups _____

Self-Care   Self-care
Ability to perform ADLs: Independent _____ Dependent _____   Feeding
Specify deficits _____   Bathing/hygiene
Discharge planning needs _____   Dressing/grooming
Toileting

PERCEIVING ▪ A pattern involving the reception of information
Self-Concept
Patient's description of self _____   Body image
Effects of illness/surgery on self-concept _____   Self-esteem
_____   Personal identity

Meaningfulness
Verbalizes hopelessness _____   Hopelessness
Verbalizes/perceives loss of control _____   Powerlessness

Fig. 16-1, cont'd

Sensory/Perception

History of restrictive environment _____

Vision impaired _____ Glasses _____ Visual

Auditory impaired _____ Hearing aid _____ Auditory

Kinesthetics impaired _____ Romberg _____ Kinesthetic

Gustatory impaired _____ Gustatory

Tactile impaired _____ Tactile

Olfactory impaired _____ Olfactory

Reflexes: grossly intact _____

EXCHANGING ▪ A pattern involving mutual giving and receiving

Circulation

Cerebral (circle appropriate response)   Cerebral tissue perfusion

Neurologic changes/symptoms _____

Pupils	Eye Opening
L 2 3 4 5 6 mm	None (1)
R 2 3 4 5 6 mm	To pain (2)
Reaction: Brisk _____	To speech (3)
Sluggish _____ Nonreactive _____	Spontaneous (4)
Best Verbal	Best Motor
No response (1)	Flaccid (1)
Incomprehensible sound (2)	Extensor response (2)
Inappropriate words (3)	Flexor response (3)
Confused conversation (4)	Semipurposeful (4)
Oriented (5)	Localized to pain (5)
	Obeys commands (6)

Glasgow Coma Scale total _____

Cardiac

Apical rate & rhythm _____ Cardiopulmonary tissue

Heart sounds/murmurs _____   perfusion

ECG _____ Fluid volume

BP: _____ Location _____   Deficit

IV fluids _____   Excess

Cardiac output

Peripheral   Peripheral tissue perfusion

Pulses: A = absent   B = bruits   D = doppler

+3 = bounding   +2 = palpable   +1 = faintly palpable

Carotid R _____ L _____	Popliteal R _____ L _____
Brachial R _____ L _____	Posterior tibial R _____ L _____
Radial R _____ L _____	Dorsalis pedis R _____ L _____

Femoral R _____ L _____   Fluid volume

Skin temp _____ Color _____   Deficit

Edema _____ Capillary refill _____   Excess

Homans' sign _____ Cardiac output

Physical Integrity

Tissue integrity _____ Rashes _____ Lesions _____ Impaired skin integrity

Petechiae _____ Bruises _____ Impaired tissue integrity

Abrasions _____ Lacerations _____

Old scars/surgical incisions _____

Localized edema _____

Generalized edema _____

Skin: Moisture _____ Color _____ Turgor _____

Fig. 16-1, cont'd

Continued.

Oxygenation

Complaints of dyspnea _____ Precipitated by _____
Orthopnea _____
Rate _____ Rhythm _____ Depth _____
Labored/unlabored (circle)
Use of accessory muscles _____
Chest expansion _____
Splinting _____
Cough: productive/nonproductive _____
Sputum: Color _____ Amount _____ Consistency _____
Breath sounds _____

Ineffective breathing patterns
Ineffective airway clearance
Impaired gas exchange

Physical Regulation

Immune
    Lymph nodes enlarged _____ Location _____

Body temperature
    Temperature _____ Route _____

Infection
Hypothermia
Hyperthermia
Ineffective thermoregulation

Nutrition

Eating patterns
    Number of meals per day _____
    Special diet _____
    Where eaten _____
    Food preferences/intolerances _____
    Food allergies _____
    Caffeine intake (coffee, tea, soft drinks, chocolate)
    _____
    Appetite changes _____
    Nausea/vomiting _____
Condition of mouth/throat _____
Dentures (upper, lower, full mouth) _____
Height _____ Weight _____
State of hydration _____
Current therapy
    NPO _____ NG suction _____
    Tube feeding _____
    TPN _____
Labs
    Na _____ K _____ CL _____ Glucose _____
    Cholesterol _____ Triglycerides _____ Fasting _____
    CBC _____
    Blood coagulation studies _____
    Serum salicylate _____ Sed. rate _____
    WBC count _____ Differential _____

Oral mucous membrane
More than body
    requirements
Less than body requirements

Elimination

Gastrointestinal/bowel
    Usual bowel habits _____
    Alterations from normal _____
    Abdominal physical examination _____
    Liver: Enlarged _____ Ascites _____
Renal/urinary
    Usual urinary pattern _____
    Alteration from normal _____
    Color _____ Catheter _____
    Urine output: 24 hour _____ Average hourly _____
    Bladder distention _____

Bowel elimination
    Constipation
    Diarrhea
    Incontinence
GI tissue perfusion

Urinary elimination
    Incontinence
    Retention

Fig. 16-1, cont'd

BUN _____ Creatinine _____ Specific gravity _____   Renal tissue perfusion
   Urine studies: Uric acid _____
   Alkaline phosphatase _____

CHOOSING ■ A pattern involving the selection of alternatives
Coping
   Patient's usual problem-solving methods _____   Ineffective individual coping
   _____   Ineffective family coping

   Family's usual problem-solving methods _____
   _____

   Patient's method of dealing with stress _____
   _____

   Family's method of dealing with stress _____
   _____

   Patient's affect _____
   Physical manifestations _____
   Coping mechanisms _____

Participation
   Compliance with past/current health care regimens _____   Noncompliance
   _____   Ineffective participation

   Willingness to comply with future health care regimen _____
   _____

Judgment
   Decision-making ability   Judgment
     Patient's perspective _____   Indecisiveness
     Others' perspectives _____

Prioritized nursing diagnosis/problem list
1. _____
2. _____
3. _____
4. _____
5. _____

Signature _____   Date _____

Fig. 16-1, cont'd

ORTHOPEDIC ASSESSMENT TOOL

Name _R.L._   Age _49_   Sex _F_
Address _15 TAYLOR ST., MIDDLETON, VA._   Telephone _636-1212_
Significant other _H.L. — HUSBAND_   Telephone _(W) 513-4500_
Date of admission _11/15_   Medical diagnosis _S/P ORIF ®ANKLE 11/13_
Allergies _CODEINE_

Nursing Diagnosis
(Potential or Altered)

COMMUNICATING ▪ A pattern involving sending messages
(Read, write, understand) English (circle) _____   Communication
Other languages _-Ø-_   Verbal
Intubated _-Ø-_   Speech impaired _-Ø-_   Nonverbal
Alternate form of communication _-Ø-_
Physical impairment affecting communication _-Ø-_

KNOWING ▪ A pattern involving the meaning associated with information
Current health problems _FX ® ANKLE, ASTHMA, HYPOTHYROID_

Current medications (steroids, ASA) _SYNTHYROID 0.1 mg PO qd, THEOPHYLLINE 200 mg PO q̄d, TYLOX ī OR ī ī q̄ 4h PRN_
Previous hospitalizations/surgeries _ORIGINAL FX AND ORIF ® ANKLE 2 d AGO (11/13); 10 YR. AGO FOR ASTHMA_
History of the following problems: Knowledge deficit
   Heart _FUNCTIONAL MURMUR — NO MEDS OR RX_
   Lung _ASTHMA SINCE CHILDHOOD_
   Gastric/duodenal ulcer _-Ø-_
   Liver _-Ø-_   Gallbladder _-Ø-_
   Kidney _-Ø-_   Urinary tract _NO BURNING OR URGENCY_
   Cerebrovascular _-Ø-_   Rheumatic fever _-Ø-_
   Thyroid _↓, SYNTHYROID_
   Diabetes _-Ø-_   Medication _-Ø-_

Risk factors	Present	Perceptions/knowledge of
1. Hypertension	(120/70)-Ø-	_YES_
2. Hyperlipidemia	-Ø-	" (LOW CHOLESTEROL)
3. Smoking	-Ø-	"
4. Obesity	-Ø-	"
5. Diabetes	-Ø-	"
6. Sedentary living	-Ø-	" (DOES EXERCISE 3X WK TILL NOW)
7. Stress	✓	" (N.B. RECENT HOSPITALIZATION, MOVE TO NEW HOUSE)
8. Alcohol use	-Ø-	"
9. Oral contraceptives	-Ø-	"
10. Family history	_NO SIGNIFICANT FAMILY HISTORY_	

Perception/knowledge of illness/tests/surgery/therapy _UNDERSTANDS OPERATIVE PROCEDURE, NEED FOR PHYS. THERAPY_
Expectations of therapy _REPAIR ANKLE_
Misconceptions _-Ø-_
Readiness to learn _YES_
   Request information concerning _1.WHEN WILL PAIN STOP? 2. USING CRUTCHES, 3. AMBULATING, 4. RETURN TO WORK_
   Educational level _H.S. COMPLETED_   Thought processes
   Learning impeded by _-Ø-_

Orientation
   Level of alertness _ALERT_   Orientation
   Orientation: Person _✓_   Place _✓_   Time _✓_   Confusion
   Appropriate behavior/communication _YES_

Fig. 16-2

Memory
Memory intact: Yes ✓ No _____ Recent ✓ Remote ✓   Memory

VALUING ▪ A pattern involving the assigning of relative worth
Religious preference *BAPTIST*   Spiritual state
Important religious practices *NO ETOH, NO TOBACCO*   Distress
Spiritual concerns *"GOD WILL HELP ME GET THROUGH THIS."*   Despair
Cultural orientation/practices *NONE SPECIAL*

RELATING ▪ A pattern involving establishing bonds
Role
  Marital status *MARRIED*   Role performance
  Age & health of significant other *49 YO HUSBAND — IN GOOD HEALTH*   Parenting
               Sexual dysfunction
  Number of children *1*   Ages *25 YO DAUGHTER*   Work
  Role/responsibilities in home *HOMEMAKER*   Family
  Financial support *HUSBAND'S + OWN SALARY, INSURANCE*   Social/leisure
  Occupation *LEGAL SECRETARY*   Family processes
    Job satisfaction/concerns *NO CONCERNS*
    Physical/mental energy expenditures *NO UNDUE EXERTION*
  Sexual relationships (satisfactory/unsatisfactory) _____   Sexuality patterns
    Physical difficulties/effects of illness related to sex *R/T FX Ⓡ ANKLE,*
    MOBILITY

Socialization
  Quality of relationships with others *"I HAVE LOTS OF FRIENDS."*   Impaired social interaction
    Patient's description *"THESE (CARDS/FLOWERS) ARE FROM FRIENDS."*
    Significant others' descriptions *"HOPE SHE'S BETTER SOON." (HUSBAND)*
    Staff observations *FAMILY, FRIENDS VISIT, GOOD SUPPORT*
    Verbalizes feelings of being alone ─⊖─   Social isolation
    Attributed to *N/A*   Social withdrawal

FEELING ▪ A pattern involving the subjective awareness of information
Comfort
  Pain/discomfort: Yes ✓ No _____
    Onset *MOVEMENT OF ANKLE*   Duration *2 DAYS*   (Comfort)
    Location Ⓡ *ANKLE* Quality *DULL*   Radiation *NO*   Pain/chronic
    Nonverbal indications: ─⊖─ Wincing ─⊖─   (Pain/acute)
      Guarding ✓ Massaging ─⊖─ Reluctance to move ✓   Discomfort
  Associated factors ─⊖─
  Aggravating factors *MOVEMENT OF LEG*
  Alleviating factors: position *ELEVATION, BED REST*
    Medications *TYLOX Ī OR ĪĪ q 4h PRN, PAIN*
    External supports *CAST c̄ BLOODY DRAINAGE*

Emotional Integrity/States
  Recent stressful life events *Ex: RECENTLY MOVED TO NEW HOUSE*   Grieving
               (Anxiety)
  Verbalizes feelings of *ANXIETY: INABILITY TO FIX HOUSE*   Fear
    Source *HOSPITALIZATION, DIFFICULTY AMBULATING*   Anger
    ("I WISH I COULD GET HOME.")   Envy
  Physical manifestations *TENSE IN BED, "STARES"*   Guilt
               Shame
               Sadness

Fig. 16-2, cont'd

Continued.

MOVING ▪ A pattern involving activity
Activity

History of physical disability *FELL AND FX'D ℝ ANKLE DURING HOUSE MOVE 11/13* （Impaired physical mobility）

Presence of: Cast ✓ _____ Braces __Ø__
 Traction __Ø__ Crutches ✓

Limitations in daily activities *↓ MOBILITY, AMBULATION(STAIRS)*   Activity intolerance
Fatigue/activity tolerance *NEEDS REST PERIODS*
Exercise habits *RAN 3X WK BEFORE FX, LITTLE EXERCISE SINCE FX*
Range of motion: Flexion ⓛ _____ Extension ⓛ） *CANNOT*
 Abduction ⓛ ✓ _____ Adduction ⓛ ✓ ｝ *ASSESS ℝ LEG*
 Rotation ⓛ ✓ _____ Sensation ⓛ ✓ ） *c̄ CAST*
Skeleton: Posture *CHANGE c̄ CRUTCHES* Symmetry *CRUTCHES*
 Gait *CRUTCHES* Appearance *CRUTCHES*
Muscles: Strength *↓ ℝ LEG* _____ Shape *ℝ IN CAST, ⓛ NORMAL*
 Movement *LIMITED IN ANTICIPATION OF PAIN*
Diagnostic findings: x-ray studies *FX REDUCED c̄ INTERNAL FIXATION*
 CT scan __Ø__ MRI __Ø__
 Myelogram __Ø__ Fluid aspiration __Ø__

Rest   Sleep pattern disturbance
Hours slept/night *7° NIGHT*   Hypersomnia
Sleep aids (pillows, meds, food) *BROUGHT OWN PILLOW*   Insomnia
Difficulty falling/remaining asleep *Ø c̄ TYLOX*   Nightmares

Recreation
Leisure activities *KNITTING, READING, TV (EXERCISE: RUNNING)*   Deficit in diversional activity
Social activities *CHURCH SOCIALS*

Environmental Maintenance
Home maintenance management
 Size & arrangement of home (stairs, bathroom) *2 FLOORS, 2 BATHROOMS,*   （Impaired home maintenance
 3 BEDROOMS Safety needs *SCATTER RUGS*   management）
 Housekeeping responsibilities *HUSBAND + DAUGHTER HELP*   Safety hazards
 Shopping responsibilities *HUSBAND + DAUGHTER HELP*

Health Maintenance
 Health insurance *BC/BS*   Health maintenance
 Regular physical checkups *LAST ONE 2 YRS AGO*

Self-Care   （Self-care）
 Ability to perform ADLs: Independent *c̄ ASSIST* Dependent _____   Feeding
 Specify deficits *WASHING, LAUNDRY (BASEMENT) BATHING, MEALS*   Bathing/hygiene
 Discharge planning needs *PHYS. THERAPY FOR ANKLE*   Dressing/grooming
                                                Toileting

PERCEIVING ▪ A pattern involving the reception of information
Self-Concept
 Patient's description of self *"THIS (FX) HAS SLOWED ME DOWN."*   Body image
 Effects of illness/surgery on self-concept *NO SIGNIFICANT OR*   Self-esteem
 LASTING EFFECT   Personal identity

Meaningfulness
 Verbalizes hopelessness __Ø__   Hopelessness
 Verbalizes/perceives loss of control *Ø (KNOWS ANKLE WILL HEAL)*   Powerlessness

Fig. 16-2, cont'd

St. Elizabeth Hospital
School of Nursing Library
1508 Tippecanoe Street
Lafayette, Indiana 47904
423-6125

Orthopedic assessment tool **269**

Sensory/Perception

History of restrictive environment ___No___

Vision impaired ___∅___ Glasses ___N/A___   Visual

Auditory impaired ___∅___ Hearing aid ___N/A___   Auditory

Kinesthetics impaired ___BED REST, CAST, CRUTCHES___ Romberg ___∅___   Kinesthetic

Gustatory impaired ___∅___   Gustatory

Tactile impaired ___∅___   Tactile

Olfactory impaired ___∅___   Olfactory

Reflexes: grossly intact ___YES___

EXCHANGING ▪ A pattern involving mutual giving and receiving

Circulation

Cerebral (circle appropriate response)   Cerebral tissue perfusion

  Neurologic changes/symptoms ___No___

Pupils	Eye Opening
L 2 3 4 (5) 6 mm	None (1)
R 2 3 4 (5) 6 mm	To pain (2)
Reaction: Brisk ✓	To speech (3)
Sluggish ___ Nonreactive ___	(Spontaneous (4))

Best Verbal	Best Motor
No response (1)	Flaccid (1)
Incomprehensible sound (2)	Extensor response (2)
Inappropriate words (3)	Flexor response (3)
Confused conversation (4)	Semipurposeful (4)
(Oriented (5))	Localized to pain (5)
	(Obeys commands (6))

Glascow Coma Scale total ___15___

Cardiac

  Apical rate & rhythm ___80 REGULAR___   Cardiopulmonary tissue

  Heart sounds (murmurs) ___SYSTOLIC, GRADE 2 (M), NORMAL S_1, S_2___   perfusion

  ECG ___NSR___   Fluid volume

  BP: ___120/70___ Location ___(R) ARM___   Deficit

  IV fluids ___∅___   Excess

    Cardiac output

    Peripheral tissue perfusion

Peripheral

  Pulses: A = absent   B = bruits   D = doppler

    +3 = bounding   +2 = palpable   +1 = faintly palpable

Carotid R ‾ L ‾	Popliteal R 2 L 2		
Brachial R ‾ L ‾	Posterior tibial R ‾ L 2		
Radial R 2 L 2	Dorsalis pedis R ‾ L 2	Fluid volume	
Femoral R ‾ L ‾		Deficit	

  Skin temp ___WARM___ Color ___PINK___   Excess

  Edema ___MILD (R) TOES___ Capillary refill ___LESS THAN 2 SEC___   Cardiac output

  Homans' sign ___∅___

Physical Integrity

Tissue integrity ___∅___ Rashes ___∅___ Lesions ___∅___   *POTENTIAL*

Petechiae ___∅___ Bruises ___TOES BRUISED FROM FRACTURE___   Impaired skin integrity

Abrasions ___∅___ Lacerations ___∅___   Impaired tissue integrity

Old scars/surgical incisions ___(R) ANKLE (UNDER CAST)___

Localized edema ___(R) TOES___

Generalized edema ___∅___

Skin: Moisture ___NOT DRY FLAKY___ Color ___PINK___ Turgor ___GOOD___

Fig. 16-2, cont'd

Continued.

Oxygenation

Complaints of dyspnea _Ø_ Precipitated by _N/A_   Ineffective breathing patterns
Orthopnea _Ø_   Ineffective airway clearance
Rate _16_ Rhythm _REGULAR_ Depth _DIAPHRAGM_   Impaired gas exchange
Labored (unlabored) (circle)
Use of accessory muscles _Ø_
Chest expansion _ADEQUATE_
Splinting _Ø_
Cough: productive/nonproductive _Ø_
Sputum: Color _N/A_ Amount _N/A_ Consistency _N/A_
Breath sounds _CLEAR_

Physical Regulation

Immune
Lymph nodes enlarged _Ø_ Location _Ø_   Infection
  Hypothermia
  Hyperthermia
Body temperature   Ineffective thermoregulation
Temperature _99² ° F_ Route _ORAL_

Nutrition

Eating patterns
Number of meals per day _3_
Special diet _Ø_
Where eaten _HOME, RESTAURANT OCCASIONALLY_
Food preferences/intolerances _LIKES CHICKEN_
Food allergies _NKA_
Caffeine intake (coffee, tea, (soft drinks,) chocolate)
DIET SODA, NONCAFFEINATED
Appetite changes _Ø_
Nausea/vomiting _Ø_
Condition of mouth/throat _HEALTHY_   Oral mucous membrane
Dentures (upper, lower, full mouth) _Ø_   More than body
Height _5'6"_ Weight _150_   requirements
State of hydration _SKIN PINK, NO DRYNESS NOTED_   Less than body requirements
Current therapy
NPO _Ø_ NG suction _Ø_
Tube feeding _Ø_
TPN _Ø_
Labs
Na _140 mEq/L_ K _4.0 mEq/L_ CL _100 mEq/L_ Glucose
Cholesterol _250 mg/dl_ Triglycerides _—_ Fasting _90 mg/dl_
CBC _HCT 46% Hgb 13 gm/dl_
Blood coagulation studies _WNL_
Serum salicylate _NOT PERFORMED_ Sed. rate _35 mm/HR (↑)_
WBC count _12 × 10³/µL ↑_ Differential _↑ NEUTROPHILS 58%_

Elimination

Gastrointestinal/bowel   Bowel elimination
Usual bowel habits _q̄ d_   (Constipation) (POTENTIAL)
Alterations from normal _Ø_   Diarrhea
Abdominal physical examination _NON TENDER_   Incontinence
Liver: Enlarged _Ø_ Ascites _Ø_   GI tissue perfusion
Renal/urinary
Usual urinary pattern _4 × d_   Urinary elimination
Alteration from normal _Ø, NO BURNING OR URGENCY_   Incontinence
Color _YELLOW, CLEAR_ Catheter _Ø_   Retention
Urine output: 24 hour _> 750 cc_ Average hourly _> 30 cc_
Bladder distention _Ø_

Fig. 16-2, cont'd

BUN *15 mg/dl* Creatinine *0.9 mg/dl* Specific gravity *1.015* _____ Renal tissue perfusion
Urine studies: Uric acid ———⟩ *WNL*
Alkaline phosphatase _____

CHOOSING ▪ A pattern involving the selection of alternatives

Coping

Patient's usual problem-solving methods *DISCUSS c̄ SPOUSE, PRAY* _____ Ineffective individual coping
Ineffective family coping

Family's usual problem-solving methods *DISCUSSION, TALK TO MINISTER*

Patient's method of dealing with stress _____
⟩ *AS ABOVE*
Family's method of dealing with stress _____

Patient's affect *TIRED (OF HOSPITALIZATION), BORED*
Physical manifestations *RESTLESSNESS, WATCHES TV*
Coping mechanisms *CONTACT MINISTER, PROVIDE RATIONALE FOR BED REST, ETC.*

Participation

Compliance with past/current health care regimens *HAS COMPLIED c̄ PRESCRIBED REGIMEN* _____ Noncompliance
Ineffective participation

Willingness to comply with future health care regimen *STATES THAT SHE WILL COMPLY*

Judgment

Decision-making ability _____ Judgment
Patient's perspective *USUALLY ADEQUATE, MORE INDECISIVE* Indecisiveness
Others' perspectives *SINCE ACCIDENT/FX (OTHER'S AGREE)*

Prioritized nursing diagnosis/problem list
1. *ALTERATION IN COMFORT R/T FRACTURED Ⓡ ANKLE*
2. *IMPAIRED PHYSICAL MOBILITY R/T FRACTURED Ⓡ ANKLE*
3. *ANXIETY ABOUT PREPARING NEW HOME R/T IMPAIRED MOBILITY*
4. *IMPAIRED HOME MAINTENANCE MANAGEMENT R/T FRACTURE*
5. _____

Signature *Patricia C. Seifert, R.N.* _____ Date *11/15* _____

Fig. 16-2, cont'd

CHAPTER 17

ONCOLOGIC ASSESSMENT TOOL

ANITA P. SHERER
PATRICIA A. BOHANNON

The Oncologic Assessment Tool was designed to assess oncologic patients with unique biopsychosocial assessment needs. The tool incorporates specific signs and symptoms pertinent to the cancer patient to facilitate identification of nursing diagnoses. It also incorporates the *Outcome Standards of Cancer Nursing Practice* developed by the Oncology Nursing Society and the American Nurses' Association. This chapter includes:

- *The way the tool was developed and refined*
- *The patient population and settings for which it applies*
- *Selected oncologic emphasis areas*
- *The way to use the tool*
- *Specific oncologic focus questions and parameters to assist the nurse in eliciting appropriate data*
- *The refined Oncology Assessment Tool*
- *A case study*
- *A completed version of the tool based on the case study*

DEVELOPMENT AND REFINEMENT OF THE TOOL

The Oncologic Assessment Tool was developed from the nursing data base prototype (see Chapter 2). Many hemodynamic monitoring and critical care variables in the prototype were replaced with in-depth integumentary and immunologic assessment variables more applicable to an oncologic assessment. Emphasis was placed on assessing the patient's pain and discomfort and any side effects of therapies. The resultant tool was then modified based on the recommendations of oncologic nurse experts. Further,

the content of this tool is supported by the literature from this field of nursing.

After the tool was developed and refined, it was clinically tested by oncologic nurse experts and clinical nurse specialists on 10 adult cancer patients receiving high-dose chemotherapy or radiation therapy in a cancer research center. The testing evaluated the adequacy of the tool in terms of flow, space for recording data, and completeness of assessment variables. Based on the results, the tool was revised.

PATIENT POPULATION AND SETTING

The Oncologic Assessment Tool was developed for use with oncologic patients needing an initial assessment for nursing care needs. It is intended for use in any inpatient hospital setting that cares for cancer patients receiving surgery, chemotherapy, or radiation therapy. The tool can easily be revised for use in outpatient settings by adapting sections to provide a screening assessment (see Chapter 4). The assessment parameters within the tool have been designed for use with adult oncologic patients. However, the tool can easily be modified for use with pediatric oncologic patients by adding growth and development and parent-child interaction assessment variables (see Chapter 21).

ONCOLOGIC EMPHASIS AREAS

Oncologic patients have specialized problems and needs. The Oncologic Assessment Tool includes appropriate assessment variables within each of the nine human response patterns of the Unitary Person Framework. The tool focuses on prevalent problems in the oncologic patient population. Table 17-1 outlines these emphasis areas.

Table 17-1

Selected oncologic emphasis areas

Patterns	Emphasis areas to determine
Communicating	Speech impairment
Valuing	Spiritual despair related to illness
	Religion and culture as support systems
Relating	Support systems
	Effect of illness and surgery on roles and relationships
Knowing	Knowledge of illness and therapy
	Orientation and memory
Feeling	Comprehensive data related to pain, nausea or vomiting, and fatigue or weakness
	Anxiety, fear, grief, and loss
Moving	Effects of illness on home maintenance
	Temporary or permanent self-care deficits
Perceiving	Effects of illness on self-concept
	Verbalizations of hopelessness and powerlessness
Exchanging	Skin and tissue integrity
	Immunologic assessment
	Changes in nutrition and elimination
Choosing	Life-style adjustments imposed by illness
	Patient's and family's adequacy in dealing with illness and surgery
	Future compliance with health care regimen

HOW TO USE THE TOOL

To use the Oncologic Assessment Tool effectively, nurses must first be familiar with the Unitary Person Framework (see Chapter 2), which provides the underlying framework for Taxonomy I. The nine human response patterns of the Unitary Person Framework serve as the major category headings for Taxonomy I and the tool. The sequence of the response patterns, as it appears in Taxonomy I, has been changed to permit a logical ordering of assessment variables. Nursing diagnoses pertinent to the oncologic patient, along with the signs and symptoms necessary to identify them, are incorporated under the appropriate human response patterns.

Nurses must also realize that this tool is very different from conventional assessment tools. As a result, nurses may encounter some initial difficulty in using it. They should remember, however, that the tool was not designed to follow the organization or content of a traditional medical data base; the data collected do not solely reflect medical patterns. Rather, this tool is used to elicit data about holistic patterns in ways not traditionally used by nurses. It provides a new method of collecting and synthesizing data and requires new thinking when processing data. This tool represents a nursing data base developed from a nursing model to permit a holistic nursing assessment to take place so nursing diagnoses can be identified.

Although nurses probably agree that a holistic nursing data base is desirable, it is realized that changing traditional assessment methods is not an easy task. For this reason, a trial usage period is recommended before any decisions about the tool's merits are made. During this period, nurses should assess 10 patients using the tool to become familiar and progressively more comfortable with its organization and data-collection methods. With experience, nurses will become accustomed to new ways of clustering and processing information. With continued use, the time necessary to complete the tool will be reduced. Most important, nurses will recognize the unique ability of the tool to elicit appropriate signs and symptoms. Nurses will discover that nursing diagnoses are easily identified when using this tool.

It is not necessary to complete the tool in one session. Priority sections can be completed during the initial assessment. Other sections or patterns can be completed within a time frame acceptable to the institution.

Nurses should be familiar with the focus questions and parameters in the next section. When assessing specific signs and symptoms to indicate a diagnosis, the nurse circles the diagnosis in the right-hand column when deviations from normal are found. A circled diagnosis does not confirm a problem but simply alerts the nurse to the possibility that it exists. After completing the tool, the nurse scans the circled problems, synthesizes the data to determine whether other clusters of signs and symptoms support a problem, and judges whether the actual or potential diagnosis is present.

Some diagnoses are repeated several times in the right-hand column. These repetitions occur only within the appropriate response pattern and are convenient for identifying certain data directly with their corresponding nursing diagnosis. These diagnoses are not absolute but focus thinking and direct detailed attention to a possible problem.

Certain signs and symptoms can indicate several diagnoses. For example, an altered 24-hour urine output can indicate impaired renal tissue perfusion or fluid volume deficit, as well as other nursing diagnoses. To avoid unnecessary repetition of assessment parameters, variables are arranged with the diagnosis most likely to result from the data assessed. Thus, data to support one diagnosis may occasionally be found in other patterns or arranged with other diagnoses. Therefore, synthesis of all data is essential.

The Oncologic Assessment Tool is not intended to be

Table 17-2
Oncologic assessment tool: focus questions and parameters

Variables	Focus questions and parameters
VALUING	
Religious leader	"Do you have a priest, pastor, or religious leader that you wish us to contact for you?"
RELATING	
Role in community	"Are you active in volunteer work, church groups, neighborhood organizations, or other social groups?"
KNOWING	
Knowledge of side effects of therapy	Is the patient likely to experience side effects from the prescribed therapy? Is the patient aware of these side effects?
Level of comprehension	Is the patient able to understand explanations given about the illness? Can the patient recall or return demonstrate knowledge about the illness?
FEELING	
Nausea/vomiting: yes/no	"Are you experiencing nausea and vomiting related to therapy (chemotherapy or radiation therapy)?"
Frequency	"How often does it occur?"
Duration	"How long does it last?"
Associated factors	"Do you associate it with anything in particular (smells or activity)?"
Aggravating factors	"Does anything make it worse?"
Alleviating factors	"Does anything make it better?"
Present management	"How is it controlled?"
Fatigue/weakness: yes/no	"Are you experiencing fatigue or weakness related to therapy (chemotherapy, radiation therapy, or immunotherapy)?"
Frequency	"How often does it occur?"
Duration	"How long does it last?"
Associated factors	"Do you associate it with anything in particular (time of day or activity)?"
Aggravating factors	"Does anything make it worse?"
Allevating factors	"Does anything make it better?"
Present management	"How do you relieve it? What helps you to overcome it?"
MOVING	
Specify deficits (temporary/permanent)	Does the patient demonstrate an inability to perform activities of daily living? Are these deficits likely to be temporary or permanent?
PERCEIVING	
Patient's description of own strengths/weaknesses	"Describe what you consider to be your own strengths as a person. Your weaknesses?"
EXCHANGING	
Physical integrity	As a result of the patient's therapy (chemotherapy, radiation therapy, or immunotherapy), are there any changes in skin or tissue integrity? Do you note any dryness, redness, breakdown areas, rashes, lesions, bruises, petechiae, or changes in pigmentation as a result of therapy? Is therapy causing hair loss (alopecia) or nosebleeds (epistaxis)?
	Has the patient's condition required surgery or an ostomy? What is the condition of the incision line or stoma?
	Because the immunosuppression associated with oncologic therapies can impair mucous membranes, does the patient's mouth and throat indicate mucositis, white patches, bleeding gums, or petechiae? Is the patient following a specific mouth care regimen related to these actual or potential problems?
	Does your assessment of the patient's perianal area reveal impairments such as erythema, ulcers, or excoriation? How is this being treated?

Table 17-2—cont'd

Oncologic assessment tool: focus questions and parameters

Variables	Focus questions and parameters
EXCHANGING—cont'd	
Physical regulation	Because of the immunosuppression associated with oncologic therapies, do the patient's laboratory values indicate significant abnormalities? Do these values indicate a potential for infection or other complications?
CHOOSING	
Necessary life-style changes due to disease	"How has this illness affected your normal life-style? How have you dealt with these changes?"
Coping mechanisms used	Does the patient express acceptance of the diagnosis? Does the patient use anger, denial, repression, rationalization, displacement, projection, bargaining, information seeking, or mental rehearsal as coping mechanisms to deal with the illness, tests, or surgery?
Patient's and family's evaluation of present coping level	"What helps you to deal with this illness? Do you feel able to handle what is happening to you? Are you having difficulty handling the stress and feelings this illness has caused? Do you feel you need help in dealing with your situation?"

the standardized and final format for assessing oncologic patients across the country. An assessment tool must meet the needs and requirements of the institutions and nurses using it. The tool is simply a working demonstration tool that is expected to be changed and revised by nurses in clinical practice. Further evaluation and refinement are necessary before adopting the tool for use in an institution. Nurses interested in changing, revising, and adapting this tool to a specific clinical setting should refer to Chapter 4. Nurses interested in adapting the tool to the pediatric oncologic setting should refer to the Pediatric Assessment Tool (see Chapter 21).

HOW TO ELICIT APPROPRIATE DATA

Because the Unitary Person Framework and the Oncologic Assessment Tool contain some terms that may be unfamiliar to nurses, specific oncologic focus questions and parameters were developed and refined to elicit information. These questions and parameters are in Table 17-2, which follows the content of the tool (Fig. 17-1). The variables in bold type in the tool are described more fully in Table 17-2. For example, the variable about the patient's evaluation of present coping level under the "choosing pattern" is in bold type. If the nurse is unsure what questions to ask about the patient's evaluation of the coping level, Table 17-2 can be used to direct the line of questioning. The questions and parameters provide clarity and guidance in eliciting data. They are not all inclusive, so nurses should not feel limited by them. There are many other ways, based on the patient's situation and condition and the nurse's skill, to elicit the information. Focus questions and parameters for other data not in bold type were presented in Chapter 3.

CASE STUDY

The case study models the process a nurse uses when assessing a patient. Based on the clustering of information obtained during assessment, the nurse formulates nursing diagnoses.

Mrs. D.M. was assessed when admitted to the oncologic unit. She underwent a mastectomy 2 years before for breast cancer and has been diagnosed with metastasis to the chest wall, lungs, and liver. She will receive high-dose chemotherapy and an autologous bone marrow transplant. Mrs. D.M. is 46 years old, married, and lives with her husband and two teenage children. The Oncologic Assessment Tool (Fig. 17-2) was used to assess Mrs. D.M.

BIBLIOGRAPHY

Belcher AE: Neoplasia. In Thompson JM et al: Clinical nursing, St Louis, 1986, The CV Mosby Co.

Brager BL and Yasko J: Care of the client receiving chemotherapy, Reston, Va, 1984, Reston Publishing Co.

Fredette SL and Gloriant FS: Nursing diagnoses in cancer chemotherapy: in theory, Am J Nurs 81:2013, 1981.

Fredette SL and Gloriant FS: Nursing diagnoses in cancer chemotherapy: in practice, Am J Nurs 81:2021, 1981.

McNally JC, Stain JC, and Sommerville ET: Guidelines for cancer nursing practice, New York, 1979, Grune & Stratton, Inc.

Oncology Nursing Society and American Nurses' Association: Outcome standards for cancer nursing practice, Kansas City, Mo, 1979, ANA, Inc.

ONCOLOGIC ASSESSMENT TOOL

Name _____ Age _____ Sex _____
Address _____ Telephone _____
Significant other _____ Telephone _____
Date of admission _____ Medical diagnosis _____
Allergies _____

Nursing Diagnosis
(Potential or Altered)

COMMUNICATING ▪ A pattern involving sending messages
Read, write, understand English (circle) _____ Communication
Other languages _____   Verbal
Speech impaired _____   Nonverbal
Alternate form of communication _____

VALUING ▪ A pattern involving the assigning of relative worth
Religious preference _____ Spiritual state
Important religious practices _____   Despair
Religious leader _____ Telephone _____   Distress
Spiritual concerns _____
Cultural orientation _____
Cultural practices _____

RELATING ▪ A pattern involving establishing bonds
Role
  Significant other _____ Role performance
  Age & health of significant other _____   Parenting
  _____   Sexual dysfunction
  Number of children _____ Ages _____   Work
  Role in home _____   Family
  Role in community _____   Social/leisure
  Financial support _____
  Occupation _____ Family processes
    Job satisfaction/concerns _____
    Physical/mental energy expenditures _____
  Sexual relationships (satisfactory/unsatisfactory) _____
    Physical difficulties/effects of illness related to sex _____ Sexuality patterns
  _____

Socialization
  Quality of relationships with others _____ Impaired social interaction
    Patient's description _____
    Significant others' descriptions _____
    Staff observations _____
  Verbalizes feelings of being alone _____ Social isolation
    Attributed to _____ Social withdrawal

KNOWING ▪ A pattern involving the meaning associated with information
Current health problems _____
_____
_____
Previous illnesses/hospitalizations/surgeries _____
_____
_____
_____
_____

Fig. 17-1

History of the following:

    Cardiac disease _____ Lung disease _____

    Liver disease _____ Renal disease _____

    Thyroid disease _____ Diabetes _____

    Hematologic disorders _____

    Musculoskeletal disorders _____

    Occupational exposures _____

    Smoking _____ Alcohol usage _____

Current medications _____   Knowledge deficit

_____

Present therapy (radiation, chemotherapy) _____

_____

Educational level _____

Perception/knowledge of illness/tests/surgery _____

_____

Expectations of therapy _____

Knowledge of side effects of therapy _____

Misconceptions _____

Readiness to learn _____

    Learning impeded by _____   Thought processes

    Level of comprehension _____

Orientation

Level of alertness _____   Orientation

Orientation: Person _____ Place _____ Time _____   Confusion

Appropriate behavior/communication _____

Memory

Memory intact: yes/no _____ Recent _____ Remote _____   Memory

FEELING ▪ A pattern involving the subjective awareness of information

Comfort

    Pain/discomfort: yes/no _____   Comfort

        Frequency _____ Location _____

        Duration _____ Quality _____ Radiation _____   Pain/chronic

        Associated factors _____

        Aggravating factors _____   Pain/acute

        Alleviating factors _____

        Present pain management _____

    Nausea/vomiting: yes/no _____

        Frequency _____ **Duration** _____

        Associated factors _____   Discomfort

        Aggravating factors _____

        Alleviating factors _____

        Present management _____

    Fatigue/weakness: yes/no _____

        Frequency _____ **Duration** _____

        Associated factors _____

        Aggravating factors _____

        Alleviating factors _____

        Present management _____

Emotional Integrity/States

    Recent stressful life events _____   Anxiety

_____   Fear

    Verbalizes feelings of fear/anxiety/loss/grief _____   Anger

        Source _____   Guilt

Fig. 17-1, cont'd

Continued.

Verbalizes other feelings _____ Shame
    Source _____ Sadness
Physical manifestations _____ Grieving

MOVING ▪ A pattern involving activity
Activity   Impaired physical mobility
History of physical disability _____ Activity intolerance
_____
Limitations in daily activities _____
_____
Exercise habits _____

Rest   Sleep pattern disturbance
Hours slept/night _____ Feels rested: yes/no _____ Hypersomnia
Sleep aids (pillows, meds, food) _____ Insomnia
Difficulty falling/remaining asleep _____ Nightmares

Recreation   Deficit in diversional activity
Leisure activities _____
Social activities _____

Environmental Maintenance
Home maintenance management
    Size & arrangement of home (stairs, bathroom) _____ Impaired home maintenance
_____   management
    Transportation _____ Safety needs _____ Safety hazards
    Home responsibilities _____
_____

Health Maintenance
Health insurance _____ Health maintenance
Regular physical checkups _____

Self-Care   Self-care
Ability to perform ADLs: Independent _____ Dependent _____   Feeding
Specify deficits (temporary/permanent) _____   Bathing/hygiene
_____   Dressing/grooming
_____   Toileting
Discharge planning needs _____
_____

PERCEIVING ▪ A pattern involving the reception of information
Self-Concept   Self-concept
Patient's description of self _____ Body image
Effects of illness/surgery on self-concept _____ Self-esteem
_____ Personal identity
_____
Patient's description of own strengths/weaknesses _____
_____

Meaningfulness
Verbalizes hopelessness _____ Hopelessness
Verbalizes/perceives loss of control _____ Powerlessness

Sensory/Perception   Sensory/perception
Glasses _____ Hearing aid _____ Visual
Deficits: specify _____ Auditory
_____ Kinesthetic
_____ Gustatory
    Tactile
    Olfactory

Fig. 17-1, cont'd

EXCHANGING ▪ **A pattern involving mutual giving and receiving**
Circulation
  Cerebral
    Neurologic changes/symptoms _____ Cerebral tissue perfusion
    _____

      Pupils   Best verbal response _____
        L 2 3 4 5 6 mm   _____
        R 2 3 4 5 6 mm   Best motor response _____
        Reaction: Brisk _____   _____
        Sluggish _____ Nonreactive _____
  Cardiac   Cardiopulmonary tissue
    Apical rate & rhythm _____ PMI _____   perfusion
    Heart sounds/murmurs _____
    BP: Sitting   Lying   Standing   Cardiac output
      R _____ L _____   R _____ L _____   R _____ L _____ Fluid volume
                                                         Deficit
  Peripheral   Excess
    Jugular venous distension: yes/no _____ R _____ L _____
    Pulses _____
    Skin temp _____ Color _____ Peripheral tissue perfusion
    Capillary refill _____ Edema _____

Physical Integrity   Impaired skin integrity
  Tissue integrity _____ **Dryness** _____ **Redness** _____ Impaired tissue integrity
  Breakdown areas/decubitus ulcers _____
  Rashes _____ **Lesions** _____ **Bruising** _____
  Petechiae _____ **Abnormal pigmentation** _____
  Surgical incision _____
  Epistaxis _____ **Alopecia** _____ **Ostomy** _____
  Venous access _____
  Oral assessment: Mucositis _____ **White patches** _____ Oral mucous membrane
    Bleeding gums _____ **Petechiae** _____
    Mouth care regimen _____
  Perianal assessment: Erythema _____ **Ulcers** _____
    Excoriation _____ **Current treatment** _____

Oxygenation
  Complaints of dyspnea _____ Precipitated by _____
  Orthopnea _____
  Rate _____ Rhythm _____ Depth _____ Ineffective breathing pattern
  Labored/unlabored (circle) Use of accessory muscles _____ Ineffective airway clearance
  Chest expansion _____ Splinting _____
  Cough: productive/nonproductive _____
  Sputum: Color _____ Amount _____ Consistency _____
  Breath sounds _____ Impaired gas exchange
  Arterial blood gases _____
  Oxygen percent and device _____

Physical Regulation
  Immune   Infection
    Lymph nodes enlarged _____ Location _____
    RBC count _____ Hemoglobin _____ Hematocrit _____
    WBC count _____ Neutrophils _____ Lymphocytes _____ Potential for injury
    Monocytes _____ Basophils _____ Eosinophils _____ Trauma
    Other _____ Platelets _____ PT _____ PTT _____
    Viral titers: EBV _____ HIV _____ Hepatitis _____ CMV _____
    Immunoglobulins: IgG _____ IgA _____ IgM _____

Fig. 17-1, cont'd

Continued.

Bone marrow: Blasts _____ Plasma _____
        Malignant cells present: yes/no _____
        Positive cultures _____   Body temperature
Body temperature   Hypothermia
    Temperature _____ Route _____   Hyperthermia
                                                            Ineffective thermoregulation

Nutrition

Eating patterns   Nutrition
    Number of meals per day _____ Where eaten _____   Fluid volume
    Special diet _____   Deficit
    Food preferences/intolerances _____   Excess
    _____
    Food allergies _____
    Fluid intake _____
    Appetite changes _____
    _____
    Taste changes _____   More than body
Height _____ Weight _____ Ideal body weight _____   requirements
Recent weight changes _____
Current therapy
    NPO _____ Current diet _____ NG suction _____   Less than body requirements
    Enteral nutrition _____ TPN _____
    IV fluids _____
Labs
    Na _____ K _____ CL _____ Glucose _____ Fasting _____
    Cholesterol _____ Triglycerides _____ Phosphorus _____
    Magnesium _____ Calcium _____ HCO$_3$ _____ Albumin _____

Elimination

GI/bowel   Bowel elimination
    Usual bowel habits _____   Constipation
    Alterations from normal _____   Diarrhea
    Frequency _____ Consistency _____ Control _____   Incontinence
    Color _____ Guaiac _____   GI tissue perfusion
    Epigastric pain _____ Difficulty swallowing _____   Impaired swallowing
    Abdominal physical examination _____
    LDH _____ SGOT _____ SGPT _____ Alkaline phosphatase _____
Renal/urinary   Urinary elimination
    Usual urinary pattern _____   Incontinence
    Alteration from normal _____   Retention
    Frequency _____ Burning _____ Control _____
    Color _____ Catheter _____
    Urine output: 24 hour _____ Average hourly _____   Renal tissue perfusion
    Bladder distention _____
    Serum: BUN _____ Creatinine _____ Specific gravity _____
    Urine studies _____
    Urine osmolality _____ Urinary sodium _____

CHOOSING ▪ A pattern involving the selection of alternatives
Coping

Past methods of dealing with stress _____   Ineffective individual coping
_____   Ineffective family coping
Necessary life-style changes due to disease _____
_____
Support systems available _____
_____

Fig. 17-1, cont'd

Coping mechanisms used _____

Patient's affect _____

Physical manifestations _____

Patient's evaluation of present coping level _____

_____

Family's evaluation of present coping level _____

_____

Participation

    Compliance with past/current health care regimens _____   Noncompliance

_____   Ineffective participation

    Willingness to comply with future health care regimen _____

_____

Judgment

    Decision-making ability   Judgment

      Patient's perspective _____   Indecisiveness

      Others' perspectives _____

Prioritized nursing diagnoses/problem list

1. _____
2. _____
3. _____
4. _____
5. _____
6. _____
7. _____
8. _____
9. _____
10. _____

Signature _____   Date _____

Fig. 17-1, cont'd

ONCOLOGIC ASSESSMENT TOOL

Name _D.M._   Age _46_   Sex _F_
Address _44 THIRD STREET, HOUSTON, TEXAS_   Telephone _445-3000_
Significant other _HUSBAND; MR. J.M._   Telephone _445-3000_
Date of admission _4/24_   Medical diagnosis _INFILTRATING DUCTAL CELL BREAST CANCER_
Allergies _BETADINE_

Nursing Diagnosis
(Potential or Altered)

COMMUNICATING ▪ A pattern involving sending messages
(Read) (write) (understand) English (circle) _____   Communication
Other languages _SPANISH_   Verbal
Speech impaired _No_   Nonverbal
Alternate form of communication _NONE_

VALUING ▪ A pattern involving the assigning of relative worth
Religious preference _CATHOLIC_   Spiritual state
Important religious practices _ATTENDS MASS WEEKLY_   Despair
Religious leader _PRIEST_   Telephone _443-3942_   Distress
Spiritual concerns _NONE EXPRESSED — HAS ROSARY IN HAND_
Cultural orientation _MEXICAN-AMERICAN_
Cultural practices _DECISIONS REGARDING CARE ARE MADE BY HUSBAND_

RELATING ▪ A pattern involving establishing bonds
Role
  Significant other _HUSBAND_   (Role performance)
  Age & health of significant other _52, NO HEALTH PROBLEMS_   Parenting
  _____   (Sexual dysfunction)
  Number of children _2_ Ages _16, 18 (JORGE & MATIAS)_   (Work)
  Role in home _WIFE, MOTHER, HOMEMAKER_   (Family)
  Role in community _VOLUNTEERS IN CHURCH ACTIVITIES_   Social/leisure
  Financial support _HUSBAND: FULL-TIME JOB_
  Occupation _PATIENT IS HOMEMAKER; HUSBAND IS BUS DRIVER_   Family processes
    Job satisfaction/concerns _CAN'T TAKE CARE OF FAMILY & HOME_
    Physical/mental energy expenditures _HOUSEWORK IS PHYSICALLY DEMANDING_
  Sexual relationships (satisfactory/(unsatisfactory))
    Physical difficulties/effects of illness related to sex _HUSBAND HAS NOT_   (Sexuality patterns)
SHOWN INTEREST SINCE MASTECTOMY 2 YRS. AGO

Socialization
  Quality of relationships with others _RELATES WELL TO SISTER_   Impaired social interaction
    Patient's description _HAS BIG FAMILY THAT HELPS HER_
    Significant others' descriptions _"WE HAVE ADJUSTED" (HUSBAND)_
    Staff observations _VERY SUPPORTIVE FAMILY_
  Verbalizes feelings of being alone _No_   Social isolation
    Attributed to _—_   Social withdrawal

KNOWING ▪ A pattern involving the meaning associated with information
Current health problems _METASTASIS TO CHEST WALL, LUNGS, & LIVER —_
ADMITTED FOR HIGH-DOSE CHEMOTHERAPY & AN AUTOLOGOUS
BONE MARROW TRANSPLANT
Previous illnesses/hospitalizations/surgeries _MASTECTOMY 2 YRS. AGO c̄_
RADIATION THERAPY. p̄ METASTASIS TO CHEST WALL WAS
FOUND 1 YEAR AGO c̄ CHEMOTHERAPY ADMINISTERED.

Fig. 17-2

History of the following:
    Cardiac disease ___*No*___ Lung disease ___*No*___
    Liver disease ___*No*___ Renal disease ___*No*___
    Thyroid disease ___*No*___ Diabetes ___*YES/CONTROLLED c̄ DIET*___
    Hematologic disorders ___*No*___
    Musculoskeletal disorders ___*No*___
    Occupational exposures ___*No KNOWN EXPOSURES*___
    Smoking ___*No*___ Alcohol usage ___*OCCASIONAL BEER*___
Current medications ___*TAMOXIFEN (NOLVADEX) 20 mg bid*___   ⟨Knowledge deficit⟩

Present therapy (radiation, chemotherapy) *HIGH-DOSE CHEMOTHERAPY &* *AUTOLOGOUS BONE MARROW TRANSPLANT*
Educational level *HIGH SCHOOL*
Perception/knowledge of illness/tests/surgery *KNOWS SHE HAS CANCER* *GROWING IN HER BODY & THERAPY IN PAST HAS NOT WORKED*
Expectations of therapy *SEES AS A CURE*
Knowledge of side effects of therapy *KNOWS TO EXPECT NAUSEA & VOMITING/ALOPECIA*
Misconceptions *THINKS BONE MARROW TRANSPLANT WILL KILL CANCER CELLS*
Readiness to learn *POOR*
    Learning impeded by *FEAR*   Thought processes
    Level of comprehension *VERY BASIC*

Orientation
Level of alertness *ALERT*   Orientation
Orientation: Person ___✓___ Place ___✓___ Time ___✓___   Confusion
Appropriate behavior/communication *APPROPRIATE*

Memory
Memory intact: yes/no *YES* ___ Recent ___✓___ Remote ___✓___   Memory

FEELING ▪ A pattern involving the subjective awareness of information
Comfort
    Pain/discomfort: yes/no *YES*   ⟨Comfort⟩
        Frequency *CONSTANT* Location *LEFT SHOULDER*
        Duration *CONSTANT* Quality *ACHING* Radiation *DOWN Ⓛ ARM*   ⟨Pain/chronic⟩
        Associated factors *MOVEMENT OF ARM*
        Aggravating factors *MOVEMENT*   Pain/acute
        Alleviating factors *RESTRICT ARM MOVEMENT*
        Present pain management *DILAUDID 2 mg PO TID*
    Nausea/vomiting: ⟨yes⟩/no *IN THE PAST*
        Frequency *q 3-4 HRS* Duration *X 2 DAYS p̄ CHEMOTHERAPY*
        Associated factors *CHEMOTHERAPY*
        Aggravating factors *SMELLS, MOVEMENT*   Discomfort
        Alleviating factors *LIE VERY STILL, ANTIEMETICS*
        Present management *NONE REQUIRED @ PRESENT*
    Fatigue/weakness: ⟨yes⟩/no *IN THE PAST*
        Frequency *CONSTANT* Duration *X 1 WK p̄ CHEMOTHERAPY*
        Associated factors *CHEMOTHERAPY*
        Aggravating factors *PHYSICAL ACTIVITY*
        Alleviating factors *REST*
        Present management *DOES NOT HAVE @ PRESENT*

Emotional Integrity/States
    Recent stressful life events *MOTHER DIED OF BREAST CANCER 5 YRS.*   Anxiety
AGO, WORRIES ABOUT EFFECT OF ILLNESS ON CHILDREN   ⟨Fear⟩
    Verbalizes feelings of ⟨fear⟩/anxiety/loss/⟨grief⟩ ___   Anger
        Source *FEARS THERAPY WILL NOT CURE CANCER; LOSS OF PRE-*   Guilt
             VIOUS LIFE-STYLE

Fig. 17-2, cont'd

Continued.

Verbalizes other feelings *SADNESS* _____
  Source *DISABILITY—UNABLE TO CARE FOR FAMILY AS "I SHOULD"*
Physical manifestations *TEARFUL ESPECIALLY WHEN DISCUSSING* _____
  CHILDREN

Shame
Sadness
Grieving

MOVING ▪ A pattern involving activity
Activity
History of physical disability *NONE* _____
_____

Impaired physical mobility
Activity intolerance

Limitations in daily activities *JUST DOES NOT HAVE THE ENERGY TO* __
COMPLETE HOUSEHOLD DUTIES
Exercise habits *NONE* _____

Rest
Hours slept/night *ABOUT 8 HRS.* Feels rested: yes/no *YES* _____
Sleep aids (pillows, meds, food) *NONE* _____
Difficulty falling/remaining asleep *No* _____

Sleep pattern disturbance
Hypersomnia
Insomnia
Nightmares

Recreation
Leisure activities *SEWS, READS* _____
Social activities *OCCASIONAL CHURCH SOCIALS, VISITS c̄ FAMILY* ____

Deficit in diversional activity

Environmental Maintenance
Home maintenance management
  Size & arrangement of home (stairs, bathroom) *2 BEDROOM APART-*
  MENT DOWNSTAIRS _____
  Transportation *CAR* _____ Safety needs *NONE* _____
  Home responsibilities *SISTERS ARE HELPING c̄ HOUSEKEEP-*
  ING, COOKING _____

Impaired home maintenance
  management
Safety hazards

Health Maintenance
Health insurance *YES — THROUGH HUSBAND'S EMPLOYER* _____
Regular physical checkups *YES — SINCE DIAGNOSIS* _____

Health maintenance

Self-Care
Ability to perform ADLs: Independent ____✓____ Dependent _____
Specify deficits (temporary/permanent) *NONE AT PRESENT* ____
_____

Self-care
  Feeding
  Bathing/hygiene
  Dressing/grooming
  Toileting

Discharge planning needs *MAY NEED HOME HEALTH CARE REFERRAL*
_____

PERCEIVING ▪ A pattern involving the reception of information
Self-Concept
Patient's description of self *"NOT WORTH MUCH LIKE I AM NOW."* ___
Effects of illness/surgery on self-concept *DECREASE IN SELF WORTH* __
BECAUSE CANNOT MEET NEEDS OF FAMILY
_____

Self-concept
Body image
Self-esteem
Personal identity

Patient's description of own strengths/weaknesses *"I AM A FIGHTER* __
AND I CAN BEAT THIS."

Meaningfulness
Verbalizes hopelessness *No* _____
Verbalizes/perceives loss of control *No* _____

Hopelessness
Powerlessness

Sensory/Perception
Glasses *No* _____ Hearing aid *No* _____
Deficits: specify *NONE* _____
_____
_____

Sensory/perception
Visual
Auditory
Kinesthetic
Gustatory
Tactile
Olfactory

Fig. 17-2, cont'd

EXCHANGING ▪ A pattern involving mutual giving and receiving

Circulation

Cerebral

Neurologic changes/symptoms _NONE_ — Cerebral tissue perfusion

Pupils
L 2 ③ 4 5 6 mm   Best verbal response _____
SPONTANEOUS
R 2 ③ 4 5 6 mm   Best motor response _____
Reaction: Brisk _✓_   _SPONTANEOUS_
Sluggish _____ Nonreactive _____

Cardiac — Cardiopulmonary tissue perfusion

Apical rate & rhythm _82 REGULAR_ PMI _4TH ICS @ MCL_
Heart sounds/murmurs _S, S₂_

BP: Sitting   Lying   Standing — Cardiac output
R _110/80_ L _120/80_   R _120/80_ L _128/80_   R __ L __ — Fluid volume
                                                                      Deficit
hx ADRIAMYCIN 1200mg CUMMULATIVE DOSE CARDIAC EJECTION   Excess
Peripheral   _FRACTION 78%_

Jugular venous distension: yes/no _NO_ ____ R __ L ____
Pulses _PALPABLE BILATERALLY_
Skin temp _WARM_ ____ Color _BROWN_ — Peripheral tissue perfusion
Capillary refill _1-2 SECONDS_ Edema _OF LEFT ARM_

Physical Integrity

Tissue integrity _IMPAIRED_ Dryness _No_ Redness _CHEST WALL_   （Impaired skin integrity）
（Breakdown areas）decubitus ulcers _CHEST WALL_   （Impaired tissue integrity）
Rashes _No_ ____ Lesions _8 NODULES_ Bruising _No_
Petechiae _No_ ____ Abnormal pigmentation _No_
Surgical incision _MASTECTOMY SCAR ⓛ CHEST WALL_
Epistaxis _No_ ____ Alopecia _No_ ____ Ostomy _No_
Venous access _DOUBLE LUMEN SUBCLAVIAN CATHETER_
Oral assessment: Mucositis _No_ ____ White patches _No_ — Oral mucous membrane
Bleeding gums _No_ ____ Petechiae _No_
Mouth care regimen _2 x DAILY c̄ TOOTHBRUSH/PASTE_
Perianal assessment: Erythema _No_ ____ Ulcers _No_
Excoriation _No_ ____ Current treatment ____

Oxygenation

Complaints of dyspnea _No_ ____ Precipitated by ____
Orthopnea _NONE_
Rate _24_ ____ Rhythm _REGULAR_ Depth _SHALLOW_   （Ineffective breathing pattern）
Labored（unlabored）(circle) Use of accessory muscles _No_   Ineffective airway clearance
Chest expansion _ASSYMETRICAL_ Splinting _PAIN IN ⓛ SHOULDER_
Cough: productive/nonproductive _No_
Sputum: Color ____ Amount ____ Consistency ____
Breath sounds _CLEAR BILATERALLY_ — Impaired gas exchange
Arterial blood gases _pH 7.35, PCO₂ 50 mmHg, PO₂ 96 mmHg, HCO₃ 24mM_
Oxygen percent and device _NONE_

Physical Regulation

Immune _HISTORY OF PREVIOUS CHEMOTHERAPY_   （POTENTIAL）
Lymph nodes enlarged _YES ♂_ ____ Location _ⓛ SUPRACLAVICULAR & AXILLARY_ （Infection）
RBC count _3.6 x 10⁶/μL_ Hemoglobin _9.0g/dl_ Hematocrit _38%_
WBC count _3.5 x 10³/μL_ Neutrophils _30%_ Lymphocytes _20%_   （Potential for injury）
Monocytes _2%_ Basophils _0.2%_ Eosinophils _2%_   Trauma
Other ____ Platelets _123,000/μL_ PT _10 SEC._ PTT _32 SEC._
Viral titers: EBV _NEG_ HIV _NEG_ Hepatitis _NEG_ CMV _POSITIVE_
Immunoglobulins: IgG _926 mg/dl_ IgA _85mg/dl_ IgM _55mg/dl_

Fig. 17-2, cont'd

Continued.

Bone marrow: Blasts ___*0*___ Plasma ___*0*___
Malignant cells present: yes/no *YES* ___
Positive cultures *NONE* ___

Body temperature
Temperature ___*98.6°F*___ Route *ORAL* ___

Body temperature
Hypothermia
Hyperthermia
Ineffective thermoregulation

Nutrition

(POTENTIAL)
(Nutrition)

Eating patterns
Number of meals per day ___*2*___ Where eaten ___*HOME*___
Special diet *(DIABETIC) ADA DIET* ___
Food (preferences)/intolerances *BEANS, TORTILLAS, RICE, CHILI,*
MEXICAN FOOD ___
Food allergies ___*NONE*___
Fluid intake *ADEQUATE* ___
Appetite changes *GOOD AT PRESENT, HOWEVER LOST 15 lbs*
WHILE ON CHEMOTHERAPY IN THE PAST ___
Taste changes *YES c̄ CHEMOTHERAPY* ___
Height *5'6"* ___ Weight *116 lbs* ___ Ideal body weight *130 lbs* ___
Recent weight changes ___*No*___

Fluid volume
    Deficit
    Excess

More than body
    requirements

Current therapy
NPO ___*No*___ Current diet *REGULAR* ___ NG suction ___*No*___
Enteral nutrition ___*No*___ TPN ___*No*___
IV fluids *D5½ NS c̄ 20 mEq KCL @ 150 cc/HR* ___

(Less than body requirements)
(POTENTIAL)

Labs
Na *130 mEq/L* K *3.6 mEq/L* CL *99 mEq/L* Glucose *120 mg/dl* Fasting *YES* ___
Cholesterol *167 mg/dl* Triglycerides *100 mg/dl* Phosphorus *3.2 mg/dl*
Magnesium *1.8 mEq/L* Calcium *8.2 mEq/L* HCO₃ *26 mM* Albumin *3.6 g/dl*

Elimination

GI/bowel
Usual bowel habits ___*1 DAILY*___
Alterations from normal *NONE @ PRESENT* ___
Frequency *DAILY* ___ Consistency *SOLID* ___ Control *GOOD* ___
Color *BROWN* ___ Guaiac *NEGATIVE* ___
Epigastric pain ___*No*___ Difficulty swallowing ___*No*___
Abdominal physical examination *NO HEPATOSPLENOMEGALY; 2+ BS ALL 4 QUADS*
LDH *125 UNITS* SGOT *30 U/ml* SGPT *34 U/ml* Alkaline phosphatase *20 IU/L*

Bowel elimination
    Constipation
    Diarrhea
    Incontinence
GI tissue perfusion
Impaired swallowing

Renal/urinary
Usual urinary pattern ___*NONE*___
Alteration from normal ___*NONE*___
Frequency *4-5 x DAILY* Burning ___*No*___ Control *GOOD* ___
Color *YELLOW CLEAR* Catheter ___*No*___
Urine output: 24 hour ___*2000 cc*___ Average hourly *400 cc/VOIDING* ___
Bladder distention ___*NONE*___
Serum: BUN *18 mg/dl* ___ Creatinine *0.8 mg/dl* ___ Specific gravity *1.005* ___
Urine studies *CREATININE CLEARANCE = 106 ml/min* ___
Urine osmolality *800 mOsm/kg H₂O* Urinary sodium *150 mEq/24HR.* ___

Urinary elimination
    Incontinence
    Retention

Renal tissue perfusion

CHOOSING ▪ A pattern involving the selection of alternatives

Coping
Past methods of dealing with stress *VERY STOIC, TRIES NOT TO SHOW*
STRESS ___
Necessary life-style changes due to disease *DECREASE IN ROLE*
FUNCTIONS ___
Support systems available *FAMILY, ESPECIALLY HUSBAND* ___

Ineffective individual coping
(Ineffective family coping)
(POTENTIAL)

Fig. 17-2, cont'd

Coping mechanisms used _ACCEPTING_

Patient's affect _APPROPRIATE_

Physical manifestations _UNCOMFORTABLE TALKING ABOUT THIS AREA; MAY NEED FURTHER ASSESSMENT AS PT. PROGRESSES_

Patient's evaluation of present coping level _OK ACCORDING TO HUSBAND (HE ANSWERED FOR HER)_

Family's evaluation of present coping level _OK ACCORDING TO HUSBAND_

Participation

Compliance with past/current health care regimens _GOOD IF SHE UNDER-STANDS_

Noncompliance

(Ineffective participation)

Willingness to comply with future health care regimen _WILLING WITH KNOWLEDGE_

(POTENTIAL)

Judgment

Decision-making ability

Patient's perspective _HUSBAND MAKES DECISIONS_

Judgment
Indecisiveness

Others' perspectives _SAME_

HUSBAND IS DECISION MAKER FOR FAMILY AS NORMAL AND EXPECTED PER CULTURAL ORIENTATION & BELIEFS

Prioritized nursing diagnoses/problem list

1. _ALTERED SELF-CONCEPT R/T BODY IMAGE CHANGES, ACTIVITY INTOLERANCE_
2. _INEFFECTIVE BREATHING PATTERN R/T (L) SHOULDER PAIN_
3. _ALTERED COMFORT R/T CHRONIC PAIN R/T TUMOR GROWTH_
4. _POTENTIAL FOR INJURY R/T IMMUNOSUPPRESSION_
5. _KNOWLEDGE DEFICIT R/T TREATMENT OUTCOME/EFFECTS OF BONE MARROW TRANSPLANT_
6. _ALTERED SEXUALITY PATTERNS R/T BODY IMAGE CHANGES, CHANGES IN MARITAL INTERACTION_
7. _ALTERED ROLE PERFORMANCE R/T ACTIVITY INTOLERANCE_
8. _FEAR, SADNESS, & GRIEVING STATES R/T UNCERTAINTY OF TREATMENT OUTCOME & LIFE STYLE CHANGES_
9. _IMPAIRED SKIN/TISSUE INTEGRITY R/T CHEST WALL ERYTHEMA & BREAKDOWN_
10. _____

Signature _Anita P. Sherer, R.N._ Date _4/22_

Fig. 17-2, cont'd

CHAPTER 18

ACQUIRED IMMUNODEFICIENCY SYNDROME ASSESSMENT TOOL

SHELIA D. BUNTON
THOMAS G. O'DONNELL

The Acquired Immunodeficiency Syndrome (AIDS) Assessment Tool was designed to assess patients with unique biopsychosocial assessment needs. It incorporates specific signs and symptoms pertinent to the AIDS patient to facilitate identification of nursing diagnoses. This chapter includes:

- *The way the tool was developed and refined*
- *The patient population and settings to which it applies*
- *Selected AIDS emphasis areas*
- *The way to use the tool*
- *Specific AIDS focus questions and parameters to assist the nurse in eliciting appropriate data*
- *The AIDS Assessment Tool*
- *A case study*
- *A completed version of the tool based on the case study*

DEVELOPMENT AND REFINEMENT OF THE TOOL

The AIDS Assessment Tool was developed from the nursing data base prototype (see Chapter 2). Many hemodynamic monitoring and critical care variables originally incorporated in the prototype were replaced with variables more applicable to an assessment of a person with AIDS. The resultant tool, which is supported by the literature from this field, was modified based on the recommendations of AIDS nurse experts.

After the tool was developed and refined, it was clinically tested by nurse experts in the field of acquired immunosuppression. The tool was tested on eight patients who had been diagnosed as having positive serum human immunodeficiency virus (HIV) results and who were seen in an intermediate care setting or clinic. Most patients were well, with little or no constitutional disease present. The testing evaluated the adequacy of the tool in terms of flow, space for recording data, and completeness of assessment variables. Based on the results, the tool was revised.

PATIENT POPULATION AND SETTING

The AIDS Assessment Tool was developed to assess the needs of adult patients being diagnosed or treated for HIV-related disorders and diseases. It was originally designed for use in the hospital because of the extensive variables included in the "exchanging pattern." The AIDS Assessment Tool may also be valuable in the outpatient setting if it is modified (see Chapter 4).

ACQUIRED IMMUNODEFICIENCY SYNDROME EMPHASIS AREAS

The person with AIDS has specialized problems and needs. The AIDS Assessment Tool, developed to include assessment variables within each of the nine human response patterns, focuses on prevalent problems among HIV-positive individuals. Table 18-1 outlines these emphasis areas.

HOW TO USE THE TOOL

To use the AIDS Assessment Tool effectively, nurses must be familiar with the nine human response patterns of the Unitary Person Framework (see Chapter 2), which provides the underlying framework for Taxonomy I. The human response patterns of the Unitary Person Framework serve as the major category headings for Taxonomy I and

Table 18-1

Selected acquired immunodeficiency syndrome emphasis areas

Patterns	Emphasis areas to determine
Communicating	Verbal and nonverbal observations
Relating	Socioeconomic status
	Co-workers' responses to disease
	Impact of disease on sexual relationships
	In-depth socialization patterns
Knowing	In-depth history, including neoplasms, infections, and risk behaviors as identified by the patient
	Patient's awareness of precautions with body fluids
Feeling	Factors used to promote comfort
	Objective and subjective observations of the patient's feelings
Moving	Examination of muscle activity and weakness
	Discussion of exercise
	Health maintenance and status of various final arrangements
Exchanging	Physical regulation and in-depth examination of immune system
Choosing	Coping behaviors and behaviors used in problem solving

the assessment tool. The sequence of the response patterns, as it appears in Taxonomy I, has been changed in this tool to permit better ordering of assessment variables. Nursing diagnoses pertinent to AIDS patients, along with the signs and symptoms necessary to identify them, have been added to the appropriate response patterns in the tool.

Nurses must also realize that this tool is very different from conventional assessment tools. As a result, nurses may encounter some initial difficulty in using it. They should remember, however, that the tool was not designed to follow the organization or content of the traditional medical data base; the data collected does not reflect solely medical patterns. Rather, the tool elicits information about holistic patterns in ways not traditionally assessed by nurses. It represents a new way of collecting and synthesizing data that requires new thinking when processing data. This tool represents a nursing data base developed from a nursing model that permits a holistic nursing assessment to take place so nursing diagnoses can be identified.

Although nurses probably agree that a holistic nursing data base would help in practice, it is realized that chang-

ing traditional assessment methods is not an easy task. For this reason, a trial usage period is recommended before nurses make any decisions about the tool's merits. During this period, nurses should assess 10 patients using the tool to become familiar and progressively more comfortable with its organization and data-collection methods. With experience, nurses will become accustomed to new ways of clustering and processing information. With continued use, the time necessary to complete the tool will be reduced. Most important, nurses will recognize the unique ability of the tool to elicit appropriate signs and symptoms. Nurses will discover that nursing diagnoses are easily identified when using the tool.

It is not necessary to complete the tool in one session. Priority sections can be completed during the initial assessment. Other sections or patterns can be completed later, within a time frame acceptable to the institution.

To elicit appropriate data, nurses should be familiar with the focus questions and parameters in the next section. When assessing specific signs and symptoms to affirm a diagnosis, the nurse circles the diagnosis in the right-hand column. The circled diagnosis dooes not confirm a problem but simply alerts the nurse to the possibility that it exists. After completing the assessment, the nurse scans the possible circled problems, synthesizes the data to determine whether other clusters of signs and symptoms support the problem, and decides whether the actual diagnosis is present.

The diagnoses in the right-hand column may be repeated in more than one place. These repetitions occur only within the appropriate response pattern and are convenient for identifying certain data directly with their nursing diagnosis. These diagnoses are not absolute but are intended to focus thinking and direct attention to collecting data concerning a possible problem.

Some signs and symptoms can indicate several diagnoses. For example, oral candidiasis can indicate infection or an alteration in the oral mucous membrane. To avoid unnecessary repetition of assessment parameters, variables are arranged with the diagnosis most likely to result from the data assessed. Thus, data to support one diagnosis may occasionally be found in other patterns or arranged with other diagnoses. Therefore, synthesis of all data is essential.

The AIDS Assessment Tool is not the standardized and final format for nationwide assessment of patients with AIDS. An assessment tool must meet the needs of the institutions and nurses using it. The AIDS Assessment Tool is simply a working demonstration tool that is expected to be changed and revised by nurses in clinical practice. Further evaluation and refinement are necessary before adopting the tool for use within a particular institution. Nurses interested in changing, revising, and adapting the tool to a specific clinical setting should refer to Chapter 4.

Table 18-2

Acquired immunodeficiency syndrome assessment tool: focus questions and parameters

Variables	Focus questions and parameters
RELATING	
Perception of co-workers' response to disease	"Are your co-workers aware of your disease?" "How have they responded to the fact that you are HIV positive?" "How do you feel about their responses?"
Impact of disease on financial status	"Is your disease creating a financial hardship?" "How will you meet your expenses while maintaining your standard of living?"
Impact of disease on sexual relationships	"Have you had a decrease in sexual activity since being identified as HIV positive?" "How does your partner feel about your being HIV positive?"
KNOWING	
History of the following neoplasms/infections	Does the patient have a history of diseases frequently experienced by AIDS patients (see list on assessment tool)?
Risk behaviors identified by	Does the patient state or demonstrate any of the behaviors that increase the risk of contracting the AIDS virus?
Expectations of therapy	"Do you believe there is a possible solution to your problem?" "What expectations do you have of your care providers?" "What do you think the results of your therapy will be?"
Memory intact	Does the patient (or significant other) acknowledge any memory loss or impaired cognitive abilities?
Recent memory	"Can you tell me what day, month, and year it is?"
Remote memory	"Can you recall the holidays we celebrated last month? In the month of _____?"
FEELING	
Verbalizes feelings	"How do you feel about past activities that have led to your hospitalization?" "Do you prefer to be alone or with others?" Does the patient verbalize fear, anxiety, fatigue, failure, or other feelings? Does the patient show subtle or overt signs of hostility, sadness, fear, frustration, or intense anxiety?
MOVING	
Muscle weakness or atrophy	"Have you noticed any decreased muscle strength, muscle control, or muscle mass?"
Patient's perception of the need to exercise	"Can you explain why it is important for you to exercise?" "What do you normally do to maintain strength and mobility?"
Desire for cardiopulmonary resuscitation	"If you quit breathing or your heart stopped beating, would you want any extraordinary measures taken to prolong your life?"
PERCEIVING	
Effects of illness on self-concept	"Has your role as a provider been affected by your disease?" "Has your disease or hospitalization interrupted your normal life-style?" "How do you feel your disease has affected your power to carry out self-imposed goals or obligations?" "How can the nursing staff help you in regaining some control over your situation?"
CHOOSING	
Patient's usual problem-solving methods	"How did you deal with previous hospitalizations?" "Do you have a plan for dealing with the future?"
Patient's method of dealing with stress	"Were you able to effectively cope with past hospitalizations?" "What coping methods did you find particularly helpful?"
Compliance with past/current health care regimens	"Do you have a plan for how you would like to participate in your health care?"
Support systems available	"Is there someone to whom you can turn to share moments of happiness, doubt, worry, or stress?" "Have you notified them? Would you like for us to notify them?"

HOW TO ELICIT APPROPRIATE DATA

Because the Unitary Person Framework and the AIDS Assessment Tool contain some terms that may be unfamiliar to nurses, specific AIDS focus questions and parameters were developed and refined to help the nurse to elicit appropriate information. These questions and parameters are in Table 18-2, which follows the content of the tool (Fig. 18-1). The variables in bold type in the tool are described in Table 18-2. For example, the variable about the patient's perception of the need to exercise under the "moving pattern" is in bold type. If nurses do not know what questions to ask about this variable, they can use Table 18-2 to direct the line of questioning. The questions and parameters are only suggestions intended to assist the nurse in focusing content when collecting data. They are not static or absolute, and nurses should not feel confined to asking only the questions or assessing only the parameters provided. There are many other ways, based on the patient's situation and condition and the nurses skill, to elicit information. Focus questions and parameters for other data not in bold type are in Chapter 3.

CASE STUDY

The case study models the process a nurse uses when assessing a patient. Based on the clustering of information obtained during assessment, the nurse formulates nursing diagnoses.

Mr. J.L. is a 36-year-old business man who was diagnosed as HIV-positive approximately 1 year ago. When admitted, he was experiencing increasing weakness and fatigue. The Acquired Immunodeficiency Syndrome Assessment Tool (Fig. 18-2) was used to assess Mr. J.L.

BIBLIOGRAPHY

DeVita VT, Hellman S, and Rosenberg SA: AIDS: etiology, diagnosis, treatment, and prevention, New York, 1985, JB Lippincott Co.

Durham J and Cohen F: The person with AIDS: nursing perspective, New York, 1987, Springer Publishing Co, Inc.

Griffin JP: Hematology and immunology: concepts for nursing, Norwalk, Conn, 1986, Appleton-Century-Crofts.

Institute of Medicine, National Academy of Science: Confronting AIDS: directions for public health, health care, and research, Washington, DC, 1986, National Academy Press.

O'Brian ME: The courage to survive, New York, 1983, Grune & Stratton, Inc.

ACQUIRED IMMUNODEFICIENCY SYNDROME ASSESSMENT TOOL

Name _____ Age _____ Sex _____
Address _____ Telephone _____
Significant other _____ Telephone _____
Date of admission _____ Medical diagnosis _____
Allergies _____

Nursing Diagnosis
(Potential or Altered)

COMMUNICATING ▪ A pattern involving sending messages

Read, write, understand English (circle) _____ Communication
Other languages _____ Interpreter needed: yes/no   Verbal
Intubated _____ Speech impaired _____   Nonverbal
Alternate form of communication _____
Verbal: thought processes _____
Nonverbal: Posture _____ Facial expressions _____
    Gestures _____ Eye contact _____

VALUING ▪ A pattern involving the assigning of relative worth

Religious preference _____   Spiritual state
Important religious practices _____   Distress
Verbalizes spiritual turmoil _____   Despair
Cultural orientation _____
Cultural practices _____

RELATING ▪ A pattern involving establishing bonds
Role

Marital status: Never married _____ Married _____ Separated _____   Role performance
    Widowed _____ Nonmarried partner _____ Divorced _____   Sexual dysfunction
Age & health of significant other _____   Work
_____   Family
                                                                        Social/leisure
Number of children _____ Ages _____   Family processes
Occupation _____ Employed/unemployed (circle)
    Socioeconomic status _____
    Job satisfaction/concerns _____
    Perception of co-workers' response to disease _____
    _____
    Financial support _____
    Impact of disease on financial status _____
    _____

Impact of disease on sexual relationships _____   Sexuality patterns
_____

Socialization
Patient's identification of significant other _____
Patient's description of relationships with
    Significant other _____   Impaired social interaction
    Family members _____
    Friends _____
Quality of relationships as described by
    Significant other _____
    Family members _____
Verbalizes feelings of being alone _____   Social isolation
    Attributed to _____   Social withdrawal
    Verbalizes need for assistance _____
    Staff observations _____

Fig. 18-1

KNOWING ▪ A pattern involving the meaning associated with information

Presenting health problems _____

_____

Current medications _____

_____

Previous illness/hospitalizations/surgery _____

History of   Knowledge deficit
   Heart disease _____ Lung disease _____
   Liver disease _____ Kidney disease _____
   Anemia _____ Other _____
   Alcohol use _____
   Substance abuse _____
   Suicide attempts _____

History of the following neoplasm/infections:
   Kaposi's sarcoma _____ Other neoplasms _____
   Pneumonia *(P. Carinii)* _____
   Herpes zoster _____ Cytomegalovirus _____
   Other viral infections _____
   Fungal infection _____ Bacterial infection _____
   Parasitic infection _____
   Other _____

Risk behaviors identified by: Patient   Nurse
   1. Homosexual/bisexual _____
   2. Intravenous drug use _____
   3. Haitian descent _____
   4. Hemophilia _____
   5. Blood product transfusion _____
   6. Heterosexual contact with high-risk persons _____
   7. Other _____   Knowledge deficit
Knowledge of disease process _____

_____

   Awareness of blood/body fluid precautions: yes/no (circle)
Knowledge of prognosis _____

_____

Expectations of therapy _____
Misconceptions _____
Readiness to learn _____
   Requesting information concerning _____
   Educational level _____   Thought processes
   Learning impeded by _____

Orientation   Orientation
Level of alertness _____   Confusion
Orientation: Person _____ Place _____ Time _____
Appropriate behavior/communication _____

Memory
Memory intact: yes/no   Recent _____ **Remote** _____   Memory

FEELING ▪ A pattern involving the subjective awareness of information
Comfort
   Pain/discomfort: yes/no   Comfort
      Onset _____ Duration _____   Pain/chronic
      Location _____ Quality _____ Radiation _____   Pain/acute
      Associated/aggravating factors _____   Discomfort
      Alleviating factors _____
      Factors used to promote comfort _____

Fig. 18-1, cont'd

Continued.

Emotional Integrity/States
   Verbalizes feelings of fear or anxiety _____

   _____

   Verbalizes other feelings _____
      Related cues: Hostility _____ Sarcasm _____
      Flippancy _____ Uncontrolled crying _____
      Dull or flat affect _____
   Verbalizes: Feeling like a failure _____
      Loss of interest in people _____
      Feeling punished _____ Denial _____

Grieving
Anxiety
Fear
Anger
Guilt
Shame
Sadness

MOVING ▪ A pattern involving activity
Activity
   History of physical disability _____

   Limitations in daily activities _____
   Verbal report of fatigue or weakness _____
   Muscle activity: gross examination _____
      Fatigue _____ Seizures _____
      Involuntary movements _____
      Gait disturbances _____
   Muscle weakness _____ Muscle atrophy _____
   Exercise program _____
      Patient's perception of the need to exercise _____

Impaired physical mobility
Activity intolerance

Rest
   Hours slept/night _____ Feels rested: yes/no
   Sleep aids (pillows, meds, food) _____
   Difficulty falling/remaining asleep _____

Sleep pattern disturbance
   Hypersomnia
   Insomnia
   Nightmares

Recreation
   Leisure activities _____
   Social activities _____

Deficit in diversional activity

Environmental Maintenance
   Home maintenance management
      Size & arrangement of home (stairs, bathroom) _____
      _____ Safety needs _____
      Housekeeping responsibilities _____

   Pets in home _____

Impaired home maintenance
   management
Safety hazards

Health Maintenance
   Health insurance: yes/no   Type: _____
   Regular physical checkups _____
      Date of last dental examination _____
   Hospital/clinic frequented for care _____
   Final arrangements complete: yes/no   Will prepared: yes/no
      Power of attorney appointed to _____
      Desire for cardiopulmonary resuscitation _____
      Other _____

Health maintenance

Self-Care
   Patient's general appearance _____
   Ability to perform ADLs: Independent _____ Dependent _____
   Specify deficits _____
   Home care planning needs _____
      Community resources available _____

Self-care
   Feeding
   Bathing/hygiene
   Dressing/grooming
   Toileting

Fig. 18-1, cont'd

PERCEIVING ▪ A pattern involving the reception of information
Self-Concept
Patient's description of self _____   Self-concept
Effects of illness on self-concept _____   Body image
_____   Self-esteem
Personal identity
Socialization

Meaningfulness
Verbalizes hopelessness _____   Hopelessness
   Inappropriate verbalizations _____   Powerlessness
Perceives/verbalizes loss of control _____   Injury
Verbalizes suicidal ideations _____

Sensory/Perception
History of restrictive environment _____   Sensory/perception
Vision: impaired _____ Glasses/contacts _____   Visual
Auditory impaired _____ Hearing aid _____ Deafness _____   Auditory
Kinesthetics impaired _____   Kinesthetic
Gustatory impaired _____   Gustatory
Tactile impaired _____   Tactile
Olfactory impaired _____   Olfactory
Reflexes: grossly intact _____

EXCHANGING ▪ A pattern involving mutual giving and receiving
Circulation
Cerebral (circle appropriate response)
   Neurologic changes/symptoms _____   Cerebral tissue perfusion

Pupils	Eye Opening
L 2 3 4 5 6 mm	None (1)
R 2 3 4 5 6 mm	To pain (2)
Reaction: Brisk _____	To speech (3)
Sluggish _____ Nonreactive _____	Spontaneous (4)

Best Verbal	Best Motor
No response (1)	Flaccid (1)
Incomprehensible sound (2)	Extensor response (2)
Inappropriate words (3)	Flexor response (3)
Confused conversation (4)	Semipurposeful (4)
Oriented (5)	Localized to pain (5)
	Obeys commands (6)

   Glascow Coma Scale total _____
Cardiac
   Apical rate & rhythm _____ PMI _____   Cardiopulmonary tissue
   Heart sounds/murmurs _____   perfusion
   BP: _____ Location _____   Cardiac output
Peripheral   Peripheral tissue perfusion
   Jugular venous distention: yes/no   R _____ L _____   Fluid volume
   Pulses: +3 = bounding   +2 = palpable   Deficit
              +1 = faintly palpable   0 = absent   Excess
   Location _____
   Skin temp _____ Color _____
   Capillary refill _____ Edema _____

Physical Integrity
   Tissue integrity: Rashes _____   Impaired skin integrity
   Lesions _____ Petechiae _____   Impaired tissue integrity
   Bruises _____ Lacerations _____   Injury
   Scars _____   Violence

Continued.

Fig. 18-1, cont'd

Oxygenation

Complaints of dyspnea _____ Precipitated by _____   Ineffective airway clearance
Orthopnea _____   Ineffective breathing patterns
Rate _____ Rhythm _____ Depth _____   Impaired gas exchange
Labored/unlabored (circle)
Use of accessory muscles _____
Chest expansion _____
Cough: productive/nonproductive _____
Sputum: Color _____ Amount _____ Consistency _____
Breath sounds _____
Arterial blood gases _____
Pulmonary function tests _____
CXR _____
Oxygen percent and device _____
Ventilator _____

Physical Regulation

Immune   Infection
  Lymph nodes enlarged _____ Location _____
  WBC count _____ Differential _____
  HIV testing: positive/negative   Date of last test _____
  T lymphocytes: OKT4 _____ OKT8 _____   Body temperature
  B lymphocytes _____   Hypothermia
Body temperature   Hyperthermia
  Temperature _____ Route _____   Ineffective thermoregulation
  Night sweats _____

Nutrition   Nutrition

Eating patterns
  Number of meals per day _____
  Special diet _____ Vitamins _____
  Where eaten _____ Eaten alone: yes/no
  Food preferences/intolerances _____
  Food allergies _____
  Fluid intake _____
  Appetite changes _____
  Nausea/vomiting/anorexia _____
Condition of mouth/throat _____   Oral mucous membrane
Oral candidiasis _____   Impaired swallowing
Height _____ Weight _____ Weight loss _____   Less than body requirements
Current therapy
  NPO _____ Tube feeding _____
  IV fluids _____
  TPN _____
Labs
  Hematocrit _____ Hemoglobin _____
  Na _____ K _____ CL _____ Glucose _____
  Alkaline phosphatase _____ Serum albumin _____
  PT _____ PTT_____

Elimination

Gastrointestinal/bowel   Bowel elimination
  Usual bowel habits _____   Constipation
  Alterations from normal: Diarrhea _____   Diarrhea
    Other _____   Incontinence
  Abdominal physical examination _____
  Perianal ulcers _____

Fig. 18-1, cont'd

Renal/urinary
    Usual urinary pattern _____   Urinary elimination
    Alteration from normal _____   Incontinence
    Color _____ Catheter _____   Retention
    Urine output: 24 hours _____ Average hourly _____
    Bladder distention _____
    External genitalia examination _____
        Presence of sores _____
        Unexplained penial/vaginal discharge _____

CHOOSING ▪ A pattern involving the selection of alternatives
Coping
    Patient's usual problem-solving methods _____   Ineffective individual coping
    _____
        Behaviors used in problem-solving: Alcohol _____   Ineffective family coping
        Smoking _____ Shopping _____
        Rituals _____ Isolation _____
        Others _____
    Family's usual problem-solving methods _____
    _____
    Patient's method of dealing with stress _____
    _____
    Family's method of dealing with stress _____
    _____
    Patient's affect: appropriate/inappropriate _____
    Physical manifestations _____
    Patient's usual defense mechanisms _____
    _____

Participation
    Compliance with past/current health care regimens _____   Noncompliance
    _____
    Support systems available _____   Ineffective participation
    Significant others' ability to support patient _____
    _____
    Family's ability to support patient _____
    _____

Judgment
    Decision-making ability _____   Judgment
        Patient's perspective _____   Indecisiveness
        Others' perspectives _____

Prioritized nursing diagnosis/problem list
1. _____
2. _____
3. _____
4. _____
5. _____

Signature _____   Date _____

Fig. 18-1, cont'd

ACQUIRED IMMUNODEFICIENCY SYNDROME ASSESSMENT TOOL

Name *J.L.* _____ Age *36* Sex *MALE* ___
Address *666 SIXTH STREET, NEW YORK, NEW YORK* ___ Telephone *555-6666* ___
Significant other *(LOVER) H.H.* _____ Telephone *SAME* ___
Date of admission *1 NOV.* _____ Medical diagnosis *HIV POSITIVE, INCREASING WEAKNESS*
Allergies *NONE* _____

Nursing Diagnosis
(Potential or Altered)

COMMUNICATING ▪ A pattern involving sending messages
(Read) (write) (understand) English (circle) _____ Communication
Other languages *NONE* _____ Interpreter needed: yes (no) Verbal
Intubated __—__ Speech impaired *No* _____ Nonverbal
Alternate form of communication *NONE* _____
Verbal: thought processes *APPROPRIATE* _____
Nonverbal: Posture *RELAXED* ___ Facial expressions *APPROPRIATE* ___
  Gestures *NONE* ___ Eye contact *YES* _____

VALUING ▪ A pattern involving the assigning of relative worth
Religious preference *METHODIST* _____ Spiritual state
Important religious practices *"NONE IN PARTICULAR"* ___ Distress
Verbalizes spiritual turmoil *"ON RARE OCCASIONS I THINK GOD'S PUNISHING ME."* Despair
Cultural orientation *AMERICAN* _____
Cultural practices *"NONE IN PARTICULAR"* _____

RELATING ▪ A pattern involving establishing bonds
Role
  Marital status: Never married _____ Married _____ Separated _____ Role performance
  Widowed _____ Nonmarried partner _____ Divorced ✓, *4 YEARS* Sexual dysfunction
  Age & health of significant other *EX-WIFE, 34 IN GOOD HEALTH; LOVER,* Work
32 EXHIBITING SIGNS OF MODERATELY ADVANCED DISEASE Family
  Number of children *2* Ages *6, 7 (2 BOYS)* Social/leisure
  Occupation *WORKS FOR COMPUTER COMPANY* Employed/unemployed (circle) Family processes
    Socioeconomic status *MIDDLE CLASS* _____
    Job satisfaction/concerns *ENJOYS JOB* _____
    Perception of co-workers' response to disease *"SOME KNOW ABOUT*
DISEASE — NO OBVIOUS CHANGES IN THEIR BEHAVIOR."
    Financial support *JOB ONLY* _____
    Impact of disease on financial status *HAS NOT NOTICED EFFECT OF*
MOUNTING MEDICAL EXPENSES AT THIS TIME
  Impact of disease on sexual relationships *"IT HAS BROUGHT US* Sexuality patterns
CLOSER TOGETHER."

Socialization
  Patient's identification of significant other *(NAME PROVIDED)* ___
  Patient's description of relationships with
    Significant other *"VERY GOOD"* _____ Impaired social interaction
    Family members *"TENSE"* _____
    Friends *"GOOD — THEY ARE UNDERSTANDING."* _____
  Quality of relationships as described by
    Significant other *N/A* _____
    Family members *(SISTER) "NOT GOOD; THE FAMILY FINDS IT DISTASTEFUL."*
  Verbalizes feelings of being alone *No* _____ Social isolation
    Attributed to __—_____ Social withdrawal
    Verbalizes need for assistance *YES, WOULD LIKE SOMEONE TO TALK TO*
  Staff observations *COMPOSED, IN CONTROL OF SITUATION* ___

Fig. 18-2

KNOWING ▪ A pattern involving the meaning associated with information

Presenting health problems *INCREASING WEAKNESS*

Current medications *MAALOX (OVER-THE-COUNTER) TAKEN AS NEEDED*

Previous illness/hospitalizations/surgery *HOSPITALIZED ABOUT 2 MONTHS AGO FOR DEHYDRATION*

History of   Knowledge deficit
- Heart disease —∅—   Lung disease —∅—
- Liver disease —∅—   Kidney disease —∅—
- Anemia —∅—   Other —∅—
- Alcohol use *YES, GLASS OF WINE WITH DINNER*
- Substance abuse *YES, AMYL NITRATE*
- Suicide attempts _____

History of the following neoplasm/infections:
- Kaposi's sarcoma *YES*   Other neoplasms —
- Pneumonia (*P. Carinii*) —
- Herpes zoster —   Cytomegalovirus *YES*
- Other viral infections —
- Fungal infection —   Bacterial infection —
- Parasitic infection —
- Other —

Risk behaviors identified by: Patient   Nurse
1. (Homosexual/bisexual) _____   ✓   ✓
2. Intravenous drug use _____   –   –
3. Haitian descent _____   –   –
4. Hemophilia _____   –   –
5. Blood product transfusion _____   –   –
6. Heterosexual contact with high-risk persons —∅—
7. Other —∅—   (Knowledge deficit)

Knowledge of disease process *HAS BASIC UNDERSTANDING OF DISEASE BUT NEEDS MORE THOROUGH TEACHING*
- Awareness of blood/body fluid precautions: (yes)/no (circle)

Knowledge of prognosis *UNDERSTANDS DISEASE HAS NO CURE*

Expectations of therapy *"THERAPY SHOULD TEMPORARILY HELP TO IMPROVE STRENGTH"*

Misconceptions *NONE*

Readiness to learn *YES, SEEKING INFORMATION*
- Requesting information concerning *DISEASE PROGRESSION*
- Educational level *COLLEGE — 4 YEARS*   Thought processes
- Learning impeded by —

Orientation   Orientation

Level of alertness *FULLY ALERT*   Confusion

Orientation: Person *YES*   Place *YES*   Time *YES*

Appropriate behavior/communication *YES*

Memory

Memory intact: (yes)/no   Recent *YES*   Remote *YES*   Memory

FEELING ▪ A pattern involving the subjective awareness of information

Comfort

Pain/discomfort: (yes)/no   Comfort
- Onset *WHEN HUNGRY* Duration *"LASTS UNTIL I EAT SOMETHING."*   Pain/chronic
- Location *ABDOMEN* Quality *WEAK–MOD.* Radiation *NO*   Pain/acute
- Associated/aggravating factors —   (Discomfort)
- Alleviating factors —
- Factors used to promote comfort *EATS SMALL, FREQUENT MEALS*

Fig. 18-2, cont'd

Continued

Emotional Integrity/States

Verbalizes feelings of fear or anxiety *FEARFUL OF FUTURE OUTCOME*

Verbalizes other feelings *GUILT FOR IGNORING "SAFE SEX" WARNING*
    Related cues: Hostility ___—___ Sarcasm _____
    Flippancy ___—___ Uncontrolled crying ___—___
    Dull or flat affect ___—___
Verbalizes: Feeling like a failure *YES*
    Loss of interest in people ___—___
    Feeling punished *YES*   Denial ___—___

Grieving
Anxiety
(Fear)
Anger
(Guilt)
Shame
Sadness

MOVING ■ A pattern involving activity

Activity

History of physical disability *No*

Limitations in daily activities *"MUST TAKE FREQUENT REST PERIODS"*
Verbal report of fatigue or weakness *YES, EASILY FATIGUED*
Muscle activity: gross examination *NORMAL*
    Fatigue *ON EXERTION* Seizures ___⊖___
    Involuntary movements ___⊖___
    Gait disturbances ___⊖___
Muscle weakness *YES*   Muscle atrophy ___⊖___
Exercise program *NONE*
    Patient's perception of the need to exercise *DOES NOT RECOGNIZE NEED FOR EXERCISE*

Impaired physical mobility
Activity intolerance

Rest

Hours slept/night *7-8 HRS.* Feels rested: (yes)/no
Sleep aids (pillows, meds, food) *I PILLOW, NO OTHER AIDS*
Difficulty falling/remaining asleep *No*

Sleep pattern disturbance
  Hypersomnia
  Insomnia
  Nightmares

Recreation

Leisure activities *READING*
Social activities *DINING OUT, VISITING c̄ FRIENDS*

Deficit in diversional activity

Environmental Maintenance

Home maintenance management
    Size & arrangement of home (stairs, bathroom) *2 BEDROOM CONDO,*
2 FLOORS   Safety needs ___—___
    Housekeeping responsibilities *MINOR REPAIRS AROUND HOUSE,*
SHARES MEAL PREPARATION & CLEANING c̄ PARTNER
Pets in home *FISH, HAS 50 GALLON TANK*

Impaired home maintenance
  management
Safety hazards

Health Maintenance

Health insurance: (yes)/no   Type: *AMERICAN LIFE INSURANCE*
Regular physical checkups *ONCE A YEAR OR AS NEEDED*
Date of last dental examination *2 MONTHS AGO*
Hospital/clinic frequented for care *SMITH HEALTH CLINIC*
Final arrangements complete: yes/(no)   Will prepared: (yes)/no
    Power of attorney appointed to *SISTER (NAME PROVIDED)*
    Desire for cardiopulmonary resuscitation *UNDECIDED*
    Other ___—___

Health maintenance

Self-Care

Patient's general appearance *NEAT, WELL GROOMED; THIN*
Ability to perform ADLs: Independent ___✓___ Dependent _____
Specify deficits *WEAKNESS, FATIGUES EASILY*
Home care planning needs *NONE AT THIS TIME*
    Community resources available ___—___

Self-care
  Feeding
  Bathing/hygiene
  Dressing/grooming
  Toileting

Fig. 18-2, cont'd

PERCEIVING ▪ A pattern involving the reception of information
Self-Concept
Patient's description of self _"I'M USUALLY A STRONG PERSON."_   Self-concept
Effects of illness on self-concept _"I FEEL AS THOUGH I'M LOSING MY_   Body image
IDENTITY."   Self-esteem
    (Personal identity)
    Socialization

Meaningfulness
Verbalizes hopelessness _No_   Hopelessness
   Inappropriate verbalizations _ø_   (Powerlessness)
Perceives/verbalizes loss of control _YES — CANNOT CONTROL PROGNOSIS_   Injury
Verbalizes suicidal ideations _No_

Sensory/Perception
History of restrictive environment _No_   Sensory/perception
Vision: impaired _YES, CORRECTED_ Glasses (contacts)   Visual
Auditory impaired _—_ Hearing aid _—_ Deafness _____   Auditory
Kinesthetics impaired _—_   Kinesthetic
Gustatory impaired _—_   Gustatory
Tactile impaired _—_   Tactile
Olfactory impaired _—_   Olfactory
Reflexes: grossly intact _FULL, PALPABLE PULSES_

EXCHANGING ▪ A pattern involving mutual giving and receiving
Circulation
Cerebral (circle appropriate response)
   Neurologic changes/symptoms _NONE_   Cerebral tissue perfusion
   Pupils   Eye Opening
     L 2 3 (4) 5 6 mm   None (1)
     R 2 3 (4) 5 6 mm   To pain (2)
     Reaction: Brisk ✓   To speech (3)
     Sluggish ____ Nonreactive ____   Spontaneous (4)
   Best Verbal   Best Motor
     No response (1)   Flaccid (1)
     Incomprehensible sound (2)   Extensor response (2)
     Inappropriate words (3)   Flexor response (3)
     Confused conversation (4)   Semipurposeful (4)
     Oriented (5)   Localized to pain (5)
                     Obeys commands (6)
   Glascow Coma Scale total _15_
Cardiac   _5TH INTERCOSTAL,_
   Apical rate & rhythm _84, REGULAR_ PMI _5cm FROM MIDLINE_   Cardiopulmonary tissue
   Heart sounds/murmurs _No MURMURS HEARD, NORMAL S₁ ₓ S₂_   perfusion
   BP: _¹¹⁸/74mmHg, SITTING_ Location _RIGHT ARM_   Cardiac output
Peripheral   Peripheral tissue perfusion
   Jugular venous distention: yes (no) R _____ L _____   Fluid volume
   Pulses: +3 = bounding   +2 = palpable   Deficit
         +1 = faintly palpable   0 = absent   Excess
     Location _2+ THROUGHOUT_
     Skin temp _WARM TO TOUCH_ Color _PALE_
     Capillary refill _LESS THAN 2 SEC._ Edema _ø_

Physical Integrity
   Tissue integrity: Rashes _ø_   Impaired skin integrity
     Lesions _ø_   Petechiae _ø_   Impaired tissue integrity
     Bruises _ø_   Lacerations _ø_   Injury
     Scars _ø_   Violence

Fig. 18-2, cont'd

Continued.

Oxygenation

Complaints of dyspnea _No_ Precipitated by _—_ Ineffective airway clearance
Orthopnea _No_ Ineffective breathing patterns
Rate _20_ Rhythm _REGULAR_ Depth _SHALLOW_ Impaired gas exchange
Labored (unlabored) (circle)
Use of accessory muscles _No_
Chest expansion _NORMAL_
Cough: productive (nonproductive) _DRY, HACKING_
Sputum: Color _—_ Amount _—_ Consistency _—_
Breath sounds _CLEAR BILATERALLY & IN ALL BASES; NO ADVENTIOUS SOUNDS_
Arterial blood gases _Ø_
Pulmonary function tests _Ø_
CXR _Ø_
Oxygen percent and device _Ø_
Ventilator _Ø_

Physical Regulation

Immune   (Infection) (POTENTIAL)
   Lymph nodes enlarged _No_ Location _—_
   WBC count _5.0 × 10³/µL_ Differential _LYMPHOCYTES = 25%_
   HIV testing: (positive) negative Date of last test _8 MARCH_
   T lymphocytes: OKT4 _DECREASED SLIGHTLY_ OKT8 _NORMAL_ Body temperature
   B lymphocytes _(PENDING)_ Hypothermia
Body temperature Hyperthermia
   Temperature _99.8°F_ Route _ORALLY_ Ineffective thermoregulation
   Night sweats _YES_

Nutrition
Nutrition

Eating patterns
   Number of meals per day _5 SMALL MEALS_
   Special diet _Ø_ Vitamins _YES_
   Where eaten _MAINLY AT HOME_ Eaten alone: yes (no)
   Food preferences/intolerances _NONE IN PARTICULAR_
   Food allergies _NONE_
   Fluid intake _APPROXIMATELY 2 LITERS/DAY_
   Appetite changes _DECREASED LATELY_
   Nausea/vomiting/anorexia _No_
Condition of mouth/throat _MUCOSA SWOLLEN_ Oral mucous membrane
Oral candidiasis _No_ Impaired swallowing
Height _6'0"_ Weight _150 #_ Weight loss _20# OVER LAST YEAR_ Less than body requirements
Current therapy
   NPO _—_ Tube feeding _—_
   IV fluids _—_
   TPN _—_
Labs
   Hematocrit _45%_ Hemoglobin _15.6 g/dl_
   Na _140 mEq/L_ K _4.8 mEq/L_ CL _96 mEq/L_ Glucose _100 mg/dl_
   Alkaline phosphatase _—_ Serum albumin _4.0 g/dl_
   PT _—_ PTT _—_

Elimination

Gastrointestinal/bowel Bowel elimination
   Usual bowel habits _ONCE A DAY_ Constipation
   Alterations from normal: Diarrhea _YES — SOMETIMES_ (Diarrhea) (POTENTIAL)
      Other _Ø_ Incontinence
   Abdominal physical examination _NO MASSES OR AREAS OF TENDERNESS, SOFT_
   Perianal ulcers _Ø_

Fig. 18-2, cont'd

Renal/urinary
    Usual urinary pattern *SEVERAL TIMES A DAY, SMALL AMOUNTS*   Urinary elimination
    Alteration from normal *⊖*   Incontinence
    Color *YELLOW/CLEAR* Catheter *⊖*   Retention
    Urine output: 24 hours *APPROX. 1000 cc* Average hourly *40 cc*
    Bladder distention *NONE*
    External genitalia examination *NO ABNORMALITIES NOTED*
        Presence of sores *NONE*
        Unexplained penial/~~vaginal~~ discharge *NO*

CHOOSING ▪ A pattern involving the selection of alternatives
Coping
Patient's usual problem-solving methods *"SIT AND THINK IT OVER"*   (Ineffective individual coping)

                                               (*POTENTIAL*)
    Behaviors used in problem-solving: Alcohol _____   Ineffective family coping
    Smoking ✔   Shopping _____
    Rituals _____ Isolation ✔
    Others _____
Family's usual problem-solving methods *"IGNORE THE PROBLEM"*

Patient's method of dealing with stress *"HOLD IT IN"*

Family's method of dealing with stress *"MY SISTER & I CAN SIT & DISCUSS THINGS — THE REST OF THE FAMILY I DON'T KNOW."*
Patient's affect: (appropriate)/inappropriate _____
Physical manifestations *⊖*
Patient's usual defense mechanisms *IS QUIET, DOES NOT BEGIN TO ARGUE WITH OTHERS*

Participation
Compliance with past/current health care regimens *PLANS TO CARE FOR SELF ACCORDING TO INFORMATION RECEIVED*   Noncompliance
Support systems available *PARTNER, FRIENDS, ONE SISTER*   Ineffective participation
Significant others' ability to support patient *PARTNER CAN GIVE ONLY LIMITED SUPPORT, FRIENDS WILL PROVIDE MUCH SUPPORT*
Family's ability to support patient *SISTER WILL PROVIDE SUPPORT, OTHER FAMILY MEMBERS WILL NOT (SISTER'S INPUT)*

Judgment
Decision-making ability _____   Judgment
    Patient's perspective *"I THINK MY DECISIONS ARE GOOD"*   Indecisiveness
    Others' perspectives *(NURSE) PT. HAS DEMONSTRATED SOUND DECISION MAKING THROUGHOUT INTERVIEW.*

Prioritized nursing diagnosis/problem list
1. *KNOWLEDGE DEFICIT RELATED TO INADEQUATE INFORMATION CONCERNING DISEASE PROCESS.*
2. *ALTERED FEAR & GUILT STATES RELATED TO FEELINGS OF PUNISHMENT & DISEASE OUTCOME.*
3. *ALTERED PERSONAL IDENTITY RELATED TO EFFECTS OF ILLNESS ON ROLE.*
4. *POWERLESSNESS RELATED TO INABILITY TO CONTROL DISEASE PROCESS.*
5. *POTENTIAL FOR INFECTION RELATED TO LOW WBC COUNT.*

Signature *Shelia Buxton, Maj., AN*   Date *1 NOV., 08.30 HRS.*

Fig. 18-2, cont'd

■ UNIT IV ■
ASSESSING PATIENTS
THROUGHOUT THE LIFE SPAN

CHAPTER 19

LABOR-DELIVERY ASSESSMENT TOOL

SHELIA D. BUNTON
CANDICE J. SULLIVAN

The Labor-Delivery Assessment Tool was designed to assess the unique biopsychosocial needs of the pregnant patient. This tool incorporates signs and symptoms pertinent to the child-bearing patient to facilitate identification of nursing diagnoses. It also incorporates the American Nurses' Association's *Standards of Maternal and Child Health Nursing Practice*. This chapter includes:

- *The way the tool was developed and refined*
- *The patient population and settings to which it applies*
- *Selected labor, delivery, and postpartum emphasis areas*
- *The way to use the tool*
- *Specific labor, delivery, and postpartum focus questions and parameters to assist the nurse in eliciting the appropriate data*
- *The Labor-Delivery Assessment Tool*
- *A case study*
- *A completed version of the tool based on the case study*

DEVELOPMENT AND REFINEMENT OF THE TOOL

The Labor-Delivery Assessment Tool was developed from the nursing data base prototype (see Chapter 2). Many hemodynamic monitoring and critical care variables originally incorporated in the prototype were replaced with variables more applicable to a labor and delivery assessment. The tool is divided into labor, delivery, and postpartum sections. Each section contains assessment parameters pertinent to that phase in the birthing process. The resul-

tant tool, supported by labor, delivery, and postpartum literature, was presented to a team of labor and delivery nurse experts.

Masters-prepared and clinically experienced nurses tested the tool on eight women in labor, delivery, recovery, and postpartum units. The patients, ranging in age from 19 to 34 years, were admitted in various stages of labor or for induction. The testing evaluated the adequacy of the tool in terms of flow, space for documenting data, and completeness of assessment variables in each phase of the birthing process. Based on the results of the testing, the tool was revised.

PATIENT POPULATION AND SETTING

The Labor-Delivery Assessment Tool assesses the needs and problems of pregnant adult patients from the labor phase through discharge and into the home. Although this tool could be used to assess pregnant teenagers, the growth and development parameters used for patients between 12 and 18 years have not been included. Because important assessment variables would be overlooked, modification of the tool to include growth and development variables is recommended when using it with this group of patients.

This tool also evaluates the status of the fetus or infant during each stage. Although no fetal or infant-related diagnoses are listed, assessment variables were included to provide a thorough maternal assessment and cues about fetal distress.

Designed for use in the hospital, the tool can be used with preterm, term, and antepartum patients admitted with or without complications of pregnancy. To avoid stress or fatigue on the patient, it may be necesssary to complete the tool in two sessions. The nurse should gather as much information as possible from the chart, spouse, or a family member before interviewing the patient.

LABOR-DELIVERY EMPHASIS AREAS

Labor, delivery, and postpartum patients have specialized problems and needs. The Labor-Delivery Assessment Tool includes appropriate assessment variables within each of the nine human response patterns and focuses on prevalent problems of the pregnant patient. Table 19-1 outlines emphasis areas for the labor, delivery, and postpartum phases.

HOW TO USE THE TOOL

To use the Labor-Delivery Tool effectively, nurses must first be familiar with the nine human response patterns of the Unitary Person Framework (see Chapter 2), which provides the underlying framework for Taxonomy I. The human response patterns of the Unitary Person Framework serve as the major category headings for Taxonomy I and the tool. The sequence of the response patterns, as it appears in Taxonomy I, has been changed in the tool to permit better ordering of assessment variables. Nursing diagnoses pertinent to pregnant patients, along with the signs and symptoms necessary to identify them, have been added to the appropriate response patterns in the tool.

Nurses must also realize that this tool is very different from conventional labor and delivery assessment tools. As a result, nurses may encounter some initial difficulty in using it. They should remember, however, that the tool was not designed to follow the organization or content of the traditional medical data base; the data collected does not reflect solely medical patterns. Rather, this tool elicits information about holistic patterns in ways not traditionally assessed by nurses. It represents a new way of collecting and synthesizing data that requires new thinking in processing data. This tool represents a nursing data base developed from a nursing model that permits a holistic nursing assessment to take place so nursing diagnoses can be identified.

Although nurses probably agree that a holistic nursing data base would help in practice, it is realized that changing traditional assessment methods is not an easy task. For this reason, a trial usage period is recommended before nurses make any decisions about the tool's merits. During this period, nurses should assess 10 patients during labor, delivery, recovery, and postpartum periods using the Labor-Delivery Assessment Tool. During this time, nurses will become familiar and progressively more comfortable with the tool's organization and data-collection methods. With experience, they will become accustomed to new ways of clustering and processing information. With continued use, the time necessary to complete the tool will be reduced. Most important, nurses will recognize the unique ability of the tool to elicit appropriate signs and symptoms.

Table 19-1
Selected labor-delivery emphasis areas

Patterns	Emphasis areas to determine
Labor Phase	
Valuing	Childbearing and child-rearing values
Relating	Parenting behavior and relationship with own parents
Knowing	Expanded maternal prenatal history
Feeling	Status of contractions
	Emotional status and fear of losing control
Moving	Environmental maintenance and post-delivery assistance
	Health maintenance and care for the newborn
Perceiving	Patient's perception of herself
Exchanging	Oxygenation and breathing pattern
	Nutrition and alteration in body weight
	Maternal and fetal predelivery evaluation
Choosing	Support systems available
Delivery Phase	
Feeling	Emotional integrity and nurse's observations
Exchanging	Alterations in comfort
	Maternal and fetal evaluations
Postpartum Phase	
Relating	Parenting, role, and family processes
Knowing	Patient's understanding of postpartum self-care, postdelivery problems, and care of the newborn
	Community resources
Feeling	Altered emotional integrity states
Exchanging	Altered maternal or infant physical integrity or regulation
	Maternal postdelivery evaluation

They will discover that nursing diagnoses are easily identified when using this tool.

It is not necessary to complete the tool in one session. Priority sections can be completed during the initial assessment. Other sections or patterns can be completed later, within a time frame acceptable to the institution. To elicit appropriate data, nurses should be familiar with the focus questions and parameters discussed in the next section. When assessing specific signs and symptoms to affirm a diagnosis, the nurse circles the diagnosis in the right-hand column. The circled diagnosis does not confirm a problem but simply alerts the nurse to the possibility that it exists.

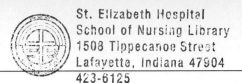

Table 19-2

Labor-delivery assessment tool: focus questions and parameters

Variables	Focus questions and parameters
Labor Phase	
VALUING	
Childbearing/rearing values	"Which childcare practices are important to you?" "How can the nursing staff assist you with these practices?" "Did you make a birth plan?" "How can we help you with your plan?"
RELATING	
Evidence of anticipatory parenting behaviors	Do parents verbalize frustration with their new role? Do parents verbalize anticipatory parenting behaviors? Do parents verbalize perceived or actual inadequacy? "Have you selected a name for your baby?" "Have you considered which method of feeding (bottle versus breast) you will use?"
Verbalized positive relationship with own parents	"Do you recall the methods of caretaking your parents used with you?" Do the parents verbalize positive feelings about their own parents? "Do you feel you will incorporate their methods in your child-care routines?" "Why or why not?"
KNOWING	
Understanding of labor, delivery, and postpartum periods	Can the patient state the events that occur in each phase? "Tell me, what do you think will happen during the_____ phase?"
MOVING	
Postdelivery assistance with responsibilities	"Will you need assistance with your routine household chores after the baby is born?" "How have you prepared for the baby?" "Is your nursery ready?" "Do you have clothes, diapers, and bottles?"
PERCEIVING	
Effects of pregnancy/delivery on self-concept	"What does this pregnancy mean to you? To you and your family?" "Has this pregnancy changed the way you feel about yourself?" "If so, in what ways?"
Verbalizes hopelessness	"Do you view this pregnancy as a difficult situation?" "Are you discouraged with the course of your pregnancy?" Does the patient exhibit crying, sad facial expressions, or an indifferent attitude? Is there a lack of effort toward delivering on the part of the patient?
Perceives/verbalizes loss of control	"Do you feel you have control over your body's actions?"
Delivery Phase	
FEELING	
Observations	Does the mother respond to the nurse's instructions? Does the mother reach out for her support person? Does the mother express relief and joy after delivery?
Postpartum Phase	
RELATING	
Diminished/inappropriate visual, tactile, or auditory stimulation of infant	Is there a lack of eye contact, smiling, gazing, or talking to the child by the parents? Do the parents "shy away" from the infant? Is the child held in the en face position? Does the mother initiate feedings? Does she prop the bottle?

Continued

Table 19-2—cont'd

Labor-delivery assessment tool: focus questions and parameters

Variables	Focus questions and parameters
RELATING—cont'd	
Verbalizes dissatisfaction/ disappointment with infant or infant's sex	Does the mother verbalize negative feelings for or about her infant? Does the mother display sadness, apathy, or ambivalence toward her infant?
FEELING	
Verbalizes positive feelings	Are the caretaking and play activities between mother and baby absent or less than expected?
Lack of contact with newborn	Does the mother refer to the infant by name and sex? Is the frequency of interactions between mother and baby less than normally expected?

After completing the assessment, the nurse scans the circled problems, synthesizes the data to determine whether other clusters of signs and symptoms support the problem, then decides whether the actual diagnosis is present.

The diagnoses in the right-hand column may be repeated in more than one place. These repetitions occur only within the appropriate response pattern and are convenient for identifying certain data directly with their corresponding nursing diagnosis. These diagnoses are not absolute but focus thinking and direct more detailed attention to collecting data about a problem.

Certain signs and symptoms can indicate several diagnoses. For example, verbalization of feelings toward the newborn can indicate altered family processes, parenting, or emotional integrity/states. To avoid unnecessary repetition of assessment parameters, variables are arranged with the diagnosis most likely to result from the data assessed. Thus, data to support a specific diagnosis may occasionally be found in other patterns or arranged with other diagnoses. Therefore, synthesis of all data is essential.

The Labor-Delivery Assessment Tool is not intended to be the standardized and final format for nationwide assessment of labor, delivery, and postpartum patients. An assessment tool must meet the needs of the institution and nurses using it. The Labor-Delivery Assessment Tool is simply a working demonstration tool that is expected to be changed and revised by nurses in clinical practice. Further evaluation and refinement are necessary before adopting the tool for use within a particular institution. Nurses interested in changing, revising, and adapting the tool to a specific clinical setting should refer to Chapter 4.

HOW TO ELICIT APPROPRIATE DATA

Because the Unitary Person Framework and the Labor-Delivery Assessment Tool contain some terms that may be unfamiliar to nurses, specific labor, delivery, and postpartum focus questions and parameters were developed and refined to help the nurse to elicit appropriate information. These questions and parameters are in Table 19-2, which follows the content of the tool (Fig. 19-1). The variables in bold type in the tool are described in Table 19-2. For example, the variable about parenting behaviors under the "relating pattern" is in bold type in the labor section of the tool. If the nurse does not know what to ask to elicit information about these behaviors, Table 19-2 can be used to direct the line of questioning. The questions and parameters are only suggestions intended to assist the nurse in focusing content when collecting data. They are neither static nor absolute. Nurses should not feel confined to asking only the questions or assessing only the parameters provided because there are many other ways, based on the patient's situation and condition and the nurse's skill, to elicit the information. Focus questions and parameters for data not in bold type are in Chapter 3.

CASE STUDY

The case study models the process a nurse uses when assessing a patient. Based on the clustering of information obtained during assessment, the nurse formulates nursing diagnoses.

Ms. P.M., 26-year-old wife of an active duty sergeant, was admitted for delivery of their first child. Her husband was out of town, and most of her relatives live in Puerto Rico. Her mother, however, was present. Before her pregnancy, Ms. P.M. was very active physically, jogging 6 to 7 miles a day. She was diagnosed as preeclamptic and has been on bed rest for several weeks. The Labor-Delivery Assessment Tool (Fig. 19-2) was used to assess Ms. P.M.

BIBLIOGRAPHY

American Nurses' Association: Standards of maternal and child health nursing practice, Kansas City, Mo, 1983, ANA, Inc.

Brown A: Social support, stress and health: a comparison of expected mothers and fathers, Nurs Res 35:72, 1986.

Humenick S: Analysis of current assessment strategies in the health care of young children and childbearing families, Norwalk, Conn, 1982, Appleton-Century-Crofts.

Klaus M and Kennell J: Parent-infant bonding, ed 2, St Louis, 1981, The CV Mosby Co.

Rubin R: Maternal identity and the maternal experience, New York, 1984, Springer, Publishing Co, Inc.

Sonstegard L, Kowalski K, and Jennings B: Women's health, vol 2, New York, 1983, Grune & Stratton, Inc.

Wright L and Leahey M: Nurses and families, Philadelphia, 1984, FA Davis Co.

LABOR-DELIVERY ASSESSMENT TOOL

Name _____ Age _21_ Sex _F_

Address _7833 SR 38 E_ _____ Telephone _____

Significant other _____ Telephone _____

Date of admission _12-12_ _____ Medical diagnosis _Pregnancy_ _____

Allergies _____

Labor Phase

Nursing Diagnosis
(Potential or Altered)

COMMUNICATING ▪ A pattern involving sending messages

Read, write, understand English (circle) _____ Communication

Other languages _____   Verbal

Speech impaired _____   Nonverbal

Alternate form of communication _____

VALUING ▪ A pattern involving the assigning of relative worth

Religious preference _____ Spiritual state

Important religious practices _____   Distress

Cultural orientation/practices _____   Despair

Childbearing/rearing values _____

_____

RELATING ▪ A pattern involving establishing bonds

Role

  Marital status _m_ _____ Sexuality patterns

  Age & health of significant other _____ Rape-trauma syndrome

  Sexual relationships (satisfactory/unsatisfactory) _____

    Fear of intercourse _____ Mistrust of men _____

    Changes in sexual behavior _____

  Physical difficulties/effects of illness on relationship ____ Sexual dysfunction

  Anticipated difficulties related to sex after delivery _____

  Role in home _____ Role performance

_____   Family

  Evidence of anticipatory parenting behaviors _____   Parenting

_____   Work

  Verbalized positive relationship with own parents _____   Social/leisure

_____ Family processes

  Number of children _____ Ages _____

  Occupation _____

    Financial support _____

    Job satisfaction/concerns _____

    Physical/mental energy expenditures _____

Socialization

  Quality of relationships with others _____ Impaired social interaction

    Patient's description _____

    Significant others' descriptions _____

    Staff observations _____

  Verbalizes feelings of being alone _____ Social isolation

  Attributed to _____ Social withdrawal

Fig. 19-1

Patterns of socialization with friends & relatives _____
_____

KNOWING ▪ A pattern involving the meaning associated with information

Gravida _____ Para _____ Premature _____ Abortion _____   Knowledge deficit
   Stillbirths _____ Caesareans _____
Onset of labor _____
Expected delivery date _____ Weeks of gestation _____
Membranes: Intact/ruptured at _____ Clear/meconium _____
Prenatal history (this pregnancy):
   Planned pregnancy: yes/no   Previous birth control _____
   Prenatal care: yes/no   Where _____ Physician _____
   Childbirth classes: When initiated _____
      Number of classes attended _____ Labor coach _____
      Complicated/uncomplicated (circle)
      Hypertension _____ Diabetes _____
      Preeclampsia _____ Venereal disease _____
      Other _____
   Plans for anesthesia _____
Previous pregnancy history: Complications _____
   Length of labor _____ Type of delivery _____
   Previous anesthesia used _____
   Weight and sex of infants _____
   Current health of other infants _____
Other significant previous illnesses/hospitalizations/surgeries:
_____
Current medications _____

Understanding of labor, delivery, & postpartum periods

Desired outcome of hospitalization (rooming in, breast feeding)
_____
Misconceptions _____
Readiness to learn _____
   Request information concerning _____
   Educational level _____   Thought processes
   Learning impeded by _____

Orientation

Level of alertness _____   Orientation
   Orientation: Person _____ Place _____ Time _____   Confused
   Appropriate behavior/communication _____

Memory

   Memory intact: yes/no   Recent _____ Remote _____   Memory

FEELING ▪ A pattern involving the subjective awareness of information
Comfort   Comfort
Onset of regular contractions _____   Pain/chronic
   Frequency _____ Quality _____   Pain/acute
   Duration _____   Discomfort
   Other pain/discomfort: yes/no
      Onset _____ Duration _____
      Location _____
      Quality _____ Radiation _____
      Associated factors _____

Continued.

Fig. 19-1, cont'd

Aggravating factors _____

Alleviating factors _____

Emotional Integrity/States

Recent stressful life events _____   Grieving

_____   Anxiety

Mothers knowledge of own birth (i.e., weight, length of labor)   Fear

_____   Anger

Verbalizes fear of losing control _____   Guilt

Verbalizes other feelings of _____   Sadness

   Source _____   Shame

_____

Physical manifestations: Crying _____ Silence _____

   Trembling hands _____ Avoids interactions with others _____

   Others _____

MOVING ▪ A pattern involving activity

Activity

History of physical disability _____   Impaired physical mobility

_____   Activity intolerance

Limitations in daily activities _____

_____

Verbal report of fatigue or weakness _____

Exercise habits _____

Rest   Sleep pattern disturbances

Hours slept/night _____ Feels rested: yes/no   Hypersomnia

Sleep aids (pillows, meds, food) _____   Insomnia

Difficulty falling/remaining asleep _____   Nightmares

Recreation

Leisure activities _____   Deficit in diversional activity

Social activities _____

Environmental Maintenance

Home maintenance management

   Size & arrangement of home (stairs, bathroom) _____

_____ Safety needs _____

   Home responsibilities (mother) _____   Impaired home maintenance

_____   management

   Home responsibilities (father) _____

_____   Safety hazards

   Home responsibilities (children) _____

_____

Postdelivery assistance with responsibilities _____

_____

Health Maintenance

Health insurance _____   Health maintenance

Regular physical checkups _____

Selected pediatrician _____

Transportation to clinic/hospital available _____

Self-Care   Self-care

Ability to perform ADLs: Independent _____ Dependent _____   Feeding

Specific deficits _____   Bathing/hygiene

Discharge planning needs _____   Dressing/grooming

                                               Toileting

Fig. 19-1, cont'd

PERCEIVING ▪ A pattern involving the reception of information
Self-Concept   Self-concept
  Patient's description of self _____   Body image
_____   Personal identity
  Effects of pregnancy/delivery on self-concept _____ Self-esteem
_____

Meaningfulness
  Verbalizes hopelessness _____   Hopelessness
    Expresses feelings of extreme discouragement &/or negative expectations _____   Powerlessness
_____
  Perceives/verbalizes loss of control _____

Sensory/Perception   Sensory/perception
  History of restrictive environment _____
  Vision impaired _____ Glasses _____   Vision
  Auditory impaired _____ Hearing aid _____   Auditory
  Kinesthetics impaired _____   Kinesthetic
  Gustatory impaired _____   Gustatory
  Tactile impaired _____   Tactile
  Olfactory impaired _____   Olfactory
  Reflexes: Biceps   R _____ L _____   Triceps R _____ L _____
          Brachioradialis R _____ L _____   Knee   R _____ L _____
          Ankle   R _____ L _____   Plantar R _____ L _____
          Clonus _____

EXCHANGING ▪ A pattern involving mutual giving and receiving
Circulation
  Cerebral
    Neurologic changes/symptoms _____   Cerebral tissue perfusion
_____   Fluid volume
    Pupils: Left 2 3 4 5 6 mm   Right 2 3 4 5 6 mm   Deficit
             Reaction: Brisk _____ Sluggish _____ Nonreactive _____   Excess
    Verbal response _____   Cardiac output
    Motor response _____   Cardiopulmonary tissue
  Cardiac   perfusion
    Heart rate & rhythm _____
    Heart sounds _____
    BP: R _____ L _____ Position _____
  Peripheral   Peripheral tissue perfusion
    Jugular vein distention: yes/no   R _____ L _____   Fluid volume
    Pulses: _____   Deficit
    Skin temp _____ Color/warmth _____ Turgor _____   Excess
    Capillary refill _____ Clubbing _____ Cardiac output
    Edema _____ Other _____

Physical Integrity
  Tissue integrity _____ Rashes _____ Lesions _____   Impaired skin integrity
    Petechiae _____ Bruising _____   Impaired tissue integrity
    Abrasions _____ Surgical incisions _____

Oxygenation
  Complaints of excessive dyspnea _____   Ineffective airway clearance
  Precipitated by _____   Ineffective breathing patterns
  Rate _____ Rhythm _____ Depth _____   Impaired gas exchange

Fig. 19-1, cont'd

Continued.

Excessively labored/unlabored (circle)
Breath sounds _____
Nasal stuffiness _____
Patient uses a breathing pattern: yes/no
   Which type: Lamaze _____ Other (list) _____

Physical Regulation
  Immune
    Lymph nodes enlarged _____ Location _____   Infection
    WBC count _____ Differential _____   Hypothermia
    Blood type _____ Rh factor _____   Hyperthermia
    Rubella titer _____ HIV titer _____   Body temperature
  Body temperature   Ineffective thermoregulation
    Temperature _____ Route _____

Nutrition   Nutrition
  Eating patterns
    Number of meals per day _____ Special diet _____
    Time of last oral intake _____ Solid intake _____
    Food preferences/intolerances _____
    Food allergies _____
    Liquid preferences/intolerances _____
    Appetite changes _____
    Anorexia/nausea/vomiting _____
  Condition of mouth/throat _____   Oral mucous membrane
  Height _____ Weight _____ Prepregnancy weight _____   More/less than body
  Weight gain during pregnancy _____   requirements
  Labs
    Hemoglobin _____ Hematocrit _____ RBC _____
    Glucose _____ Fasting: yes/no Tested at _____ weeks gestation
    1 hour postprandial glucose _____ Glucose tolerance test _____

Elimination
Gastrointestinal/bowel   Bowel elimination
  Usual bowel habits _____   Constipation
  Alterations from normal _____   Diarrhea
      Incontinence
Renal/urinary   Urinary elimination
  Usual urinary pattern _____   Incontinence
  Alteration from normal _____   Retention
  Urine: Catheter _____ Color _____   Renal tissue perfusion
    Average hourly _____ Protein _____
    Glucose _____ Acetone _____ VDRL _____
    Bladder distention _____
Maternal evaluation
  Nipple examination: Flat _____ Inverted _____
  Vaginal: LMP _____ Last PAP smear _____
      Bleeding _____ Normal show _____ Unusual _____   Impaired skin integrity
  Membranes: Intact _____ Ruptured _____   Impaired tissue integrity
    Infection
  External genitalia: Swollen _____
    Discolored _____ Lesions _____
  Cervical: Dilatation _____ Effacement _____
Fetal evaluation
  Fetal heart tone _____ Station _____
  Presentation _____ Position _____

Fig. 19-1, cont'd

Leopold's manuevers _____

Ultrasound _____

CHOOSING ▪ A pattern involving the selection of alternatives

Coping

Patient's usual problem-solving methods _____

_____

Family's usual problem-solving methods _____

_____

Patient's method of dealing with stress _____

_____

Family's method of dealing with stress _____

_____

Patient's affect _____

Physical manifestations _____

Support systems available _____

_____

Location of relatives/frequency of visits _____

_____

Location/frequency of visits of friends, others _____

_____

Ineffective individual coping
Ineffective family coping

Participation

Compliance with past/current health regimens _____

_____

Willingness to comply with future health care regimen _____

_____

Noncompliance

Ineffective participation

Judgment

Decision-making ability

Patient's perspective _____

Others' perspectives _____

Judgment
  Indecisiveness

Prioritized nursing diagnosis/problem list: labor

1. _____

2. _____

3. _____

Signature _____   Date/time _____

Delivery Phase

FEELING ▪ A pattern involving the subjective awareness of information

Comfort

Verbalizes increased pain/pressure _____

Grunting sounds _____ Other _____

Comfort
Pain
Discomfort

Emotional Integrity/States

Anxious _____

Verbalizes desire to defecate _____

_____

Observations: _____

_____

Anxiety
Fear
Shame
Guilt

Continued.

Fig. 19-1, cont'd

EXCHANGING ▪ A pattern involving mutual giving and receiving
  Maternal evaluation: cervix _____
    Observation of perineum _____
    BP & pulse (list time & recording): _____

                                  _____ _____

  Fetal evaluation: FHT (list time & recording)

                                    _____ _____

    Time of delivery: _____ Sex: _____
    Apgar score: 1 minute _____ 5 minutes _____
    Shoulder dystocia _____ Nuchal cord _____
  Placental assessment _____
  Placental abnormalities _____ Blood loss _____

Cardiopulmonary tissue
  perfusion
Impaired tissue integrity
Impaired skin integrity

Prioritized nursing diagnosis/problem list: delivery
1. _____
2. _____

Signature _____ Date/time _____

Postpartum Phase

RELATING ▪ A pattern involving establishing bonds
Role
  Observed interaction between mother, father, & infant _____
_____
  Verbalizes positive feelings _____
  Refers to infant by name _____
  Seeks eye-to-eye contact/holds, touches infant _____
  Diminished/inappropriate visual, tactile, or auditory stimulation of infant _____
_____
  Verbalizes dissatisfaction/disappointment with infant _____
_____
  Verbalizes dissatisfaction/disappointment with infant's sex _____
_____
  Verbalizes feelings of: Nervousness _____ Fatigue _____
    Tension _____ Frustration _____ Being trapped _____
    Elation _____ Hunger _____

Role performance
Family processes
  Parenting

KNOWING ▪ A pattern involving the meaning associated with information
Knowledge of self-care after hospitalization
  Breast care _____ Perineal/episiotomy care _____
  Rest periods _____ Nutrition _____ Exercise _____
  Intercourse _____ Menses/douching _____
  Emotional changes _____ Medications _____
  Bowel function _____
Knowledge of care of newborn: Feeding _____
  Care of cord _____ Bathing _____
  Sleep habits _____ Changes in stools _____
  Protection from environmental hazards (cold, sun, use of carseat, etc.) _____
Knowledge of postdelivery problems: Afterbirth pain _____
  Failure of lactation _____ Cracked nipples _____
  Breast engorgement/tenderness _____

Knowledge deficit

Fig. 19-1, cont'd

Pelvic congestion _____ Other _____

Knowledge of symptoms to report to physician _____
_____

Expresses interest in learning self-care, infant care _____
_____

Available community resources (diaper service, housekeeping, La Lache League) __
_____
_____

FEELING ▪ A pattern involving the subjective awareness of information
Comfort   Comfort
  Location _____ Character _____   Pain
  Relief measures _____   Discomfort

Emotional Integrity/States   Anxiety
  Verbalizes positive feelings _____   Anger
  Depression _____ Withdrawal _____   Guilt
  Lack of contact with newborn _____   Sadness
  How soon after delivery did mother hold infant for a prolonged period _____   Shame
  How soon after delivery did mother feed infant _____

EXCHANGING ▪ A pattern involving mutual giving and receiving
Physical Integrity
  Episiotomy _____ Suture line _____   Impaired skin integrity
  Hemorrhoids _____   Impaired tissue integrity

Physical Regulation   Injury
  Maternal blood type _____ Rh factor _____   Hyperthermia
  Infant blood type _____ Rh factor _____   Hypothermia
  RhoGAM _____   Ineffective thermoregulation
  Body temperature: Postdelivery temperature _____
  Route _____ Intervention _____

Elimination
  Genitourinary
    Bladder distention _____ Catheter _____   Urinary elimination
  Genitalia   Incontinence
    Breast: Engorgement _____ Nipples _____   Retention
    Fundus: Location _____ Tonus _____   Impaired skin integrity
    Lochia: Color _____ Amount _____ Odor _____   Impaired tissue integrity
    Perineum: Edema _____ Redness/discoloration _____
      Sutures _____

Prioritized nursing diagnosis/problem list: postpartum
  (Include problems that have continued through labor and delivery)
1. _____
2. _____
3. _____
4. _____

Signature _____   Date/time _____

Fig. 19-1, cont'd

LABOR-DELIVERY ASSESSMENT TOOL

Name *MRS. P. M.* _____ Age *26* _ Sex ____*F*____
Address *333 THIRD STREET, DENVER, COLO.* _____ Telephone *555-3333*
Significant other *HUSBAND, MR. M.; ACTIVE MILITARY DUTY* ___ Telephone *SAME*
Date of admission _____ Medical diagnosis *INTRAUTERINE PREGNANCY—36+WEEKS*
Allergies *NONE KNOWN* _____

Labor Phase

	Nursing Diagnosis (Potential or Altered)

COMMUNICATING ▪ A pattern involving sending messages
(Read) (write) (understand) English (circle) _____   Communication
Other languages ____*FLUENT SPANISH*_____   Verbal
Speech impaired ___*No*_____   Nonverbal
Alternate form of communication ___—_____

VALUING ▪ A pattern involving the assigning of relative worth
Religious preference *CATHOLIC* _____   Spiritual state
Important religious practices *WEEKLY MASS* _____   Distress
Cultural orientation/practices *SPANISH* _____   Despair
Childbearing/rearing values *WISHES TO HAVE BIRTHING ROOM DELIVERY,*
WITHOUT ANESTHESIA—"FAMILY IS THE MOST IMPORTANT THING."

RELATING ▪ A pattern involving establishing bonds
Role
  Marital status *MARRIED* _____   Sexuality patterns
  Age & health of significant other *30, GOOD HEALTH* _____   Rape-trauma syndrome

  Sexual relationships (satisfactory) (unsatisfactory) _____
    Fear of intercourse __*No*___ Mistrust of men ___*No*___
    Changes in sexual behavior *SOME WITH PREGNANCY*
  Physical difficulties/effects of illness on relationship *POSITIONS ARE*   Sexual dysfunction
  UNCOMFORTABLE
  Anticipated difficulties related to sex after delivery *NONE*

  Role in home *HUSBAND IS DOMINANT FIGURE* _____   Role performance
  _____   Family
    Evidence of anticipatory parenting behaviors *ANTICIPATES DELIVERY,*   Parenting
    HAS SELECTED NAMES FOR BABY _____   Work
    Verbalized positive relationship with own parents *CLOSE TO PARENTS,*   Social/leisure
    FEELS PARENTS RAISED HER WELL _____   Family processes
  Number of children ___*0*___ Ages ___—___
  Occupation *DEPENDENT WIFE, HUSBAND ACTIVE DUTY*
    Financial support *MILITARY PAY & BENEFITS*
    Job satisfaction/concerns ___—___
    Physical/mental energy expenditures ___—___
Socialization
  Quality of relationships with others *EXCELLENT* _____   Impaired social interaction
    Patient's description *"HAVE LOTS OF FRIENDS"*
    Significant others' descriptions ___—___
    Staff observations *RELATES WELL c̄ MOTHER & FRIENDS*
    Verbalizes feelings of being alone *YES—WANTS HUSBAND HOME*   Social isolation
    Attributed to *HUSBAND BEING OUT OF TOWN*   Social withdrawal

Fig. 19-2

Patterns of socialization with friends & relatives *FREQUENT VISITS C̄ FRIENDS & FAMILY (MOTHER)*

KNOWING ▪ A pattern involving the meaning associated with information

Gravida *1* Para *0* Premature *0* Abortion *0* (Knowledge deficit)

Stillbirths *0* Caesareans _____

Onset of labor *0900 HOURS*

Expected delivery date *25 MARCH* Weeks of gestation *36+*

Membranes: (Intact)/ruptured at _____ Clear/meconium _____

Prenatal history (this pregnancy):

Planned pregnancy: (yes)/no Previous birth control *IUD*

Prenatal care: (yes)/no Where *JACKSON HOSP.* Physician *JONES*

Childbirth classes: When initiated *10 FEB.*

Number of classes attended *5* Labor coach *MOTHER STANDING IN FOR HUSBAND*

(Complicated)/uncomplicated (circle)

Hypertension *160/110* Diabetes *—*

Preeclampsia *SEVERE* Venereal disease *—*

Other *PRETERM LABOR*

Plans for anesthesia *NONE AT THIS TIME*

Previous pregnancy history: Complications *N/A*

Length of labor *—* Type of delivery *—*

Previous anesthesia used *—*

Weight and sex of infants *—*

Current health of other infants *—*

Other significant previous illnesses/hospitalizations/surgeries:

NONE OF SIGNIFICANCE

Current medications *PRENATAL VITAMINS, 1 PO q̄d; FeSO₄ 1 PO q̄d*

Understanding of labor, delivery, & postpartum periods

PARTIAL UNDERSTANDING OF LABOR & DELIVERY; NONE OF POSTPARTUM

Desired outcome of hospitalization (rooming in, breast feeding)

WANTS HEALTHY BABY— "CAN'T THINK BEYOND LABOR AT THIS TIME"

Misconceptions *NONE*

Readiness to learn *ANXIOUS, ASKING APPROPRIATE QUESTIONS, READY TO LEARN*

Request information concerning *—*

Educational level *HIGH SCHOOL, 2 YEARS COLLEGE* Thought processes

Learning impeded by *LABOR, MAG. SULFATE INFUSION*

Orientation

Level of alertness *FULLY ALERT* Orientation

Orientation: Person *YES* Place *YES* Time *YES* Confused

Appropriate behavior/communication *YES*

Memory

Memory intact: (yes)/no Recent *YES* Remote *YES* Memory

FEELING ▪ A pattern involving the subjective awareness of information

Comfort Comfort

Onset of regular contractions *0900 HOURS* Pain/chronic

Frequency *q̄ 3 MINUTES* Quality *MODERATE* (Pain/acute)

Duration *45-60 SECONDS* Discomfort

Other pain/discomfort: (yes)/no

Onset *1030 HOURS* Duration *C̄ CONTRACTIONS 60 SECONDS OR LONGER*

Location *BACK*

Quality *INTENSE* Radiation *TO LEGS* *—*

Associated factors *VAGINAL EXAMS & PITOCIN INDUCTION*

Fig. 19-2, cont'd

Continued.

Aggravating factors *POSITION CHANGE*
Alleviating factors *PRESSURE TO BACK*

Emotional Integrity/States
Recent stressful life events *HUSBAND NOT BEING HOME FOR BIRTH OF*
THEIR FIRST CHILD   Grieving
                                                                   (Anxiety)
Mothers knowledge of own birth (i.e., weight, length of labor)   (Fear)
KNOWS OWN BIRTH WEIGHT, HAS NO OTHER DETAILS
                                                                   Anger
Verbalizes fear of losing control *"I'm AFRAID I'LL BE WILD."*   Guilt
Verbalizes other feelings of *ANXIETY*   Sadness
   Source *UNKNOWN EVENTS RELATED TO LABOR, DELIVERY,*   Shame
   AND POSTPARTUM PERIODS
Physical manifestations: Crying _____—_____ Silence _____—_____
   Trembling hands _____—_____ Avoids interactions with others _____—_____
   Others *NERVOUS PINCHING AT BED SHEETS*

MOVING ▪ A pattern involving activity
Activity
History of physical disability _____—_____   Impaired physical mobility
                                                                   Activity intolerance
Limitations in daily activities *WAS ON BED REST*

Verbal report of fatigue or weakness *FATIGUE*
Exercise habits *JOGGED 6-7 MILES/DAY UNTIL PLACED ON BED REST*

Rest
Hours slept/night *3-4* _____ Feels rested: yes (no)   Sleep pattern disturbances
Sleep aids (pillows, meds, food) *SEVERAL PILLOWS FOR SUPPORT*   Hypersomnia
Difficulty falling/(remaining) asleep *UP TO BATHROOM SEVERAL TIMES* Insomnia
                                                                      Nightmares

Recreation
Leisure activities *READ, KNIT*   Deficit in diversional activity
Social activities *VISIT c̄ FRIENDS*

Environmental Maintenance
Home maintenance management
   Size & arrangement of home (stairs, bathroom) *NO STAIRS, 1 BEDROOM,*
   SMALL HOUSE _____ Safety needs _____
   Home responsibilities (mother) *COOKING, SHOPPING, CLEANING,*   Impaired home maintenance
   CLOTHES, PAYS BILLS   management
   Home responsibilities (father) *YARD WORK, HOME & AUTO REPAIRS*
                                                                   Safety hazards
   Home responsibilities (children) _____—_____

   Postdelivery assistance with responsibilities *WILL HAVE MOTHER TO*
   ASSIST UNTIL HUSBAND RETURNS

Health Maintenance
Health insurance *MILITARY BENEFITS*
Regular physical checkups *ROUTINE PRENATAL VISITS*   Health maintenance
Selected pediatrician *(MILITARY CHOICE)*
Transportation to clinic/hospital available *YES*

Self-Care
Ability to perform ADLs: Independent ___✓___ Dependent _____   Self-care
Specific deficits _____—_____   Feeding
Discharge planning needs *NONE IDENTIFIED AT THIS TIME*   Bathing/hygiene
                                                                     Dressing/grooming
                                                                     Toileting

Fig. 19-2, cont'd

PERCEIVING ▪ A pattern involving the reception of information

Self-Concept   Self-concept
  Patient's description of self _"I LIKE MY BODY."_   Body image
  _____   Personal identity
  Effects of pregnancy/delivery on self-concept _"I'M PROUD TO BE PREGNANT."_ Self-esteem
  _____

Meaningfulness
  Verbalizes hopelessness _No_   Hopelessness
  _____
    Expresses feelings of extreme discouragement &/or negative expectations ____ Powerlessness
    _No_
  Perceives/verbalizes loss of control _No_

Sensory/Perception   Sensory/perception
  History of restrictive environment _No_
  Vision impaired _No_   Glasses _No_   Vision
  Auditory impaired _No_   Hearing aid _No_   Auditory
  Kinesthetics impaired _No_   Kinesthetic
  Gustatory impaired _No_   Gustatory
  Tactile impaired _No_   Tactile
  Olfactory impaired _No_   Olfactory
  Reflexes: Biceps   R _2+_ L _2+_   Triceps R _2+_ L _2+_
            Brachioradialis R _2+_ L _2+_   Knee   R _3+_ L _3+_
            Ankle   R _3+_ L _3+_   Plantar R _2+_ L _2+_
            Clonus _2 BEAT_

EXCHANGING ▪ A pattern involving mutual giving and receiving

Circulation
  Cerebral
    Neurologic changes/symptoms _No_   Cerebral tissue perfusion
    _____   Fluid volume
    Pupils: Left 2 ③ 4 5 6 mm   Right 2 ③ 4 5 6 mm   Deficit
                 Reaction: Brisk ✓ ___ Sluggish ____ Nonreactive ____ Excess
    Verbal response _APPROPRIATE_   Cardiac output
    Motor response _APPROPRIATE_   Cardiopulmonary tissue
  Cardiac   perfusion
    Heart rate & rhythm _100, REGULAR_
    Heart sounds _WITHIN NML. LIMITS, NO MURMURS_
    BP: R _140/90 mmHg_ L _138/92 mmHg_ Position _LYING_
  Peripheral   Peripheral tissue perfusion
    Jugular vein distention: yes (no)   R ____ L ____
    Pulses: _FULL & BOUNDING, PRESENT BUT WEAK DORSALIS PEDIS_
    Skin temp _WARM_   Color/warmth _PINK_   Turgor _NORMAL_
    Capillary refill _LESS THAN 2 SEC_ Clubbing _No_
    Edema _2+ FACIAL & LOWER EXTREM-ITIES_ Other _____

Physical Integrity
  Tissue integrity _INTACT_ Rashes _—_   Lesions _—_   Impaired skin integrity
    Petechiae _—_   Bruising _—_   Impaired tissue integrity
    Abrasions _—_   Surgical incisions _—_

Oxygenation
  Complaints of excessive dyspnea _No_   Ineffective airway clearance
  Precipitated by _—_   Ineffective breathing patterns
  Rate _18_   Rhythm _REGULAR_ Depth _NORMAL_   Impaired gas exchange

Fig. 19-2, cont'd

Continued.

Excessively labored/(unlabored)(circle)
Breath sounds *CLEAR BILATERALLY*
Nasal stuffiness —
Patient uses a breathing pattern: (yes)/no
   Which type: Lamaze ✔ Other (list)

Physical Regulation
  Immune
    Lymph nodes enlarged *No* Location —   Infection
    WBC count *10.6×10³/µL* Differential —   Hypothermia
    Blood type *O* Rh factor *POSITIVE*   Hyperthermia
    Rubella titer *POSITIVE* HIV titer *NEGATIVE*   Body temperature
  Body temperature   Ineffective thermoregulation
    Temperature *98.6°F* Route *ORAL*

Nutrition   Nutrition
  Eating patterns
    Number of meals per day *3* Special diet —
    Time of last oral intake *LAST NIGHT* Solid intake *LAST NIGHT*
    Food preferences/intolerances *NOTHING SPECIFIC*
    Food allergies *NONE*
    Liquid preferences/intolerances *NONE*
    Appetite changes *HUNGER ALL THE TIME*
    Anorexia/nausea/vomiting —
  Condition of mouth/throat *MOIST MEMBRANES, NO LESIONS*   Oral mucous membrane
  Height *5'6"* Weight *180#* Prepregnancy weight *138#* More/less than body
  Weight gain during pregnancy *42#*   requirements
  Labs
    Hemoglobin *12.6 g/dl* Hematocrit *38%* RBC *4.8×10³/µL*
    Glucose *79 mg/dl* Fasting: (yes)/no Tested at *32* weeks gestation
    1 hour postprandial glucose *120 mg/dl* Glucose tolerance test *100 mg/dl (FASTING)*

Elimination
Gastrointestinal/bowel   Bowel elimination
  Usual bowel habits *ONCE A DAY*   (Constipation)
  Alterations from normal *SLIGHTLY HARDER*   Diarrhea
                                          Incontinence
Renal/urinary   Urinary elimination
  Usual urinary pattern *FREQUENT c̄ PREGNANCY*   Incontinence
  Alteration from normal —   Retention
  Urine: Catheter *YES* Color *YELLOW, CLEAR*   Renal tissue perfusion
  Average hourly *40-50 cc* Protein *2+*
  Glucose *NEGATIVE* Acetone *NEGATIVE* VDRL *NEGATIVE*
  Bladder distention *No*
Maternal evaluation
  Nipple examination: Flat ✔ Inverted
  Vaginal: LMP *MAY* Last PAP smear *1ST CLINIC VISIT*
      Bleeding *No* Normal show ✔ Unusual *No*   Impaired skin integrity
  Membranes: Intact (Ruptured) *1200 HRS.*   Impaired tissue integrity
                                        Infection
  External genitalia: Swollen —
    Discolored — Lesions —
  Cervical: Dilatation *5 cm* Effacement *COMPLETE*
Fetal evaluation
  Fetal heart tone *140* Station *-2*
  Presentation *VERTEX* Position *OA*

Fig. 19-2, cont'd

Leopold's manuevers *VERTEX PRESENTATION, ESTIMATED FETAL WEIGHT 7-7½ lbs.*

Ultrasound *CONSISTENT c̄ DATES, ANTERIOR PLACENTA*

CHOOSING ▪ A pattern involving the selection of alternatives

Coping

Patient's usual problem-solving methods *EXPLORE POSSIBLE SOLUTIONS, SELECT MOST APPLICABLE*   Ineffective individual coping

Ineffective family coping

Family's usual problem-solving methods *SAME*

Patient's method of dealing with stress *EXERCISE, TALK TO SOMEONE*

Family's method of dealing with stress *SAME*

Patient's affect *APPROPRIATE*

Physical manifestations *NO*

Support systems available *MOTHER IS HERE*

     Location of relatives/frequency of visits *PUERTO RICO, VISIT ONCE A YEAR*

     Location/frequency of visits of friends, others *FRIENDS WITHIN A FEW MILES FROM HOME, WEEKLY VISITS*

Participation

Compliance with past/current health regimens *COMPLIANCE EVIDENT THUS FOR*   Noncompliance

Willingness to comply with future health care regimen *YES*   Ineffective participation

Judgment

     Decision-making ability   Judgment

     Indecisiveness

       Patient's perspective *"I HAVE GOOD JUDGMENT & MAKE SOUND DECISIONS."*

       Others' perspectives *DEMONSTRATES APPROPRIATE BEHAVIORAL JUDGMENT (MOTHER)*

Prioritized nursing diagnosis/problem list: labor

1. *ANXIETY & FEAR RELATED TO LABOR & ABSENCE OF HUSBAND.*
2. *ALTERED COMFORT RELATED TO PAIN OF CONTRACTIONS.*
3. *KNOWLEDGE DEFICIT RELATED TO LACK OF UNDERSTANDING OF BIRTHING PROCESS.*

Signature *Shelia Burton, Maj, AN*   Date/time *10 March, 1230 hrs.*

Delivery Phase

FEELING ▪ A pattern involving the subjective awareness of information

Comfort

     Comfort

Verbalizes increased pain/(pressure)   (Pain)

Grunting sounds *NO*   Other ____   Discomfort

Emotional Integrity/States

Anxious *TRANSITIONAL*   (Anxiety)

Verbalizes desire to defecate *YES*   Fear

     Shame

Observations: *FOLLOWS INSTRUCTIONS WELL, REQUESTING MOTHER'S ASSISTANCE WITH BREATHING.*   Guilt

Fig. 19-2, cont'd

Continued.

EXCHANGING ▪ A pattern involving mutual giving and receiving

Maternal evaluation: cervix *COMPLETELY DILATED*   *+2 STATION*

Observation of perineum *BULGING & PUSHING*

BP & pulse (list time & recording): _____

120/70 mmHg, 1200 HRS.

120/72 mmHg, 1245 HRS.

Fetal evaluation: FHT (list time & recording)

140 1200 HRS.   *↓ TO 90 c̄ CONTRACTIONS*

144 1230 HRS.

Time of delivery: *12.51 HRS.* Sex: *M*

Apgar score: 1 minute *8*   5 minutes *10*

Shoulder dystocia *NONE*   Nuchal cord *X1 LOOSE*

Placental assessment *NORMAL – DUNCAN PRESENTATION*

Placental abnormalities *NONE*   Blood loss *APPROXIMATELY 400 cc*

Cardiopulmonary tissue perfusion
Impaired tissue integrity
Impaired skin integrity

Prioritized nursing diagnosis/problem list: delivery

1. _____
2. _____

Signature *Stelia Buxton, Maj, AN*   Date/time *10 March, 1315 hrs.*

Postpartum Phase

RELATING ▪ A pattern involving establishing bonds

Role

Observed interaction between mother, (father) & infant   *ABSENT* *APPROPRIATE*

Verbalizes positive feelings *YES*

Refers to infant by name *YES*

Seeks eye-to-eye contact/holds, touches infant *YES*

Diminished/inappropriate visual, tactile, or auditory stimulation of infant *NO*

Verbalizes dissatisfaction/disappointment with infant *NO*

Verbalizes dissatisfaction/disappointment with infant's sex *NO*

Verbalizes feelings of: Nervousness —   Fatigue ✓

Tension —   Frustration —   Being trapped —

Elation ✓   Hunger ✓

Role performance
Family processes
    Parenting

KNOWING ▪ A pattern involving the meaning associated with information

Knowledge of self-care after hospitalization:

Breast care *YES*   Perineal/episiotomy care *YES*

Rest periods *YES*   Nutrition *YES*   Exercise *YES*

Intercourse *YES*   Menses/douching *YES*

Emotional changes *YES*   Medications *NO*

Bowel function *YES*

Knowledge of care of newborn: Feeding *YES*

Care of cord *YES*   Bathing *YES*

Sleep habits *NO*   Changes in stools *YES*

Protection from environmental hazards (cold, sun, use of carseat, etc.) *NO*

Knowledge of postdelivery problems: Afterbirth pain *YES*

Failure of lactation *N/A*   Cracked nipples *YES*

Breast engorgement/tenderness *YES*

Knowledge deficit

Fig. 19-2, cont'd

Pelvic congestion _N/A_ Other _—_
Knowledge of symptoms to report to physician _YES_

Expresses interest in learning self-care, infant care _YES, ASKING APPROPRI-ATE QUESTIONS DURING CLASS_
Available community resources (diaper service, housekeeping, La Lache League) _YES, WILL UTILIZE LA LACHE LEAGUE_

FEELING ▪ A pattern involving the subjective awareness of information

Comfort   Comfort
   Location _EPISIOTOMY_ Character _SORENESS_   Pain
   Relief measures _SITZ BATH_   (Discomfort)

Emotional Integrity/States   Anxiety
   Verbalizes positive feelings _YES, BUT WISHES HUSBAND WAS HERE_   Anger
   Depression _—_ Withdrawal _—_   Guilt
   Lack of contact with newborn _No_   Sadness
   How soon after delivery did mother hold infant for a prolonged period _APPROX. 1 HR_   Shame
   How soon after delivery did mother feed infant _6 HOURS_

EXCHANGING ▪ A pattern involving mutual giving and receiving

Physical Integrity
   Episiotomy _MIDLINE_ Suture line _CLEAN, CLEAR, ¢ INTACT_   Impaired skin integrity
   Hemorrhoids _ø_

Physical Regulation   Injury
   Maternal blood type _O_ Rh factor _POSITIVE_   Hyperthermia
   Infant blood type _O_ Rh factor _POSITIVE_   Hypothermia
   RhoGAM _—_   Ineffective thermoregulation
   Body temperature: Postdelivery temperature _98.6°F_
   Route _ORAL_ Intervention _—_

Elimination
   Genitourinary   Urinary elimination
     Bladder distention _No_ Catheter _—_   Incontinence
   Genitalia   Retention
     Breast: Engorgement _No_ Nipples _SORE AT TOUCHING OR RUB-BING_   Impaired skin integrity
     Fundus: Location _U-1_ Tonus _FIRM_   Impaired tissue integrity
     Lochia: Color _YELLOW/RED_ Amount _SCANT_ Odor _NONE_
     Perineum: Edema _No_ Redness/discoloration _No_
       Sutures _CLEAN ¢ INTACT_

Prioritized nursing diagnosis/problem list: postpartum
  (Include problems that have continued through labor and delivery)
1. _DISCOMFORT RELATED TO EPISIOTOMY AND SORE NIPPLES._
2. _MILD ANXIETY RELATED TO ABSENCE OF HUSBAND._
3. _KNOWLEDGE DEFICIT RELATED TO POSTPARTUM PERIOD._
4. _____

Signature _Shelia Buxton, Maj, AN_   Date/time _12 MARCH, 1600 HRS_

Fig. 19-2, cont'd

CHAPTER 20

NEONATAL ASSESSMENT TOOL

MARY TERHAAR
SHELIA D. BUNTON

The Neonatal Assessment Tool was designed to assess newborns with unique biopsychosocial assessment needs. This tool incorporates specific signs and symptoms pertinent to newborns to facilitate identification of nursing diagnoses. It also incorporates the American Nurses' Association's *Perinatal Nurse Specialist Standards*. This chapter includes:

- *The way the tool was developed and refined*
- *The patient population and settings to which it applies*
- *Selected neonatal emphasis areas*
- *How to use the tool*
- *Specific neonatal focus questions and parameters to assist the nurse in eliciting appropriate data*
- *The Neonatal Assessment Tool*
- *A case study*
- *A completed version of the tool based on the case study*

DEVELOPMENT AND REFINEMENT OF THE TOOL

The Neonatal Assessment Tool was developed from the nursing data base prototype (see Chapter 2). Many hemodynamic, neurologic, and communication variables originally incorporated in the prototype were replaced with variables more specific to the assessment of a newborn. The resultant tool, which is supported by the American Nurses' Association's standards and the literature from the field of neonatology, was then modified based on recommendations of neonatal nurse experts.

After the tool was developed and refined, it was clini-cally tested on 15 preterm and full term newborns by neonatal nurse experts and clinical nurse specialists in the healthy newborn nursery and the neonatal intensive care unit. The infants were less than 7 days old. The testing evaluated the adequacy of the tool in terms of flow, space for recording data, and sufficiency of assessment variables. Based on the results, the tool was revised.

PATIENT POPULATION AND SETTING

The Neonatal Assessment Tool was developed to assist the nurse in assessing the needs, problems, and competencies of the newborn infant. Each newborn faces the challenge of transition from intrauterine to extrauterine life. The success of this transition depends on a complex, multisystem adaptation to a new environment and a new level of independence. The complexity of the transition is augmented by preterm, postterm, or complicated birth.

This tool was designed specifically for the newborn infant in transition from intrauterine to extrauterine life. It is intended to guide the practitioner through assessment of the variables that indicate the level of maturity and the degree to which a newborn is successfully negotiating transition.

The Neonatal Assessment Tool was designed for use in the acute care setting, specifically the delivery room, the newborn nursery, or the intensive care nursery. It might be useful in the emergency room or any other setting where the nurse encounters newborn infants if it were adapted and clinically tested in these settings (see Chapter 4).

As with any assessment tool, the information produced will be most reliable when the nurse conducting the assessment is sensitive to the immediate needs of the infant. The tool has been designed so the assessment follows a logical sequence that will reduce stress for the newborn and produce organized clusters of information for the nurse. To avoid stress on the infant, it may be necessary to complete the assessment in two installments. Furthermore, some maneuvers, such as kidney palpation or eliciting nystagmus may be omitted to further reduce stress on the infant.

NEONATAL EMPHASIS AREAS

Newborns have specific problems, needs, and competencies directly related to their adaptation to extrauterine life. The Neonatal Assessment Tool includes assessment variables for the newborn and is organized using each of the nine human response patterns of the Unitary Person Framework. The tool focuses on common difficulties in adaptation. Table 20-1 outlines these emphasis areas.

HOW TO USE THE TOOL

To use the Neonatal Assessment Tool effectively, nurses must first be familiar with the Unitary Person Framework (see Chapter 2), which provides the underlying framework for Taxonomy I. The human response patterns of the Unitary Person Framework serve as the major category headings for Taxonomy I and the tool. The sequence of the response patterns, as it appears in Taxonomy I, has been changed in this tool to permit better ordering of assessment variables. Pertinent neonatal nursing diagnosis, along with clusters of signs and symptoms necessary to identify them, have been added to the appropriate human response patterns in the tool.

Nurses must also recognize that this tool is different from conventional assessment tools because it was designed to assess holistic patterns specifically. As a result, nurses may encounter some initial difficulty in using the tool. They should remember, however, that the tool was not designed to follow the organization or content of the traditional medical data base; the data collected do not solely reflect medical patterns. Rather, this tool assists nurses in eliciting data specific to holistic patterns not traditionally assessed. This tool requires new thinking and provides a new way to collect and synthesize data to permit a holistic nursing assessment to take place so specific nursing diagnoses can be identified.

Although nurses probably agree that a holistic nursing data base is desirable, it is realized that changing traditional assessment methods is a difficult task. For this reason, a trial usage period is recommended before nurses judge the tool's merits. During this trial period, nurses should assess 10 newborns using the Neonatal Assessment Tool to become more familiar and comfortable with its organization and data-collection methods. With experience, nurses will become accustomed to new ways of clustering and processing data. With continued use, the time required to complete the tool will be reduced. More important, the ability of the nurse to elicit appropriate, specific, and complex data will be recognized. Nurses will discover that nursing diagnoses are easily identified when using this tool.

It is not necessary to complete the assessment in one session. Priority sections can be completed during the initial assessment. Other sections can be completed later, within a time frame acceptable to the institution. To elicit the most helpful, accurate, and complete data, nurses should be familiar with the focus questions and parameters in the next section. When assessing specific signs and symptoms to indicate a diagnosis, the nurse circles the diagnosis in the right-hand column to indicate deviations from normal. A circled diagnosis does not confirm a prob-

Table 20-1
Selected neonatal emphasis areas

Patterns	Emphasis areas to determine
Exchanging	Extent to which prenatal factors such as nutrition, substance usage or genetic variables have influenced the integrity of the newborn
	Independent and sufficient respiratory function
	Independent and sufficient cardiovascular function
	Ability to take in sufficient nutrients to satisfy the infant's appetite and sustain growth
	Independent and sufficient elimination of body waste
	Ability to maintain body temperature within an acceptable range
Moving	The capacity for body movements appropriate to gestational age
	Ability to achieve and maintain restful states
Perceiving	Ability to take in sensory information from the environment
Feeling	Ability to express discomfort or stress
	Parents' ability to recognize the infant's discomfort or stress
Communicating	Ability to indicate availability or unavailability for social interaction
	Ability to indicate the need for assistance
Relating	Ability to initiate, maintain, and terminate satisfying interactions with parents and care givers
	Parents' ability to initiate, maintain, and terminate effective and satisfying interactions with the infant
Knowing	Parents' ability to assign meaning to the infant's needs and capabilities

Table 20-2

Neonatal assessment tool: focus questions and parameters

Variables	Focus questions and parameters
MATERNAL INFORMATION	
Substance use	Did the mother smoke, consume alcohol, or use drugs of any kind during the pregnancy?
Pregnancy complications	Was the pregnancy complicated by any medical factors?
	Is there a history of congenital anomalies or metabolic disorders?
	Was the pregnancy complicated by social factors (e.g., single mother, minimal support, or low income)?
	Was the mother able to get sufficient nourishment during the pregnancy?
EXCHANGING	
Apnea	Does the infant take in sufficient oxygen?
	Is the airway functional?
Labored/unlabored	Are the respirations easy or labored?
Breath sounds	Are breath sounds clear?
	Is air exchanging freely on auscultation?
	Is chest wall movement equal bilaterally?
Respiratory assistance	Does the infant have the energy to do the work of breathing?
	What assistance with breathing does the baby require?
Cyanosis or pallor	Is the infant able to circulate oxygen and nutrients?
	What is the quality of skin color and perfusion?
Apical rate and rhythm and PMI	What is the location and quality of the apical pulse?
Murmurs	Is there any murmur or click on auscultation?
BP, MAP, and pulse pressure	What are the systolic, diastolic, mean arterial, and pulse pressures?
Vasopressors	Does the infant require pharmacological support?
	What pharmacologic support does the infant require?
Condition of oral cavity	Is the upper GI system intact (i.e., cleft lip or palate, choanal atresia, or tracheal esophageal fistula)?
Eating patterns	Is the infant able to breast or nipple feed?
	Does the infant require nutritional supplements?
	Does the infant take in sufficient nutrients to support growth?
	What assistance does the infant require to assure adequate nutrition?
Temperature	Does the infant maintain body temperature within normal limits?
	What assistance does the infant require to maintain body temperature?
Stools	Does the infant eliminate stool without assistance?
Spontaneous urine	Does the infant void without assistance?
MOVING	
Rest	Is the infant able to quiet sufficiently to allow rest?
	What quiets the infant?
PERCEIVING	
Visual response	Does the infant blink, startle, or accelerate heart rate in response to shining of a flash light over the eyes while sleeping?
	Does the infant focus on a red ball or checkerboard pattern in bed?
	Does the infant focus on a face?
	Does the infant track a silent face?
	Does the infant brighten and attend to a face?
Auditory response	Does the infant blink, startle, or accelerate heart rate in response to a hand clap?
	Does the infant turn toward a voice?
	Does the infant brighten to a voice?
	Does the infant track a voice?

Table 20-2—cont'd

Neonatal assessment tool: focus questions and parameters

Variables	Focus questions and parameters
FEELING	
Nature of infant's cry	What is the character of the infant's cry (e.g., strong or weak, rhythmic or irregular, or high pitched or normal)?
	Does the infant have sufficient energy to cry or protest?
Associated movements	What behaviors indicate discomfort?
Parents' response to infant's pain/discomfort	Are the parents receptive and responsive to the infant's cues?
COMMUNICATION	
Infant's cry	Does the infant cry? Is the cry robust?
Time-out cues	Does the infant turn away, yawn, grunt, or cry to reset the intensity of interactions?
Self-consolation	What behavior does the infant use for self-consolation?
RELATING	
Significant others in infant's life	Does the infant have other important family (i.e., grandparents, aunts, and uncles)?
	How do the parents wish for them to be included in the care of the infant?
KNOWING	
Infant high-risk factors	"Have you given birth before?"
	"Were your previous births uncomplicated?"
	"Have any of your children expired during infancy?"
	"If so, what was the cause of death?"
Describe previous "mothering" experience	"What is your experience in caring for babies?"
VALUING	
Important religious/cultural practices	"Are there any important beliefs, customs, or religious practices to be considered in caring for your infant?"

lem but simply alerts the nurse to the possibility that it exists.

After completing the tool, the nurse scans the circled problems, synthesizes the data to determine whether other clusters of signs and symptoms support a problem, and decides whether the actual diagnosis is present.

The diagnoses in the right-hand column may be repeated in more than one place. These repetitions occur only within the appropriate response pattern and are convenient for identifying certain data directly with their corresponding nursing diagnosis. These diagnoses are not absolute but focus thinking and direct attention to collecting data concerning a possible problem.

Some signs and symptoms can indicate several diagnoses. For example, cyanosis may indicate altered cardiovascular tissue perfusion or ineffective airway clearance. To avoid unnecessary repetition of assessment parameters, variables are arranged with the diagnosis most likely to result from the data assessed. Thus, data to support one di-

agnosis may occasionally be found in other patterns or arranged with other diagnoses. Therefore, synthesis of all data is essential.

The Neonatal Assessment Tool is not intended to be the standardized and final format for nationwide assessment of newborns. An assessment tool must meet the needs of the institution and nurses using it. The Neonatal Assessment Tool is simply a working demonstration tool that is expected to be changed and revised by nurses in clinical practice. Further evaluation and refinement are necessary before adopting the tool for use within a particular institution. Nurses interested in changing, revising, and adapting the tool to a specific clinical setting should refer to Chapter 4.

HOW TO ELICIT APPROPRIATE DATA

Because the Unitary Person Framework and the Neonatal Assessment Tool contain some terms that may be unfamiliar to nurses, specific neonatal focus questions and parameters were developed and refined to help the nurse to elicit appropriate information. These questions and parameters are in Table 20-2, which follows the content of the tool (Fig. 20-1). The variables in bold type in the tool are described more fully in Table 20-2. For example, the visual response variable under the "perceiving pattern" is in bold type. If nurses do not know how to elicit this data, they can use Table 20-2 to direct observations or testing. These questions and parameters are only suggestions intended to assist the nurse in focusing content when collecting data. They are neither static nor absolute. Nurses should not feel confined to asking only the questions or assessing only the paramenters provided because there are many other ways, based on the newborn's situation and condition and the nurse's skill, to elicit the information. Questions and parameters for parent-related data not in bold type were presented in Chapter 3.

CASE STUDY

The case study models the process a nurses uses when assessing a patient. Based on the clustering of information obtained during assessment, the nurse formulates nursing diagnoses.

Baby girl C.P. was assessed in the intensive care nursery 12 hours after birth. She was born at 34 weeks gestational age. The Neonatal Assessment Tool (Fig. 20-2) was used to assess baby C.P.

BIBLIOGRAPHY

Als H, Lesler BM, Tronick E, and Brazelton TB: Manual for the assessment of preterm infants' behavior (APIB). In Fitzgerald HE, Lester BM, and Yogman MW, editors: Theory and research in behavioral pediatrics, vol 1, New York, 1982, Plenum Publishing Corp.

American Nurses' Association: Perinatal nurse specialist standards, Kansas City, Mo, 1985, ANA, Inc.

Bates B: A guide to physical examination and history taking, ed 4, Philadelphia, 1987, JB Lippincott Co.

Doenges ME, Kenty JR, and Moorehouse MF: Maternal/newborn care plans: guidelines for client care, Philadelphia, 1988, FA David Co.

Klaus M and Fanaroff AA: Care of the high risk neonate, Philadelphia, 1979, WB Saunders Co.

Klaus MH and Kennell JH: Parent-infant bonding, ed 2, St. Louis, 1982, The CV Mosby Co.

NEONATAL ASSESSMENT TOOL

Maternal information
  Name _____ Age _____ Sex _____
  Address _____ Telephone _____
  Significant other & relationship _____ Telephone _____
  Date of admission _____ Allergies _____ Dyes _____
  Gravida _____ Para _____ Abortion_____
  Medical diagnosis _____
  Substance use (circle): tobacco/alcohol/caffeine/marijuana/heroin/cocaine/other _____
  Pregnancy complications _____
  _____
  Delivery complications _____
  _____
  History: Herpes _____ Hepatitis _____ Tuberculosis _____ TORCH _____
Infant information
  Gender _____ Delivery date _____ Time of delivery _____ Type of delivery _____
  Pediatrician _____ Anesthesia used _____
  Apgar: One minute _____ Five minutes _____ Blood type _____
  Gestational age: Dates _____ Examination _____
  Birth weight _____ grams _____ pounds   AGA/SGA/LGA (circle)
  Name _____

Nursing Diagnosis
(Potential or Altered)

EXCHANGING ▪ A pattern involving mutual giving and receiving
Oxygenation
  Rate _____ Rhythm _____   Impaired gas exchange
  Apnea _____ **Labored/unlabored (circle)**
  Nasal flaring _____ Retractions _____   Ineffective breathing patterns
  Expiratory grunt _____
  Breath sounds _____   Ineffective airway clearance
  Respiratory assistance
    FIo$_2$ _____ Ambient _____ Hood _____ CPAP _____
            Prongs _____ OTT _____ NTT _____
    PIP _____ PEEP _____ IMV _____ I-time _____
  Chest tubes: yes/no   R _____ L _____
  Chest circumference _____ Clavicals intact _____
    Symmetrical chest _____ Breast tissue _____
  Blood gases: Arterial/Venous
    pH _____ Po$_2$ _____ Pco$_2$ _____ tco$_2$ _____
  Monitoring: tcPco$_2$ _____ tcPo$_2$ _____ Pulse oxygen _____
Circulation
  Cardiac   Cardiopulmonary tissue
    Cyanosis _____ **Pallor** _____   perfusion
    Apical rate _____ **Rhythm** _____ **PMI** _____   Fluid volume
    Heart sounds _____   Deficit
    Murmurs _____   Excess
    BP _____ **Location** _____   Cardiac output
    MAP _____ **Pulse pressure** _____
    Vasopressors _____
  Cerebral
    Fontanels: Anterior _____ Posterior _____ Cerebral tissue perfusion
               Findings _____

Fig. 20-1

Continued.

Pupils

    Equal _____ Brisk _____ Sluggish _____ Nonreactive _____

Fluid volume

    Deficit

Neurologic changes/symptoms _____

Excess

    Seizures _____

Cardiac output

    Posturing _____ Coma _____

Peripheral tissue perfusion

Peripheral

    Pulses: Radial _____ Posterial Tibial _____

    Brachial _____ Femoral _____

Fluid volume

    Skin temperature _____ Color _____ Jaundice _____

    Deficit

    Turgor _____ Edema _____

    Excess

    Capillary refill _____

Cardiac output

Gastrointestinal

    Liver: Palpable _____ Placement _____

GI tissue perfusion

Nutrition

Length _____ Weight _____

Less than body requirements

Facial tone _____ Facial paralysis _____

More than body

    requirements

Condition of oral cavity _____

Condition of mucous membranes _____

Oral mucous membranes

Eating patterns

    Formula _____ Breast feeding _____

    Vitamins _____ Excessive mucous _____

    Method of feed _____

    Regurgitation/vomiting _____

Parents' response to infant feeding _____

Parents' response to altered feeding patterns _____

Labs

    Na _____ K _____ CL _____ Glucose _____

    PKU _____ Other _____

    HBG _____ HCT _____ Reticulocytes _____

Physical Regulation

Immune

    WBC count _____ Differential _____

Infection

Ineffective thermoregulation

Temperature _____ **Route** _____

Hypothermia

    Open crib _____ **ISO** _____ **Warmer** _____ **ISC on** _____

Hyperthermia

Physical Integrity

Tissue integrity _____ Rashes _____ Pustules _____

Impaired skin integrity

    Petechiae _____ Lesions _____

Impaired tissue integrity

    Abrasions _____ Bruising _____

    Bleeding _____ Other _____

Distribution/placement of hair _____

Odor _____ Vernix _____

Umbilical cord: Arteries _____ Vein _____

    Clamp intact: yes/no

Arterial line _____ Venous line _____

Head circumference _____ Forceps _____

    Caput succedaneum _____ Cephalohematoma _____

    Molding _____ Other _____

Elimination

Bowel

    Abdominal physical examination _____

Bowel patterns

    Redness _____ Distention _____

    Constipation

    Tenderness _____ Rigidity _____

    Diarrhea

    Loops _____ Imperforate anus _____

Fig. 20-1, cont'd

Bowel sounds _____

Stools: Time of first _____ Color/normal _____

Stool pattern _____

Abnormalities _____

Genitourinary

First voiding _____ Urine color _____   Urinary patterns

Spontaneous urine _____   Retention

Stream _____

Genitalia examination: Male _____ Female _____ Ambiguity ___

Male: Position of urethral opening _____

Testes descended _____ Palpable _____

Tip of glands: Hypospadias _____ Epispadias _____

Female: Vaginal discharge _____

Vulva _____ Labia _____

MOVING ▪ A pattern involving activity
Activity

General appearance _____

Tremors _____ Paralysis _____ Limpness _____

Injuries _____

Muscle tone & strength: Arms   R   L   Legs   R   L   Impaired physical mobility

Intact   ____   ____   ____   ____

Tone _____

Activity _____

Other _____

Hands: Number of digits   R _____ L _____

Anomalies _____

Feet: Number of digits   R _____ L _____

Anomalies _____

Hips: Abduct/adduct _____

Posterior thigh skin folds (symmetrical) _____

Leg length (symmetrical) _____

Anomalies _____

Spine: Anomalies _____

Dimples, cysts, protrusions _____

Comparison use of all extremities _____

Reflexes: Babinski _____

Moro _____

Rooting _____

Sucking _____

Grasping _____

Stepping _____

Other _____

Awake states: Active alert _____ Quiet alert _____

Crying _____ Drowsy _____

Rest

Sleep pattern _____   Sleep pattern disturbances

Sleep states: Quiet _____ Active _____

Deep _____ Light _____

PERCEIVING ▪ A pattern involving the reception of information
Sensory/Perception

    Sensory/perception

Visual response _____   Visual

Blinks to light shown at eyes while sleeping _____

Brightens to faces _____ Follows faces _____

Fig. 20-1, cont'd

Continued.

Gazes at inanimate black & white checkerboard _____

Auditory response _____ Auditory

Startles to loud noise _____ Attends to voice _____

Brightens to voice _____ Follows voice _____ Tactile

Tactile response _____

Proprioreceptive _____

Nystagmus to spinning _____ Brightens when vertical _____

FEELING ▪ A pattern involving the subjective awareness of information

Comfort Comfort

Pain/discomfort Pain/chronic

Nature of infant's cry _____ Pain/acute

Associated movements _____ Discomfort

Aggravating factors _____

Emotional Integrity/States

Parents' response to infant's pain/discomfort _____ Anxiety

_____ Fear

COMMUNICATION ▪ A pattern involving sending messages

Infant's cry: Strong _____ Weak _____ Communication

Constant _____ Absent _____ Nonverbal

High pitched _____ Other _____

Infant's states

Predominate sleep state: Light sleep _____

Deep sleep _____ Drowsy _____

Predominate waking state: Quiet alert _____ Active alert _____

Infant's tone: Flaccid _____ Rigid/tense _____ Normal _____

Infant's motor activity: Smooth _____ Twitchy _____

Calm _____ Active _____ Frantic _____

Time-out cues: Yawn _____ Eye aversion _____ Hiccup _____ Fuss _____

Sneeze _____ Close eyes _____ Salute _____ Finger splay _____

Self-consolation: Hand to face _____ Hand to mouth _____

Suck _____ Grasp _____ Foot brace _____ Hold on ____

Hand clasp _____ Foot clasp _____

Parents' response to infant's cry _____

Eye contact _____ Tactile response _____

RELATING ▪ A pattern involving establishing bonds

Role

Marital status of parents _____ Family processes

Age and health of mother _____

Age and health of father _____

Number of siblings _____ Ages _____

Recognized family friends for support _____

Significant others in infant's life _____ Role performance

Mother's initial response to child _____

Mother's response to infant cues _____

Father's initial response to child _____ Parenting

Father's response to infant cues _____

Observed interaction between mother, father, & infant _____

En face _____ Eye contact _____

Fig. 20-1, cont'd

Occupation of parents: Mother _____ Father _____
   Job satisfaction/concerns _____
   Expresses physical/mental energy expenditures of job _____
_____

KNOWING ▪ A pattern involving the meaning associated with information
Infant high-risk factors: family history of   Knowledge deficit
   SIPS _____ Prematurity _____ Other _____
Mother's understanding of infant risk factors _____
_____

Description of previous "mothering" experience _____
_____

VALUING ▪ A pattern involving the assigning of relative worth
Religious preference _____   Spiritual state
Cultural orientation _____
Important religious/cultural practices related to newborns _____
_____
Significant religious person _____
   Phone number _____

CHOOSING ▪ A pattern involving the selection of alternatives
Coping
   Mother's usual problem-solving methods _____   Ineffective individual coping
_____   Ineffective family coping
   Family's usual problem-solving methods _____
_____
   Mother's method of dealing with stress _____
_____
   Family's method of dealing with stress _____
_____

Prioritized nursing diagnosis/problem list
1. _____
2. _____
3. _____
4. _____

Signature _____   Date _____

Fig. 20-1, cont'd

NEONATAL ASSESSMENT TOOL

Maternal information

Name _R.P._   Age _22_   Sex _F_

Address _5 FIFTH AVE., CONCORD, MAINE_   Telephone _555-555_

Significant other & relationship _HUSBAND, MR. P._   Telephone _SAME_

Date of admission _1 MAY_   Allergies _RAGWEED_   Dyes _—_

Gravida _i_   Para _O_   Abortion _0_

Medical diagnosis _PRETERM LABOR_

Substance use (circle): tobacco/alcohol/caffeine/marijuana/heroin/cocaine/other _NONE_

Pregnancy complications _PRETERM LABOR, PREMATURE RUPTURE OF MEMBRANES; ANTIBIOTICS_
X 48 HOURS AND BETADEXAMETHASONE x iii

Delivery complications _—_

History: Herpes _—_   Hepatitis _—_   Tuberculosis _—_   TORCH _—_

Infant information

Gender _F_   Delivery date _3 MAY_   Time of delivery _0620_   Type of delivery _SVD_

Pediatrician _SMITH_   Anesthesia used _LOCAL_

Apgar: One minute _7_   Five minutes _9_   Blood type _A+_

Gestational age: Dates _34_   Examination _34_

Birth weight _2640_   grams _—_   pounds   (AGA)/SGA/LGA (circle)

Name _C.P._

Nursing Diagnosis
(Potential or Altered)

EXCHANGING ▪ A pattern involving mutual giving and receiving
Oxygenation

Rate _68_   Rhythm _RAPID & REGULAR_

Apnea _0_   (Labored)/unlabored (circle)

Nasal flaring _MODERATE_   Retractions _SUBSTERNAL & INTERCOSTAL_

Expiratory grunt _MILD_

Breath sounds _FINE RALES IN LOWER LOBES_

Respiratory assistance

   FIo_2 _40%_   Ambient _____   Hood _✓_   CPAP _____

   Prongs _____   OTT _____   NTT _____

   PIP _0_   PEEP _0_   IMV _0_   I-time _0_

Chest tubes: yes/(no)   R _____   L _____

Chest circumference _30 cm_   Clavicals intact _YES_

   Symmetrical chest _YES_   Breast tissue _NML._

Blood gases: Arterial/Venous

   pH _7.38_ Po_2 _86 mmHg_ Pco_2 _37 mmHg_ tco_2 _21 mmHg_

   Monitoring: $tcPco_2$ _—_ $tcPo_2$ _92_   Pulse oxygen _—_

Circulation

Cardiac

   Cyanosis _CIRCUMORAL c̄ STRESS_   Pallor _YES_

   Apical rate _152_   Rhythm _REGULAR_   PMI _ACTIVE_ (L)

   Heart sounds _WITHIN NORMAL LIMITS_

   Murmurs _0_

   BP _46/22 mmHg_   Location (R) _ARM_

   MAP _34 mm Hg_   Pulse pressure _23 mmHg_

   Vasopressors _0_

Cerebral

   Fontanels: Anterior _SOFT-FLAT_   Posterior _SOFT-FLAT_

   Findings _WITHIN NORMAL LIMITS_

Nursing diagnoses (right column):

(Impaired gas exchange)

(Ineffective breathing patterns)

Ineffective airway clearance

Cardiopulmonary tissue
   perfusion
Fluid volume
   Deficit
   Excess
Cardiac output

Cerebral tissue perfusion

Fig. 20-2

Pupils   Cerebral tissue perfusion

Equal ✓   Brisk ✓   Sluggish _____   Nonreactive _____   Fluid volume

Neurologic changes/symptoms _Ө_____   Deficit

     Seizures _Ө_____   Excess

     Posturing _Ө_____ Coma _Ө_____   Cardiac output

Peripheral   Peripheral tissue perfusion

     Pulses: Radial _STRONG THROUGHOUT_ Posterial Tibial _PRESENT, STRONG_

         Brachial _PRESENT, STRONG_   Femoral _PRESENT, STRONG_   Fluid volume

     Skin temperature _WARM_   Color _PINK_   Jaundice _Ө_____   Deficit

         Turgor _WITHIN NORMAL LIMITS_ Edema _ORBITAL_   Excess

         Capillary refill _GOOD, < 2 SECONDS_   Cardiac output

Gastrointestinal

     Liver: Palpable _YES_   Placement _AT SUBCOSTAL MARGIN_   GI tissue perfusion

Nutrition

Length _50 cm_   Weight _2640 g_   (Less than body requirements)

Facial tone _GOOD-EQUAL_ Facial paralysis _Ө_____   More than body

Condition of oral cavity _INTACT_   requirements

Condition of mucous membranes _PINK, MOIST_   Oral mucous membranes

Eating patterns

     Formula __—__   Breast feeding _✓ (POST NPO)_

     Vitamins __—__   Excessive mucous _____

     Method of feed _NPO SECONDARY TO HYDRATION VIA UMBILICAL ARTERY CATHETER_

     Regurgitation/vomiting _Ө_____

Parents' response to infant feeding _NA AT PRESENT_

Parents' response to altered feeding patterns __—__

Labs

Na _136 mEq/L_   K _4.5 mEq/L_   CL _98 mEq/L_   Glucose _100 mg/dl_

PKU _2 WKS. P̄ BIRTH_   Other __—__

HBG _18.0 g/dl_   HCT _48%_   Reticulocytes _NA_

IV FLUIDS: D₁₀ c̄ HEPARIN AT 2 cc/HR, D₁₀ AT 4 cc/HR.

Physical Regulation

Immune   Infection

     WBC count _5.0×10³/µL_ Differential _NORMAL_   (Ineffective thermoregulation)

Temperature _98.4° F_   Route _AXILLARY_   Hypothermia

     Open crib _____ ISO _✓_   Warmer _____ ISC on _98.4° F_   Hyperthermia

Physical Integrity

Tissue integrity _INTACT_   Rashes _Ө_____   Pustules _Ө_____   Impaired skin integrity

     Petechiae _Ө_____   Lesions _Ө_____   Impaired tissue integrity

     Abrasions _Ө_____   Bruising _Ө_____

     Bleeding _Ө_____   Other _Ө_____

Distribution/placement of hair _LIGHT GENERALIZED HAIR_

Odor _Ө_____   Vernix _YES_

Umbilical cord: Arteries _2_   Vein _1_

     Clamp intact: yes (no) _UMBILICAL ARTERY CATHETER_

Arterial line _✓_   Venous line _✓_

Head circumference _32 cm_   Forceps _Ө_____

     Caput succedaneum _Ө_____   Cephalohematoma _Ө_____

     Molding _Ө_____   Other _Ө_____

Elimination

Bowel   Bowel patterns

     Abdominal physical examination _WITHIN NORMAL LIMITS_   Constipation

         Redness _Ө_____   Distention _Ө_____   Diarrhea

         Tenderness _Ө_____   Rigidity _Ө_____

         Loops _Ө_____   Imperforate anus _Ө_____

Fig. 20-2, cont'd

Continued.

Bowel sounds *ACTIVE IN ALL QUADRANTS*
Stools: Time of first *20 MINUTES* Color/normal *MECONIUM, NORMAL*
Stool pattern *NOT DETERMINED*
Abnormalities *∅*

Genitourinary
First voiding *2 HOURS p̄ DELIVERY* Urine color *CLEAR-YELLOW*   Urinary patterns
Spontaneous urine *YES*   Retention
Stream *UNREMARKABLE*
Genitalia examination: Male *∅* Female *WNL* Ambiguity *∅*
Male: Position of urethral opening *—*
Testes descended *—* Palpable *—*
Tip of glands: Hypospadias *—* Epispadias *—*
Female: Vaginal discharge *SLIGHTLY CREAMY*
Vulva *WNL* Labia *WNL*

MOVING ▪ A pattern involving activity
Activity
General appearance *LARGELY SMOOTH MOVEMENTS x4 EXTREMITIES*
Tremors *FINE* Paralysis *∅* Limpness *∅*
Injuries *∅*

Muscle tone & strength: Arms   R   L   Legs   R   L   Impaired physical mobility
Intact   ✓   ✓   ✓   ✓
Tone *GOOD*
Activity *SQUIRMS, SOME STARTLES, MOSTLY SMOOTH MOVEMENTS*
Other *IV IN (R) HAND → IMMOBILIZED ON IV BOARD*
Hands: Number of digits   R *5*   L *5*
Anomalies *∅*
Feet: Number of digits   R *5*   L *5*
Anomalies *∅*
Hips: Abduct/adduct *WNL*
Posterior thigh skin folds (symmetrical) *YES*
Leg length (symmetrical) *YES*
Anomalies *∅*
Spine: Anomalies *∅*
Dimples, cysts, protrusions *∅*
Comparison use of all extremities
Reflexes: Babinski *⊕*
Moro *⊕*
Rooting *⊕*
Sucking *⊕* *UNCOORDINATED*
Grasping *⊕* *STRONG*
Stepping *NOT ELICITED — IN OXIHOOD*
Other *∅*
Awake states: Active alert *⊕* Quiet alert *⊕*
Crying *⊕* Drowsy *⊕*

Rest
Sleep pattern *SLEEPS LIGHTLY — AROUSES EASILY*   Sleep pattern disturbances
Sleep states: Quiet *⊕* Active *⊕*
Deep *⊕* Light *⊕*

PERCEIVING ▪ A pattern involving the reception of information   Sensory/perception
Sensory/Perception
Visual response *APPROPRIATE*   Visual
Blinks to light shown at eyes while sleeping *xii*
Brightens to faces *⊕* Follows faces *UNABLE TO ELICIT*

Fig. 20-2, cont'd

Gazes at inanimate black & white checkerboard ⊕_____
Auditory response *APPROPRIATE*_____ Auditory
   Startles to loud noise ___⊕____ Attends to voice ___⊕____
   Brightens to voice ____⊕____ Follows voice *UNABLE TO ELICIT*_____ Tactile
Tactile response *QUIETS TO TOUCH*_____
Proprioreceptive *UNABLE TO ELICIT*_____
   Nystagmus to spinning ___—___ Brightens when vertical ___—___

FEELING ▪ A pattern involving the subjective awareness of information
Comfort ⟨Comfort⟩
  Pain/discomfort Pain/chronic
    Nature of infant's cry *VIGOROUS, RHYTHMATIC*_____ Pain/acute
    Associated movements *GRIMACE, FISTING*_____ Discomfort
    Aggravating factors *PAIN, LOUD NOISES, STARTLE*_____

Emotional Integrity/States
   Parents' response to infant's pain/discomfort *Mom ᵥ DAD TOUCH, STROKE,* Anxiety
*ᵥ SPEAK SOFTLY TO BABY*_____ Fear

COMMUNICATION ▪ A pattern involving sending messages
Infant's cry: Strong ___⊕____ Weak _____ Communication
   Constant _____ Absent _____ Nonverbal
   High pitched _____ Other *WNL*_____
Infant's states
   Predominate sleep state: Light sleep ___⊕____
    Deep sleep _____ Drowsy _____
   Predominate waking state: Quiet alert _____ Active alert ___⊕____
Infant's tone: Flaccid _____ Rigid/tense _____ Normal ___⊖___
Infant's motor activity: Smooth *PREDOMINANT* Twitchy ⊕ *WHEN STRESSED*
   Calm ___⊕____ Active ___⊕____ Frantic ___—___
   Time-out cues: Yawn _____ Eye aversion _____ Hiccup _____ Fuss ___⊕____
   Sneeze _____ Close eyes _____ Salute _____ Finger splay _____
   Self-consolation: Hand to face ___⊕____ Hand to mouth ___⊕____
   Suck ___⊕____ Grasp ___⊕____ Foot brace ___⊕____ Hold on ⊕
   Hand clasp ___⊖____ Foot clasp ___⊖____
Parents' response to infant's cry *SOOTHING*_____
   Eye contact ___⊕____ Tactile response ___⊕____

RELATING ▪ A pattern involving establishing bonds
Role
  Marital status of parents *MARRIED 2 YEARS*_____ Family processes
   Age and health of mother *22 HEALTHY*_____
   Age and health of father *23 HEALTHY*_____
  Number of siblings ___⊖____ Ages ___—___
  Recognized family friends for support *MATERNAL ᵥ PATERNAL*
GRAND PARENTS, SIBLINGS
  Significant others in infant's life *SAME*_____ Role performance
  Mother's initial response to child *WEEPY, SMILING*_____
  Mother's response to infant cues *Mom FINDS HER BABY AMAZING*

  Father's initial response to child *DAD TOUCHES LIGHTLY*_____ Parenting
  Father's response to infant cues *LOOKS FOR HELP*_____
  Observed interaction between mother, father, & infant *Mom ᵥ DAD SIT*
QUIETLY TOUCHING, TALKING TO BABY
   En face ___⊕____ Eye contact ___⊕____

Fig. 20-2, cont'd

Continued.

Occupation of parents: Mother ___∅___ Father _SALES_
   Job satisfaction/concerns _RELATIVELY NEW JOB (1 YEAR)_
   Expresses physical/mental energy expenditures of job _BOSS IS SUPPOR-_
TIVE

KNOWING ▪ A pattern involving the meaning associated with information
   Infant high-risk factors: family history of _____   Knowledge deficit
      SIDS ___∅___ Prematurity ___∅___ Other _____
   Mother's understanding of infant risk factors _"I AM WORRIED THAT SHE_
IS SO SMALL."
   Description of previous "mothering" experience _POSITIVE EXPERIENCE,_
CARING FOR 2 NIECES (HOLDING, DIAPERING, FEEDING)

VALUING ▪ A pattern involving the assigning of relative worth
   Religious preference _ROMAN CATHOLIC_   Spiritual state
   Cultural orientation _HISPANIC_
   Important religious/cultural practices related to newborns _BAPTISM_

   Significant religious person _PARISH PRIEST_
      Phone number _555-1212_

CHOOSING ▪ A pattern involving the selection of alternatives
Coping
   Mother's usual problem-solving methods _"TALK c̄ HUSBAND OR DISCUSS_   Ineffective individual coping
PROBLEM c̄ SISTER"   Ineffective family coping
   Family's usual problem-solving methods _"I'M JUST QUIET, THINK IT_
OUT." (FATHER)
   Mother's method of dealing with stress _"I CRY, TALK c̄ MY SISTER."_

   Family's method of dealing with stress _"I EXERCISE, BASKETBALL_
MAINLY, IT REALLY HELPS." (FATHER)

Prioritized nursing diagnosis/problem list
1. _IMPAIRED GAS EXCHANGE RELATED TO PUMONARY IMMATURITY_
2. _ALTERED NUTRITION (LESS THAN BODY REQUIREMENTS) RELATED TO PREMATURITY, DYSPNEA, &_
                                                                          NPO STATUS
3. _INEFFECTIVE THERMOREGULATION RELATED TO PREMATURITY_
4. _ALTERED COMFORT RELATED TO THERAPEUTIC INTERVENTIONS_
   ASSOCIATED WITH CARE
Signature _Mary Terhaar, RN_   Date _3 MAY, 1830 HOURS_

Fig. 20-2, cont'd

CHAPTER 21

PEDIATRIC ASSESSMENT TOOL

ANITA P. SHERER
MARY FRAN HAZINSKI

The Pediatric Assessment Tool was designed to assess pediatric patients with unique biopsychosocial assessment needs. The tool incorporates signs and symptoms pertinent to the pediatric patient to facilitate identification of nursing diagnoses. It also incorporates the *Standards of Maternal and Child Health Nursing Practice* developed by the American Nurses' Association. This chapter includes:

- *The way the tool was developed and refined*
- *The patient population and settings to which it applies*
- *Selected pediatric emphasis areas*
- *The way to use the tool*
- *Specific pediatric focus questions and parameters to assist the nurse in eliciting appropriate data*
- *The Pediatric Assessment Tool*
- *A case study*
- *A completed version of the tool based on the case study*

DEVELOPMENT AND REFINEMENT OF THE TOOL

The Pediatric Assessment Tool was developed from the nursing data base prototype (see Chapter 2). Many cardiovascular and hemodynamic monitoring variables originally incorporated in the prototype were deleted and replaced with growth and development assessment variables more applicable to a pediatric assessment. Emphasis was placed on assessing the child's response to illness and hospitalization, parent-child interaction, family stressors, and deficits in growth and development. The resultant tool was then modified based on the recommendations of pediatric nurse experts. Further, the content of this tool is supported by the literature from this field of nursing.

After the tool was developed and refined, it was clinically tested by pediatric nurse experts and clinical nurse specialists on 10 patients in a pediatric intensive care unit and a general pediatric unit of a tertiary medical center. The testing evaluated the adequacy of the tool in terms of flow, space for recording data, and completeness of assessment variables. Based on the results, the tool was revised.

PATIENT POPULATION AND SETTING

The Pediatric Assessment Tool was developed for use in any inpatient setting with pediatric patients requiring an initial assessment to determine their nursing care needs. The tool can be used for children from ages 1 to 12. Although the Pediatric Assessment Tool can be used with infants, the testing process revealed that a separate, more specific tool would be beneficial to that age group. Such a tool would allow the deletion of unnecessary variables and the inclusion of more specific parental-bonding and infancy assessment variables. Nurses interested in developing an infant assessment tool should refer to the Neonatal Assessment Tool (see Chapter 20) as a guide for revisions.

The Pediatric Assessment Tool can be used in general pediatric units and pediatric critical care settings. If the tool will be used primarily in pediatric intensive care units, nurses may wish to add hemodynamic monitoring variables and delete some psychosocial variables. To adapt the tool to such a setting, nurses should refer to Chapter 4. The Pediatric Assessment Tool can also be used in an outpatient setting by adapting certain sections of the tool to provide a screening assessment (see Chapter 4).

PEDIATRIC EMPHASIS AREAS

Pediatric patients have specialized problems and needs. The Pediatric Assessment Tool includes appropriate assessment variables within each of the nine human response patterns of the Unitary Person Framework. The tool focuses on prevalent problems in this patient population. Table 21-1 outlines these emphasis areas.

HOW TO USE THE TOOL

To use the Pediatric Assessment Tool effectively, nurses must first be familiar with the Unitary Person Framework (see Chapter 2), which provides the underlying framework for Taxonomy I. The nine human response patterns of the Unitary Person Framework serve as the major category headings for Taxonomy I and the tool. The sequence of the response patterns, as it appears in Taxonomy I, has been changed in the tool to permit a more logical ordering of assessment variables. Nursing diagnoses pertinent to pediatric patients, along with the signs and symptoms necessary to identify them, are incorporated under the appropriate human response pattern.

Nurses must also realize that this tool is very different from conventional assessment tools. As a result, nurses may have some initial difficulty in using it. They should remember, however, that the tool was not designed to follow the organization or content of a traditional medical data base; the data collected do not solely reflect medical patterns. Rather, this tool elicits data about holistic patterns in ways not traditionally assessed by nurses. It provides a new method of collecting and synthesizing data and requires new thinking when processing data. This tool represents a nursing data base developed from a nursing model to permit a holistic nursing assessment to take place so nursing diagnoses can be identified.

Although nurses probably agree that a holistic nursing data base is desirable, it is realized that changing traditional assessment methods is not an easy task. For this reason, a trial usage period is recommended before any decisions about the tool's merits are made. During this period, nurses should assess 10 patients using the tool to become familiar and progressively more comfortable with its organization and data-collection methods. With experience, nurses will become accustomed to new ways of clustering and processing information. With continued use, the time necessary to complete the tool will be reduced. Most important, nurses will recognize the unique ability of the tool to elicit appropriate signs and symptoms. Nurses will discover that nursing diagnoses are easily identified when using the tool.

It is not necessary to complete the tool in one session. Priority sections can be completed during the initial assessment. Other sections or patterns can be completed later, within a time frame acceptable to the institution. To elicit appropriate data, nurses should be familiar with the focus questions and parameters in the next section. When assessing specific signs and symptoms to indicate a diagnosis, the nurse circles the diagnosis in the right-hand column when deviations from normal are found. A circled diagnosis does not confirm a problem but simply alerts the nurse to the possibility that it exists. After completing the tool, the nurse scans the circled problems, synthesizes the data to determine whether other clusters of signs and symptoms support a problem, and decides whether the actual or potential diagnosis is present.

Some diagnoses are repeated several times in the right-hand column. These repetitions occur only within the appropriate response pattern and are convenient for identifying certain data directly with their corresponding nursing diagnosis. These diagnoses are not absolute but focus thinking and direct more detailed attention to a problem.

Some signs and symptoms can indicate several diagnoses. For example, particular financial stressors can indicate altered role performance and ineffective family coping. To avoid unnecessary repetition of assessment parameters, variables are arranged with the diagnosis most likely to result from the data assessed. Thus, data to support one diagnosis may occasionally be found in other patterns or arranged with other diagnoses. Therefore, synthesis of all data is essential.

Table 21-1
Selected pediatric emphasis areas

Patterns	Emphasis areas to determine
Communicating	Language skills
	Speech impairment
Valuing	Religion and culture as support systems
Relating	Family processes
	Personal and social skills
Knowing	Child's and parents' learning needs
Feeling	Comprehensive data related to pain
	Child's emotional state
Moving	Limitations in daily activities
	Gross motor and fine motor skills
	Sleep patterns
	Recreational activities
	Self-care abilities
Perceiving	Effects of illness or surgery on self-concept
	Sensory-perceptual deficits
Exchanging	Physical examination for children
	Nutritional assessment
Choosing	Child's and family's adequacy in dealing with stress
	Child's reaction to illness and hospitalization
	Future compliance with health care regimen

Table 21-2

Pediatric assessment tool: focus questions and parameters

Variables	Focus questions and parameters
RELATING	
Particular financial stressors	To parent: "Are you having any particular financial problems at this time? Is _____ 's illness causing any financial problems? Do you need help with these problems?"
Home behavior problems	To parent: "Are you having any problems managing _____ at home? Does _____ follow instructions and obey commands?"
Appropriateness of discipline methods	To parent: "How do you discipline _____? How does _____ react? Does this method work? Who usually disciplines_____?" Does the discipline method seem unusually harsh or lenient? Does the child's reaction seem appropriate?
Parents' verbalized extreme/inappropriate feelings	Do the parents voice extreme levels of anger or frustration that seem inappropriate for the situation? Do the parents verbalize feeling "trapped"? Are the parents' comments appropriate to the situation?
Parent-child interaction: appropriate/ inappropriate	How does the child interact with the parents? Do the parents talk to the child? Look at the child? Touch the child? Play with the child? Does the interaction between parents and child seem appropriate for the situation?
School problems	To parent: "Is _____ having any problems in school? Does _____ get along with classmates? Has _____ been disciplined for misbehavior in school? Do you expect this illness to have an effect on _____'s school performance or attendance?"
KNOWING	
Communicable diseases	To parent: "Has _____ ever had measles, mumps, chickenpox, or rubella?"
MOVING	
Child's responsibilities in home	To parent: "Does _____ have any duties or chores at home?" Do these duties seem appropriate for the child's age and health status?
Meets growth and developmental milestones	Does the child's developmental skill level confirm that growth and developmental milestones are being met?
Parents' perceptions	To parent: "Do you feel that _____ is growing and developing normally?"
PERCEIVING	
Effects of illness/surgery on self-concept	To child: "Since you've been sick, are you able to play like you did before? Can you run or play games like before? Is there anything you can't do? Do these changes make you upset or angry?" To parent: "How has _____'s illness changed _____? Has it made a difference in _____'s behavior? How do you think _____ feels about these changes?"
Reflexes	Are the child's reflexes normal, hyperreflexive, or hyporeflexive? Specify.
EXCHANGING	
Pulses	Are the child's peripheral pulses palpable bilaterally? If no, specify.
Abnormalities	Is the child overweight or underweight? Is a dietitian's consultation needed?
CHOOSING	
Special toy	To parent: "Does _____ have a special toy, blanket, or bottle to keep nearby?"
Parent's perception of child's/family's coping level	To parent: "What helps you and your family to deal with this illness? Do you feel able to deal with what is happening to _____? Are you having difficulty handling the stress and feelings this illness has caused? Do you feel you need help in dealing with your situation? How do you think _____ is dealing with the illness? How do you think we can help _____?"

Although the variable concerning altered growth and development is under the "moving pattern" in Taxonomy I, it pertains to many areas, including communication, socialization, activity, recreation, and self-care. Therefore, this nursing diagnosis appears within each of these areas.

The Pediatric Assessment Tool is not intended to be the standardized and final format for assessment of pediatric patients across the country. An assessment tool must meet the needs and requirements of the institutions and nurses using it. The Pediatric Assessment Tool is simply a working demonstration tool that is expected to be changed and revised by nurses in clinical practice. Further evaluation and refinement are necessary before adopting the tool for use within an institution. Nurses interested in changing, revising, and adapting the tool to a specific clinical setting should refer to Chapter 4.

HOW TO ELICIT APPROPRIATE DATA

Because the Unitary Person Framework and the Pediatric Assessment Tool contain some terms that may be unfamiliar to nurses, specific pediatric focus questions and parameters were developed and refined to elicit appropriate information. These questions and parameters are in Table 21-2, which follows the content of the Pediatric Assessment Tool (Fig. 21-1). The variables in bold type in the tool are described more fully in Table 21-2. For example, the variable concerning appropriateness of discipline methods under the "relating pattern" is in bold type. If the nurse does not know what to ask to determine whether the parents' discipline methods are appropriate, Table 21-2 can be used to direct the line of questioning. The focus questions and parameters provide clarity and guidance when eliciting data. They are not all inclusive, so nurses should not feel limited by them. Many other questions can be used, based on the patient's situation and condition and the nurse's skill, to elicit the appropriate information. Focus questions and parameters for data not in bold type were presented in Chapter 3.

CASE STUDY

The case study models the process a nurse uses when assessing a patient. Based on the clustering of information obtained during assessment, the nurse formulates nursing diagnoses.

C.J. was assessed when admitted to a pediatric unit. C.J. was admitted after a surgical resection for a Wilms' tumor. He has been diagnosed with liver metastasis and was admitted for chemotherapy. C.J. is 8 years old and lives with his parents. The Pediatric Assessment Tool (Fig. 21-2) was used to assess him.

BIBLIOGRAPHY

American Nurses' Association: Standards of maternal and child health nursing practice, Kansas City, Mo, 1983, ANA, Inc.

Axton SE: Neonatal and pediatric care plans, Baltimore, 1986, Williams & Wilkins.

Greenburg C: Nursing care planning guide for children, Baltimore, 1988, Williams & Wilkins.

Hazinski MF, editor: Nursing care of the critically ill child, St Louis, 1984, The CV Mosby Co.

Johanson BC, Hoffmeister D, Wells SJ, and Dungca CU, editors: Standards for critical care, ed 3, St Louis, 1988, The CV Mosby Co.

PEDIATRIC ASSESSMENT TOOL

Name _____ Nickname _____ Age _____ Sex _____
Address _____ Telephone _____
Significant other _____ Telephone _____
Birthdate _____ Date of admission _____ Medical diagnosis _____
Allergies: Drugs _____ Other _____
Pediatrician _____ Informant _____

Nursing Diagnosis
(Potential or Altered)

COMMUNICATING ▪ A pattern involving sending messages
Read, write, understand English (circle) _____ Communication
Other languages _____ Language skills normal for age: yes/no   Verbal
Speech impaired _____   Nonverbal
Communicates by: Key words _____ Gestures _____ Growth and development
  Other _____

VALUING ▪ A pattern involving the assigning of relative worth
Religious preference _____ Baptized _____ Spiritual state
Important religious practices _____   Distress
Cultural orientation _____   Despair
Significant cultural practices _____

RELATING ▪ A pattern involving establishing bonds
Role
  Father: Age _____ Health _____ Occupation _____
  Mother: Age _____ Health _____ Occupation _____
  Marital status _____ Role performance
  Foster/adoptive parents _____   Parenting
  Primary care taker for child _____
  Number of siblings _____ Ages & health _____
  _____
  Particular financial stressors _____
  Parents' descriptions of child's temperament _____ Family processes
  Home behavior problems _____
  Appropriateness of discipline methods _____
  Parents' verbalized extreme/inappropriate feelings _____
  _____
  Parent-child interaction: appropriate/inappropriate _____

Socialization
  Peer interaction _____ Pets _____ Impaired social interaction
    Child's description _____
    Parents' descriptions _____
    Staff observations _____
  Personal/social skills normal for age: yes/no _____ Growth and development
  School grade _____ Performance _____ Attendance _____
    Problems _____ Social isolation
  Verbalizes feelings of being alone _____ Social withdrawal
    Attributed to _____

KNOWING ▪ A pattern involving the meaning associated with information
Current health problems _____
_____

Fig. 21-1

Continued.

Previous illnesses/hospitalizations/surgeries _____
_____
_____
_____

Communicable diseases _____
Family history of the following:
   Cardiovascular disease _____ Lung disease _____
   Cancer _____ Liver disease _____ Diabetes _____
   Renal disease _____ Epilepsy _____ TB _____
   Bleeding disorders _____ Anemia _____ Sickle cell _____
Perinatal history: Pregnancy complications _____
   Birth history _____ Birth weight _____
Current medications _____
_____

Knowledge of illness/planned tests/surgery
  Child _____
    Misconceptions _____
    Readiness to learn _____
    Learning impeded by _____
  Parents _____
    Misconceptions _____
    Readiness to learn _____
    Learning impeded by _____

Knowledge deficit

Thought processes

Orientation
  Confusion

Memory

FEELING ▪ A pattern involving the subjective awareness of information
Comfort
  Pain/discomfort: yes/no _____ Described by: parents/child (circle)
    Onset _____ Location _____
    Duration _____ Quality _____ Radiation _____
    Associated factors _____
    Aggravating factors _____
    Alleviating factors _____

Comfort
  Pain/chronic
  Pain/acute
  Discomfort

Emotional Integrity/States
  Recent stressful life events _____
  _____ Child's reaction _____
  Child verbalizes feelings of _____
    Source _____
    Physical manifestations _____
  History of child abuse, rape, neglect _____

Anxiety
Fear
Grieving
Anger
Guilt
Shame
Sadness
Potential for violence
Rape-trauma syndrome

MOVING ▪ A pattern involving activity
Activity
  History of physical disability/limitations in daily activities
  _____
  Prosthetic devices (crutches, walker) _____
  Gross motor/fine motor skills normal for age: yes/no _____
  Exercise habits/play activities _____

Impaired physical mobility
Activity intolerance
Growth and development

Rest
  Sleep patterns _____
  Bedtime rituals (pacifier, bottle) _____
  Difficulties (enuresis) _____

Sleep pattern disturbance

Fig. 21-1, cont'd

Recreation
    Leisure activities _____ Favorite toys _____   Deficit in diversional activity
    Social activities _____ Normal for age _____   Growth and development
    Favorite TV programs _____ Sports _____
    Child's responsibilities in home _____

Environmental Maintenance
    Home maintenance management   Impaired home maintenance
        Size & arrangement of home (stairs, bathroom) _____   management
        _____ Safety needs _____   Safety hazards
        Neighborhood: presence/safety of play areas _____
        _____
        Parental home management problems _____
        Discharge planning needs _____
    _____

Health Maintenance
    Health insurance _____   Health maintenance
    Regular physical checkups _____
    Immunization status _____

Self-Care   Self-care
    ADL performance: Child performs ADLs independently at age-appropriate level: Feeding
        yes/no _____ Problems _____   Bathing/hygiene
    _____   Dressing/grooming
    Needs help with _____   Toileting
    Meets growth and developmental milestones _____   Growth and development
    Parents' perceptions _____

PERCEIVING ▪ A pattern involving the reception of information
Self-Concept   Self-concept
    Physical appearance/grooming _____
    Child's description of self _____   Body image
    Effects of illness/surgery on self-concept _____   Self-esteem
    _____   Personal identity

Sensory/Perception   Sensory/perception
    Vision/hearing normal: yes/no _____ Deficits _____   Visual
    _____   Auditory
    Movement/sensation normal: yes/no _____ Deficits _____   Kinesthetic
    _____   Gustatory
    Reflexes: _____   Tactile
    Olfactory

EXCHANGING ▪ A pattern involving mutual giving and receiving
Circulation
    Cerebral   Cerebral tissue perfusion
        Neurologic changes/symptoms _____
        _____
        Pupils
          L 2 3 4 5 6 mm   Reaction: Brisk _____
          R 2 3 4 5 6 mm   Sluggish _____ Nonreactive _____
        Level of alertness _____
    Cardiac
        PMI _____ Apical rate & rhythm _____   Cardiopulmonary tissue
        Heart sounds/murmurs _____   perfusion
        Dysrhythmias _____   Cardiac output
        BP: R _____ L _____ Position: _____

Continued.

Fig. 21-1, cont'd

Peripheral
Pulses _____   Fluid volume
  Skin color _____ Jaundice _____   Deficit
  Skin temp _____ Turgor _____   Excess
  Capillary refill _____ Edema _____   Peripheral tissue perfusion

Physical Integrity

	Description	Location	Distribution

Impaired skin integrity
Rashes _____   Impaired tissue integrity
Lesions _____
Petechiae _____
Bruising _____
Abrasions/lacerations _____
Surgical incision _____

Oxygenation   Ineffective breathing pattern
Complaints of dyspnea _____ Precipitated by _____
Rate _____ Rhythm _____ Depth _____
Labored/unlabored (circle) Nasal flaring, retractions _____   Ineffective airway clearance
Apnea _____ Chest expansion _____
Cough: productive/nonproductive _____   Impaired gas exchange
Sputum: Color _____ Amount _____ Consistency _____
Breath sounds _____
Arterial blood gases _____
Oxygen percent and device _____
Ventilator _____

Physical Regulation
Immune
  Lymph nodes enlarged _____ Location _____   Infection
  WBC count _____ Differential _____   Body temperature
  RBC count _____ Hemoglobin _____ Hematocrit _____ ESR _____   Hypothermia
  Culture & sensitivity: source _____   Hyperthermia
Altered body temperature   Ineffective thermoregulation
  Temperature _____ Route _____

Nutrition
Eating patterns
  Feeding type _____ Pattern _____   Nutrition
  Special diet _____ Vitamins _____   More than body
  Food preferences _____   requirements
  Food intolerances/allergies _____   Less than body requirements
  Appetite changes _____
  Nausea/vomiting _____   Fluid volume
  Daily fluid intake _____   Deficit
  Eating problems _____   Excess
  How handled _____   Oral mucous membrane
Height _____ Weight _____ Recent weight changes _____
Abnormalities _____
Condition of mouth/throat _____
Braces _____ Retainer _____ Loose teeth _____
Current therapy
  NPO _____ NG suction _____
  Tube feeding _____ TPN _____
  IV fluids _____
Labs
  Na _____ K _____ CL _____ Glucose _____ Fasting _____

Fig. 21-1, cont'd

Elimination
  GI/bowel   Bowel elimination
    Usual bowel habits _____   Constipation
    Alterations from normal _____   Diarrhea
    Words for defecation _____   Incontinence
    Abdominal physical examination _____   GI tissue perfusion
  Renal/genitourinary
    Usual urinary pattern _____   Urinary elimination
    Alteration from normal _____   Incontinence
    Words for urination _____   Retention
    Color _____ Catheter _____   Enuresis
    Urine output: 24 hour _____ Average hourly _____   Renal tissue perfusion
    Bladder distention _____   Menstrual patterns
    Serum BUN _____ Creatinine _____ Specific gravity _____
    Urine studies _____
    Menses: Began _____ Frequency _____ Duration _____
    Last menstrual period _____ Problems _____

CHOOSING ■ A pattern involving the selection of alternatives
Coping
  Child's usual reaction to stress _____ Ineffective individual coping

  _____
  Family's method of dealing with stress _____

  _____
  Child's reaction to illness _____
  Child's previous tolerance to separation _____ Ineffective family coping
  Special toy _____
  Child's affect _____
  Parents' perceptions of child's/family's coping level

  _____

Participation
  Compliance with past/current health care regimens _____ Noncompliance
  _____ Ineffective participation
  Willingness to comply with future health care regimen _____

  _____

Prioritized nursing diagnosis/problem list
1. _____
2. _____
3. _____
4. _____
5. _____
6. _____
7. _____
8. _____

Signature _____ Date _____

Fig. 21-1, cont'd

PEDIATRIC ASSESSMENT TOOL

Name _C. J._ _____ Nickname _____ Age _8_ ____ Sex _M_ _____
Address _77 SEVENTH STREET, NASHVILLE, TENNESSEE_ _____ Telephone _771-1000_ _____
Significant other _MOM & DAD_ _____ Telephone _771-1000_ _____
Birthdate _2/1/1980_ _____ Date of admission _2/3_ _____ Medical diagnosis _WILMS' TUMOR c̄ METASTASIS_
Allergies: Drugs _PHENERGAN/ADRIAMYCIN_ _____ Other _____
Pediatrician _DR. T._ _____ Informant _MOTHER_ _____

Nursing Diagnosis
(Potential or Altered)

COMMUNICATING ▪ A pattern involving sending messages
(Read) (write) (understand) English (circle) _____ Communication
Other languages _-Ø-_ _____ Language skills normal for age: (yes)/no Verbal
Speech impaired _No_ _____ Nonverbal
Communicates by: Key words _____ Gestures _____ Growth and development
   Other _SENTENCES, NORMAL SPEECH PATTERN, QUIET - DOESN'T TALK MUCH_

VALUING ▪ A pattern involving the assigning of relative worth
Religious preference _PRESBYTERIAN_ ____ Baptized _@ BIRTH_ _____ Spiritual state
Important religious practices _NONE EXPRESSED_ _____ Distress
Cultural orientation _SOUTHERN CAUCASIAN_ _____ Despair
Significant cultural practices _NONE EXPRESSED_ _____

RELATING ▪ A pattern involving establishing bonds
Role
   Father: Age _50_ _____ Health _GOOD_ _____ Occupation _EXTERMINATOR_
   Mother: Age _43_ _____ Health _GOOD_ _____ Occupation _MACHINE OPERATOR_
   Marital status _MARRIED_ _____ Role performance
   Foster/adoptive parents _No_ _____ Parenting
   Primary care taker for child _MOTHER_ _____
   Number of siblings _4_ ____ Ages & health _2 BROTHERS - 27 & 26 BOTH GOOD HEALTH; 2 SISTERS — 24 & 21 BOTH GOOD HEALTH_
   Particular financial stressors _No - BOTH PARENTS c̄ INSURANCE THRU WORK_
   Parents' descriptions of child's temperament _FIESTY_ _____ Family processes
   Home behavior problems _No_ _____
   Appropriateness of discipline methods _WITHDRAWAL OF PRIVILEGES - APPROPRIATE_
   Parents' verbalized extreme/inappropriate feelings _No_ _____
   _____
   Parent-child interaction: (appropriate)/inappropriate _____

Socialization _SCHOOLMATES_
   Peer interaction _PLAYS c̄ NEIGHBORS. →_ Pets _2 DOGS_ _____ Impaired social interaction
      Child's description _"I GET ALONG OK c̄ MY FRIENDS."_
      Parents' descriptions _"PLAYS WELL c̄ OTHER KIDS" (MOM)_
      Staff observations _GOOD INTERACTION c̄ PARENTS, OTHER PATIENTS_
   Personal/social skills normal for age: yes/no _YES_ _____ Growth and development
   School grade _2ND_ Performance _GOOD_ ____ Attendance _GOOD BEFORE ILLNESS_
      Problems _NONE — MAY HAVE DIFFICULTY IF CONTINUES TO MISS_ Social isolation
   Verbalizes feelings of being alone _No_ _____ _SCHOOL D/T ILLNESS_ Social withdrawal
      Attributed to _—_ _____

KNOWING ▪ A pattern involving the meaning associated with information
Current health problems _ADMITTED FOR CHEMOTHERAPY_
_____

Fig. 21-2

Previous illnesses/hospitalizations/surgeries *RECENT SURGICAL RESECTION OF WILMS' TUMOR*

Communicable diseases *HAS HAD CHICKENPOX, MEASLES*
Family history of the following: *GRANDFATHER*
  Cardiovascular disease *MI-PATERNAL* Lung disease *No*
  Cancer *No* Liver disease *No* Diabetes *MATERNAL GRANDMOTHER/GRANDFATHER*
  Renal disease *MATERNAL UNCLE* Epilepsy *No* TB *No*
  Bleeding disorders *No* Anemia *No* Sickle cell *No*
Perinatal history: Pregnancy complications *NONE*
  Birth history *NORMAL 3 COMPLICATIONS* Birth weight *8 lbs*
Current medications *NONE*   (Knowledge deficit) (CHILD)

Knowledge of illness/planned tests/surgery   Thought processes
  Child *"I HAVE TO GET STUCK c̄ NEEDLES."*
    Misconceptions *RELATES PAIN AS PUNISHMENT SOMETIMES*   Orientation
    Readiness to learn *FAIR*   Confusion
    Learning impeded by *FATIGUE*
  Parents *UNDERSTAND DISEASE ∨ NEED FOR CHEMOTHERAPY*
    Misconceptions *NONE*   Memory
    Readiness to learn *HIGH*
    Learning impeded by *ANXIETY*

FEELING ▪ A pattern involving the subjective awareness of information
Comfort
  Pain/discomfort: yes/no *YES* Described by: parents (child) (circle)   (Comfort)
    Onset *CONTINUOUS* Location *(R) SIDE OF ABDOMEN*   Pain/chronic
    Duration *CONSTANT* Quality *DULL* Radiation *No*   (Pain/acute)
    Associated factors *NAUSEA RELIEVED BY COMPAZINE*   Discomfort
    Aggravating factors *RUNNING, MOVEMENT*
    Alleviating factors *SITTING QUIETLY*

Emotional Integrity/States   Anxiety
  Recent stressful life events *HOSPITALIZATION, SURGERY*   (Fear)
  _____ Child's reaction *CRIED, BECAME QUIETER*   Grieving
  Child verbalizes feelings of *FEAR*   Anger
    Source *AFRAID OF PROCEDURES — WILL RESIST*   Guilt
    Physical manifestations *↑HEART RATE, STRUGGLING*   Shame
  History of child abuse, rape, neglect *No*   Sadness
                                                             Potential for violence
                                                             Rape-trauma syndrome

MOVING ▪ A pattern involving activity
Activity
  History of physical disability/limitations in daily activities   Impaired physical mobility
  CAN'T RUN OR PLAY HARD SINCE HIS ILLNESS   (Activity intolerance)
  Prosthetic devices (crutches, walker) *No*   Growth and development
  Gross motor/fine motor skills normal for age: yes/no *YES*
  Exercise habits/play activities *RIDES BIKE, RUNS AROUND*

Rest
  Sleep patterns *SLEEPS NORMALLY 8P-6A*   Sleep pattern disturbance
  Bedtime rituals (pacifier, bottle) *MOM READS BEDTIME STORY*
  Difficulties (enuresis) *No*

Fig. 21-2, cont'd

Continued.

Recreation

Leisure activities *MONOPOLY, TV, CARDS* Favorite toys *CARS* — Deficit in diversional activity

Social activities *PLAYS C NEIGHBORS* Normal for age *YES* — Growth and development

Favorite TV programs *"ALF"* Sports *FOOTBALL*

Child's responsibilities in home *EMPTIES TRASH, CLEANS ROOM*

Environmental Maintenance

Home maintenance management — Impaired home maintenance

Size & arrangement of home (stairs, bathroom) *TRAILER* — management

_____ Safety needs *NONE* — Safety hazards

Neighborhood: presence/safety of play areas *OUT IN COUNTRY —*
PRIVATE ROAD NEAR TRAILER

Parental home management problems *NONE*

Discharge planning needs *MAY NEED SOCIAL SERVICE CONSULT*
FOR TRANSPORTATION FOR CHEMO, MAY NEED TUTOR

Health Maintenance

Health insurance *YES* — Health maintenance

Regular physical checkups *YES*

Immunization status *UP-TO-DATE*

Self-Care — Self-care

ADL performance: Child performs ADLs independently at age-appropriate level: — Feeding

yes/no *YES* Problems *NONE* — Bathing/hygiene

_____ — Dressing/grooming

Needs help with *NONE OTHER THAN WHEN FATIGUED R/T ILLNESS/CHEMO* — Toileting

Meets growth and developmental milestones *YES* — Growth and development

Parents' perceptions *APPROPRIATE FOR AGE*

PERCEIVING ▪ A pattern involving the reception of information — (POTENTIAL)

Self-Concept — (Self-concept)

Physical appearance/grooming *TYPICAL BOY—UNCONCERNED ABOUT APPEARANCE*

Child's description of self *"I DON'T KNOW."(PT) "HAPPY BOY"(MOTHER)* — Body image

Effects of illness/surgery on self-concept *"I CAN'T RUN NOW." (PT.) SEEMS* — Self-esteem

QUIETER & UPSET ABOUT NOT BEING ABLE TO RUN— "THE OTHER — Personal identity

KIDS TREAT HIM DIFFERENTLY NOW, I THINK." (MOTHER)

Sensory/Perception — Sensory/perception

Vision/hearing normal: yes/no *YES* Deficits *NONE* — Visual

_____ — Auditory

Movement/sensation normal: yes/no *YES* Deficits *NONE* — Kinesthetic

_____ — Gustatory

Reflexes: *NORMAL* — Tactile

— Olfactory

EXCHANGING ▪ A pattern involving mutual giving and receiving

Circulation

Cerebral

Neurologic changes/symptoms *NONE* — Cerebral tissue perfusion

_____

Pupils

L 2 ③ 4 5 6 mm   Reaction: Brisk ✓

R 2 ③ 4 5 6 mm   Sluggish _____ Nonreactive _____

Level of alertness *ALERT, ORIENTED*

Cardiac

PMI *APEX* Apical rate & rhythm *90 REGULAR* — Cardiopulmonary tissue

Heart sounds/murmurs *S_1 & S_2* — perfusion

Dysrhythmias *NONE (hx OF PVCs)* — Cardiac output

BP: R *$^{114}/_{60}$* L *$^{116}/_{60}$* Position: *LYING*

Fig. 21-2, cont'd

Peripheral
Pulses *PALPABLE BILATERALLY*   Fluid volume
Skin color *PINK*   Jaundice *NO*   Deficit
Skin temp *WARM*   Turgor *GOOD*   Excess
Capillary refill *BRISK, <2 SEC* Edema *—*   Peripheral tissue perfusion

Physical Integrity

	Description	Location	Distribution	
Rashes	*NONE*			Impaired skin integrity
Lesions	*NONE*			Impaired tissue integrity
Petechiae	*NONE*			
Bruising	*NONE*			
Abrasions/lacerations	*NONE*			
Surgical incision	*ABDOMEN R/T NEPHRECTOMY — HEALING WELL*			

Oxygenation

Complaints of dyspnea *No*   Precipitated by *—*   Ineffective breathing pattern
Rate *24*   Rhythm *REGULAR*   Depth *DEEP*
Labored/(unlabored) (circle) Nasal flaring, retractions *NONE*   Ineffective airway clearance
Apnea *No*   Chest expansion *SYMMETRICAL*
Cough: productive/nonproductive *NONE*   Impaired gas exchange
Sputum: Color ___ Amount ___ Consistency *—*
Breath sounds *CLEAR BILATERALLY*
Arterial blood gases *—*
Oxygen percent and device *—*
Ventilator *—*

Physical Regulation

Immune
Lymph nodes enlarged *No*   Location *No*   (Infection) (POTENTIAL)
WBC count *9.54 x10³/μL*   Differential *—*   Body temperature
RBC count *2.71x10⁶/μL* Hemoglobin *8.1g/dl* Hematocrit *27.8%* ESR *—*   Hypothermia
Culture & sensitivity: source *THROAT — PENDING*   Hyperthermia
Altered body temperature   Ineffective thermoregulation
Temperature *99°F*   Route *ORAL*

Nutrition

Eating patterns
Feeding type *SOLIDS*   Pattern *6 SMALL MEALS*   Nutrition
Special diet *No*   Vitamins *No*   More than body
Food preferences *HOT DOGS, PIZZA, PEANUT BUTTER, POPSICLES*   requirements
Food intolerances/allergies *No*   Less than body requirements
Appetite changes *CAN'T EAT MUCH @ ONE TIME R/T ABDOMINAL PAIN*
Nausea/vomiting *YES*   Fluid volume
Daily fluid intake *1000 CC*   Deficit
Eating problems *No*   Excess
How handled *— SMALL MEALS*   (Oral mucous membrane)
Height *5' 1"*   Weight *31 Kg*   Recent weight changes *—*
Abnormalities *—*
Condition of mouth/throat *2 SMALL, WHITE PATCHES BACK OF MOUTH*
Braces *No*   Retainer *No*   Loose teeth *No*
Current therapy
NPO *No*   NG suction *No*
Tube feeding *No*   TPN *No*
IV fluids *D₅W @ KVO*
Labs
Na *131 mEq/L* K *3.2 mEq/L* CL *85 mEq/L* Glucose *118 mg/dl* Fasting *No*

Fig. 21-2, cont'd

Continued.

Elimination

GI/bowel

Usual bowel habits *NORMALLY CONTROLLED — ONCE A DAY*

Alterations from normal *No*

Words for defecation *"BATHROOM — #2"*

Abdominal physical examination *LIVER ENLARGED, ABDOMEN RIGID*

Renal/genitourinary

Usual urinary pattern *6-8 TIMES/DAY*

Alteration from normal *No*

Words for urination *"NEED TO PEE"*

Color *YELLOW, CLEAR* Catheter *No*

Urine output: 24 hour *1550* Average hourly *≈75*

Bladder distention *No*

Serum BUN *25mg/dl* Creatinine *0.5mg/dl* Specific gravity *1.015*

Urine studies *24 HR URINE FOR CREATININE CLEARANCE, LYTES, PROTEIN, OSMOLALITY IN PROGRESS*

Menses: Began *N/A* Frequency *N/A* Duration *N/A*

Last menstrual period *N/A* Problems *N/A*

Bowel elimination
- Constipation
- Diarrhea
- Incontinence
- GI tissue perfusion

Urinary elimination
- Incontinence
- Retention
- Enuresis
- Renal tissue perfusion
- Menstrual patterns

CHOOSING ▪ A pattern involving the selection of alternatives

Coping

Child's usual reaction to stress *CRIES*

Family's method of dealing with stress *Mom & DAD TALK TO EACH OTHER & FRIENDS*

Child's reaction to illness *"HANGING IN THERE" (MOTHER)*

Child's previous tolerance to separation *FAIR c̄ PREVIOUS HOSPITALIZATIONS*

Special toy *DUMP TRUCK — LIKES TO KEEP c̄ HIM*

Child's affect *APPROPRIATE*

Parents' perceptions of child's/family's coping level
FEELS THEY ARE HANDLING ILLNESS OK — NO HELP NEEDED EXCEPT CONTINUED SUPPORT

Ineffective individual coping

Ineffective family coping

Participation

Compliance with past/current health care regimens *GOOD*

Willingness to comply with future health care regimen *PARENTS INTEND COMPLIANCE*

Noncompliance
Ineffective participation

Prioritized nursing diagnosis/problem list
1. *ALTERED COMFORT R/T ACUTE ABDOMINAL PAIN*
2. *POTENTIAL FOR INFECTION*
3. *ALTERED ORAL MUCOUS MEMBRANE R/T WHITE PATCHES IN MOUTH*
4. *KNOWLEDGE DEFICIT (CHILD) R/T DISEASE PROCESS, PROCEDURES*
5. *ACTIVITY INTOLERANCE R/T FATIGUE, ANEMIA, PAIN 2° ILLNESS*
6. *FEAR R/T MEDICAL PROCEDURES*
7. *POTENTIAL ALTERED SELF-CONCEPT*
8.

Signature *Anita P. Sherer, R.N.* Date *6/27*

Fig. 21-2, cont'd

CHAPTER 22

ADOLESCENT ASSESSMENT TOOL

ANITA P. SHERER
MARY FRAN HAZINSKI

The Adolescent Assessment Tool was designed for adolescent patients with unique biopsychosocial assessment needs. The tool incorporates signs and symptoms pertinent to adolescent patients to facilitate identification of nursing diagnoses. It also incorporates the *Standards of Maternal and Child Health Nursing Practice* developed by the American Nurses' Association. This chapter includes:

- *The way the tool was developed and refined*
- *The patient population and settings to which it applies*
- *Selected adolescent emphasis areas*
- *The way to use the tool*
- *Specific adolescent focus questions and parameters to assist the nurse in eliciting appropriate data*
- *The Adolescent Assessment Tool*
- *A case study*
- *A completed version of the tool based on the case study*

DEVELOPMENT AND REFINEMENT OF THE TOOL

The Adolescent Assessment Tool was developed from the nursing data base prototype (see Chapter 2). Many cardiovascular and hemodynamic monitoring variables originally incorporated in the prototype were deleted and replaced with growth and development assessment variables more applicable to an adolescent assessment. Emphasis was placed on assessing the adolescent's response to illness and hospitalization, parent-adolescent interaction, family stressors, and deficits in growth and development. The resultant tool was then modified based on the recommendations of pediatric nurse experts. Further, the content of this tool was supported by the literature from this field of nursing.

After the tool was developed and refined, it was clinically tested by pediatric nurse experts and clinical nurse specialists on 10 adolescent patients in a pediatric intensive care unit and a general pediatric unit of a tertiary medical center. The testing evaluated the adequacy of the tool in terms of flow, space for recording data, and completeness of assessment variables. Based on the results, the tool was revised.

PATIENT POPULATION AND SETTING

The Adolescent Assessment Tool was developed for use in any inpatient setting with adolescent patients requiring an initial assessment to determine their nursing care needs. The tool is designed for use with adolescents from age 12 to 18.

The Adolescent Assessment Tool can be used in general pediatric units and in pediatric critical care settings. If the tool is to be used primarily in a pediatric intensive care unit, nurses may wish to add hemodynamic monitoring variables and delete some psychosocial variables. To adapt the tool to such a setting, nurses should refer to Chapter 4. The Adolescent Assessment Tool can also be used in an outpatient setting by adapting certain sections to provide a screening assessment (see Chapter 4).

ADOLESCENT EMPHASIS AREAS

Adolescent patients have specialized problems and needs. The Adolescent Assessment Tool includes appropriate assessment variables within each of the nine human response patterns of the Unitary Person Framework. The tool focuses on prevalent problems in the adolescent patient population. Table 22-1 outlines these emphasis areas.

HOW TO USE THE TOOL

To use the Adolescent Assessment Tool effectively, nurses must first be familiar with the Unitary Person Framework (see Chapter 2), which provides the framework for Taxonomy I. The nine human response patterns of the Unitary Person Framework serve as the major category headings for Taxonomy I and the tool. The sequence of the response patterns, as it appears in Taxonomy I, has been changed in the tool to permit a more logical ordering of assessment variables. Nursing diagnoses pertinent to adolescent patients, along with the signs and symptoms necessary to identify them, are incorporated under the appropriate human response pattern.

Nurses must also realize that this tool is very different from conventional assessment tools. As a result, nurses may have some initial difficulty in using it. They should remember, however, that the tool was not designed to follow the organization or content of a traditional medical data base; the data collected do not solely reflect medical patterns. Rather, this tool elicits data about holistic patterns in ways not traditionally assessed by nurses. It provides a new method of collecting and synthesizing data and requires new thinking in processing data. This tool represents a nursing data base developed from a nursing model to permit a holistic nursing assessment to take place so nursing diagnoses can be identified.

Although nurses probably agree that a holistic nursing data base is desirable, changing traditional assessment methods is not an easy task. For this reason, a trial usage period is recommended before any decisions about the tool's merits are made. During this period, nurses should assess 10 patients using the Adolescent Assessment Tool to become familiar and progressively more comfortable with its organization and data-collection methods. With experience, nurses will become accustomed to new ways of clustering and processing information. With continued use, the time necessary to complete the tool will be reduced. Most important, nurses will recognize the unique ability of the tool to elicit appropriate signs and symptoms. Nurses will discover that nursing diagnoses are easily identified when using this tool.

It is not necessary to complete the tool in one session. Priority sections can be completed during the initial assessment. Other sections or patterns can be completed later, within a time frame acceptable to the institution.

To elicit appropriate data, nurses should be familiar with the focus questions and parameters in the next section. When assessing specific signs and symptoms to indicate a diagnosis, the nurse circles the diagnosis in the right-hand column when deviations from normal are found. A circled diagnosis does not confirm a problem but simply alerts the nurse to the possibility that it exists. After completing the tool, the nurse scans the circled problems, synthesizes the data to determine whether other clusters of signs and symptoms support the problem, and decides whether the actual or potential diagnosis is present.

Some diagnoses are repeated several times in the right-hand column. These repetitions occur only within the appropriate response pattern and are convenient for identifying data directly with their corresponding nursing diagnosis. These diagnoses are not absolute but focus thinking and direct more detailed attention to a possible problem.

Certain signs and symptoms can indicate several diagnoses. For example, perception of own sexuality can indicate altered sexuality patterns or knowledge deficit related to sexuality. To avoid unnecessary repetition of assessment parameters, variables are arranged with the diagnosis most likely to result from the data assessed. Thus, data to support one diagnosis may occasionally be found in other patterns or arranged with other diagnoses. Therefore, synthesis of all data is essential.

Although altered growth and development is under the "moving pattern" in Taxonomy I, it pertains to many other areas, including communication, socialization, activity,

---

Table 22-1
Selected adolescent emphasis areas

Patterns	Emphasis areas to determine
Communicating	Speech impairment
Valuing	Religion and culture as support systems
Relating	Family processes
	Parent-adolescent relationship
	Perceptions of sexuality
	Peer relationships
Knowing	Adolescent's and parents' learning needs
Feeling	Comprehensive data related to pain
	Adolescent's emotional state
Moving	Limitations in daily activities
	Recreational activities
	Self-care abilities
Perceiving	Effects of illness or surgery on self-concept
Exchanging	Physical examination for adolescents
	Nutritional assessment
Choosing	Adolescent's and family's adequacy in dealing with stress
	Adolescent's reaction to illness and hospitalization
	Adolescent's response to maturational crises
	Future compliance with health care regimen

recreation, and self-care. Therefore, this nursing diagnosis appears within each of these areas.

The Adolescent Assessment Tool is not intended to be the standardized and final format for assessment of adolescent patients across the country. An assessment tool must meet the needs and requirements of the institutions and nurses using it. The Adolescent Assessment Tool is simply a working demonstration tool that is expected to be changed and revised by nurses in clinical practice. Further evaluation and refinement are necessary before adopting the tool for use within an institution. Nurses interested in changing, revising, and adapting the tool to a specific clinical setting should refer to Chapter 4.

HOW TO ELICIT APPROPRIATE DATA

Because the Unitary Person Framework and the Adolescent Assessment Tool contain some terms that may be unfamiliar to nurses, specific adolescent focus questions and parameters were developed and refined to elicit appropriate information. These questions and parameters are in Table 22-2, which follows the content of the Adolescent Assessment Tool (Fig. 22-1). The variables in bold type in the tool are described more fully in Table 22-2. For example the variable concerning the patient's description of abilities and relationships under the "perceiving pattern" is in bold type. If the nurse does not know what to ask to elicit this information, Table 22-2 can be used to direct the line of

Table 22-2
Adolescent assessment tool: focus questions and parameters

Variables	Focus questions and parameters
RELATING	
Particular financial stressors	To parent: "Are you having any financial problems at this time? Is _____'s illness causing financial problems? Do you need help with these problems?"
Home behavior problems	To parent: "Do you have problems managing _____ at home? Does _____ follow instructions and obey commands?"
Appropriateness of discipline methods	To parent: "How do you discipline _____? How does _____ react? Does this method work? Who usually disciplines _____?" Does the discipline method seem unusually harsh or lenient? Does the adolescent's reaction seem appropriate?
Verbalized extreme/inappropriate feelings	Do the parents voice extreme levels of anger or frustration that seem inappropriate for the situation? Do the parents verbalize feeling "trapped"? Are the parents' comments appropriate to the situation?
Observed parent-adolescent interaction	How does the adolescent interact with the parents? Do the parents and adolescent talk to each other? Do they maintain eye contact? Do the parents touch the adolescent? Is the nonverbal communication between the parents and adolescent positive or negative? Does the interaction between the parents and adolescent seem appropriate for the situation?
Perception of own sexuality	To adolescent: "Are you attracted to or do you like the opposite sex?"
Emotional responses to sexuality	To adolescent: "How do you feel about liking boys or girls? Is it hard for you to talk about this?"
School problems	To adolescent: "Are you having any problems in school? Do you get along with your classmates? Have you been disciplined for misbehavior in school? Do you expect this illness to have an effect on your school performance and attendance?"
KNOWING	
Communicable diseases	To adolescent (or parent): "Have you (has _____) ever had measles, mumps, chickenpox, or rubella?"

Continued.

Table 22-2—cont'd

Adolescent assessment tool: focus questions and parameters

Variables	Focus questions and parameters
MOVING	
Responsibilities in home	To adolescent: "Do you have any duties or chores at home?" Do these duties seem appropriate for the adolescent's age and health status?
Meets growth and developmental milestones	Does the assessment of the adolescent's developmental skill level confirm that growth and developmental milestones are being met?
Parents' perceptions	To parent: "Do you feel that _____ is growing and developing normally?"
PERCEIVING	
Patient's description of abilities/ relationships	To adolescent: "What kinds of things do you feel you are good at? Are there things you aren't good at? How do you feel about your relationships with your friends and family? Are these relationships what you want them to be?"
Effects of illness/surgery on self-concept	To adolescent: "How has this illness or surgery affected you? Has it changed how you feel about yourself?"
Reflexes	Are the patient's reflexes normal, hyperreflexive, or hyporeflexive? Specify.
EXCHANGING	
Pulses	Are the patient's peripheral pulses palpable bilaterally? If no, specify.
Abnormalities	Is the patient overweight or underweight? Is a dietitian's consultation needed?
Eating problems	Does the patient have a problem with eating?
Patient's perception	To adolescent: "Do you have any problems with eating? Do you feel you eat too much or too little? How do you feel about these problems? Is there anything that makes you want to eat more or less?
Parents' perception	To parent: "Does _____ have any problems with eating? What do you think causes these problems?"
CHOOSING	
Patient's coping response to	
Adolescence	"When someone is your age, there are a lot of changes happening to and around them. How do you feel about these changes?"
Peer pressure	"Do you feel pressure from your friends to do things or act a certain way? How do you react to this? How do you feel about this?"
School	"Are there pressures at school that are hard to deal with? What do you do about these?"
Physical changes	"You are changing physically. How do you feel about these changes? Do they embarrass you?"
Other	"Are there other things that are difficult for you to deal with? How do you handle them?"

questioning. The questions and parameters provide clarity and guidance in eliciting data. They are not all inclusive, so nurses should not feel limited by them. Many other questions, based on the patient's situation and condition and the nurse's skill, could be asked to elicit the information. Questions and parameters for data not in bold type were presented in Chapter 3.

CASE STUDY

The case study models the process a nurse uses when assessing a patient. Based on the clustering of information obtained during assessment, the nurse formulates nursing diagnoses.

R.C. was assessed when admitted to a pediatric unit. He had a surgical correction at age 2 for transposition of the great vessels and has been admitted to undergo cardiac catheterization. R.C. is 15 years old and lives with his grandmother. The Adolescent Assessment Tool (Fig. 22-2) was used to assess him.

BIBLIOGRAPHY

American Nurses' Association: Standards of maternal and child health nursing practice, Kansas City, Mo, 1983, ANA, Inc.

Axton SE: Neonatal and pediatric care plans, Baltimore, 1986, Williams & Wilkins.

Greenburg C: Nursing care planning guide for children, Baltimore, 1988, Williams & Wilkins.

Hazinski MF, editor: Nursing care of the critically ill child, St Louis, 1984, The CV Mosby Co.

Johanson BC, Hoffmeister D, Wells SJ, and Dungca CU, editors: Standards for critical care, ed 3, St Louis, 1988, The CV Mosby Co.

ADOLESCENT ASSESSMENT TOOL

Name _____ Nickname _____ Age _____ Sex _____
Address _____ Telephone _____
Significant other _____ Telephone _____
Birthdate _____ Date of admission _____ Medical diagnosis _____
Allergies: Drugs _____ Other _____
Pediatrician _____ Informant _____

Nursing Diagnosis
(Potential or Altered)

COMMUNICATING ▪ A pattern involving sending messages
Read, write, understand English (circle) _____   Communication
Other languages _____ Language skills normal for age: yes/no   Verbal
Speech impaired _____   Nonverbal
Communicates by: Key words _____ Gestures _____   Growth and development
    Other _____

VALUING ▪ A pattern involving the assigning of relative worth
Religious preference _____ Baptized _____   Spiritual state
Important religious practices _____   Distress
Cultural orientation _____   Despair
Significant cultural practices _____

RELATING ▪ A pattern involving establishing bonds
Role
Parents
    Father: Age _____ Health _____ Occupation _____   Role performance
    Mother: Age _____ Health _____ Occupation _____   Parenting
    Marital status _____
    Foster/adoptive parents _____   Family processes
    Primary care taker for patient _____
    Number of siblings _____ Ages & health _____
_____
    Particular financial stressors _____
    Parents' descriptions of patient's temperament _____   Sexuality patterns
    Home behavior problems _____
    Appropriateness of discipline methods _____
    Perception of relationship with adolescent _____
    Verbalized extreme/inappropriate feelings _____
    Observed parent-adolescent interaction _____
Adolescent
    Perception of relationship with parents _____
    Description of own temperament _____
    Perception of discipline methods _____
    Perception of own sexuality _____
    Emotional responses to sexuality _____

Socialization
    Description of peer interaction _____   Impaired social interaction
        Relationship with boyfriend/girlfriend _____   Growth and development
        Parents' descriptions _____
        Staff observations _____
    Personal/social skills normal for age: yes/no _____
    School grade _____ Performance _____ Attendance _____
    Problems _____

Fig. 22-1

Verbalizes feelings of being alone ———————————————————— Social isolation
  Atrributed to ———————————————————————————— Social withdrawal

KNOWING ▪ A pattern involving the meaning associated with information
Current health problems ————————————————————————
————————————————————————————————————

Previous hospitalizations/surgeries ——————————————————
————————————————————————————————————
————————————————————————————————————

Communicable diseases ————————————————————————
Family history of the following
  Cardiovascular disease ——————— Lung disease ———————————— Knowledge deficit
  Cancer ——————— Liver disease ——————— Diabetes ———————
  Renal disease ——————— Epilepsy ——————— TB ———————
  Bleeding disorders ——————— Anemia ——————— Sickle cell ———————
  Current medications ———————————————————————
————————————————————————————————————

Adolescent
  Smoking ——————— Alcohol ———————————————————
  Drugs: type & frequency ——————————————————————
  Sexually active ——————— Contraceptives ———————————————
  Identified learning needs ——————————————————————
Knowledge of illness/planned tests/surgery
  Adolescent ———————————————————————————— Thought processes
    Misconceptions ———————————————————————— Orientation
    Readiness to learn ——————————————————————— Confusion
    Learning impeded by ———————————————————————
  Parent ——————————————————————————— Memory
    Misconceptions ————————————————————————
    Readiness to learn ———————————————————————
    Learning impeded by ———————————————————————

FEELING ▪ A pattern involving the subjective awareness of information
Comfort
  Pain/discomfort: yes/no ——— Comfort
    Onset ——————— Location ——————————————— Pain/chronic
    Duration ——————— Quality ——————— Radiation ——————— Pain/acute
    Associated factors ————————————————————— Discomfort
    Aggravating factors —————————————————————
    Alleviating factors —————————————————————

Emotional Integrity/States   Anxiety
  Recent stressful life events ———————————————————— Fear
——————————————————— Reaction ——————————— Grieving
  Verbalizes feelings of ———————————————————————— Anger
    Source ——————————————————————————— Guilt
    Physical manifestations ———————————————————— Shame
  History of child abuse, rape, neglect ——————————————— Sadness
     Potential for violence
     Rape-trauma syndrome

MOVING ▪ A pattern involving activity
Activity
  History of physical disability/limitations in daily activities   Impaired physical mobility
————————————————————————————————— Activity intolerance
  Prosthetic devices (crutches, walker) ——————————————— Growth and development
  Gross motor/fine motor skills normal for age: yes/no ———————

Fig. 22-1, cont'd

Continued.

Exercise habits _____ Impaired physical mobility
Effect of current illness/injury on normal activities _____ Activity intolerance
_____

Rest
Sleep patterns _____ Sleep pattern disturbance
Difficulties _____

Recreation
Leisure activities _____ Deficit in diversional activity
Social activities _____ Growth and development
Responsibilities in home _____
Employment _____

Environmental Maintenance
Home maintenance management
    Size & arrangement of home (stairs, bathroom) _____ Impaired home maintenance
_____ Safety needs _____   management
    Neighborhood: safety concerns _____ Safety hazards
    Parental home management problems _____
    Discharge planning needs _____

Health Maintenance
    Health insurance _____ Health maintenance
    Regular physical checkups _____
    Immunization status _____

Self-Care
Ability to perform ADLs: Independent _____ Dependent _____   Self-care
Specify deficits _____   Feeding
_____   Bathing/hygiene
_____   Dressing/grooming
Meets growth and developmental milestones _____   Toileting
Parents' perceptions _____ Growth and development

PERCEIVING ▪ A pattern involving the reception of information
Self-Concept
Physical appearance/grooming _____ Self-concept
Patient's description of self _____
Patient's description of abilities/relationships _____ Body image
_____ Self-esteem
Effects of illness/surgery on self-concept _____ Personal identity
_____

Sensory/Perception
Vision/hearing normal: yes/no _____ Specify deficits _____ Sensory/perception
_____ Visual
Movement/sensation normal: yes/no _____ Specify deficits _____ Auditory
_____ Kinesthetic
Reflexes _____ Gustatory
                                                       Tactile
                                                       Olfactory

EXCHANGING ▪ A pattern involving mutual giving and receiving
Circulation
Cerebral
    Neurologic changes/symptoms _____ Cerebral tissue perfusion
_____

    Pupils
       L 2 3 4 5 6 mm   Reaction: Brisk _____
       R 2 3 4 5 6 mm   Sluggish _____ Nonreactive _____
    Level of alertness _____

Fig. 22-1, cont'd

Cardiac
PMI _____ Apical rate & rhythm _____   Cardiopulmonary tissue
Heart sounds/murmurs _____   perfusion
Dysrhythmias _____   Cardiac output
BP: R _____ L _____ Position: _____

Peripheral   Fluid volume
Pulses _____   Deficit
Skin color _____ Jaundice _____   Excess
Skin temp _____ Turgor _____   Peripheral tissue perfusion
Capillary refill _____ Edema _____

Physical Integrity

	Description	Location	Distribution
Rashes			

       Impaired skin integrity
Rashes _____   Impaired tissue integrity
Lesions _____
Petechiae _____
Bruising _____   Potential for injury
Abrasions/lacerations _____
Surgical incision _____
Other _____

Oxygenation

Complaints of dyspnea _____ Precipitated by _____   Ineffective breathing pattern
Rate _____ Rhythm _____ Depth _____   Ineffective airway clearance
Labored/unlabored (circle)   Chest expansion _____   Impaired gas exchange
Cough: productive/nonproductive _____
Sputum: Color _____ Amount _____ Consistency _____
Breath sounds _____
Arterial blood gases _____
Oxygen percent and device _____
Ventilator _____

Physical Regulation

Immune
    Lymph nodes enlarged _____ Location _____   Infection
    WBC count _____ Differential _____   Body temperature
    RBC count _____ Hemoglobin _____ Hematocrit _____ ESR _____   Hypothermia
    Culture & sensitivity: source _____   Hyperthermia
Altered body temperature   Ineffective thermoregulation
    Temperature _____ Route _____

Nutrition

Eating patterns   Nutrition
    Number of meals per day _____ Special diet _____   More than body
    Food preferences _____   requirements
    Food intolerances/allergies _____
    Appetite changes _____
    Nausea/vomiting _____   Less than body requirements
    Daily fluid intake _____
Height _____ Weight _____ Recent weight changes _____
Abnormalities _____   Oral mucous membrane
Eating problems _____ Anorexia _____ Bulemia _____
    How handled _____
Patient's perception _____   Fluid volume
Parents' perceptions _____   Deficit
Condition of mouth/throat _____   Excess
Braces _____ Retainer _____ Loose teeth _____
Current therapy
    NPO _____ NG suction _____

Fig. 22-1, cont'd

Continued.

Tube feeding _____ TPN _____
IV fluids _____
Labs
  Na _____ K _____ CL _____ Glucose _____ Fasting _____

Elimination
GI/bowel
  Usual bowel habits _____
  Alterations from normal _____
  Abdominal physical examination _____

Renal/genitourinary
  Usual urinary pattern _____
  Alteration from normal _____
  Color _____ Catheter _____
  Urine output: 24 hour _____ Average hourly _____
  Bladder distention _____
  Serum BUN _____ Creatinine _____ Specific gravity _____
  Urine studies _____
  Menses: Began _____ Frequency _____ Duration _____
  Last menstrual periods _____ Problems _____

Bowel elimination
  Constipation
  Diarrhea
  Incontinence
GI tissue perfusion
Urinary elimination
  Incontinence
  Retention
Renal tissue perfusion

Menstrual patterns

CHOOSING ▪ A pattern involving the selection of alternatives
Coping
Patient's usual reaction to stress _____
_____
Family's method of dealing with stress _____
_____
Patient's reaction to illness _____
_____
Previous reaction to hospitalization _____
Previous experiences away from home _____
_____
Patient's affect _____
Patient's coping response to: Adolescence _____
_____
  Peer pressure _____
  School _____
  Physical changes _____ **Other** _____

Ineffective individual coping
Ineffective family coping

Participation
Compliance with past/current health care regimens _____
_____
Willingness to comply with future health care regimen _____
_____

Noncompliance
Ineffective participation

Prioritized nursing diagnoses/problem list
1. _____
2. _____
3. _____
4. _____
5. _____
6. _____
7. _____
8. _____

Signature _____ Date _____

Fig. 22-1, cont'd

ADOLESCENT ASSESSMENT TOOL

Name *R.C.* Nickname *—* Age *15* Sex *M*
Address *88 EIGHTH STREET, NASHVILLE, TENNESSEE* Telephone *772-2000*
Significant other *GRANDMOTHER* Telephone *772-2000*
Birthdate *6/3/73* Date of admission *12/2* Medical diagnosis *TRANSPOSITION OF GREAT*
Allergies: Drugs *NKA* Other *VESSELS*
Pediatrician *DR. C. & DR. P.* Informant *PATIENT & GRANDMOTHER*

Nursing Diagnosis
(Potential or Altered)

COMMUNICATING ■ A pattern involving sending messages
(Read,)(write,)(understand) English (circle) _____ Communication
Other languages *No* Language skills normal for age:(yes)/no   Verbal
Speech impaired *No* Nonverbal
Communicates by: Key words _____ Gestures _____ Growth and development
 Other *NORMAL SPEECH PATTERN*

VALUING ■ A pattern involving the assigning of relative worth
Religious preference *BAPTIST* Baptized *YES @ BIRTH* Spiritual state
Important religious practices *CHURCH/SUNDAY SCHOOL EVERY WEEK* Distress
Cultural orientation *CAUCASIAN* Despair
Significant cultural practices *NONE IN PARTICULAR*

RELATING ■ A pattern involving establishing bonds
Role
Parents
 Father: Age *35* Health *GOOD* Occupation *ELECTRICIAN* Role performance
 Mother: Age *35* Health *GOOD* Occupation *BEAUTICIAN* Parenting
 Marital status *DIVORCED — MOTHER NOT IN PICTURE*
 Foster/adoptive parents *GRANDMOTHER HAS CUSTODY — AGE 55* Family processes
 Primary care taker for patient *GRANDMOTHER*
 Number of siblings *1* Ages & health *13 — GOOD HEALTH*

 Particular financial stressors *No*
 Parents' descriptions of patient's temperament *EVEN TEMPERED* Sexuality patterns
 Home behavior problems *No*
 Appropriateness of discipline methods *WITHDRAWAL OF PRIVILEGES — APPROPRIATE*
 Perception of relationship with adolescent *GOOD — INTERACTS WELL*
 Verbalized extreme/inappropriate feelings *No*
 Observed parent-adolescent interaction *SUPPORTIVE POSITIVE INTERACTION*
Adolescent
 Perception of relationship with parents *GOOD c̄ GRANDMOTHER*
 Description of own temperament *"PRETTY COOL"*
 Perception of discipline methods *FAIR*
 Perception of own sexuality *"I LIKE GIRLS."*
 Emotional responses to sexuality *EMBARRASSED*

Socialization
 Description of peer interaction *HAS LOTS OF FRIENDS* Impaired social interaction
  Relationship with boyfriend/girlfriend *GOOD RELATIONSHIP c̄ GIRLFRIEND* Growth and development
  Parents' descriptions *"GETS ALONG WELL c̄ OTHERS." (GRANDMOTHER)*
  Staff observations *INTERACTS WELL c̄ PEERS & STAFF*
 Personal/social skills normal for age: yes/no *YES*
 School grade *11* Performance *A's & B's* Attendance *GOOD*
  Problems *NONE*

Fig. 22-2

Continued.

Verbalizes feelings of being alone _No_ .... Social isolation
  Atrributed to ___—___ .... Social withdrawal

KNOWING ▪ A pattern involving the meaning associated with information
Current health problems _ADMITTED FOR CARDIAC CATH — PT HAS hx_
OF TRANSPOSITION OF GREAT VESSELS, MITRAL INSUFFICIENCY
Previous hospitalizations/surgeries _SURGERY FOR SHUNT @ 2 mos OF_
AGE, SURGICAL CORRECTION OF TRANSPOSITION @ 2 YRS OF AGE,
CARDIAC CATH @ AGE 12
Communicable diseases _CHICKENPOX, MEASLES IN CHILDHOOD_
Family history of the following
  Cardiovascular disease _No_   Lung disease _No_
  Cancer _No_   Liver disease _No_   Diabetes _No_   (Knowledge deficit)
  Renal disease _No_   Epilepsy _No_   TB _No_
  Bleeding disorders _No_   Anemia _No_   Sickle cell _No_
Current medications _DIGOXIN 0.125 mg qd, LASIX 20 mg qd_

Adolescent
  Smoking _No_   Alcohol _No_
  Drugs: type & frequency _No_
  Sexually active _No_   Contraceptives _No_
  Identified learning needs _NONE – EMBARRASSED TO DISUSS THIS_
Knowledge of illness/planned tests/surgery   _HEART DISEASE."_
  Adolescent _"PEOPLE c̄ HIGH CHOLESTEROL ∨ NO EXERCISE HAVE_ .... Thought processes
    Misconceptions _"ALL PEOPLE c̄ BAD HEART DISEASE DIE."_ .... Orientation
    Readiness to learn _WANTS TO LEARN ABOUT CATH BUT IS SCARED_   Confusion
    Learning impeded by _ANXIETY_
  Parent _UNDERSTANDS PROCEDURE ∨ ITS RATIONALE_ .... Memory
    Misconceptions _NONE_
    Readiness to learn _GOOD_
    Learning impeded by _MILD ANXIETY_

FEELING ▪ A pattern involving the subjective awareness of information
Comfort
  Pain/discomfort: yes/no _No_ .... Comfort
    Onset _____ Location _____ .... Pain/chronic
    Duration _____ Quality _____ Radiation _____ .... Pain/acute
    Associated factors _____ .... Discomfort
    Aggravating factors _____
    Alleviating factors _____

Emotional Integrity/States   (Anxiety)
  Recent stressful life events _COMING TO HOSPITAL_ .... Fear
  _____ Reaction _NERVOUSNESS_ .... Grieving
  Verbalizes feelings of _ANXIETY_ .... Anger
    Source _FEARS HE WILL DIE DURING CATH_ .... Guilt
    Physical manifestations _SWEATING, ↑ HEART RATE_ .... Shame
  History of child abuse, rape, neglect _No_ .... Sadness
                                    Potential for violence
                                    Rape-trauma syndrome

MOVING ▪ A pattern involving activity
Activity
  History of physical disability/limitations in daily activities .... Impaired physical mobility
  DOES NOT PLAY CONTACT SPORTS R/T HEART CONDITION .... (Activity intolerance) (POTENTIAL)
  Prosthetic devices (crutches, walker) _No_ .... Growth and development
  Gross motor/fine motor skills normal for age: yes/no _YES_

Fig. 22-2, cont'd

Exercise habits *PHYSICAL ED @ SCHOOL, LIKES BASEBALL*   Impaired physical mobility
Effect of current illness/injury on normal activities *NO ANTICIPATED*   Activity intolerance
CHANGES

Rest
Sleep patterns *7-8 HRS/NIGHT*   Sleep pattern disturbance
Difficulties *NONE*

Recreation
Leisure activities *READS, COLLECTS BUTTERFLIES*   Deficit in diversional activity
Social activities *CHURCH, BASEBALL, HANGS OUT c̄ FRIENDS*   Growth and development
Responsibilities in home *CLEANS ROOM, EMPTIES TRASH, mows LAWN*
Employment *NO*

Environmental Maintenance
Home maintenance management
  Size & arrangement of home (stairs, bathroom) *2 STORY HOUSE c̄ BATH*   Impaired home maintenance
ON BOTH LEVELS   Safety needs *NONE IDENTIFIED*   management
  Neighborhood: safety concerns *NONE*   Safety hazards
  Parental home management problems *NONE*
  Discharge planning needs *NO IDENTIFIED NEEDS @ THIS TIME*

Health Maintenance
  Health insurance *GRANDMOTHER'S WORK*   Health maintenance
  Regular physical checkups *YES*
  Immunization status *UP-TO-DATE*

Self-Care
  Ability to perform ADLs: Independent ___✓___ Dependent _____   Self-care
  Specify deficits *NONE*   Feeding
                                                                      Bathing/hygiene
  _____   Dressing/grooming
  Meets growth and developmental milestones *YES*   Toileting
  Parents' perceptions *"HE'S NORMAL FOR HIS AGE." (GRANDMOTHER)*   Growth and development

PERCEIVING ▪ A pattern involving the reception of information
Self-Concept   Self-concept
  Physical appearance/grooming *NEAT/CLEAN*
  Patient's description of self *"PRETTY GOOD GUY"*   Body image
  Patient's description of abilities/relationships *LOTS OF FRIENDS THAT*   Self-esteem
  HE DOES THINGS WITH   Personal identity
  Effects of illness/surgery on self-concept *WORRIED ABOUT "DYING*
  DURING THE CATH"

Sensory/Perception   Sensory/perception
  Vision/hearing normal: yes/no *YES* Specify deficits ___—___   Visual
                                                                      Auditory
  Movement/sensation normal: yes/no *YES* Specify deficits ___—___   Kinesthetic
                                                                      Gustatory
  Reflexes *NORMAL*   Tactile
                                                                      Olfactory

EXCHANGING ▪ A pattern involving mutual giving and receiving
Circulation
Cerebral
  Neurologic changes/symptoms *NO CHANGES*   Cerebral tissue perfusion

  Pupils
    L 2 ③ 4 5 6 mm   Reaction: Brisk ___✓___
    R 2 ③ 4 5 6 mm   Sluggish _____ Nonreactive _____
    Level of alertness *ALERT, TALKATIVE*

Continued.

Fig. 22-2, cont'd

Cardiac
PMI _APEX_ Apical rate & rhythm _100 REGULAR_   Cardiopulmonary tissue perfusion
Heart sounds/murmurs _II/vi HOLOSYSTOLIC (m) AT LLSB WITH RADIATION_ Cardiac output
Dysrhythmias _NO_   _TO (L) AXILLA)_
BP: R _110/72_ L _—_ Position: _SITTING_   _((L) PULSE THREADY/ABSENT AS ARTERY TAKEN FOR SHUNT)_
Peripheral   Fluid volume
Pulses _PALPABLE BILATERALLY EXCEPT (L) ARM R/T SHUNT_   Deficit
Skin color _WARM_ Jaundice _NO_   Excess
Skin temp _PINK_ Turgor _GOOD_   (Peripheral tissue perfusion)
Capillary refill _BRISK<2SEC_ Edema _NO_

Physical Integrity

	Description	Location	Distribution	
Rashes	_No_			Impaired skin integrity
Lesions	_No_			Impaired tissue integrity
Petechiae	_No_			
Bruising	_No_			Potential for injury
Abrasions/lacerations	_No_			

Surgical incision _WELL-HEALED MIDSTERNAL SCAR & (L) THORACOTOMY SCAR_
Other _WELL-HEALED (L) ARM SCAR_

Oxygenation
Complaints of dyspnea _No_ Precipitated by _—_   Ineffective breathing pattern
Rate _20_ Rhythm _REGULAR_ Depth _NORMAL_   Ineffective airway clearance
Labored/(unlabored) (circle) Chest expansion _SYMMETRICAL_   Impaired gas exchange
Cough: productive/nonproductive _No_
Sputum: Color _—_ Amount _—_ Consistency _—_
Breath sounds _CLEAR BILATERALLY_
Arterial blood gases _—_
Oxygen percent and device _—_
Ventilator _—_

Physical Regulation
Immune
Lymph nodes enlarged _No_ Location _—_   Infection
WBC count _5.5x10³/μl_ Differential _NOT DONE_   Body temperature
RBC count _4.6x10⁶/μl_ Hemoglobin _8g/dl_ Hematocrit _48%_ ESR _—_   Hypothermia
Culture & sensitivity: source _—_   Hyperthermia
Altered body temperature   Ineffective thermoregulation
Temperature _98°F_ Route _ORAL_

Nutrition
Eating patterns   (Nutrition)
Number of meals per day _3+ SNACK_ Special diet _No_   More than body
Food preferences _LIKES HAMBURGERS & FRIES_   requirements
Food intolerances/allergies _NONE_
Appetite changes _No_
Nausea/vomiting _No_   (Less than body requirements)
Daily fluid intake _8 GLASSES MILK/COKE/WATER/JUICE A DAY_
Height _5'6"_ Weight _100_ Recent weight changes _No_
Abnormalities _BELOW IDEAL BODY WEIGHT_   Oral mucous membrane
Eating problems _No_ Anorexia _No_ Bulemia _No_
How handled _—_
Patient's perception _—_   Fluid volume
Parents' perceptions _—_   Deficit
Condition of mouth/throat _Good_   Excess
Braces _No_ Retainer _No_ Loose teeth _No_
Current therapy
NPO _No_ NG suction _No_

Fig. 22-2, cont'd

Tube feeding _No_   TPN _No_
IV fluids _D₅ W @ KVO WILL BE STARTED BEFORE CATH_
Labs
  Na _136 mEq/L_ K _3.6 mEq/L_ CL _100 mEq/L_ Glucose _120 mg/dl_ Fasting _No_

Elimination
GI/bowel   Bowel elimination
  Usual bowel habits _↑ BM/DAY_   Constipation
  Alterations from normal _No_   Diarrhea
  Abdominal physical examination _⊕ BS IN ALL 4 QUADS; FLAT, NON-_   Incontinence
                                    TENDER   GI tissue perfusion

Renal/genitourinary   Urinary elimination
  Usual urinary pattern _VOIDS 3-4 x/DAY_   Incontinence
  Alteration from normal _No_   Retention
  Color _YELLOW CLEAR_   Catheter _No_   Renal tissue perfusion
  Urine output: 24 hour _3-4 x/DAY_ Average hourly _—_
  Bladder distention _No_   Menstrual patterns
  Serum BUN _8 ml/dl_ Creatinine _0.2 mg/dl_ Specific gravity _1.005_
  Urine studies _—_
  Menses: Began _N/A_ Frequency _N/A_ Duration _N/A_
  Last menstrual periods _N/A_ Problems _N/A_

CHOOSING ■ A pattern involving the selection of alternatives
Coping
Patient's usual reaction to stress _BITES FINGER NAILS_   Ineffective individual coping
                                        Ineffective family coping
Family's method of dealing with stress _TALK ABOUT PROBLEMS_

Patient's reaction to illness _SCARED OF UPCOMING CATH_

Previous reaction to hospitalization _DOESN'T LIKE HOSPITALS_
Previous experiences away from home _3 HOSPITALIZATIONS,_
SPENDS NIGHT C̄ FRIENDS
Patient's affect _APPROPRIATE_
Patient's coping response to: Adolescence _"I'M DOING OK. SOMETIMES_
MY FRIENDS ACT KIND OF WEIRD."
Peer pressure _"NO, I DO WHAT I WANT TO."_
School _"SOMETIMES IT'S HARD TO DO ALL MY SCHOOLWORK."_
Physical changes _"I DON'T_ Other _"HAVING THIS HEART PROBLEM-_
        KNOW—OK"   _I GET SCARED."_

Participation
Compliance with past/current health care regimens _COMPLIANT_   Noncompliance
                                        Ineffective participation
Willingness to comply with future health care regimen _INTENDS TO_
COMPLY

Prioritized nursing diagnoses/problem list
1. _ANXIETY R/T IMPENDING CARDIAC CATH_
2. _KNOWLEDGE DEFICIT R/T DISEASE PROCESS, CARDIAC CATH_
3. _ALTERED NUTRITION: LESS THAN BODY REQUIREMENTS R/T LOW BODY WEIGHT_
4. _ALTERED PERIPHERAL TISSUE PERFUSION R/T ℗ ARM SHUNT_
5. _POTENTIAL ACTIVITY INTOLERANCE R/T ANEMIA_
6. _____
7. _____
8. _____

Signature _Anita P. Shever, R.N._   Date _6/29_

Fig. 22-2, cont'd

CHAPTER 23

GERONTOLOGIC ASSESSMENT TOOL

PATRICIA C. SEIFERT
MARIE LOOBY

The Gerontologic Assessment Tool was designed to assess eiderly patients with unique biopsychosocial assessment needs. The tool incorporates signs and symptoms pertinent to elderly patients to facilitate identification of nursing diagnoses. It also incorporates the American Nurses' Association's *Standards of Gerontologic Nursing Practice*. This chapter includes:

- *The way the tool was developed and refined*
- *The patient populations and settings to which it applies*
- *Selected gerontologic emphasis areas*
- *The way to use the tool*
- *Specific gerontologic focus questions and parameters to assist the nurse in eliciting appropriate data*
- *The Gerontologic Assessment Tool*
- *A case study*
- *A completed version of the tool based on the case study*

DEVELOPMENT AND REFINEMENT OF THE TOOL

The Gerontologic Assessment Tool was developed from the nursing data base prototype (see Chapter 2). Many hemodynamic monitoring and critical care variables originally incorporated in the prototype were deleted and replaced with specific variables more applicable to gerontologic assessment. The resultant tool was modified based on the recommendations of gerontologic nurse experts. Further, the content of the tool is supported by the literature from this field of nursing.

After the tool was developed and refined, it was clini-cally tested by gerontologic nurse experts and clinical nurse specialists on 10 patients in acute care medical and surgical units. All patients were 60 years of age or older, with several problems or medical diagnoses. Many patients were chronically ill with acute exacerbations of previous problems or the development of new ones. The testing evaluated the adequacy of the tool in terms of flow, space for recording data, and completeness of assessment variables. Based on the results, the tool was revised.

PATIENT POPULATION AND SETTING

The Gerontologic Assessment Tool was developed to assess the needs and problems of elderly patients, 60 years and older, who may have multisystem problems. It was designed for use in the hospital or home care, long-term care, or adult day-care settings. It is intended for use with stable patients. To avoid fatiguing elderly patients, it may be necessary to complete the assessment tool in two sessions, preferably within 24 hours. Depending on the patient's degree of orientation, the family or significant other may provide necessary data.

GERONTOLOGIC EMPHASIS AREAS

Gerontologic patients have specialized problems and needs. The Gerontologic Assessment Tool includes appropriate assessment variables within each of the nine human response patterns of the Unitary Person Framework. The tool focuses on prevalent problems among elderly patients. Table 23-1 outlines these emphasis areas.

HOW TO USE THE TOOL

To use the Gerontologic Assessment Tool effectively, nurses must first be familiar with the Unitary Person

Table 23-1

Selected gerontologic emphasis areas

Patterns	Emphasis areas to determine
Communicating	Physical impairment affecting communication
	Expressive versus receptive aphasia
Valuing	Important religious or cultural practices
Relating	Role in home
	Physical and mental energy expenditures
	Physical difficulties and effects of illness on relationships
	Recent losses
	Quality of relationship with others
Choosing	Compliance with past and current health regimens
	Family support available
	Decision-making ability
Knowing	Current health problems
	Previous accidents or injuries
	Current medications or prescriptions
	Level of alertness and memory
Feeling	Pain or discomfort
	Recent stressful life events
Moving	Use of devices and limitations in daily activities
	Resources available
	Home maintenance management and housekeeping responsibilities
	Ability to perform activities of daily living
Perceiving	History of restrictive environment
Exchanging	Neurologic and cardiac changes and symptoms
	Tissue integrity: falls, accidents, and skin condition
	Eating patterns and dentures
	Usual bowel habits and urinary patterns

Framework (see Chapter 2), which provides the underlying framework of Taxonomy I. The nine human response patterns of the Unitary Person Framework serve as the major category headings for Taxonomy I and the tool. The sequence of the response patterns, as it appears in Taxonomy I, has been changed in the tool to permit a more logical ordering of assessment variables. Nursing diagnoses pertinent to gerontologic patients, along with the signs and symptoms necessary to identify them, are incorporated under the appropriate human response patterns.

Nurses must also realize that this tool is very different from conventional assessment tools. As a result, nurses may have some initial difficulty in using it. They should remember, however, that the tool was not designed to follow the organization or content of a traditional medical data base; the data collected do not solely reflect medical patterns. Rather, this tool elicits data about holistic patterns in ways not traditionally assessed by nurses. It provides a new method of collecting and synthesizing data and requires new thinking when processing data. This tool represents a nursing data base developed from a nursing model to permit a holistic nursing assessment to take place so nursing diagnoses can be identified.

Although nurses probably agree that a holistic nursing data base is desirable, it is realized that changing traditional assessment methods is not an easy task. For this reason, a trial usage period is recommended before any decisions about the tool's merits are made. During this period, nurses should assess 10 elderly patients using the tool to become familiar and progressively more comfortable with its organization and data-collection methods. With experience, nurses will become accustomed to new ways of clustering and processing information. With continued use, the time necessary to complete the tool will be reduced. Most important, nurses will recognize the unique ability of the tool to elicit appropriate signs and symptoms. Nurses will discover that nursing diagnoses are easily identified when using this tool.

It is not necessary to complete the tool in one session. Priority sections can be completed during the initial assessment. Other sections or patterns can be completed later, within a time frame acceptable to the institution.

To elicit appropriate data, nurses should be familiar with the focus questions and parameters in the next section. When assessing specific signs and symptoms to indicate a diagnosis, the nurse circles the diagnosis in the right-hand column when deviations from normal are found. A circled diagnosis does not confirm a problem but simply alerts the nurse to the possibility that it exists. After completing the tool, the nurse scans the circled problems, synthesizes the data to determine whether other clusters of signs and symptoms support a problem, and decides whether the actual or potential diagnosis is present.

Some diagnoses are repeated several times in the right-hand column. These repetitions occur only within the appropriate response pattern and are convenient for identifying certain data directly with their corresponding nursing diagnosis. These diagnoses are not absolute but focus thinking and direct more detailed attention to a possible problem.

Certain signs and symptoms can indicate several diagnoses. For example, fever can indicate infection and ineffective thermoregulation. To avoid unnecessary repetition of assessment parameters, variables are arranged with the diagnosis most likely to result from the data assessed. Thus, data to support one diagnosis may occasionally be

Table 23-2
Gerontologic assessment tool: focus questions and parameters

Variables	Focus questions and parameters
COMMUNICATING	
Physical impairment affecting communications	Does arthritis inhibit writing or phoning?
Expressive versus receptive aphasia	Does the patient exhibit expressive or receptive aphasia? (See Chapter 25.)
VALUING	
Important religious or cultural practices	Has patient requested a rabbi, priest, or minister? Are there age-related cultural practices?
RELATING	
Role in home	Is the patient capable of performing duties at home (cooking, cleaning, and managing finances)? Is the patient responsible for others?
Physical/mental energy expenditure	"Do you find your job, housework, or volunteer, or church work too demanding?" "Are you frequently tired? When? Why?"
Recent losses	"Have you had any recent major losses that you fret or worry about?"
CHOOSING	
Compliance with past/current health care regimens	Are there age-related difficulties such as forgetfulness or impaired mobility?
Family support available	"If you feel sick or are out of food or medicine, who is available to help you?" To family member: "What would you do if _____ (patient) were sick or out of food or medicine?"
Decision-making ability	To patient: "What would you do if you felt sick?"
KNOWING	
Current health problems	"Tell me what ails you now."
Previous accidents/injuries	Have the patient describe recent accidents or injuries (e.g., burns or bruises).
Current medications	"What medicines do you take on your own (that your physician didn't order)?" "What medicines has your physician ordered?"
Level of alertness	"Can you tell me today's date and day, the time, and where we are? Is it hard to think clearly?" Is patient alert, lethargic, stuporous, or comatose?
Memory intact	"Have you found it difficult to remember events lately?" Does the family report losses in the patient's memory?
FEELING	
Pain/discomfort	"How does pain affect your activities of daily living?" "What activities have you changed because of your pain?" "Why do you think you have this pain? What causes it?" "Is the pain tolerable or intolerable?"
Recent stressful life events	"How do you feel about yourself? Your situation? Recent events?"
MOVING	
Use of devices	Is a device such as a walker, cane, or wheel chair useful for ambulation or mobility?
Limitations in daily activities	"Are you able to get in and out of bed or a chair? Do you need human or mechanical help?"
Resources available	What community or church resources are available to the patient and family?
Home maintenance management	Are there safety hazards in the home (stairs, kitchen, and bathroom)?
Housekeeping responsibilities	Is the patient able to keep up with housekeeping chores? Is help available?
Ability to perform ADLs	"Are you able to bathe, groom, dress, feed yourself? Do these things with help?"

Table 23-2—cont'd
Gerontologic assessment tool: focus questions and parameters

Variables	Focus questions and parameters
PERCEIVING	
History of restricted environments	Has the patient recently experienced any restrictive situations or environments (e.g., intensive care, traction, confining illness, institutionalization, hospice)?
EXCHANGING	
Neurologic changes/symptoms	Are there signs or symptoms of altered cerebral tissue perfusion (forgetfulness, headaches, fainting, loss of vision, confusion, and numbness)?
History of falls/accidents	"Have you had any recent falls or accidents? Can you describe why you fell? Were you dizzy? Did you have trouble seeing? Could you call for help?"
	Is there any evidence of skin breakdown, bed sores, rashes, or injuries?
Eating patterns	What are the patient's food preferences?
Dentures	Is mastication a problem? Is a special diet needed?
Usual bowel habits	Assess the number and consistency of bowel movements. Does the patient use laxatives? How often?
Usual urinary patterns	"Are you ever unable to hold urine when you sneeze, cough, or laugh?"
	Assess for frequency, urgency, and burning.

found in other patterns or arranged with other diagnoses. Therefore, synthesis of all data is essential.

The Gerontologic Assessment Tool is not intended to be the standardized and final format for assessment of elderly patients across the country. An assessment tool must meet the needs of the institutions and nurses using it. The Gerontologic Assessment Tool is simply a working demonstration tool that is expected to be changed and revised by nurses in clinical practice. Further evaluation and refinement are necessary before adapting the tool for use in an institution. Nurses interested in changing, revising, and adapting the tool to a specific clinical setting should refer to Chapter 4.

HOW TO ELICIT APPROPRIATE DATA

Because the Unitary Person Framework and the Gerontologic Assessment Tool contain some terms that may be unfamiliar to nurses, specific gerontologic focus questions and parameters were developed and refined to elicit appropriate information. These questions and parameters are in Table 23-2, which follows the content of the tool (Fig. 23-1). The variables in bold type in the tool are described more fully in Table 23-2. For example, the variable about a restricted history of environments under the "perceiving pattern" is in bold type. If the nurse does not know what to ask to elicit this information, Table 23-2 can be used to direct the line of questioning. The questions and parameters provide clarity and guidance when eliciting data. They are not all inclusive, so nurses should not feel limited by them. There are many other ways, based on the patient's situation and condition and

the nurses's skill, to elicit the information. Focus questions and parameters for data not in bold type were presented in Chapter 3.

CASE STUDY

The case study models the process a nurse uses when assessing a patient. Based on the clustering of information obtained during assessment, the nurse formulates nursing diagnoses.

Mrs. L.M. was assessed in the hospital after an aortic valve replacement. She is 77 years old, widowed, and lives alone. The Gerontologic Assessment Tool (Fig. 23-2) was used to assess Mrs. L.M.

BIBLIOGRAPHY

American Nurses' Association: Standards of gerontological nursing practice, Kansas City, Mo, 1976, ANA, Inc.

Bates B: A guide to physical examination, Philadelphia, 1983, JB Lippincott Co.

Carnevali D and Patrick M: Nursing management for the elderly, Philadelphia, 1986, JB Lippincott Co.

Ebersole P and Hess P: Toward healthy aging: human needs and nursing response, ed 3, St Louis, 1989, The CV Mosby Co.

Eliopolous C: Health assessment of the older adult, Menlo Park, Calif, 1984, Addison-Wesley Publishing Co, Inc.

Gress L and Bahr Sr R: The aging person: a holistic perspective, St Louis, 1984, The CV Mosby Co.

Steffl B: Handbook of gerontological nursing, New York, 1984, Van Nostrand Reinhold Co, Inc.

GERONTOLOGIC ASSESSMENT TOOL

Name _____ Age _____ Sex _____
Address _____ Telephone _____
Significant other _____ Telephone _____
Date of admission _____ Medical diagnosis _____
Allergies _____ Historical source _____

Nursing Diagnosis
(Potential or Altered)

COMMUNICATING ▪ A pattern involving sending messages
Read, write, understand English (circle) _____ Communication
Other languages _____   Verbal
Intubated _____ Speech impaired _____   Nonverbal
Alternate form of communication _____
Physical impairment affecting communications _____
   Expressive versus receptive aphasia _____

VALUING ▪ A pattern involving the assigning of relative worth
Religious preference _____ Spiritual state
Important religious practices _____   Distress
Cultural orientation _____   Despair
Important cultural practices (i.e., food, treatment) _____
_____

RELATING ▪ A pattern involving establishing bonds
Role   Role performance
  Marital status _____   Parenting
  Age & health of significant other _____   Sexual dysfunction
  With whom do you live? _____   Work
  Number of children _____ Ages _____   Family
  Addresses of children _____   Social/leisure
  Pets _____
  Role in home _____   Family processes
  Financial support _____
  Occupation _____ Retired _____
  Job satisfaction/concerns _____
  Volunteer work _____
  Physical/mental energy expenditures (work, home, volunteering)
  _____
  Sexual relationships (satisfactory/unsatisfactory) _____ Sexuality patterns
    Physical difficulties/effects of illness on relationships
  _____
  Recent losses (role, functional ability, home, significant others) _____
Socialization
  Quality of relationships with others _____   Impaired social interaction
    Patient's description _____
    Significant others' descriptions _____
    Staff observations _____
  Verbalizes feelings of being alone _____ Depressed _____ Social isolation
    Attributed to _____   Social withdrawal
  Social status _____

Fig. 23-1

CHOOSING ▪ A pattern involving the selection of alternatives
Coping
Patient's usual problem-solving methods _____
_____
Family's usual problem-solving methods _____
_____
Patient's method of dealing with stress _____
_____
Family's method of dealing with stress _____
_____
Patient's affect _____
Physical manifestations _____

Ineffective individual coping
Ineffective family coping

Participation
Compliance with past/current health regimens _____
_____
Willingness to comply with future health care regimen _____
_____
Family support available _____
Other resources available _____

Noncompliance
Ineffective participation

Judgment
Decision-making ability
Patient's perspective _____
Others' perspectives _____

Judgment
  Indecisiveness

KNOWING ▪ A pattern involving the meaning associated with information
Current health problems _____
_____
Previous illness/hospitalizations/surgeries _____
_____

Knowledge deficit

Previous accidents/injuries _____
History of the following:
Heart disease _____ CHF _____ Peripheral vascular _____
Rheumatic fever _____ HTN _____ Lung disease _____
Bronchitis _____ Asthma _____ TB _____
Pneumonia _____ Influenza _____ Liver _____
Gallbladder _____ Kidney _____
Cerebrovascular _____ Stroke _____ Seizures _____
Thyroid _____ Gout _____
Cancer _____ Anemia _____
Prostate _____ Diabetes _____
Alzheimer's disease _____ Osteoarthritis _____
Rheumatoid arthritis _____ Osteoporosis _____
Cataract _____ Glaucoma _____
Smoking _____ Alcohol _____ Psychiatric illness _____
Family health history _____

Thought processes

Orientation
Confusion
Memory

Current medications:	Dose	Route	Frequency
Over-the-counter			

Continued.

Fig. 23-1, cont'd

Prescription

_____

_____

_____

_____

_____

_____

Immunization status _____

Knowledge/perception of illness _____

Knowledge/perception of planned therapy _____

Expectations of therapy _____

Misconceptions _____

Readiness to learn _____   Thought processes

   Request information concerning _____

   Educational level _____

   Learning impeded by _____

Orientation

Level of alertness _____   Orientation

Orientation: Person _____ Place _____ Time _____   Confusion

Appropriate behavior/communication _____

Memory

Memory intact: yes/no   Recent _____ Remote _____   Memory

FEELING ▪ A pattern involving the subjective awareness of information

Comfort

  Pain/discomfort: yes/no   Comfort

    Onset _____ Duration _____   Pain/chronic

    Location _____ Quality _____ Radiation _____   Pain/acute

    Associated factors _____   Discomfort

    Aggravating factors _____

    Alleviating factors (meds, TENS) _____

    Claudication _____

Emotional Integrity/States

  Emotional status: Angry _____ Denial _____ Depressed _____   Grieving

    Cooperative _____ Other _____   Anxiety

  Recent stressful life events _____   Fear

_____   Anger

  Verbalizes feelings of _____   Guilt

    Source _____   Shame

  Physical manifestations (of fear, anger) _____   Sadness

_____   Violence

  Evidence of aggression: Toward self _____

    Toward others _____ Toward environment _____

  Does patient desire counseling? _____

MOVING ▪ A pattern involving activity

Activity

  Ambulation _____ OOB/transferring _____   Impaired physical mobility

  Assistance _____

  History of physical disability _____

_____

Fig. 23-1, cont'd

Use of devices (protheses, cane, wheel chair) _____ Activity intolerance

Limitations in daily activities _____

Verbal report of fatigue or weakness _____
Exercise habits _____

Rest
  Hours slept/night _____ Feels rested: yes/no   Sleep pattern disturbances
  Sleep aids (pillows, meds, food) _____   Hypersomnia
  Difficulty falling/remaining asleep _____   Insomnia
                          Nightmares

Recreation
  Leisure activities _____   Deficit in diversional activity
  Social activities _____
Resources available (community, church) _____

Environmental Maintenance
  Home maintenance management   Impaired home maintenance
    Size & arrangement of home (stairs, bathroom) _____   management
    _____ Safety needs _____   Safety hazards
  Transportation available _____
  Housekeeping responsibilities _____

Health Maintenance
  Health insurance _____   Health maintenance
  Regular physical checkups _____
  Date of last checkup: Rectal _____
    Female: PAP _____ Pelvic _____ Breast _____
        Self-breast _____ Onset of menopause _____   Menstrual patterns
    Male: Testicular _____ BPH _____

Self-Care
  Ability to perform ADLs: Independent _____ Dependent _____   Self-care
  Specific deficits _____   Feeding
  Discharge planning needs: _____   Bathing/hygiene
  Referrals _____   Dressing/grooming
  Community resources available _____   Toileting
  Financial management _____ Taking medications _____

PERCEIVING ▪ A pattern involving the reception of information
Self-Concept   Self-concept
  Patient's description of self _____   Body image
  Effects of illness/surgery on self-concept _____   Self-esteem
                          Personal identity

Meaningfulness
  Verbalizes hopelessness _____   Hopelessness
  Perceives/verbalizes loss of control _____   Powerlessness

Sensory/Perception
  History of restricted environments _____   Sensory/perception
  Vision impaired _____ Glasses _____   Visual
  Auditory impaired _____ Hearing aid _____   Auditory
  Kinesthetic impaired _____   Kinesthetic
  Gustatory impaired _____   Gustatory

Fig. 23-1, cont'd

Continued.

Tactile impaired _____   Tactile
Olfactory impaired· _____   Olfactory
Reflexes: grossly intact _____
Evidence of: Inattentiveness _____ Distractibility _____   Attention
     Hyperalertness _____ Selective attention _____
     Unilateral neglect _____

EXCHANGING ▪ A pattern involving mutual giving and receiving
Circulation
Cerebral   Cerebral tissue perfusion
Neurologic changes/symptoms _____

Pupils	Eye opening
L 2 3 4 5 6 mm	None (1)
R 2 3 4 5 6 mm	To pain (2)
Reaction: Brisk _____	To speech (3)
Sluggish _____. Nonreactive _____	Spontaneous (4)

Best Verbal   Best Motor   Fluid volume
   No response (1)   Flaccid (1)   Deficit
   Incomprehensible sound (2)   Extensor response (2)   Excess
   Inappropriate words (3)   Flexor response (3)   Cardiac output
   Confused conversation (4)   Semipurposeful (4)
   Oriented (5)   Localized to pain (5)
                                 Obeys commands (6)

Glasgow Coma Scale total _____
Neurologic deficits _____ Etiology _____
CT scan _____ MRI _____
Cardiac   Cardiopulmonary tissue
Apical rate & rhythm _____ PMI _____   perfusion
Heart sounds/murmurs _____   Fluid volume
Dysrhythmias _____   Deficit
Pacemaker _____   Excess
BP: _____   Cardiac output
                                            Peripheral tissue perfusion

Peripheral
   Jugular venous distention: yes/no   R _____ L _____
   Pulses: A = absent   B = bruits   D = doppler
       +3 = bounding   +2 = palpable   +1 = faintly palpable

Carotid	R _____ L _____	Popliteal	R _____ L _____	Fluid volume
Brachial	R _____ L _____	Posterior tibial	R _____ L _____	Deficit
Radial	R _____ L _____	Dorsalis pedis	R _____ L _____	Excess
Femoral	R _____ L _____			

Skin temp _____ Color/warmth _____ Turgor _____
Capillary refill _____ Clubbing _____   Cardiac output
Edema _____
Appearance of skin on lower extremities _____

Physical Integrity
Tissue integrity: Rashes _____ Lesions _____   Impaired skin integrity
Petechiae _____ Bruises _____   Impaired tissue integrity
Abrasions _____ Surgical incisions _____
Decubitus ulcers _____ Skin turgor _____   Injury
Pigmentation _____   Trauma
History of falls/accidents _____

Fig. 23-1, cont'd

Oxygenation

Complaints of dyspnea _____ Precipitated by _____
Orthopnea _____
Rate _____ Rhythm _____ Depth _____
Labored/unlabored (circle)
Use of accessory muscles _____
Chest expansion _____ Splinting _____
Cough: productive/nonproductive _____
Sputum: Color _____ Amount _____ Consistency _____
Breath sounds _____

Ineffective airway clearance
Ineffective breathing patterns
Impaired gas exchange

Physical Regulation

Immune
   Lymph nodes enlarged _____ Location _____
   WBC count _____ Differential _____
   Temperature _____ Route _____

Body temperature
Infection
Hypothermia
Hyperthermia
Ineffective thermoregulation

Nutrition
Eating patterns

   Number of meals per day _____
   Special diet _____ Snacks _____
   Where eaten _____ Typical 24-hour intake _____

   Food preferences/intolerances _____
   Food allergies _____
   Caffeine intake (coffee, tea, soft drinks) _____
   Appetite changes _____
   Anorexia/nausea/vomiting _____
   Diverticulitis _____ Ulcers _____
Condition of mouth/tongue _____
Dentures _____ Last dental examination _____
Height _____ Weight _____ Recent weight changes _____
Current therapy
   NPO _____ NG suction _____
   Enteral nutrition _____ TPN _____
   Vitamins _____
   IV fluids _____
Labs (list date)
   Hemoglobin _____ Hematocrit _____ RBC _____
   Na _____ K _____ CL _____ Glucose _____
   Cholesterol _____ Triglycerides _____ Fasting _____
   Other _____

Nutrition

Oral mucous membrane
Less/more than body
  requirements

Fluid volume
  Deficit
  Excess

Elimination

GI/bowel
Usual bowel patterns _____
Alterations from normal (ostomy) _____
Abdominal physical examination: Appearance _____
   Bowel sounds _____ Palpable organs _____
   Ascites _____ Tenderness _____
   Distention _____
Rectal examination: Impaction _____ Mass _____
   Hemorrhoids _____ Blood in stool _____
Remedies used (e.g., antacids) _____
   Indigestion _____ Abdominal pain _____

Bowel elimination
  Constipation
  Diarrhea
  Incontinence
GI tissue perfusion

Fig. 23-1, cont'd

Continued.

Renal/urinary

Usual urinary pattern _____

Alteration from normal (ostomy) _____

Bladder distention _____

Color _____ Odor _____ Blood _____ Catheter _____

Urine output: 24 hour _____ Average hourly _____

Serum BUN _____ Serum creatinine _____

Specific gravity _____

Urinary elimination
Incontinence
Retention

Renal tissue perfusion

Prioritized nursing diagnosis/problem list

1. _____
2. _____
3. _____
4. _____
5. _____

Signature _____ Date _____

Fig 23-1, cont'd

GERONTOLOGIC ASSESSMENT TOOL

Name _L.M._   Age _77_   Sex _F_

Address _50 SOUTH ST., SPRINGFIELD, MA._   Telephone _312 - 5551_

Significant other _DAUGHTER_   Telephone _312 - 0992_

Date of admission _12/6_   Medical diagnosis _S/P AORTIC VALVE REPLACEMENT (12/2)_

Allergies _NKA_   Historical source _PT., DAUGHTER, CHART_

Nursing Diagnosis
(Potential or Altered)

COMMUNICATING ▪ A pattern involving sending messages

(Read) (write) (understand) English (circle) _____   Communication

Other languages _Ø_   Verbal

Intubated _Ø_   Speech impaired _Ø_   Nonverbal

Alternate form of communication _Ø_

Physical impairment affecting communications _(DENTURES)_

   Expressive versus receptive aphasia _Ø_

VALUING ▪ A pattern involving the assigning of relative worth

Religious preference _ROMAN CATHOLIC_   Spiritual state

Important religious practices _MASS q SUNDAY_   Distress

Cultural orientation _WHITE, MIDDLE CLASS_   Despair

Important cultural practices (i.e., food, treatment) _NO SPECIAL PRACTICES VERBALIZED_

RELATING ▪ A pattern involving establishing bonds

Role

(Role performance)

   Marital status _WIDOW X 3 YRS._   Parenting

   Age & health of significant other _50 yo DAUGHTER, GOOD HEALTH_   Sexual dysfunction

   With whom do you live? _ALONE_   Work

   Number of children _4_ Ages _50♀, 48♂, 45♀, 43♂_   Family

   Addresses of children _DTR: 100 MAIN ST., SPRINGFIELD_   Social/leisure

   Pets _Ø_

   Role in home _HOMEMAKER_   Family processes

   Financial support _ABOUT $800/mo. + SAVINGS_

   Occupation _HOMEMAKER_   Retired _N/A_

   Job satisfaction/concerns _Ø_

   Volunteer work _Ø_

   Physical/mental energy expenditures (work, home, volunteering)
   LITTLE ENERGY EXPENDED, RARELY GOES OUT

   Sexual relationships (satisfactory/unsatisfactory) _"INACTIVE"_   Sexuality patterns

     Physical difficulties/effects of illness on relationships
     HARDER TO SOCIALIZE

   Recent losses (role) (functional ability) (home) (significant others) _HOME NOW THREATENED, HAS RESOLVED GRIEF OF HUSBAND'S DEATH_

Socialization

   Quality of relationships with others _MAINLY c̄ CHILDREN_   (Impaired social interaction)

     Patient's description _"I DON'T REALLY HAVE FRIENDS ANYMORE."_

     Significant others' descriptions _DTR AGREES, CONCERNED ABOUT ISOLATION_

     Staff observations _ONLY DTR VISITS_

   Verbalizes feelings of being alone _No_   Depressed _No_   (Social isolation)

   Attributed to _Ø_   Social withdrawal

   Social status _MIDDLE CLASS_

Fig. 23-2

Continued.

CHOOSING ▪ A pattern involving the selection of alternatives
Coping

Patient's usual problem-solving methods *"OFTEN DENIES EXISTENCE OF PROBLEM, IN PAST ABLE TO COPE" (PER DTR)*

Family's usual problem-solving methods *TALK, MAKE PLANS, REVISE AS NEEDED — ESPECIALLY c̄ DTR*

Patient's method of dealing with stress *WORRIES OCCASIONALLY, OFTEN DENIES, TALKS TO DTR*

Family's method of dealing with stress *TALKING, "TAKING A BREAK" FROM THE STRESSOR (DTR)*

Patient's affect *PLEASANT, UNCONCERNED*

Physical manifestations *NO UNUSUAL MANNERISMS*

(Ineffective individual coping)
Ineffective family coping

Participation

Compliance with past/current health regimens *POOR IN PAST YEAR SECONDARY TO ↓ MEMORY AND ↓ ATTENTION*

Willingness to comply with future health care regimen *WILLING TO TRY, ACKNOWLEDGES SHE NEEDS SUPERVISION*

Family support available *DTR AND SONS*

Other resources available *DAY-CARE, CHURCH (ST. JOHN'S)*

Noncompliance
Ineffective participation

Judgment

Decision-making ability
Patient's perspective *CAN MAKE DECISIONS*
Others' perspectives *"CONFUSED" (DTR)*

(Judgment
Indecisiveness)

KNOWING ▪ A pattern involving the meaning associated with information

Current health problems *AORTIC VALVE DISEASE (AVR 12/2), TROUBLE c̄ MEMORY; AGITATED AT NIGHT; HYPERTENSION, HYPOTHYROID, DIABETES, UNSTEADY GAIT*

(Knowledge deficit)

Previous illness/hospitalizations/surgeries *3-4 HOSPITALIZATIONS FOR CHF (AORTIC STENOSIS); APPENDECTOMY (CAN'T RECALL DATES)*

Previous accidents/injuries *FELL p̄ SYNCOPAL EPISODE IN HOSPITAL*

(Thought processes)

History of the following:

Heart disease _✓_ CHF _✓_ Peripheral vascular _Ø_
Rheumatic fever _Ø_ HTN _✓_ Lung disease _Ø_
Bronchitis _Ø_ Asthma _Ø_ TB _Ø_
Pneumonia _✓_ Influenza _Ø_ Liver _Ø_
Gallbladder _Ø_ Kidney _Ø_
Cerebrovascular _RISK_ Stroke _Ø_ Seizures _Ø_
Thyroid _✓ (HYPO)_ Gout _Ø_
Cancer _Ø_ Anemia _Ø_
Prostate _NA_ Diabetes _✓ NEW ONSET_
Alzheimer's disease _Ø_ Osteoarthritis _Ø_
Rheumatoid arthritis _Ø_ Osteoporosis _Ø_
Cataract _Ø_ Glaucoma _Ø_
Smoking _Ø_ Alcohol _RARE_ Psychiatric illness _Ø_

Orientation
Confusion
Memory

Family health history *FATHER: ↓ MI (50 yo) SIBLINGS: HEART, CVA*

Current medications:	Dose	Route	Frequency
Over-the-counter			
ASA	_250 mg_	_P.O._	_qd_

Fig. 23-2, cont'd

Prescription

REG. INSULIN ON SLIDING SCALE   *MACRODANTIN 100mg PO q A.M.*

MELLARIL 25 mg PO TID   *KCL 40 mEq PO qd*

APRESOLINE 25mg PO q 8°   *COLACE ↑ qd*

SYNTHYROID 0.1 mg PO qd

DIGOXIN   0.125 mg PO qd   *(PT. COULD NOT STATE*

LASIX   40 mg PO qd   *MEDS/DOSAGES)*

Immunization status *CAN'T RECALL*

Knowledge/perception of illness *POOR, ONLY KNOWS "HAD SURGERY TO FIX HEART."*

Knowledge/perception of planned therapy *"TO GET BETTER" "TO RECOVER FROM SURGERY"*

Expectations of therapy *"TO FEEL BETTER"*

Misconceptions *SOMETIMES THINKS SHE IS AT HOME*

Readiness to learn *SEEMS INTERESTED, BUT ↓ ATTENTION*   ⬭ Thought processes

   Request information concerning *NONE REQUESTED*

   Educational level *HIGH SCHOOL*

   Learning impeded by *↓ ATTENTION, ↓ MEMORY, CONFUSION, RECUPERATION*

Orientation

Level of alertness *ALERT, BUT CONFUSED AT TIMES*   Orientation

Orientation: Person ✓   Place *USUALLY* Time *USUALLY*   ⬭ Confusion

Appropriate behavior/communication *APPROPRIATE, BUT SOMETIMES CONFUSED*

Memory

Memory intact: ⬭yes/no   Recent *OCCASIONAL* Remote *USUALLY*   Memory

   CONFUSION   ACCURATE

FEELING ▪ A pattern involving the subjective awareness of information

Comfort

   Pain/discomfort: yes⬭no *STERNAL INCISION "ITCHES"*   Comfort

   Onset *N/A*   Duration *N/A*   Pain/chronic

   Location *N/A*   Quality *N/A*   Radiation *N/A*   Pain/acute

   Associated factors *N/A*   Discomfort

   Aggravating factors *N/A*

   Alleviating factors (meds, TENS) *N/A*

   Claudication ⊖

Emotional Integrity/States

   Emotional status: Angry ⊖   Denial ✓   Depressed ⊖   Grieving

   Cooperative *YES*   Other *CONFUSED*   Anxiety

   Recent stressful life events *SURGERY, FUNCTIONAL DIFFICULTIES*   Fear

             Anger

   Verbalizes feelings of *(DENIES PROBLEMS)*   Guilt

   Source *PT.*   Shame

   Physical manifestations (of ~~fear, anger~~) *DENIAL: CONTINUES*   Sadness

   PRACTICES THAT PLACE HER AT RISK   Violence

   Evidence of aggression: Toward self ⊖

   Toward others ⊖   Toward environment ⊖

   Does patient desire counseling? *NOT REQUESTED*

MOVING ▪ A pattern involving activity

Activity

   Ambulation ✓   OOB/transferring ✓   ⬭ Impaired physical mobility

   Assistance *YES*   ⬭ *SAFETY HAZARD*

   History of physical disability *UNSTEADY GAIT*

Fig. 23-2, cont'd

Continued.

Use of devices (protheses, cane, wheel chair) *WALKER*   Activity intolerance

Limitations in daily activities *NONE TILL NOW — GAIT PROBLEM NEW*
Verbal report of (fatigue) or weakness *OCCASIONALLY*
Exercise habits *WALKS IN APT., ERRANDS TO STORE*

Rest
Hours slept/night *5-6°/NIGHT* Feels rested: (yes) no *SOMETIMES*   Sleep pattern disturbances
Sleep aids (pillows, meds, food) *MELLARIL FOR AGITATION*   Hypersomnia
Difficulty falling/remaining asleep *WHEN AGITATED*   Insomnia
                                                                            Nightmares

Recreation
Leisure activities *TV, READS*   Deficit in diversional activity
Social activities *FAMILY VISITS*
Resources available (community, church) *(DOESN'T USE)*

Environmental Maintenance
Home maintenance management   Impaired home maintenance
   Size & arrangement of home (stairs, bathroom) *Sm. 1 BEDROOM APT.,*   management
   IN DISARRAY PER DTR. _____ Safety needs *CLUTTER IN APT.*   (Safety hazards)
   Transportation available *DTR*
   Housekeeping responsibilities *ALL, BUT CAN'T KEEP UP*

Health Maintenance
Health insurance *MEDICARE*   Health maintenance
Regular physical checkups *YES*
Date of last checkup: Rectal *11/87*
   Female: PAP *11/87* ___ Pelvic *11/87* ___ Breast *11/87*
      Self-breast *No* ___ Onset of menopause *14 yo*   Menstrual patterns
   Male: Testicular *N/A* ___ BPH *N/A*

Self-Care
Ability to perform ADLs: Independent *EATING* ___ Dependent *✓* :   Self-care
~~Specific deficits~~ *NEEDS ASSIST. c̄ BATHING, TOILET, DRESSING*   Feeding
Discharge planning needs: *HOME CARE*   (Bathing/hygiene
Referrals *HOME CARE, VISITING NURSES*   Dressing/grooming
Community resources available *CENTER, FAMILY, CHURCH*   Toileting)
Financial management *NEEDS ASSIST.* Taking medications *NEEDS ASSIST.*

PERCEIVING ▪ A pattern involving the reception of information
Self-Concept
Patient's description of self *HAPPY*   Self-concept
Effects of illness/surgery on self-concept *NONE*   Body image
                                                                            Self-esteem
                                                                            Personal identity

Meaningfulness
Verbalizes hopelessness *No*   Hopelessness
Perceives/verbalizes loss of control *No*   Powerlessness

Sensory/Perception
History of restricted environments *NO*   Sensory/perception
Vision impaired *OK c̄ GLASSES* Glasses *✓*   Visual
Auditory impaired *SLIGHT* ___ Hearing aid *∅*   Auditory
Kinesthetic impaired *USES WALKER, OCCASIONALLY UNSTEADY*   (Kinesthetic)
Gustatory impaired *No*   Gustatory

Fig. 23-2, cont'd

Tactile impaired __No__   Tactile
Olfactory impaired __No__   Olfactory
Reflexes: grossly intact __YES__
Evidence of: Inattentiveness __SOMETIMES__ Distractibility __SOMETIMES__   (Attention)
  Hyperalertness __No__ Selective attention __SOMETIMES__
  Unilateral neglect __No__

EXCHANGING ▪ A pattern involving mutual giving and receiving

Circulation

Cerebral   Cerebral tissue perfusion
Neurologic changes/symptoms __UNSTEADY GAIT, MILD APRAXIA__

Pupils	Eye opening
L 2 ③ 4 5 6 mm	None (1)
R 2 ③ 4 5 6 mm	To pain (2)
Reaction: Brisk ✓	To speech (3)
Sluggish ___ Nonreactive ___	Spontaneous (④)

Best Verbal	Best Motor	
No response (1)	Flaccid (1)	Fluid volume
Incomprehensible sound (2)	Extensor response (2)	Deficit
Inappropriate words (3)	Flexor response (3)	Excess
Confused conversation (④)	Semipurposeful (4)	Cardiac output
Oriented (5)	Localized to pain (5)	
	Obeys commands (⑥)	

Glasgow Coma Scale total __14__
Neurologic deficits __CONFUSION__ Etiology __SURGERY, BED REST__
CT scan __FRONTAL ATROPHY__ MRI __⊖__

Cardiac   Cardiopulmonary tissue perfusion
  Apical rate & rhythm __108/min NSR__ PMI __5TH ICS-MCL__
  Heart sounds/murmurs __(PIG VALVE); NORMAL S₁ ʋS₂__   Fluid volume
  Dysrhythmias __⊖__   Deficit
  Pacemaker __⊖__   Excess
  BP: __100/70 (Ⓛ ARM SITTING)__   Cardiac output
     Peripheral tissue perfusion

  Peripheral
    Jugular venous distension: yes/ⓝⓞ   R __⊖__ L __⊖__
    Pulses: A = absent   B = bruits   D = doppler
      +3 = bounding   +2 = palpable   +1 = faintly palpable

Carotid R __2+__ L __2+__		Popliteal R __2+__ L __2+__	Fluid volume
Brachial R __|__ L __|__		Posterior tibial R __|__ L __|__	Deficit
Radial R __↓__ L __↓__		Dorsalis pedis R __↓__ L __↓__	Excess
Femoral R __↓__ L __↓__			

    Skin temp __WARM__ Color/warmth __PINK__ Turgor __FAIR__
    Capillary refill __LESS THAN 2 SEC__ Clubbing __⊖__   Cardiac output
    Edema __⊖__
    Appearance of skin on lower extremities __INTACT, PINK__

Physical Integrity

Tissue integrity: Rashes __⊖__ Lesions __⊖__   Impaired skin integrity
Petechiae __⊖__ Bruises __⊖__   Impaired tissue integrity
Abrasions __⊖__ Surgical incisions __HEALING STERNAL INCISION__
Decubitus ulcers __⊖__ Skin turgor __FAIR__   Injury
Pigmentation __NO UNUSUAL COLORING__   Trauma
History of falls/accidents __FELL X1 IN HOSPITAL—NO INJURY SUSTAINED__

Fig. 23-2, cont'd

Continued.

Oxygenation

Complaints of dyspnea __⊖__ Precipitated by __N/A__   Ineffective airway clearance
Orthopnea __⊖__   Ineffective breathing patterns
Rate __18/MIN__ Rhythm __WNL__ Depth __WNL__   Impaired gas exchange
Labored (unlabored) (circle)
Use of accessory muscles __NO__
Chest expansion __WNL__ Splinting __⊖__
Cough: productive (nonproductive) __ENCOURAGED TO COUGH; DEEP BREATHE__
Sputum: Color __⊖__ Amount __⊖__ Consistency __⊖__
Breath sounds __CLEAR__

Physical Regulation

Immune   Body temperature
  Lymph nodes enlarged __⊖__ Location __⊖__   Infection
  WBC count __6.5×10³/µL__ Differential __WNL__   Hypothermia
  Temperature __98.4° F__ Route __ORAL__   Hyperthermia
   Ineffective thermoregulation

Nutrition

Eating patterns   Nutrition
  Number of meals per day __3⁺ SNACKS__
  Special diet __↓Na, ↓FAT__ Snacks __YES; CHEESE/CRACKERS__
  Where eaten __HOME__ Typical 24-hour intake __CEREAL OR EGG,__
  __JUICE, COFFEE, TOAST; SANDWICH, SOUP; FROZEN DINNERS__
  Food preferences/intolerances __⊖__
  Food allergies __NKA__
  Caffeine intake ((coffee) (tea,) soft drinks) __1-2/d__
  Appetite changes __NO__
  Anorexia/nausea/vomiting __NO__
  Diverticulitis __NO__ Ulcers __NO__
Condition of mouth/tongue __WNL__   Oral mucous membrane
Dentures __YES (UPPER)__ Last dental examination __YRS AGO__   Less/more than body
Height __5' 4"__ Weight __135 lbs__ Recent weight changes __NO__   requirements
Current therapy
  NPO __⊖__ NG suction __⊖__   Fluid volume
  Enteral nutrition __⊖__ TPN __⊖__   Deficit
  Vitamins __⊖__   Excess
  IV fluids __⊖__
Labs
  Hemoglobin __11.6 g/dl__ Hematocrit __38%__ RBC __4.6×10⁶/µL__
  Na __137 mEq/L__ K __4.5 mEq/L__ CL __101 mEq/L__ Glucose __256 mg/dl__
  Cholesterol __⊖__ Triglycerides __⊖__ Fasting __YES__
  Other __CHECK BLOOD SUGAR FOR INSULIN DOSE__

Elimination

GI/bowel   Bowel elimination
  Usual bowel patterns __q̄d – qod__   Constipation
  Alterations from normal (ostomy) __⊖__   Diarrhea
  Abdominal physical examination: Appearance __PROTUBERANT__   Incontinence
    Bowel sounds __2+__ Palpable organs __⊖__   GI tissue perfusion
    Ascites __⊖__ Tenderness __⊖__
    Distention __⊖__
  Rectal examination: Impaction __⊖__ Mass __⊖__
    Hemorrhoids __⊖__ Blood in stool __⊖__
  Remedies used (e.g., antacids) __COLACE T̄ qd__
    Indigestion __⊖__ Abdominal pain __⊖__

Fig. 23-2, cont'd

Renal/urinary
    Usual urinary pattern _q 3-4°_
    Alteration from normal (ostomy) _∅_
    Bladder distention _∅_
    Color _YELLOW/CLEAR_ Odor _∅_ Blood _∅_ Catheter _d/c 2d POST. OR._
    Urine output: 24 hour _1.5-2L_ Average hourly _> 30 cc_
    Serum BUN _25 mg/dl_ Serum creatinine _1.0 mg/dl_
    Specific gravity _1.015_

Urinary elimination
    Incontinence
    Retention

Renal tissue perfusion

Prioritized nursing diagnosis/problem list
1. _CONFUSION R/T BED REST, SURGERY (? MEDS, BYPASS)_
2. _ALTERATIONS IN SELF-CARE R/T FATIGUE, SURGERY_
3. _KNOWLEDGE DEFICIT R/T CONFUSION ABOUT MEDS & SURGERY_
4. _SAFETY HAZARDS R/T IMPAIRED MOBILITY, CONFUSION_
5. _IMPAIRED SOCIAL INTERACTION R/T FEW OUTSIDE INTERESTS, FRIENDS._
Signature _Patricia C. Seifert, R.N._ Date _12/6_

Fig 23-2. cont'd

■ UNIT V ■
ASSESSING REHABILITATION PATIENTS

CHAPTER 24

CARDIAC REHABILITATION
ASSESSMENT TOOL

ANITA P. SHERER
POLLY RYAN

The Cardiac Rehabilitation Assessment Tool was designed to assess stable cardiovascular rehabilitation patients with unique biopsychosocial assessment needs. The tool incorporates signs and symptoms pertinent to cardiovascular rehabilitation patients to facilitate identification of nursing diagnoses. It also incorporates the *Standards of Cardiovascular Nursing Practice* developed by the American Nurses' Association and the American Heart Association Council on Cardiovascular Nursing. This chapter includes:

- *The way the tool was developed and refined*
- *The patient population and settings to which it applies*
- *Selected cardiac rehabilitation emphasis areas*
- *The way to use the tool*
- *Specific cardiac rehabilitation focus questions and parameters to assist the nurse in eliciting appropriate data*
- *The Cardiac Rehabilitation Assessment Tool*
- *A case study*
- *A completed version of the tool based on the case study*

DEVELOPMENT AND REFINEMENT OF THE TOOL

The Cardiac Rehabilitation Assessment Tool was developed from the nursing data base prototype (see Chapter 2). Many hemodynamic monitoring and critical care variables originally incorporated in the prototype were deleted and replaced with variables more appropriate to a cardiovascu-

lar rehabilitation assessment. The resultant tool was then modified based on the recommendations of cardiac rehabilitation nurse experts. Further, the content of the tool is supported by the literature from this field of nursing.

After the tool was developed and refined, it was clinically tested by cardiac rehabilitation nurse experts and clinical nurse specialists on 10 adult patients participating in Phases I, II, and III of cardiac rehabilitation programs. The testing evaluated the adequacy of the tool in terms of flow, space for recording data, and completeness of assessment variables. Based on the results, the tool was revised.

PATIENT POPULATION AND SETTING

The Cardiac Rehabilitation Assessment Tool was developed to assess the biopsychosocial needs of patients who have cardiovascular conditions such as hypertension, angina pectoris, myocardial infarction, and those who have undergone cardiac surgery. The tool was developed for use in outpatient cardiac rehabilitation programs but could easily be adapted for use in inpatient cardiac rehabilitation by modifying the physical assessment variables for this setting.

CARDIAC REHABILITATION EMPHASIS AREAS

Cardiac rehabilitation patients have specialized problems and needs. The Cardiac Rehabilitation Assessment Tool includes appropriate assessment variables for each of the nine human response patterns of the Unitary Person Framework. The tool focuses on prevalent problems in the cardiac rehabilitation patient population. Table 24-1 outlines these emphasis areas.

Table 24-1
Selected cardiac rehabilitation emphasis areas

Patterns	Emphasis areas to determine
Valuing	Spiritual despair related to cardiovascular illness
	Religion and culture as support systems
Relating	Support systems
	Effect of illness or surgery on roles and relationships
Knowing	Cardiovascular risk factors
	Learning needs related to life-style changes
	Understanding of illness and therapy
Feeling	Comprehensive data related to pain
	Anxiety, fear, grief, or loss
Moving	Activity tolerance
	Effects of illness or surgery on home maintenance (housekeeping and shopping)
Perceiving	Effects of illness or surgery on self-concept
	Locus of control
Exchanging	Cardiovascular physical assessment
Choosing	Patient's and family's adequacy in dealing with problems and stress
	Degree of future compliance with health care regimen
	Decision-making ability

HOW TO USE THE TOOL

To use the Cardiac Rehabilitation Assessment Tool effectively, nurses must first be familiar with the Unitary Person Framework (see Chapter 2), which provides the underlying framework for Taxonomy I. The nine human response patterns of the Unitary Person Framework serve as the major category headings for Taxonomy I and the tool. The sequence of the response patterns, as it appears in Taxonomy I, has been changed in the tool to permit a more logical ordering of assessment variables. Nursing diagnoses pertinent to the cardiac rehabilitation patient, along with the signs and symptoms necessary to identify them, are incorporated under the appropriate human response patterns.

Nurses must also realize that this tool is very different from conventional assessment tools. As a result, nurses may have some initial difficulty in using it. They should remember, however, that the tool was not designed to follow the organization or content of a traditional medical data base; the data collected do not solely reflect medical patterns. Rather, this tool elicits data about holistic patterns in ways not traditionally assessed by nurses. It pro-

vides a new method of collecting and synthesizing data and requires new thinking when processing data. This tool represents a nursing data base developed from a nursing model to permit a holistic nursing assessment to take place so nursing diagnoses can be identified.

Although nurses probably agree that a holistic nursing data base is desirable, it is realized that changing traditional assessment methods is not an easy task. For this reason, a trial usage period is recommended before any decisions about the tool's merits are made. During this period, nurses should assess 10 patients using the tool to become familiar and progressively more comfortable with its organization and data-collection methods. With experience, nurses will become accustomed to new ways of clustering and processing information. With continued use, the time necessary to complete the tool will be reduced. Most important, nurses will recognize the unique ability of the tool to elicit appropriate signs and symptoms. Nurses will discover that nursing diagnoses are easily identified when using this tool.

It is not necessary to complete the tool in one session. Priority sections can be completed during the initial assessment. Other sections or patterns can be completed within a time frame acceptable to the institution.

To elicit appropriate data, nurses should be familiar with the focus questions and parameters in the next section. When assessing specific signs and symptoms, the nurse circles the diagnosis in the right-hand column when deviations from normal are found. A circled diagnosis does not confirm a problem but simply alerts the nurse to the possibility that it exists. After completing the tool, the nurse scans the circled problems, synthesizes the data to determine whether other clusters of signs and symptoms support the problem, and decides whether the actual or potential diagnosis is present.

Some diagnoses are repeated several times in the right-hand column. These repetitions occur only within the appropriate response pattern and are convenient for identifying certain data directly with their corresponding nursing diagnosis. These diagnoses are not absolute but focus thinking and direct more detailed attention to a problem.

Certain signs and symptoms can indicate several diagnoses. For example, edema can indicate altered cardiac output and fluid volume excess. To avoid unnecessary repetition of assessment parameters, variables are arranged with the diagnosis most likely to result from the data assessed. Thus, data to support one diagnosis may occasionally be found in other patterns or arranged with other diagnoses. Therefore, synthesis of all data is essential.

The Cardiac Rehabilitation Assessment Tool is not intended to be the standardized and final format for assessment of cardiovascular patients across the country. An assessment tool must meet the needs and requirements of the institutions and nurses using it. The Cardiac Rehabilitation

Table 24-2
Cardiac rehabilitation assessment tool: focus questions and parameters

Variables	Focus questions and parameters
COMMUNICATING	
Inconsistent statements and/or behavior	Are the patient's comments appropriate to the conversation? Do they pertain to the immediate question or comment? Are the patient's behavior and verbal comments consistent?
KNOWING	
Difficulties taking medications	Most people have difficulty taking their medications all the time. Some people have trouble when they are away from home or on weekends; tell me when you have difficulty taking your medications."
Method of organizing medications	"How do you organize your medications?"
Patient's perceived risk factors	"What do you think caused your heart condition?"
Normal BP range	"When your blood pressure is checked, what are the usual readings? Have you ever been told you have high blood pressure?"
Exercise habits	"Do you exercise regularly? What type of exercise? How far and fast do you _____? How long does it take you to _____ (walk or bike) that far? How many times per week?"
Learning needs (assess for each risk factor)	"Do you have anything you feel you need or would like to learn about _____?" Does the patient demonstrate a lack of knowledge about certain topics or areas? Does the patient ask questions about a particular subject? Is the patient able to answer questions about the topic in question?
Description of daily intake	"Can you describe a typical day's meals and snacks?"
Glucose monitoring method	"Do you monitor your blood sugar level at home? How (by a glucometer or by testing urine)?"
Degree of diabetic control	"Do you feel your diabetes is well controlled? How many insulin reactions have you had in the past month? What is your average blood sugar?"
Method of monitoring exercise tolerance	"How do you monitor your tolerance to exercise (by symptoms or by monitoring pulse rate)?"
Understanding of disease	"Describe what _____ (a heart attack or heart surgery) is."
Expectations of treatment	"How do exercise, diet, and medications affect your heart? How will this exercise program help you?"
Rehabilitation goals	"What do you expect to gain from participating in this program?"
Preferred method of learning	"How do you prefer to learn? By written material or verbal explanations? (This question can help to identify the patient's reading ability.)
MOVING	
Verbal report of fatigue/ weakness interfering with exercise	"Does anything interfere with your normal exercise routine (i.e., fatigue or weakness)?"
PERCEIVING	
Patient's description of own strengths/weaknesses	"Describe your strengths as a person. Your weaknesses."
Patient's perception of health/ illness	"Tell me what has happened to you. What do you think caused this? What do you think will happen now? How serious do you feel this is? Do you feel you are able to influence your health through your actions, or do you feel your health is subject to fate?"
Patient's perception of life-style changes	"Do you feel that the life-style changes you need to make to reduce your risk of further heart disease are very restrictive or too difficult?"
CHOOSING	
Adequacy of social support available	"Do you have a specific person that you feel comfortable being around and talking with? Do you have family members or friends that you rely on to help you and support you when you need it?" Does the patient's support system seem adequate for the situation?

Assessment Tool is simply a working demonstration tool that is expected to be changed and revised by nurses in clinical practice. Further evaluation and refinement are necessary before adopting the tool for use in an institution. Nurses interested in changing, revising, and adapting this tool to a specific clinical setting should refer to Chapter 4.

HOW TO ELICIT APPROPRIATE DATA

Because the Unitary Person Framework and the Cardiac Rehabilitation Assessment Tool contain some terms that may be unfamiliar to nurses, specific cardiac rehabilitation focus questions and parameters were developed to elicit the information. These questions and parameters are in Table 24-2, which follows the content of the Cardiac Rehabilitation Assessment Tool (Fig. 24-1). The variables in bold type in the tool are described more fully in Table 24-2. For example, the variable about the degree of diabetic control under the "knowing pattern" is in bold type. If the nurse does not know what to ask to elicit this information, Table 24-2 can be used to direct the line of questioning. The questions and parameters provide clarity and guidance when eliciting data. They are not all inclusive, so nurses should not feel limited by them. Many other questions, based on the patient's situation and condition and the nurse's skill, could be asked to elicit the information. Questions and parameters for other data not in bold type were presented in Chapter 3.

CASE STUDY

The case study models the process a nurse uses when assessing a patient. Based on the clustering of information obtained during assessment, the nurse formulates nursing diagnoses.

Mrs. G.H. was assessed before beginning a Phase II cardiac rehabilitation program. She is 62 years old and suffered a myocardial infarction two months before. The Cardiac Rehabilitation Assessment Tool (Fig. 24-2) was used to assess Mrs. G.H.

BIBLIOGRAPHY

American Nurses' Association and the American Heart Association Council on Cardiovascular Nursing: Standards of cardiovascular nursing practice, Kansas City, Mo, 1981, ANA, Inc.

DiMatteo MR and DiNicola DD: Achieving patient compliance: the psychology of the medical practitioner's role, New York, 1982, Pergamon Press, Inc.

Frenn M, Borgeson D, Lee H, and Simandl G: Life-style changes in a cardiac rehabilitation program: a client perspective, J Cardiovasc Nurs 3(2):43, 1989.

Guzzetta CE and Dossey BM: Cardiovascular nursing: bodymind tapestry, St Louis, 1984, The CV Mosby Co.

Hurst JW: The heart, ed 6, New York, 1986, McGraw-Hill Inc.

Pender NJ: Health promotion in nursing practice, ed 2, Norwalk, Conn, 1987, Appleton & Lange.

Redman BK: The process of patient education, ed 6, St Louis, 1988, The CV Mosby Co.

Ryan P: Strategies for motivating life-style change, J Cardiovasc Nurs 1:54, 1987.

Underhill S, Woods S, Sivarajan E, and Halpenny CJ: Cardiac nursing, Philadelphia, 1982, JB Lippincott Co.

Wenger NK and Hellerstein HK: Rehabilitation of the coronary patient, ed 2, New York, 1984, John Wiley & Sons, Inc.

CARDIAC REHABILITATION ASSESSMENT TOOL

Name _____ Age _____ Sex _____
Address _____ Telephone _____
Significant other _____ Telephone _____
Date of admission _____ Medical diagnosis _____
Allergies _____

Nursing Diagnosis
(Potential or Altered)

COMMUNICATING ▪ A pattern involving sending messages
Read, write, understand English (circle) _____   Communication
Other languages: read, write, understand (circle) _____   Verbal
Speech impaired by dyspnea _____ Other _____   Nonverbal
Alternate form of communication _____
Difficulty expressing self verbally _____
Inconsistent statements and/or behavior _____

VALUING ▪ A pattern involving the assigning of relative worth
Religious preference _____   Spiritual state
Important religious practices _____   Distress
Spiritual concerns _____   Despair
Cultural orientation _____
Cultural practices _____

RELATING ▪ A pattern involving establishing bonds
Role
  Marital status _____   Role performance
  How long married/divorced/widowed _____   Parenting
  Age & health of significant other _____   Sexual dysfunction
  Number of children _____ Ages _____   Work
  Role in home _____   Family
  Financial support _____   Social/leisure
  Occupation _____   Family processes
    Job satisfaction/concerns _____
    _____
    Physical/mental energy expenditures _____
    _____
  Sexual relationships (satisfactory/unsatisfactory) _____
    Physical difficulties/effects of illness related to sex _____   Sexuality patterns
    _____

Socialization
  Quality of relationships with others _____   Impaired social interaction
    Patient's description _____   Social isolation
    Significant others' descriptions _____   Social withdrawal
    Staff observations _____
  Verbalizes feelings of being alone _____
    Attributed to _____

KNOWING ▪ A pattern involving the meaning associated with information
Cardiovascular history _____   Knowledge deficit
_____
_____
Previous illnesses/hospitalizations/surgeries _____

Fig. 24-1

Continued.

Other health problems _____

_____

Current medications   Knowledge deficit

Drug   Dosage   Times taken   Side effects

_____   _____   _____   _____

_____   _____   _____   _____

_____   _____   _____   _____

_____   _____   _____   _____

_____   _____   _____   _____

_____   _____   _____   _____

Difficulties taking medications _____

Method of organizing medications _____

Patient's perceived risk factors _____

Actual risk factors

  Hypertension: Diagnosed when _____ **Normal BP range** _____

    Controlled by _____ Regular BP checkups _____

    Low-sodium diet _____ **Exercise habits** _____

    Learning needs _____

  Hyperlipidemia: At present _____ Past history _____

    Cholesterol _____ Triglycerides _____ HDL _____ LDL _____

    Dietary habits _____ Knowledge of diet _____

    Exercise habits _____

    Learning needs _____

  Smoking: At present: _____ Past history _____

    _____ packs/day   Number of years _____ When stopped _____

    Previous attempts to quit _____ Complicated by _____

    Plans for cessation _____

    Learning needs _____

  Obesity: yes/no _____ Recent weight changes _____

    Previous dieting methods _____ Problems _____

    Description of daily intake _____

    Learning needs _____

  Diabetes: Type _____ Controlled by _____

    Most recent fasting glucose _____ Regular checkups _____

    Glucose monitoring method _____ ADA diet _____

    Degree of diabetic control _____

    Learning needs _____

  Sedentary living: Exercise habits _____

    Type _____ Frequency _____ Duration _____

    Method of monitoring exercise tolerance _____

    Learning needs _____

  Stress: Patient's description of stressors: Home _____

    Work _____ Social _____ Other _____

    Present/past management methods _____

    Effectiveness _____ Knowledge of other methods _____

    Learning needs _____

  Alcohol use: _____ Drinks/day Type _____

    Present/past excessive usage _____

    Plans for cessation _____

    Assistance/support available _____

    Learning needs _____

  Oral contraceptives: Type _____ How long taken _____

  Family history of cardiovascular disease, diabetes _____

Educational level _____

Understanding of disease _____

Fig. 24-1, cont'd

Expectations of treatment _____
Rehabilitation goals _____
Misconceptions _____
Learning needs _____
Preferred method of learning _____
Readiness to learn as indicated by questions _____
   Eye contact _____ Body language _____
   Learning impeded by _____   Thought processes
Memory intact: yes/no _____ Recent _____ Remote _____   Memory

FEELING ▪ A pattern involving the subjective awareness of information
Comfort   Comfort
   Pain/discomfort: yes/no _____
      Patient's perception of etiology of pain: Angina _____
      Incisional _____ Other _____
      Frequency _____ Location _____   Pain/chronic
      Duration _____ Quality _____ Radiation _____   Pain/acute
      Associated factors _____
      Aggravating factors _____   Discomfort
      Alleviating factors _____

Emotional Integrity/States
   Recent stressful life events _____   Anxiety
   _____   Fear
   Verbalizes feelings _____   Anger
      Source _____   Guilt
      _____   Shame
      Physical manifestations _____   Sadness
      _____   Grieving

MOVING ▪ A pattern involving activity
Activity
   History of physical disability _____   Impaired physical mobility
   _____   Activity intolerance
   Limitations in daily activities _____
   _____

   Verbal report of fatigue/weakness interfering with exercise _____
   _____
   Favorite sports activities _____

Rest
   Hours slept/night _____ Feels rested: yes/no _____   Sleep pattern disturbance
   Sleep aids (pillows, meds, food) _____
   Difficulty falling/remaining asleep _____

Recreation
   Leisure activities _____   Deficit in diversional activity
   Social activities _____

Environmental Maintenance
   Home maintenance management   Impaired home maintenance
      Size & arrangement of home (stairs, bathroom) _____   management
      _____ Safety needs _____   Safety hazards
      Home responsibilities _____
      _____

Health Maintenance
   Health insurance _____   Health maintenance
   Regular physical checkups _____

Fig. 24-1, cont'd

Continued.

Self-Care
  Ability to perform ADLs: Independent _____ Dependent _____
  Specify deficits _____
  _____

Self-care
  Feeding
  Bathing/hygiene
  Dressing/grooming
  Toileting

PERCEIVING ▪ A pattern involving the reception of information
Self-Concept
  Patient's description of self _____
  Effects of illness/surgery on self-concept _____
  _____

Self-concept
Body image
Self-esteem
Personal identity

  Patient's description of own strengths/weaknesses _____
  _____
  Patient's perception of health/illness _____
  Patient's perception of life-style changes _____

Meaningfulness
  Verbalizes hopelessness _____
  Verbalizes/perceives loss of control _____
  Verbalizes grief related to loss of health _____

Hopelessness
Powerlessness

Sensory/Perception
  Sensory/perceptual deficits: Specify _____
  _____
  Glasses _____ Hearing Aid _____

Sensory/perception
Visual
Auditory
Kinesthetic
Olfactory
Gustatory
Tactile

EXCHANGING ▪ A pattern involving mutual giving and receiving
Circulation
  Cerebral
    Level of alertness _____
    Neurologic changes/symptoms _____
    Appropriate examination _____
  Cardiac
    PMI _____ Pacemaker _____
    Apical rate & rhythm _____
    Heart sounds/murmurs _____
    Dysrhythmias _____
    BP: R _____ L _____ Position: _____
  Peripheral
    Jugular venous distention: yes/no _____ R _____ L _____
    Pulses _____
    Skin temp _____ Color _____
    Capillary refill _____ Clubbing _____
    Edema _____ Claudication _____

Cerebral tissue perfusion

Cardiopulmonary tissue
  perfusion
Cardiac output

Fluid volume
  Deficit
  Excess

Peripheral tissue perfusion

Physical Integrity
  Tissue integrity _____ Surgical incision _____
  Abnormalities: specify _____

Impaired skin integrity
Impaired tissue integrity

Oxygenation
  Respiratory pattern _____
  Abnormalities _____
  Breath sounds _____

Ineffective airway clearance
Ineffective breathing pattern
Impaired gas exchange

Fig. 24-1, cont'd

Nutrition
Eating patterns
Number of meals per day _____ Where eaten _____   Nutrition
Special diet _____   More than body
Food preferences/intolerances/allergies _____   requirements
Caffeine intake (coffee, tea, soft drinks, chocolate)

_____
Appetite changes _____
Height _____ Weight _____ Ideal body weight _____   Less than body requirements
Body fat measurements _____

Elimination
Bowel   Bowel elimination
Abnormal bowel patterns _____   GI tissue perfusion
Urinary   Urinary elimination
Abnormal urinary patterns _____   Renal tissue perfusion

CHOOSING ▪ A pattern involving the selection of alternatives
Coping
Patient's usual problem-solving methods _____   Ineffective individual coping
_____   Ineffective family coping
Family's usual problem-solving methods _____
_____
Patient's method of dealing with stress _____
_____
Family's method of dealing with stress _____
_____
Patient's affect _____
Physical manifestations _____
Coping mechanisms used _____
Adequacy of social support available _____

Participation
Compliance with past/current health care regimens _____   Noncompliance
_____   Ineffective participation
Willingness to comply with future health care regimen _____
_____

Judgment
Decision-making ability   Judgment
Patient's perspective _____   Indecisiveness
Others' perspectives _____

Prioritized nursing diagnosis/problem list
1. _____
2. _____
3. _____
4. _____
5. _____
6. _____
7. _____
8. _____
9. _____
10. _____

Signature _____   Date _____

Fig. 24-1, cont'd

CARDIAC REHABILITATION ASSESSMENT TOOL

Name _G.H._   Age _62_   Sex _F_

Address _99 Ninth Street, Milwaukee, Wisconsin_   Telephone _999-1000_

Significant other _Daughter — C.J._   Telephone _999-1000_

Date of admission _12/15_   Medical diagnosis _Myocardial Infarction 10/1 (Anterior MI)_

Allergies _NKA_

Nursing Diagnosis
(Potential or Altered)

COMMUNICATING ▪ A pattern involving sending messages

Read, write, (understand) English (circle) _Daughter reads and writes_   (Communication)

Other languages: read, write, understand (circle) _No_   Verbal

Speech impaired by dyspnea _No_   Other _No_   (Nonverbal)

Alternate form of communication _—_

Difficulty expressing self verbally _No difficulty_

Inconsistent statements and/or behavior _No_

VALUING ▪ A pattern involving the assigning of relative worth

Religious preference _Presbyterian_   Spiritual state

Important religious practices _Attends Bible study & evening church_   Distress

Spiritual concerns _Nothing specific_   _meetings_   Despair

Cultural orientation _American Caucasian_

Cultural practices _Nothing specific_

RELATING ▪ A pattern involving establishing bonds

Role

   Marital status _Divorced_   (Role performance)

   How long married/divorced/widowed _10 yrs._   Parenting

   Age & health of significant other _Lives c̄ daughter — 40 good health_   Sexual dysfunction

   Number of children _3_ Ages _Son-43; daughter-40; son-38_   (Work)

   Role in home _Grandmother — assists c̄ housework_   Family

   Financial support _On Title 19_   Social/leisure

   Occupation _Unemployed x6 mos. Was factory worker_   Family processes

     Job satisfaction/concerns _Very upset over recent job loss. Lack_
of money increases dependency on daughter. "I don't know what to do with my time."

     Physical/mental energy expenditures _Job was physically demanding_
and tiring. Unemployment has been a big stressor for her.

   Sexual relationships (satisfactory/unsatisfactory) _—_

     Physical difficulties/effects of illness related to sex _Not sexually_   Sexuality patterns
active @ this time

Socialization

   Quality of relationships with others _Good in general_   Impaired social interaction

     Patient's description _Good c̄ children/grandchildren/friends_   Social isolation

     Significant others' descriptions _Daughter reports good relationship_   Social withdrawal

     Staff observations _Pleasant loving interaction between pt. & family_

   Verbalizes feelings of being alone _No_

     Attributed to _—_

KNOWING ▪ A pattern involving the meaning associated with information

Cardiovascular history _"I had a heart attack in October." "Then they_   Knowledge deficit
said I had heart failure too." Cath showed 2 vessel disease
c̄ 100% proximal LAD lesion & 50% mid-RCA lesion. To be treated c̄ medications & exercise

Previous illnesses/hospitalizations/surgeries _Aortic valve replacement_
_in 1980_

Fig. 24-2

Other health problems _COPD (MILD)_
_____

Current medications

Knowledge deficit

Drug	Dosage	Times taken	Side effects
COUMADIN	2.5 mg	qod – 8 A.M.	BRUISES EASILY
LASIX	20 mg	qd – 8 A.M.	OCC. LEG CRAMPS – TAKES KCL
MICRO K	10 mEq	BID – 8 A.M. & 8 P.M.	
DIGOXIN	0.125 mg	qd – 8 A.M.	
VASOTEC	10 mg	qd – 8 A.M.	

Difficulties taking medications _SOMETIMES FORGETS PILLS IN EVENING_
Method of organizing medications _PUTS ONE DAY'S PILLS IN CUP IN A.M._
Patient's perceived risk factors _HTN, SMOKING_

Actual risk factors

Hypertension: Diagnosed when _1974_ Normal BP range _130/70 – 150/90_
   Controlled by _MEDS_ Regular BP checkups _SOMETIMES_
   Low-sodium diet _DOESN'T FOLLOW_ Exercise habits _FAIR – WALKS 2-3x/WK_
   Learning needs _IMPORTANCE OF LOW Na DIET & REGULAR CHECKUPS_
Hyperlipidemia: At present _YES_ Past history _YES x 5 YRS_
   Cholesterol _228 mg/dl_ Triglycerides _190 mg/dl_ HDL _—_ LDL _—_
   Dietary habits _HIGH FAT INTAKE_ Knowledge of diet _POOR_
   Exercise habits _WALK 2-3 x PER WEEK_
   Learning needs _NEEDS DIET INSTRUCTION_
Smoking: At present: _YES_ Past history _—_
   _1_ packs/day Number of years _40_ When stopped _STILL SMOKING_
   Previous attempts to quit _x 2_ Complicated by _UNDER STRESS → STARTS BACK_
   Plans for cessation _WOULD LIKE TO QUIT – WANTS HELP_
   Learning needs _ASSISTANCE IN ARRANGING SMOKING CESSATION CLASSES_
Obesity: yes/no _No_ Recent weight changes _—_
   Previous dieting methods _—_ Problems _—_
   Description of daily intake _—_
   Learning needs _—_
Diabetes: Type _No_ Controlled by _—_
   Most recent fasting glucose _—_ Regular checkups _—_
   Glucose monitoring method _—_ ADA diet _—_
   Degree of diabetic control _—_
   Learning needs _—_
Sedentary living: Exercise habits _MOSTLY SEDENTARY – WAS ACTIVE c̄ JOB_
   Type _WALKING_ Frequency _2-3x/WK_ Duration _15 MIN._
   Method of monitoring exercise tolerance _SYMPTOMS → FATIGUE/ANGINA_
   Learning needs _IMPROVE CONSISTENT ADHERENCE, PULSE MONITORING_
Stress: Patient's description of stressors: Home _LIMITED IN DOING HOUSEWORK_
   Work _UNEMPLOYED_ Social _—_ Other _—_
   Present/past management methods _KEPT BUSY c̄ CHORES/NEEDLEWORK_
   Effectiveness _FAIR_ Knowledge of other methods _ABSENT_
   Learning needs _STRESS MANAGEMENT TECHNIQUES_
Alcohol use: _No_ Drinks/day Type _—_
   Present/past excessive usage _—_
   Plans for cessation _—_
   Assistance/support available _—_
   Learning needs _—_
Oral contraceptives: Type _No_ How long taken _—_
Family history of cardiovascular disease, diabetes _FATHER c̄ HTN & MI_
   MOTHER c̄ CVA
Educational level _FINISHED 6TH GRADE_
Understanding of disease _"I LOST PART OF MY HEART"_

Fig. 24-2, cont'd

Continued.

Expectations of treatment *"EXERCISE WILL FIX MY HEART."*
Rehabilitation goals *WANTS TO GET STRONGER*
Misconceptions *FEELS EXERCISE PROGRAM WILL CURE HEART DISEASE*
Learning needs *TEACHING R/T ETIOLOGY OF CAD/MI/RISK FACTORS*
Preferred method of learning *VERBAL EXPLANATIONS, DISCUSSION*
Readiness to learn as indicated by questions *GOOD QUESTIONS/COMMENTS*
   Eye contact *OK*   Body language *POSITIVE — APPROPRIATE*
   Learning impeded by *EDUCATIONAL LEVEL — INABILITY TO READ*   Thought processes
Memory intact: yes/no *YES* Recent ✔   Remote ✔   Memory

FEELING ▪ A pattern involving the subjective awareness of information
Comfort   (Comfort)
   Pain/discomfort: yes/no *YES*
      Patient's perception of etiology of pain: Angina ✔
      Incisional ―――― Other ――――
      Frequency *2-3x/WK* Location *MID-CHEST AREA*   (Pain/chronic)
      Duration *3-5 MIN* Quality *PRESSURE* Radiation Ⓛ *ARM*   Pain/acute
      Associated factors *SOB*   *ING HAIR*
      Aggravating factors *WALKING FAST, CLIMBING STAIRS, VACUUMING, FIX-*   Discomfort
      Alleviating factors *RESTING, TAKING SUBLINGUAL NTG*

Emotional Integrity/States
   Recent stressful life events *LOSS OF FULL-TIME JOB AND ASSOCIATED*   (Anxiety)
HEALTH INSURANCE, HEART ATTACK & HOSPITALIZATION   Fear
   Verbalizes feelings *ANXIETY*   Anger
     Source *LOSS OF INCOME, PRESENT HEALTH STATE*   Guilt
                                             Shame
     Physical manifestations *TEARFUL WHEN DISCUSSING THIS. WRINGS*   Sadness
HANDS, FIDGETS   Grieving

MOVING ▪ A pattern involving activity
Activity
   History of physical disability *NONE*   Impaired physical mobility
                                          (Activity intolerance)
   Limitations in daily activities *ANGINA/SOB Ē FAST WALKS & CLIMBING*
STAIRS, CAN'T DO HOUSEWORK SOMETIMES, CAN'T FIX OWN HAIR SOMETIMES
   Verbal report of fatigue/weakness interfering with exercise *HAS TO STOP AND*
REST EVERY 5 MIN. WHEN WALKING, CAN CLIMB ONLY 3 STAIRS BETWEEN REST PERIODS
   Favorite sports activities *NONE*

Rest
   Hours slept/night *8* Feels rested: yes/no *YES*   Sleep pattern disturbance
   Sleep aids (pillows, meds, food) *NONE*
   Difficulty falling/remaining asleep *NONE*

Recreation
   Leisure activities *TV, SEWING*   Deficit in diversional activity
   Social activities *VISITING Ē FAMILY/CHURCH ACTIVITIES*

Environmental Maintenance
   Home maintenance management   Impaired home maintenance
      Size & arrangement of home (stairs, bathroom) *2ND FLOOR APT ONE*   management
LEVEL/MEDIUM SIZE Safety needs *NONE*   Safety hazards
      Home responsibilities *HELPS DAUGHTER BY DUSTING, WASHING*
DISHES, LIGHT MEALS

Health Maintenance
   Health insurance *LOST HEALTH INSURANCE Ē JOB*   Health maintenance
   Regular physical checkups *RAN OUT OF MEDS & HAD NO FOLLOW UP*
FOR 4 MONTHS UNTIL HAD MI. NOW RECEIVING SOCIAL SERVICE ASSISTANCE

Fig. 24-2, cont'd

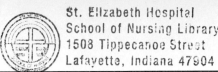

Self-Care
Ability to perform ADLs: Independent ✓ Dependent _____
Specify deficits _—_____

_____

Self-care
Feeding
Bathing/hygiene
Dressing/grooming
Toileting

PERCEIVING ▪ A pattern involving the reception of information
Self-Concept
Patient's description of self _"I'M EASY GOING/A HARD WORKER "___
Effects of illness/surgery on self-concept _"I'M JUST NOT THE SAME_
PERSON — I CAN'T DO AS MUCH AS I USED TO."
Patient's description of own strengths/weaknesses _"I'VE ALWAYS BEEN ABLE_
TO TAKE CARE OF MYSELF. I'M IMPATIENT."
Patient's perception of health/illness _FEELS LIMITED SINCE MI_
Patient's perception of life-style changes _DIFFICULT TO MAKE ALL THE_
CHANGES

Self-concept
Body image
Self-esteem
Personal identity

Meaningfulness
Verbalizes hopelessness _No_____
Verbalizes/perceives loss of control _CAN'T CONTROL UNEMPLOYMENT_
Verbalizes grief related to loss of health _Yes_____

Hopelessness
(Powerlessness)

Sensory/Perception _"DIDN'T KNOW WHERE TO TURN" UNTIL RECEIVED_
Sensory/perceptual deficits: Specify _NONE   SOCIAL SERVICE ASSISTANCE_

_____
Glasses _YES_____ Hearing Aid ___No_____

Sensory/perception
Visual
Auditory
Kinesthetic
Olfactory
Gustatory
Tactile

EXCHANGING ▪ A pattern involving mutual giving and receiving
Circulation
Cerebral
Level of alertness _ALERT_____
Neurologic changes/symptoms _NONE_____
Appropriate examination _—_____

Cerebral tissue perfusion

Cardiac
PMI _5TH ICS @ MCL_ Pacemaker _No_____
Apical rate & rhythm _86 REGULAR_____
Heart sounds/murmurs _NORMAL S_1 & S_2____
Dysrhythmias _RARE PVC_____
BP: R _124/70_ L _128/74_ Position: _SITTING_____
Peripheral
Jugular venous distention: yes/no _No___ R _—_ L _—_
Pulses _PALPABLE BILATERALLY_____
Skin temp _WARM___ Color _PINK_____
Capillary refill _GOOD, < 1-2 SECS_ Clubbing _NEGATIVE_
Edema _SLIGHT PEDAL_____ Claudication _NONE_____

Cardiopulmonary tissue
perfusion
Cardiac output

Fluid volume
Deficit
Excess

Peripheral tissue perfusion

Physical Integrity
Tissue integrity _INTACT___ Surgical incision _OLD WELL-HEALED_
Abnormalities: specify _NONE_____ _STERNOTOMY_

Impaired skin integrity
Impaired tissue integrity

Oxygenation
Respiratory pattern _REGULAR, UNLABORED, 20_____
Abnormalities _OCCASIONAL PRODUCTIVE COUGH_____
Breath sounds _CLEAR BILATERALLY_____

Ineffective airway clearance
Ineffective breathing pattern
Impaired gas exchange

Fig. 24-2, cont'd

Continued.

Nutrition
Eating patterns
Number of meals per day ___3___ Where eaten ___HOME___
Special diet ___No___
Food preferences/intolerances/allergies ___NO MILK___
Caffeine intake (coffee, tea, soft drinks, chocolate)
___2-3 CUPS COFFEE/DAY___
Appetite changes ___NONE___
Height ___5' 4"___ Weight ___124 lbs.___ Ideal body weight ___120 lbs.___
Body fat measurements ___NOT MEASURED AS OF YET___

Nutrition

More than body
requirements

Less than body requirements

Elimination
Bowel
Abnormal bowel patterns ___NO PROBLEMS___
Urinary
Abnormal urinary patterns ___NO PROBLEMS___

Bowel elimination
GI tissue perfusion
Urinary elimination
Renal tissue perfusion

CHOOSING ▪ A pattern involving the selection of alternatives
Coping
Patient's usual problem-solving methods ___POOR PROBLEM SOLVING___
___SKILLS R/T HEALTH CARE NEEDS — REQUIRES ASSISTANCE___
Family's usual problem-solving methods ___SOMETIMES TALKS OVER___
___PROBLEM ∨ TRIES TO SOLVE IT___
Patient's method of dealing with stress ___SOMETIMES IGNORES___
___PROBLEM, KEEPS BUSY___
Family's method of dealing with stress ___PULLS TOGETHER ∨ HELPS___
___EACH OTHER___
Patient's affect ___PLEASANT, COOPERATIVE___
Physical manifestations ___BODY LANGUAGE SUGGESTS NERVOUSNESS IN DISCUSSING THIS___
Coping mechanisms used ___DENIAL___
Adequacy of social support available ___DAUGHTER/GRANDCHILDREN/SONS SUPPORTIVE___

(POTENTIAL)
(Ineffective individual coping)
Ineffective family coping

Participation
Compliance with past/current health care regimens ___DOES WELL WITH___
___BASIC INSTRUCTIONS___
Willingness to comply with future health care regimen ___ANTICIPATE SOME___
___DIFFICULTIES FOLLOWING HEALTH CARE REGIMEN___

(Noncompliance) (POTENTIAL)
Ineffective participation

Judgment
Decision-making ability
Patient's perspective ___FEELS ABLE TO MAKE DECISIONS — OFTEN___ ASKS CHILDREN
Others' perspectives ___NEEDS ASSISTANCE c̄ HEALTH CARE DECISIONS___

(Judgment)
Indecisiveness

Prioritized nursing diagnosis/problem list
1. ___KNOWLEDGE DEFICIT R/T RISK FACTOR MODIFICATIONS ∨ DISEASE PROCESS___
2. ___ACTIVITY INTOLERANCE R/T ANGINA ∨ DYSPNEA___
3. ___ANXIETY R/T LOSS OF INCOME ∨ PRESENT HEALTH STATE___
4. ___POTENTIAL FOR NONCOMPLIANCE___
5. ___ALTERED SELF-CONCEPT R/T CHANGES IN HEALTH STATE___
6. ___ALTERED ROLE PERFORMANCE R/T WORK D/T UNEMPLOYMENT___
7. ___ALTERED COMFORT R/T CHRONIC PAIN D/T ANGINA___
8. ___POWERLESS R/T UNEMPLOYMENT___
9. ___POTENTIAL INEFFECTIVE INDIVIDUAL COPING___
10. ___ALTERED NONVERBAL COMMUNICATION R/T INABILITY TO READ ∨ WRITE___
Signature ___Anita P. Shرer, R.N.___ Date ___5/20___

Fig. 24-2, cont'd

CHAPTER 25

STROKE REHABILITATION ASSESSMENT TOOL

ANITA P. SHERER
HELEN A. BOZZO

The Stroke Rehabilitation Assessment Tool was designed to assess stable cerebrovascular accident (CVA) patients with unique biopsychosocial assessment needs. The tool incorporates signs and symptoms pertinent to CVA patients to facilitate identification of nursing diagnoses. It also incorporates the *Standards of Rehabilitation Nursing Practice* developed by the American Nurses' Association and the Association of Rehabilitation Nurses. This chapter includes:

- *The way the tool was developed and refined*
- *The patient population and settings to which it applies*
- *Selected stroke rehabilitation emphasis areas*
- *The way to use the tool*
- *Specific stroke rehabilitation focus questions and parameters to assist the nurse in eliciting appropriate data*
- *The Stroke Rehabilitation Assessment Tool*
- *A case study*
- *A completed version of the tool based on the case study*

DEVELOPMENT AND REFINEMENT OF THE TOOL

The Stroke Rehabilitation Assessment Tool was developed from the nursing data base prototype (see Chapter 2). Many hemodynamic monitoring and critical care variables originally incorporated in the prototype were replaced with in-depth musculoskeletal, neurologic, and self-care assessment variables more applicable to a stroke rehabilitation assessment. Emphasis was placed on the patient's patterns and habits before and after the disability, as well as on communication and sensory-perceptual deficits. The resultant tool was then modified based on the recommendations of stroke rehabilitation nurse experts. Further, the content of this tool is supported by the literature from this field of nursing.

After the tool was developed and refined, it was clinically tested by stroke rehabilitation nurse experts and clinical nurse specialists on 10 adult patients, ages 57 to 86, in rehabilitation units of acute care hospitals and in comprehensive rehabilitation hospitals. All patients had suffered CVAs and were being assessed for rehabilitation potential. Some patients were assessed when admitted to the rehabilitation units in acute care hospitals or before referral to other facilities; others were assessed when admitted to the comprehensive rehabilitation facility. The testing evaluated the adequacy of the tool in terms of flow, space for recording data, and completeness of assessment variables. Based on the results, the Stroke Rehabilitation Assessment Tool was revised.

PATIENT POPULATION AND SETTING

The Stroke Rehabilitation Assessment Tool was developed for use with stable CVA patients requiring assessment to determine their rehabilitation potential and nursing care needs. The tool can be used in many rehabilitation settings, including comprehensive rehabilitation facilities, rehabilitation or CVA units in acute care hospitals, rehabilitation units in nursing homes, or outpatient rehabilitation centers serving CVA patients. The tool could easily be revised for use in home health care though adjustments in assessment parameters would need to be made. The tool is intended for use with stable patients recovering from

CVAs regardless of causes. For patients with severe communication deficits, the family or significant other may provide necessary information.

STROKE REHABILITATION EMPHASIS AREAS

Stroke rehabilitation patients have specialized problems and needs. The Stroke Rehabilitation Assessment Tool includes appropriate assessment variables within each of the nine human response patterns of the Unitary Person Framework. The tool focuses on prevalent problems in the stroke rehabilitation patient population. Table 25-1 outlines these emphasis areas.

HOW TO USE THE TOOL

To use the Stroke Rehabilitation Assessment Tool effectively, nurses must first be familiar with the Unitary Person Framework (see Chapter 2), which provides the underlying framework for Taxonomy I. The nine human response patterns of the Unitary Person Framework serve as the major category headings for Taxonomy I and the tool. The sequence of the response patterns, as it appears in Taxonomy I, has been changed in the tool to permit a more logical ordering of assessment variables. Nursing diagnoses pertinent to stroke rehabilitation patients, along with the signs and symptoms necessary to identify them, are incorporated under the appropriate human response pattern.

Nurses must also realize that this tool is very different from conventional assessment tools. As a result, nurses may have some initial difficulty in using it. They should remember, however, that the tool was not designed to follow the organization or content of a traditional medical data base. The data collected do not solely reflect medical patterns. Rather, this tool elicits data about holistic patterns in ways not traditionally assessed by nurses. It provides a new method of collecting and synthesizing data and requires new thinking when processing data. This tool represents a nursing data base developed from a nursing model to permit a holistic nursing assessment to take place so nursing diagnoses can be identified.

Although nurses probably agree that a holistic nursing data base is desirable, it is realized that changing traditional assessment methods is not an easy task. For this reason, a trial usage period is recommended before any decisions about the tool's merits are made. During this period, nurses should assess 10 patients using the tool to become familiar and progressively more comfortable with its organization and data-collection methods. With experience, nurses will become accustomed to new ways of clustering and processing information. With continued use, the time necessary to complete the tool will be reduced. Most important, nurses will recognize the unique ability of the tool to elicit appropriate signs and symptoms. Nurses will discover that nursing diagnoses are easily identified when using this tool.

It is not necessary to complete the tool in one session. Priority sections can be completed during the initial assessment. Other sections or patterns can be completed later, within a time frame acceptable to the institution. To elicit appropriate data, nurses should be familiar with the focus questions and parameters in the next section. When assessing specific signs and symptoms to indicate a diagnosis, the nurse circles the diagnosis in the right-hand column when deviations from normal are found. A circled diagnosis does not confirm a problem but alerts the nurse to the possibility that it exists. After completing the tool, the nurse scans the circled problems, synthesizes the data to determine whether other clusters of signs and symptoms support a problem, and decides whether the actual or potential diagnosis is present.

Some diagnoses are repeated several times in the right-hand column. These repetitions occur only within the appropriate response pattern and are convenient for identifying certain data directly with their corresponding nursing diagnosis. These diagnoses are not absolute but focus thinking and direct more detailed attention to a problem.

Certain signs and symptoms can indicate several diagnoses. For example, altered skin color can indicate im-

Table 25-1
Selected stroke rehabilitation emphasis areas

Patterns	Emphasis areas to determine
Communicating	Aphasia
Valuing	Spiritual despair related to stroke
	Religion and culture as support systems
Relating	Support systems
	Effect of disability on roles and relationships
Knowing	Cardiovascular risk factors
	Orientation and memory
Feeling	Comprehensive data related to pain
	Anxiety, fear, grief, or loss
	Emotional lability
Moving	Effects of stroke on home maintenance
	Musculoskeletal examination
	Self-care deficits
Perceiving	Sensory-perceptual deficits
	Effects of stroke on self-concept
Exchanging	Neurologic assessment
	Safety concerns
	Changes in nutrition and elimination related to stroke
Choosing	Patient's and family's adequacy in dealing with problems and stress
	Future compliance with health care regimen

Table 25-2

Stroke rehabilitation assessment tool: focus questions and parameters

Variables	Focus questions and parameters
COMMUNICATING	
Handedness	"Are you right- or left-handed?"
Aphasia	Is aphasia present? If yes, what type?
Expressive	Can the patient name common objects? Does the patient use gestures to convey needs? Is the patient's speech halting or non fluent? Does the patient demonstrate an awareness of a speech problem?
Receptive	Does the patient follow 1- or 2-step commands, repeat, or require gestures to follow commands? Is the patient's speech smooth or fluent, yet lack meaning or substance?
Symptoms of right hemisphere disorder	Does the patient exhibit verbose, tangential conversation, have difficulty understanding figurative language (proverbs and idioms), or lack emotional expression facially or verbally?
RELATING	
Effects of disability on role in home	"How has your stroke changed your responsibilities in your home and your role as spouse or parent? Has your stroke changed your relationship with your spouse or significant other? Do you feel able to carry out what is normally expected of you at home? How do you feel about these changes?"
Quality of relationship with others	Will the patient's communication deficits impair social interaction?
KNOWING	
Learning impeded by	Does the patient have aphasia, decreased attention span, apraxia, poor insight, or concrete thinking with inability to problem solve?
FEELING	
Verbalizes feelings of grief or loss	Does your knowledge of the patient's predisability life-style and current stroke deficits lead you to conclude that grieving is present or anticipated?
Displays inappropriate emotional responses (lability)	Does the patient demonstrate inappropriate emotional reactions (smiling one monent and crying the next or reacting unusually to comments)?
MOVING	
Performs volitional movements	Is the patient unable to execute a motor act on command (stick out tongue or wash face) (apraxia)?
Involuntary movements present	Does the patient exhibit uncontrollable movements? Tremors?
Safety precautions needed	Does the patient's musculoskeletal status indicate possible safety hazards (falls)?
Orthotic devices in use	Does the patient use a cane, walker, or splint?
PERCEIVING	
Abnormal head posture	Is the patient's head held in a fixed position (left or right)? Can a neutral head position be obtained?
Attention shown to affected side	Can the patient identify or touch the affected extremities and protect these extremities during movement?
Attention shown to environment	Does the patient attend to persons or objects in the environment on the affected side or require cueing to focus on a particular part of the environment?
Ability to focus on tasks/topics	Is the patient easily distracted by environmental stimuli? Does the patient require excessive cueing to complete or sequence a task properly?
Insight about stroke deficits/limitations	Does the patient realize what can and cannot be done because of the stroke?
EXCHANGING	
Awareness/nonawareness of new limitations	Does the patient's expression of capabilities and actions correlate accurately with stroke-related deficits? Is impulsiveness, diminished judgment, or decreased insight present?
Presence of "wet voice"	Does the patient's voice indicate excessive secretions?
Oral management of food/liquids	Does the patient have difficulty controlling the rate, bolus size, and quantity of foods and fluids taken? Is a gag reflex present? Does the patient drool food or liquids?
Choking/coughing/pocketing of food	Is there any choking or coughing when the patient attempts to swallow? Is food cleared from the cheek or retained on the affected side of the mouth?

paired peripheral tissue perfusion and impaired skin integrity. To avoid unnecessary repetition of assessment parameters, variables are arranged with the diagnosis most likely to result from the data assessed. Thus, data to support one diagnosis may occasionally be found in other patterns or arranged with other diagnoses. Therefore, synthesis of all data is essential.

The Stroke Rehabilitation Assessment Tool is not intended to be the standardized and final format for assessment of stroke patients across the country. An assessment tool must meet the needs and requirements of the institutions and nurses using it. The Stroke Rehabilitation Assessment Tool is simply a working demonstration tool that is expected to be changed and revised by nurses in clinical practice. Further evaluation and refinement are necessary before adopting the tool for use in an institution. Nurses interested in changing, revising, and adapting this tool to a specific clinical setting should refer to Chapter 4.

HOW TO ELICIT APPROPRIATE DATA

Because the Unitary Person Framework and the Stroke Rehabilitation Assessment Tool contain some terms that may be unfamiliar to nurses, specific stroke rehabilitation focus questions and parameters were developed to elicit appropriate information. These questions and parameters are in Table 25-2, which follows the content of the tool (Fig. 25-1). The variables in bold type in the tool are described more fully in Table 25-2. For example, the variable concerning aphasia under the "communicating pattern" is in bold type. If the nurse does not know how to assess for aphasia, Table 25-2 can be used to focus the assessment. The questions and parameters provide clarity and guidance when eliciting data. They are not all inclusive, so nurses should not feel limited by them. Many

other questions, based on the patient's situation and condition and the nurse's skill, could be used to elicit the information. Questions and parameters for data not in bold type were presented in Chapter 3.

CASE STUDY

The case study models the process a nurse uses when assessing a patient. Based on the clustering of information obtained during assessment, the nurse formulates nursing diagnoses.

Mrs. S.R. was assessed in the hospital after a left-sided CVA to determine her rehabilitation potential. She is 61 years old, married, and lives with her husband. Her recent CVA had left her with aphasia, so her husband served as a source of information. The Stroke Rehabilitation Assessment Tool (Fig. 25-2) was used to assess Mrs. S.R.

BIBLIOGRAPHY

American Nurses' Association and Association of Rehabilitation Nurses: Standards of rehabilitation nursing practice, Kansas City, Mo, 1986, ANA, Inc.

Brandstater ME and Basmajian JV: Stroke rehabilitation, Baltimore, 1987, Williams & Wilkins.

Norman S and Baratz R: Understanding aphasia, Am J Nurs 79:2135, 1979.

O'Brien MT and Pallett PJ: Total care of the stroke patient, Boston, 1978, Little, Brown & Co, Inc.

Pimental PA: Alteration in communication, Nurs Clin North Am 21:321, 1986.

Shapless JW: Mossman's a problem-oriented approach to stroke rehabilitation, ed 2, Springfield, 1982, Charles C Thomas, Publisher.

Tilton CN and Maloof M: Diagnosing the problem in stroke, Am J Nurs 82:596, 1982.

STROKE REHABILITATION ASSESSMENT TOOL

Name _____ Age _____ Sex _____
Address _____ Telephone _____
Significant other _____ Telephone _____
Date of admission _____ Medical diagnosis _____
Allergies _____

Nursing Diagnosis
(Potential or Altered)

COMMUNICATING ▪ A pattern involving sending messages
Prior ability to read, write, understand English (circle) _____   Communication
Other languages _____   Verbal
Educational level _____ **Handedness** _____   Nonverbal
Present reading ability _____ Writing ability _____
Aphasia _____ **Expressive** _____ **Receptive** _____
Speech impaired _____
Alternate form of communication _____
Symptoms of right hemisphere disorder _____

VALUING ▪ A pattern involving the assigning of relative worth
Religious preference _____   Spiritual state
Important religious practices _____   Distress
Spiritual concerns _____   Despair
Cultural orientation _____
Cultural practices _____

RELATING ▪ A pattern involving establishing bonds
Role
  Marital status _____   Role performance
  Age/health/location of significant other _____   Parenting
  _____   Sexual dysfunction
  Number of children _____ Ages _____   Work
  Effects of disability on role in home _____   Family
  _____
  Financial support _____   Social/leisure
  Occupation _____   Family processes
    Job satisfaction/concerns _____
    Physical/mental energy expenditures _____
  Sexual relationships (satisfactory/unsatisfactory) _____   Sexuality patterns
    Difficulties related to sex _____
    _____
  Effects of disability on sexuality _____

Socialization
  Quality of relationships with others _____   Impaired social interaction
    Patient's description _____
    Significant others' descriptions _____   Social isolation
    _____   Social withdrawal
  Staff observations _____
  Verbalizes feelings of being alone _____
    Attributed to _____

KNOWING ▪ A pattern involving the meaning associated with information
Cerebrovascular history _____
_____

Continued.

Fig. 25-1

Previous illness/hospitalization/surgeries _____

Other current health problems _____

Current medications _____   Knowledge deficit

Risk factors: Hypertension _____ Hyperlipidemia _____ Smoking _____
    Obesity _____ Diabetes _____ Stress _____ Alcohol usage _____
    Sedentary living _____ Oral contraceptives _____
    Family history _____
Perceptions of disability _____

Expectations of therapy _____

Misconceptions _____
Readiness to learn _____
   Learning impeded by _____   Thought processes

Orientation
Orientation: Person _____ Place _____ Time _____   Orientation
Level of awareness/understanding _____   Confusion
Safety concerns/needs _____

Memory
Memory intact: yes/no _____ Recent _____ Remote _____   Memory

FEELING ▪ A pattern involving the subjective awareness of information
Comfort
  Pain/discomfort: yes/no _____   Comfort
    Frequency _____ Duration _____   Pain/chronic
    Location _____ Quality _____ Radiation _____   Pain/acute
    Associated factors _____
    Aggravating factors _____   Discomfort
    Alleviating factors _____

Emotional Integrity/States
  Recent stressful life events _____   Anxiety
  _____   Fear
  Verbalizes feelings _____   Anger
    Source _____   Guilt
  _____   Shame
    Physical manifestations _____   Sadness
  _____   Grieving
  Verbalizes feelings of grief or loss _____   Dysfunctional
  _____   Anticipatory
  Displays inappropriate emotional responses (lability) _____

MOVING ▪ A pattern involving activity
Rest
  Hours slept/night _____ Perception of adequacy _____   Sleep pattern disturbance
  Sleep aids (pillows, meds, food) _____   Hypersomnia
  Difficulty falling/remaining asleep _____   Insomnia
    Nightmares

Recreation
  Leisure activities _____   Deficit in diversional activity
  Social activities _____

Fig. 25-1, cont'd

Environmental Maintenance

Home maintenance management   Impaired home maintenance
   Size & arrangement of home (stairs, bathroom) _____   management
_____   Safety hazards

   Transportation _____
   Home responsibilities _____
_____

   Assistance available _____

Health Maintenance   Health maintenance

Health insurance _____
Regular physical checkups _____
Access to health care _____

Activity

Strength: RUE _____ RLE _____ LUE _____ LLE _____   Impaired physical mobility
ROM: RUE _____ RLE _____ LUE _____ LLE _____
Tone: RUE _____ RLE _____ LUE _____ LLE _____
Coordination—finger-nose: Right _____ Left _____
Performs volitional movement _____
Involuntary movements present (describe) _____
Balance impaired _____ Sitting _____ Standing _____
Transfers: Dependent _____ Independent _____ Assist _____
Bed Mobility: Dependent _____ Independent _____ Assist _____
Endurance for activity _____   Activity intolerance
Predisability ambulation status _____   Safety hazards
Present ambulation status _____ Aids _____
Safety precautions needed _____
Orthotic devices in use _____

Self-Care

ADL performance: Independent   Dependent   Assist (specify type)   Self-care
           Feeding: _____ _____ _____   Feeding
          Bathing: _____ _____ _____   Bathing/hygiene
          Hygiene: _____ _____ _____   Dressing/grooming
  Dressing: Upper: _____ _____ _____   Toileting
           Lower: _____ _____ _____
        Toileting: _____ _____ _____
    Taking meds: _____ _____ _____

PERCEIVING ▪ A pattern involving the reception of information

Sensory/Perception   Sensory/perception

History of restricted environment _____
Vision impaired _____ Glasses _____   Visual
   Patient's description of vision (double, blurred, tearing)   Auditory
_____   Kinesthetic

   Visual field cut _____ Right _____ Left _____   Tactile
   EOM impaired (describe) _____   Olfactory
   Ptosis _____ Nystagmus _____   Gustatory
   Ability to identify common objects (agnosia) _____
Auditory impaired _____ Hearing aid _____
Kinesthetics (position sense) impaired _____
Tactile impaired _____
Reflexes impaired _____
Other _____

Attention   Unilateral neglect
Abnormal head posture _____   Distractibility
Attention shown to affected side _____   Inattention

Fig. 25-1, cont'd

Continued.

Attention shown to environment _____   Unilateral neglect
Ability to focus on task/topics _____   Distractibility
Insight about stroke deficits/limitations _____   Inattention
_____

Self-Concept   Self-concept
Patient's description of self _____   Body image
Effects of disability on self-concept _____   Self-esteem
_____   Personal identity
Concerns related to body image/personal identity _____
_____
Patient's description of own strengths/weaknesses _____
_____

Meaningfulness
Verbalizes hopelessness _____   Hopelessness
Verbalizes/perceives loss of control _____   Powerlessness

EXCHANGING ▪ A pattern involving mutual giving and receiving
Circulation
Cerebral   Cerebral tissue perfusion
  Results of tests (CT, MRI, EEG) _____
  Present neurologic deficits _____
    Cranial nerve impairment _____
    Gag reflex _____ Facial droop _____
  Seizure history/precautions _____
  Anticoagulation therapy _____ Protime _____
  BP: Sitting   Lying   Standing   Fluid volume
     R ____ L ____   R ____ L ____   R ____ L ____   Deficit
                                                 Excess
Cardiac   Cardiopulmonary tissue
  Apical rate & rhythm _____ Pacemaker _____   perfusion
  Heart sounds/murmurs _____   Cardiac output
  Dysrhythmias _____
Peripheral
  Pulses: A = absent   P = palable   B = bruits   Peripheral tissue perfusion
  Carotid   R ____ L ____   Radial   R ____ L ____
  Brachial R ____ L ____   Dorsalis pedis R ____ L ____
  Skin temp _____ Color _____ Capillary refill _____
  Edema (location) _____   Cardiac output
    Management (elevate, glove) _____

Physical Integrity
Tissue integrity
    Impaired _____ Rashes _____ Lesions _____   Impaired skin integrity
    Petechiae _____ Bruises _____   Impaired tissue integrity
    Skin turgor _____ Other (Specify) _____
    Past history/treatment of skin breakdown _____
    Present pressure sores (site/grade) _____
_____
    Current treatment _____
Potential for Injury   Potential for injury
  Awareness/nonawareness of new limitations (circle) _____
  Safety concerns _____

Oxygenation
Complaints of dyspnea _____ Precipitated by _____   Ineffective breathing pattern
Rate _____ Rhythm _____ Depth _____ Labored/unlabored   Impaired gas exchange
Chest expansion _____   Ineffective airway clearance

Fig. 25-1, cont'd

Cough: productive/nonproductive _____   Ineffective breathing pattern
Sputum: Color _____ Amount _____ Consistency _____   Impaired gas exchange
Need for suction (frequency) _____   Ineffective airway clearance
Presence of "wet voice" _____
Breath sounds _____
Oxygen percent and device _____

Physical Regulation
Hormonal/metabolic patterns   Hormonal/metabolic patterns
   Menstrual period (frequency/duration) _____   Menstrual pattern
   Last menstrual period _____

Nutrition
Eating patterns   Nutrition
   Number of meals per day _____   More than body
   Special diet _____   requirements
   Tube feeding/NG/gastrostomy _____   Less than body requirements
   Food preferences/intolerances/allergies _____
   Daily fluid intake _____   Fluid volume
   Appetite changes _____   Deficit
   Nausea/vomiting _____   Excess
   Oral management of food/liquids _____
   Choking/coughing/pocketing of food _____   Impaired swallowing
Condition of mouth/throat _____   Oral mucous membrane
Height _____ Weight _____ Ideal body weight: _____
Labs
   Na _____ K _____ CL _____ Glucose _____ Fasting _____

Elimination
Bowel   Bowel elimination
   Predisability bowel habits (frequency/adjuncts) _____   Diarrhea
      Constipation
   Defecation problems _____   Incontinence
   Methods of control _____   GI tissue perfusion
   Abdominal physical examination _____
Urinary   Urinary elimination
   Predisability urinary patterns/problems _____   Incontinence
      Retention
   Current problems/patterns _____
     Frequency _____ Urgency _____ Incontinence _____   Renal tissue perfusion
     Retention _____ Burning _____ Small quantity _____
   Methods of control: Diapers _____ Foley: _____ Size _____
     Intermittent cath _____ Frequency _____
   Urine output: 24 hour _____ Specific gravity _____
     BUN _____ Creatinine _____ Other _____
   Bladder distention _____ Color _____
   Infection: _____ Temperature _____ Route _____   Infection
     Urine C&S results _____   Body temperature

CHOOSING ■ A pattern involving the selection of alternatives
Coping
Patient's usual problem-solving methods _____   Ineffective individual coping
    Ineffective family coping

Family's usual problem-solving methods _____

Patient's method of dealing with stress _____

Fig. 25-1, cont'd

Continued.

Family's method of dealing with stress _____

_____

Patient's affect _____

Physical manifestations _____

Coping mechanisms used _____

Support systems/resources _____

Participation

Compliance with past/current health care regimens _____   Noncompliance

_____   Ineffective participation

Willingness to comply with future health care regimen _____

_____

Judgment

Decision-making ability   Judgment

Patient's perspective _____   Indecisiveness

Others' perspectives _____

Prioritized nursing diagnoses/problem list

1. _____

2. _____

3. _____

4. _____

5. _____

6. _____

7. _____

8. _____

9. _____

10. _____

Signature _____   Date _____

Fig. 25-1, cont'd

STROKE REHABILITATION ASSESSMENT TOOL

Name _S.R._   Age _61_   Sex _F_
Address _22 TWENTY-FIFTH STREET, GREENVILLE, S.C._   Telephone _243-3000_
Significant other _HUSBAND — T.R.   DAUGHTER— L.C._   Telephone _243-3000_
Date of admission _12/4_   Medical diagnosis _LEFT-SIDED CVA WITH APHASIA_
Allergies _NKA_

Nursing Diagnosis
(Potential or Altered)

COMMUNICATING ▪ A pattern involving sending messages
Prior ability to (read) (write,) (understand) English (circle) ___   (Communication)
Other languages _NONE_   (Verbal)
Educational level _10TH GRADE_ Handedness _RIGHT_   (Nonverbal)
Present reading ability _IMPAIRED_ Writing ability _IMPAIRED_
Aphasia _YES_   Expressive _YES_   Receptive _YES_
Speech impaired _YES, DYSARTHRIA_
Alternate form of communication _GESTURES_
Symptoms of right hemisphere disorder _NONE_

VALUING ▪ A pattern involving the assigning of relative worth
Religious preference _BAPTIST_   Spiritual state
Important religious practices _NONE_   Distress
Spiritual concerns _NONE_   Despair
Cultural orientation _BLACK AMERICAN_
Cultural practices _NONE_

RELATING ▪ A pattern involving establishing bonds
Role
Marital status _MARRIED_   (Role performance)
Age/health/location of significant other _HUSBAND 70-RECOVERING FROM_   Parenting
HIP SURGERY/LIVES IN LOCAL AREA c̄ PT   Sexual dysfunction
Number of children _1_ Ages _45-DAUGHTER LIVES c̄ PT. & HUSBAND_   Work
Effects of disability on role in home _PREVIOUS ROLE AS HOMEMAKER —_   (Family)
NOW ACTIVITIES LIMITED DUE TO STROKE
Financial support _PENSION_   Social/leisure
Occupation _RETIRED - CLEANING LADY X40 YRS_   Family processes
  Job satisfaction/concerns ___
  Physical/mental energy expenditures ___
Sexual relationships (satisfactory)(unsatisfactory) _(PER HUSBAND)_   Sexuality patterns
  Difficulties related to sex ___
  CAN'T ASSESS D/T APHASIA
  Effects of disability on sexuality ___

Socialization
Quality of relationships with others _"GOOD IN GENERAL"(PER HUSBAND)_   (Impaired social interaction)
  Patient's description _CAN'T ASSESS D/T APHASIA_
  Significant others' descriptions _"GOOD, CLOSE RELATIONSHIPS c̄ FAMILY_   Social isolation
& FRIENDS" (HUSBAND)   Social withdrawal
  Staff observations _FLAT AFFECT s̄ CHANGE WHEN INTERACTING c̄ FAMILY_
Verbalizes feelings of being alone ___
  Attributed to ___

KNOWING ▪ A pattern involving the meaning associated with information
Cerebrovascular history _SUDDEN ONSET (R) SIDED WEAKNESS,_
INABILITY TO SPEAK → (L) CVA

Fig. 25-2   *Continued.*

Previous illness/hospitalization/surgeries _HTN_

Other current health problems _NEUROGENIC BLADDER, PULMONARY EMBOLUS_

Current medications _CATAPRES 0.1mg BID, ELAVIL 2.5mg TID, COUMADIN 5mg qd_   Knowledge deficit

Risk factors: Hypertension _✓_ Hyperlipidemia _—_ Smoking _—_
Obesity _✓_ Diabetes _—_ Stress _—_ Alcohol usage _—_
Sedentary living _✓_ Oral contraceptives _—_
Family history _HTN_
Perceptions of disability _____

Expectations of therapy _____ _CAN'T ASSESS D/T APHASIA_

Misconceptions _____
Readiness to learn _ATTEMPTS TO PARTICIPATE_
  Learning impeded by _SEVERE EXPRESSIVE APHASIA & POSSIBLE ORAL APRAXIA_   (Thought processes)

Orientation
Orientation: Person _✓_ Place _✓_ Time _No_   (Orientation)
Level of awareness/understanding _ALERT, DECREASED UNDERSTANDING_   Confusion
Safety concerns/needs _UNABLE TO EXPRESS NEEDS ADEQUATELY, @ RISK FOR UNSAFE ACTIONS_

Memory
Memory intact: yes/no _APHASIC_ Recent _—_ Remote _—_   (Memory)

FEELING ▪ A pattern involving the subjective awareness of information
Comfort
  Pain/discomfort: yes/no _No_   Comfort
    Frequency _—_ Duration _—_   Pain/Chronic
    Location _—_ Quality _—_ Radiation _—_   Pain/Acute
    Associated factors _—_
    Aggravating factors _—_   Discomfort
    Alleviating factors _—_

Emotional Integrity/States
  Recent stressful life events _NEW STROKE c̄ SIGNIFICANT COMMUNICATION PROBLEMS, HUSBAND'S SURGERY_   Anxiety
                              Fear
  Verbalizes feelings ____   Anger
    Source ____ _CAN'T ASSESS D/T APHASIA_   Guilt
                              Shame
  Physical manifestations _SAD EXPRESSION/FRUSTRATION PRESENT_ (Sadness)
                              Grieving
  Verbalizes feelings of grief or loss _—_   Dysfunctional
                              Anticipatory
  Displays inappropriate emotional responses (lability) _No_

MOVING ▪ A pattern involving activity
Rest
  Hours slept/night _8HRS_ Perception of adequacy _—_   Sleep pattern disturbance
  Sleep aids (pillows, meds, food) _____   Hypersomnia
  Difficulty falling/remaining asleep _NONE (PER HUSBAND)_   Insomnia
                              Nightmares

Recreation
  Leisure activities _KNITTING, SEWING_   (Deficit in diversional activity)
  Social activities _VERY INVOLVED IN CHURCH ACTIVITIES_   (POTENTIAL)

Fig. 25-2, cont'd

Environmental Maintenance
Home maintenance management
Size & arrangement of home (stairs, bathroom) *IST FLOOR APT WITHOUT STEPS*
Transportation *HUSBAND DRIVES HER*
Home responsibilities *PRIMARY HOMEMAKER — COOKING CLEANING HUSBAND DOES SHOPPING. DAUGHTER/GRANDDAUGHTER HELP BUT BOTH WORK*
Assistance available *DAUGHTER/GRANDDAUGHTER*

(Impaired home maintenance management)
Safety hazards

Health Maintenance
Health insurance *AETNA*
Regular physical checkups *YES*
Access to health care *GOOD*

Health maintenance

Activity
Strength: RUE *2/5 PASSIVE* RLE *2/5 PASSIVE* LUE *5/5 ACTIVE* LLE *5/5 ACTIVE*
ROM: RUE *nml* RLE *nml* LUE *nml* LLE *nml*
Tone: RUE *SL. SPASTICITY* RLE *SL. SPASTICITY* LUE *nml* LLE *nml*
Coordination—finger-nose: Right *NOT TESTED* Left *nml*
Performs volitional movement *CAN'T DO ORAL MOTOR ACTS ON COMMAND*
Involuntary movements present (describe) *NONE*
Balance impaired *YES* Sitting *POOR* Standing *NOT TESTED*
Transfers: Dependent ___ Independent ___ Assist *MODERATE*
Bed Mobility: Dependent ___ Independent *TO (R)* Assist *TO (L) — MODERATE*
Endurance for activity *TIRES EASILY*
Predisability ambulation status *nml*
Present ambulation status *NONAMBULATORY* Aids ___—___
Safety precautions needed *POSEY VEST @ NIGHT*
Orthotic devices in use *SPLINT — (R) FOREARM*

(Impaired physical mobility)

Activity intolerance
Safety hazards

Self-Care
ADL performance:	Independent	Dependent	Assist (specify type)
Feeding:			✓ SET UP
Bathing:		✓ LOWER	✓ SET UP/CUE FOR UPPER
Hygiene:			✓ SET UP
Dressing: Upper:		✓	
Lower:		✓	
Toileting:		✓	
Taking meds:		✓	

Self-care
(Feeding)
(Bathing/hygiene)
(Dressing/grooming)
(Toileting)

PERCEIVING ▪ A pattern involving the reception of information
Sensory/Perception
History of restricted environment *ICU x 7 DAYS*
Vision impaired *No* Glasses *YES*
Patient's description of vision (double, blurred, tearing) *CAN'T ASSES D/T APHASIA*
Visual field cut *No* Right ___—___ Left ___—___
EOM impaired (describe) *No*
Ptosis *No* Nystagmus *No*
Ability to identify common objects (agnosia) *ABSENT*
Auditory impaired *No* Hearing aid *No*
Kinesthetics (position sense) impaired *(R) EXTREMITIES — ABSENT*
Tactile impaired *YES — TOUCH/PAIN APPEAR IMPAIRED*
Reflexes impaired *DECREASED (R) PLANTAR REFLEX*
Other ___

Sensory/perception
Visual
Auditory
Kinesthetic
Tactile
Olfactory
Gustatory

Attention
Abnormal head posture *No*
Attention shown to affected side *ATTENDS WELL*

Unilateral neglect
Distractibility
Inattention

Fig. 25-2, cont'd

Continued.

Attention shown to environment _ATTENDS WELL_   Unilateral neglect
Ability to focus on task/topics _DECREASED D/T APHASIA_   Distractibility
Insight about stroke deficits/limitations _CAN'T ASSESS D/T APHASIA_   Inattention

Self-Concept

Patient's description of self _"WARM, CARING, VERY ACTIVE LADY" (HUSBAND)_   Self-concept
         Body image
Effects of disability on self-concept _APHASIA_   Self-esteem
         Personal identity

Concerns related to body image/personal identity _"CAN'T TALK"_
(HUSBAND)

Patient's description of own strengths/weaknesses _APHASIC_

Meaningfulness

Verbalizes hopelessness _____ ⎞ _CAN'T ASSESS_   Hopelessness
Verbalizes/perceives loss of control ___ ⎠   Powerlessness

EXCHANGING ▪ A pattern involving mutual giving and receiving

Circulation

Cerebral   Cerebral tissue perfusion
  Results of tests (CT, MRI, EEG) _CT → (L) BASAL GANGLIA INFARCT_
  Present neurologic deficits _APHASIA, APRAXIA, (R) EXTREMITIES PARESIS_
    Cranial nerve impairment _CRANIAL NERVE 7 OUT ON (R) FACE_
    Gag reflex _⊕_   Facial droop _⊕ ON (R)_
  Seizure history/precautions _NONE_
  Anticoagulation therapy _YES, COUMADIN_ Protime _20 SEC_
  BP: Sitting   Lying   Standing   Fluid volume
    R _120/80_ L _122/78_   R _132/82_ L _130/80_   R ___ L ___   Deficit
         Excess

Cardiac   Cardiopulmonary tissue
  Apical rate & rhythm _84 REGULAR_ Pacemaker _No_   perfusion
  Heart sounds/murmurs _NORMAL S₁ S₂_   Cardiac output
  Dysrhythmias _NONE_

Peripheral
  Pulses: A = absent   P = palable   B = bruits   Peripheral tissue perfusion
  Carotid   R _P_ L _P_   Radial   R _P_ L _P_
  Brachial   R _P_ L _P_   Dorsalis pedis R _P_ L _P_
  Skin temp _WARM, DRY_ Color _PINK_ Capillary refill _GOOD, < 2 SEC_
  Edema (location) _R UE_   Cardiac output
    Management (elevate, glove) _ELEVATE_

Physical Integrity

Tissue integrity
  Impaired _No_ Rashes _—_ Lesions _—_   Impaired skin integrity
  Petechiae _—_ Bruises _—_   Impaired tissue integrity
  Skin turgor _GOOD_ Other (Specify) _—_
  Past history/treatment of skin breakdown _NONE_
  Present pressure sores (site/grade) _NONE_

  Current treatment _—_
Potential for Injury   (Potential for injury)
  Awareness/(nonawareness) of new limitations (circle) _____
  Safety concerns _DECREASED UNDERSTANDING CREATES POTENTIAL_
    FOR UNSAFE ACTS

Oxygenation

Complaints of dyspnea _No_ Precipitated by _—_   Ineffective breathing pattern
Rate _20_ Rhythm _REGULAR_ Depth _SHALLOW_ Labored/(unlabored)   Impaired gas exchange
Chest expansion _FAIR_   Ineffective airway clearance

Fig. 25-2, cont'd

Cough: productive (nonproductive) _____ | Ineffective breathing pattern
Sputum: Color __—__ Amount __—__ Consistency __—__ | Impaired gas exchange
Need for suction (frequency) _NO_ _____ | Ineffective airway clearance
Presence of "wet voice" _____ _NO_ _____
Breath sounds _CLEAR_ _____
Oxygen percent and device _NONE_ _____

Physical Regulation

Hormonal/metabolic patterns | Hormonal/metabolic patterns
  Menstrual period (frequency/duration) _MENOPAUSE COMPLETE AGE 54_ | Menstrual pattern
  Last menstrual period _AGE 54_ _____

Nutrition

  Eating patterns | (Nutrition / More than body /   requirements)
    Number of meals per day _3_ | Less than body requirements
    Special diet _2 gm SODIUM DIET_ _____
    Tube feeding/NG/gastrostomy _NONE_ | (POTENTIAL)
    Food preferences/intolerances/allergies _NONE_ | (Fluid volume /   Deficit)
    Daily fluid intake _INADEQUATE SINCE STROKE_
    Appetite changes _DECREASED SINCE STROKE_
    Nausea/vomiting _NONE_ | Excess
    Oral management of food/liquids _DIFFICULTY SWALLOWING — APRAXIA_
    Choking/coughing (pocketing of food) _IN RIGHT CHEEK_ | (Impaired swallowing)
    Condition of mouth/throat _nml_ | Oral mucous membrane
    Height _5'2"_ Weight _165 lbs_ Ideal body weight: _115 lbs_
    Labs
    Na _140 mEq/L_ K _4.2 mEq/L_ CL _100 mEq/L_ Glucose _120 mg/dl_ Fasting _YES_

Elimination

  Bowel | Bowel elimination
    Predisability bowel habits (frequency/adjuncts) _EVERY MORNING c̄_ | Diarrhea
    OCCASIONAL LAXATIVES | (Constipation)
    Defecation problems _CONSTIPATION_ | Incontinence
    Methods of control _DULCOLAX SUPPOSITORY q̄od SINCE STROKE_ | GI tissue perfusion
    Abdominal physical examination _SOFT; 2 ⊕ BS IN ALL 4 QUADS_
  Urinary | Urinary elimination
    Predisability urinary patterns/problems _4-5 X / DAY_ | (Incontinence)
    _____ | Retention
    Current problems/patterns _FREQUENT USE OF BEDPAN_
    Frequency __—__ Urgency __—__ Incontinence _✓ REFLEX_ | Renal tissue perfusion
    Retention __—__ Burning __—__ Small quantity __—__
    Methods of control: Diapers _@ NIGHT_ Foley: __—__ Size __—__
    Intermittent cath __—__ Frequency __—__
    Urine output: 24 hour _≈ 1000 cc_ Specific gravity _1.012_
    BUN _18 mg/dl_ Creatinine _1.4 mg/dl_ Other _CYSTOGRAM PENDING_
    Bladder distention _NO_ Color _YELLOW, CLEAR_
    Infection: _NO_ Temperature _97.8°F_ Route _ORAL_ | Infection
    Urine C&S results _TO BE OBTAINED_ | Body temperature

CHOOSING ▪ A pattern involving the selection of alternatives

Coping

  Patient's usual problem-solving methods _CAN'T ASSESS_ | Ineffective individual coping
  _____ | Ineffective family coping
  Family's usual problem-solving methods _HUSBAND STATES THAT HE + PT_
  TALK PROBLEMS OVER, DISCUSS SOLUTIONS, + PICK BEST ONE
  Patient's method of dealing with stress _CAN'T ASSESS_

Fig. 25-2, cont'd

Continued.

Assessing rehabilitation patients

Family's method of dealing with stress *HUSBAND STATES THAT THEY USUALLY TRY TO PUT PROBLEMS/STRESS IN PERSPECTIVE*

Patient's affect *FLAT — DEPRESSION SUSPECTED*

Physical manifestations *SLOW TO INITIATE*

Coping mechanisms used *CAN'T ASSESS*

Support systems/resources *SUPPORTIVE HUSBAND/DAUGHTER/GRANDDAUGHTER*

Participation

Compliance with past/current health care regimens *GOOD*　　　　　　　Noncompliance
　　　　　　　　　　　　　　　　　　　　　　　　　　　　　　　　　　　　　Ineffective participation

Willingness to comply with future health care regimen *ANTICIPATE GOOD COMPLIANCE*

Judgment

Decision-making ability　　　　　　　　　　　　　　　　　　　　　　Judgment

　Patient's perspective *? IMPAIRED — DIFFICULT TO ASSESS*　　　　Indecisiveness

　Others' perspectives *REPORT PT AS GOOD DECISION MAKER IN PAST*

Prioritized nursing diagnoses/problem list

1. *ALTERED VERBAL/NONVERBAL COMMUNICATION R/T APHASIA, DYSARTHRIA*
2. *IMPAIRED PHYSICAL MOBILITY R/T ⓇSIDED WEAKNESS*
3. *ALTERED SELF-CARE R/T DISABILITY*
4. *ALTERED THOUGHT PROCESSES R/T CHANGES IN MEMORY, ORIENTATION*
5. *IMPAIRED SWALLOWING R/T APRAXIA*
6. *ALTERED URINARY/BOWEL ELIMINATION R/T REFLEX INCONTINENCE, CONSTIPATION*
7. *POTENTIAL FOR INJURY R/T STROKE DEFICITS*
8. *ALTERED ROLE PERFORMANCE R/T ACTIVITY LIMITATIONS IMPOSED BY DISABILITY*
9. *IMPAIRED SOCIAL INTERACTION R/T COMMUNICATION DEFICITS*
10. *SADNESS R/T DISABILITY, COMMUNICATION DEFICITS*
11. *ALTERED NUTRITION: MORE THAN BODY REQUIREMENTS R/T INCREASED BODY WEIGHT*

Signature *Anita P. Shener, R.N.*　　　　　　　　Date *6/6*

Fig. 25-2, cont'd

CHAPTER 26

SPINAL CORD INJURY REHABILITATION ASSESSMENT TOOL

ANITA P. SHERER
SUSAN M. BRADY

The Spinal Cord Injury Rehabilitation Assessment Tool was designed to assess stable patients with spinal cord injuries who have unique biopsychosocial assessment needs. The tool incorporates signs and symptoms pertinent to the patient with a spinal cord injury to facilitate identification of nursing diagnoses. It also incorporates the *Standards of Rehabilitation Nursing Practice* developed by the American Nurses' Association and the Association of Rehabilitation Nurses. This chapter includes:

- *The way the tool was developed and refined*
- *The patient population and settings to which it applies*
- *Selected spinal cord injury rehabilitation emphasis areas*
- *The way to use the tool*
- *Specific spinal cord injury rehabilitation focus questions and parameters to assist the nurse in eliciting appropriate data*
- *The Spinal Cord Injury Rehabilitation Assessment Tool*
- *A case study*
- *A completed version of the tool based on the case study*

DEVELOPMENT AND REFINEMENT OF THE TOOL

The Spinal Cord Injury Rehabilitation Assessment Tool was developed from the nursing data base prototype (see Chapter 2). Many hemodynamic monitoring and critical care variables originally incorporated in the prototype were deleted and replaced with in-depth musculoskeletal, neurologic, and self-care assessment variables more applicable to a spinal cord injury rehabilitation assessment. The resultant tool was then modified based on the recommendations of nurse experts in spinal cord injury rehabilitation. Further, the content of this tool is supported by the literature from this field of nursing.

After the tool was developed and refined, it was clinically tested by spinal cord injury rehabilitation nurse experts and clinical nurse specialists on 10 patients, ages 19 to 60, in rehabilitation units of acute care hospitals and in comprehensive rehabilitation facilities. All patients had suffered spinal cord injuries, and most had been injured two or three months before and were being assessed for rehabilitation potential when entering the comprehensive rehabilitation settings. Some patients with spinal cord injuries acquired long before entering the facilities were assessed in acute care hospitals where they had been admitted for a related problem. The testing evaluated the adequacy of the tool in terms of flow, space for recording data, and completeness of assessment variables. Based on the results, the tool was revised.

PATIENT POPULATION AND SETTING

The Spinal Cord Injury Rehabilitation Assessment Tool was developed for use with stable patients with spinal cord injuries who require assessment to determine their rehabilitation potential and nursing care needs. The tool was developed for use in any rehabilitation setting caring for patients with spinal cord injuries. Such settings include comprehensive rehabilitation facilities or rehabilitation units in acute care hospitals.

SPINAL CORD INJURY REHABILITATION EMPHASIS AREAS

Spinal cord injury rehabilitation patients have specialized problems and needs. The Spinal Cord Injury Rehabilitation Assessment Tool includes appropriate assessment variables within each of the nine human response patterns of the Unitary Person Framework. The tool focuses on prevalent problems in the spinal cord injury rehabilitation patient population. Table 26-1 outlines these emphasis areas.

HOW TO USE THE TOOL

To use the Spinal Cord Injury Rehabilitation Assessment Tool effectively, nurses must first be familiar with the Unitary Person Framework (see Chapter 2), which provides the underlying framework for Taxonomy I. The nine human response patterns of the Unitary Person Framework serve as the major category headings for Taxonomy I and the tool. The sequence of the response patterns, as it appears in Taxonomy I, has been changed in the tool to permit a more logical ordering of assessment variables. Nursing diagnoses pertinent to the patients with spinal cord injuries, along with the signs and symptoms necessary to identify them, are incorporated under the appropriate human response patterns.

Nurses must also realize that this tool is very different from conventional assessment tools. As a result, nurses may have some initial difficulty in using it. They should remember, however, that this tool was not designed to follow the organization or content of a traditional medical data base; the data collected do not solely reflect medical patterns. Rather, this tool elicits data about holistic patterns in ways not traditionally assessed by nurses. It provides a new method of collecting and synthesizing data and requires new thinking when processing data. This tool represents a nursing data base developed from a nursing model to permit a holistic nursing assessment to take place so nursing diagnoses can be identified.

Although nurses probably agree that a holistic nursing data base is desirable, it is realized that changing traditional assessment methods is not an easy task. For this reason, a trial usage period is recommended before any decisions about the tool's merits are made. During this period, nurses should assess 10 patients using the tool to become familiar and progressively more comfortable with its organization and data-collection methods. With experience, nurses will become accustomed to new ways of clustering and processing information. With continued use, the time necessary to complete the tool will be reduced. Most important, nurses will recognize the unique ability of the tool to elicit appropriate signs and symptoms. Nurses will discover that nursing diagnoses are easily identified when using the tool.

It is not necessary to complete the tool in one session. Priority sections can be completed during the initial assessment. Other sections or patterns can be completed later, within a time frame acceptable to the institution.

To elicit appropriate data, nurses should be familiar with the focus questions and parameters in the next section. When assessing specific signs and symptoms to indicate a diagnosis, the nurse circles the diagnosis in the right-hand column when deviations from normal are found. A circled diagnosis does not confirm a problem but simply alerts the nurse to the possibility that it exists. After completing the tool, the nurse scans the circled problems, synthesizes the data to determine whether other clusters of signs and symptoms support a problem, and decides whether the actual or potential diagnosis is present.

Some diagnoses are repeated several times in the right-hand column. These repetitions occur only within the appropriate response pattern and are convenient for identifying certain data directly with their corresponding nursing diagnosis. These diagnoses are not absolute but focus thinking and direct more detailed attention to a problem.

Certain signs and symptoms can indicate several diagnoses. For example, recent stressful life events can indicate anxiety and ineffective individual coping. To avoid unnecessary repetition of assessment parameters, variables are arranged with the diagnosis most likely to result from

Table 26-1

Selected spinal cord injury rehabilitation emphasis areas

Patterns	Emphasis areas to determine
Communicating	Speech impairment
Valuing	Spiritual despair related to spinal cord injury
	Religion and culture as support systems
Relating	Support systems
	Effect of injury on roles and relationships
Knowing	Understanding of injury and therapy
	Orientation and memory
Feeling	Comprehensive data related to pain
	Anxiety, fear, grief, or loss
Moving	Musculoskeletal examination
	Effects of injury on home maintenance
	Self-care deficits
Perceiving	Effects of injury on self-concept
Exchanging	Skin integrity
	Changes in elimination related to injury
Choosing	Patient's and family's adequacy in dealing with problems and stress
	Future compliance with health care regimen

the data assessed. Thus, data to support one diagnosis may occasionally be found in other patterns or arranged with other diagnoses. Therefore, synthesis of all data is essential.

The Spinal Cord Injury Rehabilitation Assessment Tool is not intended to be the standardized and final format for nationwide assessment of patients with spinal cord injuries. An assessment tool must meet the needs and requirements of the institutions and nurses using it. The Spinal Cord Injury Rehabilitation Assessment Tool is simply a

working demonstration tool that is expected to be changed and revised by nurses in clinical practice. Further evaluation and refinement are necessary before adopting the tool for use in an institution. Nurses interested in changing, revising, and adapting this tool to a specific clinical setting should refer to Chapter 4.

HOW TO ELICIT APPROPRIATE DATA

Because the Unitary Person Framework and the Spinal Cord Injury Rehabilitation Assessment Tool contain some

Table 26-2
Spinal cord injury rehabilitation assessment tool: focus questions and parameters

Variables	Focus questions and parameters
RELATING	
Role in home	"How has your injury changed your responsibilities in your home and your relationship with your spouse or significant other? How do you feel about these changes?"
Physical difficulties/effects of injury related to sex	"Do you expect any problems related to sexuality or sexual functioning?" For males: "Do you have erections? Do they last long enough for intercourse?" For females: "Have you menstruated since your injury?"
KNOWING	
Understanding of injury	"Can you tell me what you know about your injury? How has it affected you?"
Expectations of therapy	"What skills do you expect to gain from participating in this program (i.e., transferring independently or feeding self)?"
Rehabilitation goals	"What do you think participating in this program will do for you?"
Level of comprehension	Is the patient able to understand explanations about the injury and recovery? Can the patient recall or return demonstrate knowledge about the injury?
MOVING	
Accessibility of home/ community	"Is your home accessible? What changes are needed? Is your community accessible? Grocery stores? Restaurants?"
Transportation	"How do you plan to get around your community? Public transportation? Car with hand controls or van with wheelchair lift?"
Modifications needed	What modifications are necessary to make the patient's home and community accessible?
Home responsibilities	"Before your injury, what activities were you responsible for in your home (i.e., meal preparation, cleaning, or shopping)?" Will the patient be able to return to these activities after rehabilitation?
Assistance available	Are there resources (friends and family) available to assist the patient with these activities? What other resources will be needed?
Present legal proceedings	Is the patient involved in any legal proceedings related to the injury or accident that may affect rehabilitation (i.e., stressors for the patient or financial concerns)?
PERCEIVING	
Effects of injury on self-concept	"What does this injury mean to you? Has it changed how you feel about yourself? What do you think will happen to you now? How do you feel about the changes in your life this injury has caused?"
Concerns related to body image	"Has your thinking about different parts of your body changed since your injury?"
Patient's description of own strengths/weaknesses	"Describe your strengths as a person. Your weaknesses."
EXCHANGING	
Intravenous pyelogram	"Have you had an x-ray examination of your kidneys?"
Urodynamic evaluation	"Have you had a test to measure the pressures in your bladder?"

terms that may be unfamiliar to nurses, specific spinal cord injury rehabilitation focus questions and parameters were developed and refined to elicit appropriate information. These questions and parameters are in Table 26-2, which follows the content of the tool (Fig. 26-1). The variables in bold type in the tool are described in Table 26-2. For example, the variable about present legal proceedings under the "moving pattern" is in bold type. If the nurse does not know what to ask to elicit this information, Table 26-2 can be used to direct the line of questioning. The questions and parameters provide clarity and guidance when eliciting data. They are not all inclusive, so nurses should not feel limited by them. Many other questions, based on the patient's situation and condition and the nurse's skill, could be used to elicit the information. Questions and parameters for data not in bold type were presented in Chapter 3.

CASE STUDY

The case study models the process a nurse uses when assessing a patient. Based on the clustering of information obtained during assessment, the nurse formulates nursing diagnoses.

Mr. S.P., a 19-year-old patient with C-5 quadriplegia, was assessed when admitted to a rehabilitation facility to determine his rehabilitation potential. He is single, a sophomore in college, and was injured in a car accident 3 months before. The Spinal Cord Injury Rehabilitation Assessment Tool (Fig. 26-2) was used to assess Mr. S.P.

BIBLIOGRAPHY

American Nurses' Association and Association of Rehabilitation Nurses: Standards of rehabilitation nursing practice, Kansas City, Mo, 1986, ANA, Inc.

Hanak M and Scott A: Spinal cord injury: an illustrated guide for health care professionals, New York, 1988, Springer Publishing Co, Inc.

Hickey J: The clinical practice of neurological and neurosurgical nursing, Philadelphia, 1981, JB Lippincott Co.

Martin N, Holt N, and Hicks D, editors: Comprehensive rehabilitation nursing, New York, 1981, McGraw-Hill, Inc.

Persaud D and Stowe K, editors: Spinal cord injury: educational guidelines for professional nursing practice, New York, 1987, American Association of Spinal Cord Injury Nurses (AASCIN).

Zejdlik C: Management of spinal cord injury, Monterey, Calif, 1983, Wadsworth, Inc.

SPINAL CORD INJURY REHABILITATION ASSESSMENT TOOL

Name _____ Age _____ Sex _____
Address _____ Telephone _____
Significant other _____ Telephone _____
Date of admission _____ Medical diagnosis _____
_____
Allergies _____
Level of injury _____ Date of injury _____
Cause of injury _____

Nursing Diagnosis
(Potential or Altered)

COMMUNICATING ▪ A pattern involving sending messages
Read, write, understand English (circle) _____ Communication
Other languages _____ Speech impaired _____ Verbal
Family's understanding of English _____ Nonverbal

VALUING ▪ A pattern involving the assigning of relative worth
Religious preference _____ Spiritual state
Important religious practices _____ Despair
Spiritual concerns _____ Distress
Cultural orientation _____
Cultural practices _____

RELATING ▪ A pattern involving establishing bonds
Role
  Marital status _____ Role performance
  Age & health of significant other _____ Parenting
  _____ Sexual dysfunction
  Number of children _____ Ages _____ Work
  Number of siblings _____ Ages _____ Family
  Role in home _____ Social/leisure
  Financial support _____
  Occupation _____ Family processes
    Job satisfaction/concerns _____
    Physical/mental energy expenditures _____
  Sexual relationships (satisfactory/unsatisfactory) _____
  Physical difficulties/effects of injury related to sex _____ Sexuality patterns
  _____

Socialization
  Quality of relationships with others _____ Impaired social interaction
    Patient's description _____
    Significant others' descriptions _____
    Staff observations _____
  Verbalizes feelings of being alone _____ Social isolation
    Attributed to _____ Social withdrawal

KNOWING ▪ A pattern involving the meaning associated with information
Current health problems _____
_____
_____
Previous hospitalizations/illnesses/surgeries _____
_____
Previous participation in rehabilitation programs _____
_____
Current medications _____ Knowledge deficit
_____

Fig. 26-1

Continued.

Smoking ＿＿＿＿＿＿ Alcohol usage ＿＿＿＿＿＿＿ Drug usage ＿＿＿＿＿＿＿ Knowledge deficit
Educational level ＿＿＿＿＿＿＿＿＿＿＿＿＿＿＿＿＿＿＿＿＿＿＿＿＿＿＿
Understanding of injury ＿＿＿＿＿＿＿＿＿＿＿＿＿＿＿＿＿＿＿＿＿
＿＿＿＿＿＿＿＿＿＿＿＿＿＿＿＿＿＿＿＿＿＿＿＿＿＿＿＿＿＿＿＿＿＿＿

Expectations of therapy ＿＿＿＿＿＿＿＿＿＿＿＿＿＿＿＿＿＿＿＿＿
Misconceptions ＿＿＿＿＿＿＿＿＿＿＿＿＿＿＿＿＿＿＿＿＿＿＿＿＿＿ Thought processes
Rehabilitation goals ＿＿＿＿＿＿＿＿＿＿＿＿＿＿＿＿＿＿＿＿＿＿＿
Readiness to learn ＿＿＿＿＿＿＿＿＿＿＿＿＿＿＿＿＿＿＿＿＿＿＿＿＿
   Learning impeded by ＿＿＿＿＿＿＿＿＿＿＿＿＿＿＿＿＿＿＿＿
＿＿＿＿＿＿＿＿＿＿＿＿＿＿＿＿＿＿＿＿＿＿＿＿＿＿＿＿＿＿＿＿＿＿＿

   Level of comprehension ＿＿＿＿＿＿＿＿＿＿＿＿＿＿＿＿＿＿＿

Orientation   Orientation
Level of alertness ＿＿＿＿＿＿＿＿＿＿＿＿＿＿＿＿＿＿＿＿＿＿＿＿＿   Confusion
Orientation: Person ＿＿＿＿＿＿ Place ＿＿＿＿＿＿ Time ＿＿＿＿＿＿   LOC

Memory
Memory intact: yes/no ＿＿＿ Recent ＿＿＿＿＿＿ Remote ＿＿＿＿＿＿ Memory

FEELING ▪ A pattern involving the subjective awareness of information
Comfort
  Pain/discomfort: yes/no ＿＿＿＿＿＿＿   Comfort
    Frequency ＿＿＿＿＿ Location ＿＿＿＿＿＿＿＿＿＿＿   Pain/chronic
    Duration ＿＿＿＿＿ Quality ＿＿＿＿＿ Radiation ＿＿＿＿   Pain/acute
    Associated factors ＿＿＿＿＿＿＿＿＿＿＿＿＿＿＿＿＿＿   Discomfort
    Aggravating factors ＿＿＿＿＿＿＿＿＿＿＿＿＿＿＿＿＿＿
    Alleviating factors ＿＿＿＿＿＿＿＿＿＿＿＿＿＿＿＿＿＿

Emotional Integrity/States
  Recent stressful life events ＿＿＿＿＿＿＿＿＿＿＿＿＿＿＿＿ Anxiety
＿＿＿＿＿＿＿＿＿＿＿＿＿＿＿＿＿＿＿＿＿＿＿＿＿＿＿＿＿＿＿＿＿ Fear
  Verbalizes feelings ＿＿＿＿＿＿＿＿＿＿＿＿＿＿＿＿＿＿＿＿ Anger
    Source ＿＿＿＿＿＿＿＿＿＿＿＿＿＿＿＿＿＿＿＿＿＿＿＿ Guilt
＿＿＿＿＿＿＿＿＿＿＿＿＿＿＿＿＿＿＿＿＿＿＿＿＿＿＿＿＿＿＿＿＿ Shame
    Physical manifestations ＿＿＿＿＿＿＿＿＿＿＿＿＿＿＿＿ Sadness
＿＿＿＿＿＿＿＿＿＿＿＿＿＿＿＿＿＿＿＿＿＿＿＿＿＿＿＿＿＿＿＿＿ Grieving

MOVING ▪ A pattern involving activity
Activity
  Skeletal stabilization (type) ＿＿＿＿＿＿＿＿＿＿＿＿＿＿＿＿ Impaired physical mobility
＿＿＿＿＿＿＿＿＿＿＿＿＿＿＿＿＿＿＿＿＿＿＿＿＿＿＿＿＿＿＿＿＿
  Activity tolerance/endurance ＿＿＿＿＿＿＿＿＿＿＿＿＿＿＿ Activity intolerance
＿＿＿＿＿＿＿＿＿＿＿＿＿＿＿＿＿＿＿＿＿＿＿＿＿＿＿＿＿＿＿＿＿
  Prosthetic/orthotic devices ＿＿＿＿＿＿＿＿＿＿＿＿＿＿＿＿＿
＿＿＿＿＿＿＿＿＿＿＿＿＿＿＿＿＿＿＿＿＿＿＿＿＿＿＿＿＿＿＿＿＿
  Previous exercise habits ＿＿＿＿＿＿＿＿＿＿＿＿＿＿＿＿＿＿
  Range of motion examination ＿＿＿＿＿＿＿＿＿＿＿＿＿＿＿＿
  Balance impaired ＿＿＿＿＿＿ Sitting ＿＿＿＿＿＿＿＿＿＿＿
  Transfers: Dependent ＿＿＿ Independent ＿＿＿ Assist ＿＿＿＿
  Bed mobility: Dependent ＿＿＿ Independent ＿＿＿ Assist ＿＿＿
  Safety precautions needed ＿＿＿＿＿＿＿＿＿＿＿＿＿＿＿＿＿
  Reflexes: Biceps   R ＿＿ L ＿＿   Triceps R ＿＿ L ＿＿
        Brachioradialis R ＿＿ L ＿＿   Knee   R ＿＿ L ＿＿
        Ankle   R ＿＿ L ＿＿   Plantar R ＿＿ L ＿＿
        Ankle clonus   R ＿＿ L ＿＿   Nuchal rigidity ＿＿＿＿

Rest
  Hours slept/night ＿＿＿ Feels rested: yes/no ＿＿＿＿＿＿＿ Sleep pattern disturbance
  Sleep aids (pillows, meds, food) ＿＿＿＿＿＿＿＿＿＿＿＿＿＿
  Difficulty falling/remaining asleep ＿＿＿＿＿＿＿＿＿＿＿＿＿

Fig. 26-1, cont'd

Recreation
Leisure activities _____   Deficit in diversional activity
Social activities _____

Environmental Maintenance
Home maintenance management   Impaired home maintenance
  Accessibility of home/community _____   management
_____
  Transportation _____   Safety hazards
  Modifications needed _____
  Home responsibilities _____
_____
  Assistance available _____

Health Maintenance
Health insurance _____   Health maintenance
Regular physical checkups _____
Access to health care _____
Present legal proceedings _____

Self-Care

ADL performance:	Independent	Dependent	Assist (specify type)	Self-care
Feeding:	_____	_____	_____	Feeding
Bathing:	_____	_____	_____	Bathing/hygiene
Hygiene:	_____	_____	_____	
Dressing: Upper:	_____	_____	_____	Dressing/grooming
Lower:	_____	_____	_____	
Toileting:	_____	_____	_____	Toileting
Transfers:	_____	_____	_____	

Medication
  Administration: _____   _____   _____
Difficulty swallowing _____   Impaired swallowing
Discharge planning needs _____
_____
_____

PERCEIVING ▪ A pattern involving the reception of information
Self-Concept   Self-concept
Patient's description of self _____   Body image
Effects of injury on self-concept _____   Self-esteem
_____   Personal identity
_____
Concerns related to body image _____
_____
Patient's description of own strengths/weaknesses _____
_____

Meaningfulness
Verbalizes hopelessness _____   Hopelessness
Verbalizes/perceives loss of control _____   Powerlessness

Sensory/Perception   Sensory/perception
History of restricted environment _____   Visual
Vision impaired _____ Glasses _____   Auditory
Auditory impaired _____ Hearing aid _____   Tactile
Tactile impaired _____   Kinesthetic
Other _____   Gustatory
     Olfactory

Fig. 26-1, cont'd

Continued.

EXCHANGING ▪ A pattern involving mutual giving and receiving

Circulation

Cerebral   Cerebral tissue perfusion

    Neurologic changes/symptoms _____ Cardiopulmonary tissue

Cardiac   perfusion

    Apical rate & rhythm _____

    BP: Sitting   Lying   Cardiac output

        R _____ L _____   R _____ L _____   Peripheral tissue perfusion

Peripheral

    History of thrombophlebitis _____

    Jugular venous distention: yes/no _____ R _____ L _____

    Skin temp _____ Color _____ Cardiac output

    Capillary refill _____ Edema _____ Fluid volume

    Pulses _____   Deficit

                                                                    Excess

Physical Integrity

Tissue integrity _____ Rashes _____ Lesions _____ Impaired skin integrity

    Petechiae _____ Bruises _____ Impaired tissue integrity

    Skin turgor _____ Other (specify) _____ Potential for injury

    Past history/treatment of skin breakdown _____

    Pressure sores (site/grade) _____

    _____

    Treatment _____

Oxygenation

Complaints of dyspnea _____ Precipitated by _____ Ineffective breathing pattern

History of pulmonary embolus _____ Ineffective airway clearance

Rate _____ Rhythm _____ Depth _____

Labored/unlabored (circle) Use of accessory muscles _____

Chest expansion _____

Cough: productive/nonproductive _____

Sputum: Color _____ Amount _____ Consistency _____

Assistive cough _____ Chest physical therapy _____

Breath sounds _____ Impaired gas exchange

Nutrition   Nutrition

Eating patterns   More than body

    Number of meals per day _____ Where eaten _____   requirements

    Special diet _____ Less than body requirements

    Food preferences/intolerances/allergies _____ Fluid volume

    Daily fluid intake _____   Deficit

    Appetite changes _____   Excess

    Nausea/vomiting _____

Condition of mouth/throat _____

Height _____ Weight _____ Ideal body weight _____ Oral mucous membrane

Elimination

GI/bowel   Bowel elimination

    Usual bowel program _____   Constipation

    Abdominal physical examination _____   Diarrhea

                                                               Incontinence

                                                           GI tissue perfusion

Renal/urinary   Urinary elimination

    Bladder drainage: Catheter (size/type) _____   Incontinence

        Condom catheter (type) _____   Retention

        Intermittent catheterization (frequency) _____

    24-hour urine output _____ Urine color _____

    Serum: BUN _____ Creatinine _____ Specific gravity _____ Renal tissue perfusion

Fig. 26-1, cont'd

Intravenous pyelogram _____   Infection
Urodynamic evaluation _____   Body temperature
Infection: Present _____ Past history _____   Hypothermia
   Urine C&S results _____   Hyperthermia
   Temperature _____ Route _____   Ineffective thermoregulation

CHOOSING ▪ A pattern involving the selection of alternatives
Coping
   Patient's usual problem-solving methods _____   Ineffective individual coping
   _____   Ineffective family coping
   Family's usual problem-solving methods _____
   _____
   Patient's method of dealing with stress _____
   _____
   Family's method of dealing with stress _____
   _____
   Patient's affect _____
   Physical manifestations _____
   Coping mechanisms used _____
   Support systems/resources _____

Participation
   Compliance with past/current health care regimens _____   Noncompliance
   _____
   Willingness to comply with future health care regimen _____
   _____

Judgment
   Decision-making ability   Judgment
      Patient's perspective _____   Indecisiveness
      Others' perspectives _____

Prioritized nursing diagnosis/problem list
1. _____
2. _____
3. _____
4. _____
5. _____
6. _____
7. _____
8. _____

Signature _____   Date _____

Fig. 26-1, cont'd

SPINAL CORD INJURY REHABILITATION ASSESSMENT TOOL

Name _S.P._ _____ Age _19_ Sex _M_

Address _67 SIXTH STREET, CAMDEN, NEW JERSEY_ _____ Telephone _667-7000_

Significant other _PARENTS: MR. & MRS. P._ _____ Telephone _667-7000_

Date of admission _1/8_ _____ Medical diagnosis _QUADRIPLEGIC_

Allergies _NKA_

Level of injury _C-5_ _____ Date of injury _11/3_

Cause of injury _CAR ACCIDENT_

Nursing Diagnosis
(Potential or Altered)

COMMUNICATING ▪ A pattern involving sending messages

(Read,)(write,)(understand) English (circle) _____ Communication

Other languages _NONE_ Speech impaired _NO_ — Verbal

Family's understanding of English _EXCELLENT_ — Nonverbal

VALUING ▪ A pattern involving the assigning of relative worth

Religious preference _CATHOLIC_ _____ Spiritual state

Important religious practices _MASS/SACRAMENTS_ — Despair

Spiritual concerns _NONE_ — Distress

Cultural orientation _IRISH AMERICAN_

Cultural practices _NOTHING SPECIFIC_

RELATING ▪ A pattern involving establishing bonds

Role

Marital status _SINGLE_ _____ Role performance

Age & health of significant other _PARENTS — LATE 40'S IN GOOD_ — Parenting

HEALTH — (Sexual dysfunction)

Number of children _0_ Ages _—_ — Work

Number of siblings _2_ Ages _BROTHER-23, SISTER-25_ — Family

Role in home _YOUNGEST SON_ — Social/leisure

Financial support _PARENTS_

Occupation _STUDENT - SOPHOMORE IN COLLEGE — FULL TIME_ — Family processes

  Job satisfaction/concerns _WANTS TO FINISH COLLEGE_

  Physical/mental energy expenditures _STUDYING — STRESSFUL "A LOT OF PRESSURE"_

Sexual relationships (satisfactory)(unsatisfactory) _IN PAST_

  Physical difficulties/effects of injury related to sex _CHANGES IN ABILITY/_ — Sexuality patterns

OPPORTUNITY DOES HAVE REFLEX ERECTIONS

Socialization

Quality of relationships with others _GOOD IN GENERAL_ — Impaired social interaction

  Patient's description _GOOD - LOTS OF FRIENDS; SUPPORTIVE FAMILY_

  Significant others' descriptions _PARENTS STATE GOOD RELATIONSHIP_ — (POTENTIAL)

  Staff observations _EXCELLENT INTERACTIONS - USES HUMOR A LOT_

Verbalizes feelings of being alone _YES_ — (Social isolation)

  Attributed to _INJURY/HOSPITALIZATION_ — Social withdrawal

KNOWING ▪ A pattern involving the meaning associated with information

Current health problems _QUESTIONABLE NECK STABILITY — MAY RE-_
QUIRE SURGERY; SEVERE SPASTICITY — C5 QUADRIPLEGIA

Previous hospitalizations/illnesses/surgeries _APPENDECTOMY_

Previous participation in rehabilitation programs _NONE_

Current medications _MOTRIN 300mg q6h, AMPHOJEL 600mg QID pc &_ — Knowledge deficit
hs, COLACE 50mg qd, VITAMIN C 50mg qd, MULTIVITAMIN 1 TAB qd

Fig. 26-2

Smoking __No__ Alcohol usage __5-6 BEERS/WK__ Drug usage __No__   Knowledge deficit

Educational level __COLLEGE - 2 YRS__

Understanding of injury __KNOWS THERE HAS BEEN DAMAGE TO SPINAL__ __CORD· MAY NOT WALK AGAIN__   PROPULSION

Expectations of therapy __INDEPENDENT FEEDING, SELF-CARE, WHEELCHAIR__ Thought processes

Misconceptions __NONE - STILL HAS HOPE HE'LL WALK BUT ACCEPTS IT AS UNREALISTIC__

Rehabilitation goals __TO INCREASE GENERAL MOBILITY__

Readiness to learn __EXCELLENT - DEMONSTRATED BY QUESTIONS/COMMENTS__

  Learning impeded by __No__

  Level of comprehension __GOOD__

Orientation   Orientation

Level of alertness __ALERT__   Confusion

Orientation: Person __✓__   Place __✓__   Time __✓__   LOC

Memory

Memory intact: yes/no __YES__ Recent __✓__   Remote __✓__   Memory

FEELING ▪ A pattern involving the subjective awareness of information

Comfort

  Pain/discomfort: yes/no __YES__   (Comfort)

    Frequency __CONTINUOUS__ Location __NECK__   (Pain/chronic)

    Duration __CONTINUOUS__ Quality __DULL, ACHING__ Radiation __SHOULDERS__   Pain/acute

    Associated factors __SPASTICITY · CONTRACTURES__   Discomfort

    Aggravating factors __STAYING IN ONE POSITION TOO LONG__

    Alleviating factors __POSITION CHANGES, ROM__

Emotional Integrity/States

  Recent stressful life events __INJURY · HOSPITALIZATION__   (Anxiety)

     Fear

  Verbalizes feelings __ANXIETY; GRIEF; ANGER__   (Anger)

    Source __FEARS HE WILL STOP BREATHING; ACCIDENT · PARALY-__   Guilt

    __SIS; PARALYSIS · "CAN'T WALK AGAIN"__   Shame

    Physical manifestations __TEARFUL @ TIMES; YELLS @ FRIENDS·__   Sadness

    __FAMILY; MOOD SWINGS__   (Grieving)

MOVING ▪ A pattern involving activity

Activity

  Skeletal stabilization (type) __HALO VEST__   (Impaired physical mobility)

  Activity tolerance/endurance __SIT UP IN WHEELCHAIR × 2 HRS__   Activity intolerance

  Prosthetic/orthotic devices __WHEELCHAIR, SPLINTS, UNIVERSAL__ __CUFF, AUTOMATIC PAGE-TURNER, ELASTIC STOCKINGS__

  Previous exercise habits __JOGGED 5 MILES/DAY, PLAYED BASEBALL__

  Range of motion examination __SEVERE SPASTICITY__

  Balance impaired __YES__ Sitting __YES__

  Transfers: Dependent __✓__ Independent _____ Assist _____

  Bed mobility: Dependent __✓__ Independent _____ Assist _____

  Safety precautions needed __SIDE RAILS__

  Reflexes: Biceps R __+1__ L __+1__   Triceps R __0__ L __0__

      Brachioradialis R __0__ L __0__   Knee R __0__ L __0__

      Ankle R __0__ L __0__   Plantar R __0__ L __0__

      Ankle clonus R __0__ L __0__   Nuchal rigidity __DUE TO__ __STABILIZATION__

Rest

  Hours slept/night __7__ Feels rested: yes/no __YES__   Sleep pattern disturbance

  Sleep aids (pillows, meds, food) __NONE__

  Difficulty falling/remaining asleep __NONE__

Fig. 26-2, cont'd

Continued.

Recreation

Leisure activities *READS SCIENCE FICTION, TV*   Deficit in diversional activity

Social activities *LISTENS TO MUSIC c̄ FRIENDS*

Environmental Maintenance

Home maintenance management   *POTENTIAL*

Accessibility of home/community *HOME — 2ND FLOOR WALKUP — NOT*   Impaired home maintenance management

ACCESSIBLE. GROCERY STORES/RESTAURANTS/CHURCH ACCESSIBLE

Transportation *PUBLIC TRANSPORTATION ACCESSIBLE.*   Safety hazards

Modifications needed *WILL NEED ACCESSIBLE ENTRANCE TO HOME, ? CAR*

Home responsibilities *YARDWORK, CLEANED ROOM — UNABLE TO DO THESE ACTIVITIES NOW*

Assistance available *PARENTS, SIBLINGS, FRIENDS*

Health Maintenance

Health insurance *BLUE CROSS / BLUE SHIELD*   Health maintenance

Regular physical checkups *FAIRLY REGULAR IN PAST*

Access to health care *GOOD, NO ANTICIPATED PROBLEMS*

Present legal proceedings *PRESENTLY INVOLVED IN LAWSUIT RE: ACCIDENT*

Self-Care

ADL performance:	Independent	Dependent	Assist (specify type)	
Feeding:		✓	*CAN FEED SELF IF FOOD IS CUT*	Self-care
Bathing:		✓	*WASHES FACE*	Feeding
Hygiene:		✓	*BRUSHES TEETH*	Bathing/hygiene
Dressing: Upper:		✓		Dressing/grooming
Lower:		✓	*NEEDS ASSISTANCE*	
Toileting:		✓	*DEVICES FOR ABOVE*	Toileting
Transfers:		✓		

Medication

Administration: ✓

Difficulty swallowing *NO*   Impaired swallowing

Discharge planning needs *① FIND ACCESSIBLE HOUSING OR CONTRACT FOR ADAPTATION IN CURRENT HOUSING ② PROVIDE TRAINING FOR ATTENDANT (FAMILY MEMBER OR PAID HELP) ③ VOCATIONAL/EDUCATIONAL EVALUATION — INVESTIGATE ACCESSIBLE COLLEGES*

PERCEIVING ▪ A pattern involving the reception of information

Self-Concept

Patient's description of self *"I LIKE TO LAUGH A LOT."*   Self-concept / Body image

Effects of injury on self-concept *"I'M STILL THE SAME PERSON EVEN THOUGH I'M PARALIZED." "I'M TRYING TO DEAL WITH IT."*   Self-esteem / Personal identity

Concerns related to body image *"I THINK PEOPLE LOOK AT ME DIFFERENTLY." "MAYBE THEY THINK I LOOK STRANGE."*

Patient's description of own strengths/weaknesses *"I KEEP A POSITIVE ATTITUDE & AM ABLE TO LAUGH A LOT AT MYSELF." "I'M IMPATIENT A LOT."*

Meaningfulness

Verbalizes hopelessness *NO "THINGS WILL WORK OUT."*   Hopelessness

Verbalizes/perceives loss of control *YES "NO ONE LISTENS TO WHAT I THINK." "THEY THINK I CAN'T DO ANYTHING."*   Powerlessness

Sensory/Perception

History of restricted environment *ICU x 1 MONTH*   Sensory/perception / Visual

Vision impaired *NO* Glasses *NO*   Auditory

Auditory impaired *NO* Hearing aid *NO*   Tactile

Tactile impaired *YES — SENSATION ONLY TO SHOULDER AREA, HEAD,*   Kinesthetic

Other *NECK*   Gustatory / Olfactory

Fig. 26-2, cont'd

EXCHANGING ▪ **A pattern involving mutual giving and receiving**
Circulation
Cerebral   Cerebral tissue perfusion
  Neurologic changes/symptoms *NONE OTHER THAN INJURY*   Cardiopulmonary tissue
Cardiac   perfusion
  Apical rate & rhythm *74 REGULAR*
  BP: Sitting   Lying   Cardiac output
         R *128/80* L *130/70*   R *114/70* L *116/74*   Peripheral tissue perfusion
Peripheral
  History of thrombophlebitis *NO*
  Jugular venous distention: yes/no *NO*   R *—*   L *—*
  Skin temp *WARM, DRY* Color *PINK*   Cardiac output
  Capillary refill *GOOD, <2SEC* Edema *NONE*   Fluid volume
  Pulses *PALPABLE BILATERALLY*   Deficit
                                                                                                  Excess
                                                                                               (POTENTIAL)
Physical Integrity
  Tissue integrity *INTACT* Rashes *NONE* Lesions *NONE*   (Impaired skin integrity)
  Petechiae *NONE* Bruises *NONE*   Impaired tissue integrity
  Skin turgor *GOOD* Other (specify) *—*   (Potential for injury)
  Past history/treatment of skin breakdown *NONE*
  Pressure sores (site/grade) *REDDENED AREAS ON BOTH ELBOWS*

  Treatment *ELBOW PADS*

Oxygenation
  Complaints of dyspnea *NO* Precipitated by *—*   Ineffective breathing pattern
  History of pulmonary embolus *NO*   Ineffective airway clearance
  Rate *24* Rhythm *REGULAR* Depth *SHALLOW*
  Labored/(unlabored)(circle) Use of accessory muscles *NO*
  Chest expansion *SYMMETRICAL*
  Cough: productive/(nonproductive) *POOR*
  Sputum: Color *—* Amount *—* Consistency *—*
  Assistive cough *YES* Chest physical therapy *YES*
  Breath sounds *CLEAR*   Impaired gas exchange

Nutrition   (Nutrition)
  Eating patterns   More than body
    Number of meals per day *3* Where eaten *LUNCH/DINNER DINING*   requirements
    Special diet *NO*   *ROOM*   (Less than body requirements)
    Food preferences/intolerances/allergies *NONE*   Fluid volume
    Daily fluid intake *3 LITERS*   Deficit
    Appetite changes *NO*   Excess
    Nausea/vomiting *NO*
  Condition of mouth/throat *nml — INTACT*
  Height *5'10"* Weight *140* Ideal body weight *166*   Oral mucous membrane

Elimination
  GI/bowel   (Bowel elimination)
    Usual bowel program *QOD IN A.M., GLYCERIN SUPPOSITORY, COLACE* Constipation
    Abdominal physical examination *SOFT, ⊕ BS IN ALL 4 QUADS*   Diarrhea
                                                                                              (Incontinence)
                                                                                              GI tissue perfusion
  Renal/urinary   (Urinary elimination)
    Bladder drainage: Catheter (size/type) *—*   (Incontinence)
      Condom catheter (type) *—*   Retention
      Intermittent catheterization (frequency) *q 4h*
    24-hour urine output *3400cc* Urine color *CLEAR YELLOW*
    Serum: BUN *12 mg/dl* Creatinine *0.7 mg/dl* Specific gravity *1.025*   Renal tissue perfusion

Fig. 26-2, cont'd

Continued.

Intravenous pyelogram *NORMAL*   Infection
Urodynamic evaluation *PENDING*   Body temperature
Infection: Present ___*No*___ Past history *UTI – E. COLI 2 mos. AGO*   Hypothermia
  Urine C&S results *NEGATIVE*   Hyperthermia
  Temperature *98.4° F* ___ Route *ORAL*   Ineffective thermoregulation

CHOOSING ▪ A pattern involving the selection of alternatives
Coping
Patient's usual problem-solving methods *TALKS c̄ PARENTS/FRIENDS*   Ineffective individual coping
                                                                       Ineffective family coping

Family's usual problem-solving methods *DISCUSSES PROBLEMS/CON-FLICTS OPENLY*

Patient's method of dealing with stress *USES HUMOR, SITS QUIETLY & LISTENS TO MUSIC, SOMETIMES GETS ANGRY*

Family's method of dealing with stress *DISCUSSION – PULL TOGETHER TO WORK THINGS OUT*

Patient's affect *APPROPRIATE*
Physical manifestations *MOOD CHANGES – APPROPRIATE*
Coping mechanisms used *ANGER, DENIAL*
Support systems/resources *FAMILY, FRIENDS*

Participation
Compliance with past/current health care regimens *GOOD COMPLIANCE*   Noncompliance

Willingness to comply with future health care regimen *EXPECT COMPLIANCE*

Judgment
Decision-making ability   Judgment
  Patient's perspective *"I CAN MAKE MY OWN DECISIONS"*   Indecisiveness
  Others' perspectives *GOOD*

Prioritized nursing diagnosis/problem list
1. *BOWEL/URINARY INCONTINENCE R/T SPINAL CORD INJURY*
2. *IMPAIRED PHYSICAL MOBILITY R/T SPINAL CORD INJURY*
3. *ALTERED SELF-CARE R/T PARALYSIS*
4. *ALTERED SELF-CONCEPT R/T BODY IMAGE CHANGES & SEXUAL DYSFUNCTION*
5. *ANXIETY, GRIEVING, & ANGER STATES R/T ACCIDENT & PARALYSIS*
6. *POWERLESSNESS R/T LACK OF INVOLVEMENT IN DECISION-MAKING SINCE ACCIDENT*
7. *ALTERED COMFORT R/T CHRONIC NECK & SHOULDER PAIN*
8. *ALTERED NUTRITION: LESS THAN BODY REQUIREMENTS R/T LOW BODY WEIGHT*

Signature *Anita P. Shrer, R.N.*   Date *5/10*

Fig. 26-2, cont'd

APPENDIX I

TAXONOMY I REVISED (JUNE, 1988)

Pattern 1	**EXCHANGING**
1.1.2.1	Altered nutrition: more than body requirements
1.1.2.2	Altered nutrition: less than body requirements
1.1.2.3	Altered nutrition: potential for more than body requirements
1.2.1.1	Potential for infection
1.2.2.1	Potential altered body temperature
†1.2.2.2	Hypothermia
1.2.2.3	Hyperthermia
1.2.2.4	Ineffective thermoregulation
*1.2.3.1	Dysreflexia
‡1.3.1.1	Constipation
*1.3.1.1.1	Perceived constipation
*1.3.1.1.2	Colonic constipation
‡1.3.1.2	Diarrhea
‡1.3.1.3	Bowel incontinence
1.3.2	Altered patterns of urinary elimination
1.3.2.1.1	Stress incontinence
1.3.2.1.2	Reflex incontinence
1.3.2.1.3	Urge incontinence
1.3.2.1.4	Functional incontinence
1.3.2.1.5	Total incontinence
1.3.2.2	Urinary retention
‡1.4.1.1	Altered (specify type) tissue perfusion (renal, cerebral, cardiopulmonary, gastrointestinal, peripheral)
1.4.1.2.1	Fluid volume excess
1.4.1.2.2.1	Fluid volume deficit (1)
1.4.1.2.2.1	Fluid volume deficit (2)
1.4.1.2.2.2	Potential fluid volume deficit
‡1.4.2.1	Decreased cardiac output
1.5.1.1	Impaired gas exchange
1.5.1.2	Ineffective airway clearance
1.5.1.3	Ineffective breathing pattern

From the North American Nursing Diagnosis Association, St. Louis, 1988.
*New diagnostic categories approved 1988
†Revised diagnostic categories approved 1988
‡Categories with modified label terminology

1.6.1	Potential for injury
1.6.1.1	Potential for suffocation
1.6.1.2	Potential for poisoning
1.6.1.3	Potential for trauma
*1.6.1.4	Potential for aspiration
*1.6.1.5	Potential for disuse syndrome
1.6.2.1	Impaired tissue integrity
‡1.6.2.1.1	Altered oral mucous membrane
1.6.2.1.2.1	Impaired skin integrity
1.6.2.1.2.2	Potential impaired skin integrity

Pattern 2   **COMMUNICATING**

2.1.1.1	Impaired verbal communication

Pattern 3   **RELATING**

3.1.1	Impaired social interaction
3.1.2	Social isolation
‡3.2.1	Altered role performance
3.2.1.1.1	Altered parenting
3.2.1.1.2	Potential altered parenting
3.2.1.2.1	Sexual dysfunction
3.2.2	Altered family processes
*3.2.3.1	Parental role conflict
3.3	Altered sexuality patterns

Pattern 4   **VALUING**

4.1.1	Spiritual distress (distress of the human spirit)

Pattern 5   **CHOOSING**

5.1.1.1	Ineffective individual coping
5.1.1.1.1	Impaired adjustment
*5.1.1.1.2	Defensive coping
*5.1.1.1.3	Ineffective denial
5.1.2.1.1	Ineffective family coping: disabling
5.1.2.1.2	Ineffective family coping: compromised
5.1.2.2	Family coping: potential for growth
5.2.1.1	Noncompliance (specify)
*5.3.1.1	Decisional conflict (specify)
*5.4	Health-seeking behaviors (specify)

Pattern 6   **MOVING**

6.1.1.1	Impaired physical mobility
6.1.1.2	Activity intolerance
*6.1.1.2.1	Fatigue
6.1.1.3	Potential activity intolerance
6.2.1	Sleep pattern disturbance
6.3.1.1	Diversional activity deficit
6.4.1.1	Impaired home maintenance management
6.4.2	Altered health maintenance
‡6.5.1	Feeding self-care deficit
6.5.1.1	Impaired swallowing

*6.5.1.2	Ineffective breastfeeding
‡6.5.2	Bathing/hygiene self-care deficit
‡6.5.3	Dressing/grooming self-care deficit
‡6.5.4	Toileting self-care deficit
6.6	Altered growth and development

Pattern 7   **PERCEIVING**

‡7.1.1	Body image disturbance
‡†7.1.2	Self-esteem disturbance
*7.1.2.1	Chronic low self-esteem
*7.1.2.2	Situational low-self esteem
‡7.1.3	Personal identity disturbance
7.2	Sensory/perceptual alterations (specify) (visual, auditory, kinesthetic, gustatory, tactile, olfactory)
7.2.1.1	Unilateral neglect
7.3.1	Hopelessness
7.3.2	Powerlessness

Pattern 8   **KNOWING**

8.1.1	Knowledge deficit (specify)
8.3	Altered thought processes

Pattern 9   **FEELING**

‡9.1.1	Pain
9.1.1.1	Chronic pain
9.2.1.1	Dysfunctional grieving
9.2.1.2	Anticipatory grieving
9.2.2	Potential for violence: self-directed or directed at others
9.2.3	Post-trauma response
9.2.3.1	Rape-trauma syndrome
9.2.3.1.1	Rape-trauma syndrome: compound reaction
9.2.3.1.2	Rape-trauma syndrome: silent reaction
9.3.1	Anxiety
9.3.2	Fear

APPENDIX II

SELECTED NORMAL LABORATORY VALUES

ABBREVIATIONS USED IN TABLES

<	= less than	mg	= milligram	ng	= nanogram
>	= greater than	ml	= milliliter	pg	= picogram
dl	= 100 ml	mM	= millimole	μEq	= microequivalent
g	= gram	mm Hg	= millimeters of mercury	μg	= microgram
IU	= International Unit	mIU	= milliInternational Unit	μIU	= microInternational Unit
kg	= kilogram	mOsm	= milliosmole	μL	= microliter
mEq	= milliequivalent	mμ	= millimicron	μU	= microunit

Table 1
Whole blood, serum, and plasma chemistry

| Component | System | Typical reference intervals | | |
		Conventional units	Factor*	Recommended SI units†
Acetone				
Qualitative	Serum	Negative	—	Negative
Albumin				
Quantitative	Serum	3.2-4.5 g/dl (salt fraction-ation)	10	32-45 g/L
Amylase	Serum	60-160 Somogyi units/dl	1.85	111-296 U/L
Barbiturates	Serum, plasma, or whole blood	Negative	—	Negative
Base excess	Whole blood			
Male		−3.3 to + 1.2 mEq/L	1	−3.3 to + 1.2 mmol/L
Female		−2.4 to + 2.3 mEq/L		−2.4 to + 2.3 mmol/L
Base, total	Serum	145-160 mEq/L	1	145-160 mmol/L
Bicarbonate	Plasma	21-28 mM	1	21-28 mmol/L
Bilirubin, total	Serum	0.1-1.2 mg/dl	17.1	1.7-20.5 μmol/L
Blood gases				
pH	Whole blood	7.38-7.44 (arterial)	1	7.38-7.44
		7.36-7.41 (venous)		7.36-7.41
P_{CO_2}	Whole blood	35-40 mm Hg (arterial)	0.133	4.66-5.32 kPa
		40-45 mm Hg (venous		5.32-5.99 kPa
P_{O_2}	Whole blood	95-100 mm Hg (arterial)	0.133	12.64-13.30 kPa
Calcium, total	Serum	4.6-5.5 mEq/L	0.5	23-28 mmol/L

Adapted from Henry JB: Todd-Sanford-Davidsohn clinical diagnosis and management by laboratory methods, ed 17, Philadelphia, 1984, WB Saunders Co.

*Factor, Number factor (note that units are not presented).

†Value in SI units, Value in conventional units × factor.

‡From Report of the National Cholesterol Education Program Expert Panel on Detection, Evaluation, and Treatment of High Blood Cholesterol in Adults; Arch Intern Med 148:36, 1988.

Table 1—cont'd

Whole blood, serum, and plasma chemistry

Component	System	Typical reference intervals		
		Conventional units	Factor*	Recommended SI units†
Carbon dioxide (CO₂ content)	Whole blood (arterial)	19-24 mM	1	19-24 mmol/L
	Plasma or serum (arterial)	21-28 mM		21-28 mmol/L
Carbon dioxide	Whole blood (venous)	22-26 mM	1	22-26 mmol/L
	Plasma or serum (venous)	24-30 mM		24-30 mmol/L
CO₂ partial pressure (Pco₂)	Whole blood (arterial)	35-40 mm Hg	0.133	4.66-5.32 kPa
Chloride	Serum	95-103 mEq/L	1	95-103 mmol/L
Cholesterol, total‡	Serum	<200 mg/dl (varies with diet, sex, and age)	0.026	< 5.2 mmol/L
Creatine kinase (CK)	Serum			
	Male	55-170 U/L at 37° C	1	55-170 U/L at 37° C
	Female	30-135 U/L at 37° C	1	30-135 U/L at 37° C
Creatinine	Serum or plasma	0.6-1.2 mg/dl (adult)	88.4	53-106 µmol/L
		0.3-0.6 mg/dl (children <2 yr)		27-54 µmol/L
Creatinine clearance (endogenous)	Serum or plasma and urine			
	Male	107-139 ml/min	0.0167	1.78-2.32 ml/sec
	Female	87-107 ml/min		1.45-1.79 ml/sec
Cytomegalo virus (CMV) titer	Serum	None		
Electrophoresis, protein	Serum	Percent		Fraction of total protein
Albumin		52%-65% of total protein	0.01	0.52-0.65
Alpha-1		2.5%-5.0% of total protein	0.01	0.025-0.05
Alpha-2		7.0%-13.0% of total protein	0.01	0.07-0.13
Beta		8.0%-14.0% of total protein	0.01	0.08-0.14
Gamma		12.0%-22.0% of total protein	0.01	0.12-0.22
		Concentration		
Albumin		3.2-5.6 g/dl	10	32-56 g/L
Alpha-1		0.1-0.4 g/dl		1-4 g/L
Alpha-2		0.4-1.2 g/dl		4-12 g/L
Beta		0.5-1.1 g/dl		5-11 g/L
Gamma		0.5-1.6 g/dl		5-16 g/L
Fibrinogen	Plasma	200-400 mg/dl	0.01	2.00-4.00 g/L
Gamma globulin	Serum	0.5-1.6 g/dl	10	5-16 g/L
Globulins, total	Serum	2.3-3.5 g/dl	10	23-35 g/L
Glucose, fasting	Serum or plasma	70-110 mg/dl	0.055	3.85-6.05 mmol/L
Glucose tolerance				
Oral	Serum or plasma			
Fasting		70-110 mg/dl	0.055	3.85-6.05 mmol/L
30 min		30-60 mg/dl above fasting		1.65-3.30 mmol/L above fasting
60 min		20-50 mg/dl above fasting		1.10-2.75 mmol/L above fasting
120 min		5-15 mg/dl above fasting		0.28-0.83 mmol/L above fasting
180 min		Fasting level or below		Fasting level or below
Intravenous	Serum or plasma			
Fasting		70-110 mg/dl		3.85-6.05 mmol/L
5 min		Maximum of 250 mg/dl		Maximum of 13.75 mmol/L

Continued

Table 1—cont'd
Whole blood, serum, and plasma chemistry

Component	System	Typical reference intervals		
		Conventional units	Factor*	Recommended SI units†
	60 min	Significant decrease		Significant decrease
	120 min	Below 120 mg/dl		Below 6.60 mmol/L
	180 min	Fasting level		Fasting level
Glucose 6-phosphate dehydrogenase (G6PD)	Erythocytes	250-500 units/10^6 cells	1	250-500 μunits/cells
Hemoglobin	Whole blood			
	Female	12.0-16.0 g/dl	10	120-160 mmol/L
	Male	13.5-18.0 g/dl		135-180 mmol/L
Immunoglobulins	Serum			
IgG		800-1801 mg/dl	0.01	8.0-18.0 g/L
IgA		113-563 mg/dl		1.1-5.6 g/L
IgM		54-222 mg/dl		0.54-2.2 g/L
IgD		0.5-3.0 mg/dl	10	5.0-30 mg/L
IgE		0.01-0.04 mg/dl		0.1-0.4 mg/L
Insulin	Plasma			
	Bioassay	11-240 μIU/ml	0.0417	0.46-10.00 μg/L
	Radioimmunoassay	4-24 μIU/ml		0.17-1.00 μg/L
Insulin tolerance (0.1 unit/kg)	Serum			
	Fasting	Glucose of 70-110 mg/dl	0.055	Glucose of 3.85-6.05 mmol/L
	30 min	Fall to 50% of fasting level	0.01	Fall to 0.5 of fasting level
	90 min	Fasting level		Fasting level
Iron, total	Serum	60-150 μg/dl	0.179	11-27 μmol/L
Iron binding capacity	Serum	250-400 μg/dl	0.179	54-64 μmol/L
Iron saturation	Serum	20%-55%	0.01	Fraction of total iron binding capacity: 0.20-0.55
Ketone bodies	Serum	Negative	—	Negative
17-Ketosteroids	Plasma	25-125 μg/dl	0.01	0.25-1.25 mg/L
Lactic acid (as lactate)	Whole blood			
	Venous	5-20 mg/dl	0.111	0.6-2.2 mmol/L
	Arterial	3-7 mg/dl		0.3-0.8 mmol/L
Lactate dehydrogenase (LDH)	Serum	(Lactate → pyruvate) 80-120 units at 30° C	0.48	38-62 U/L at 30° C
Lactate dehydrogenase isoenzymes	Serum			
LDH$_1$ (anode)		17%-27%	0.01	0.17-0.27
LDH$_2$		27%-37%		0.27-0.37
LDH$_3$		18%-25%		0.18-0.25
LDH$_4$		3%-8%		0.03-0.08
LDH$_5$ (cathode)		0%-5%		0.00-0.05
Lead	Whole blood	0-50 μg/dl	0.048	0-2.4 μmol/L
Lipids, total	Serum	400-800 mg/dl	0.01	4.00-8.00 g/L
Cholesterol‡		< 200 mg/dl	0.026	< 5.2 mmol/L
Triglycerides		10-190 mg/dl	0.109	1.09-20.71 mmol/L
Phospholipids		150-380 mg/dl	0.01	1.50-380 g/L

Table 1—cont'd
Whole blood, serum, and plasma chemistry

Component	System	Typical reference intervals		
		Conventional units	Factor*	Recommended SI units†
Fatty acids (free)		9.0-15.0 mM/L	1	9.0-15.0 mmol/L
		300-480 μEq/L	0.01	300-480 μmol/L
Phospholipid phosphorus		8.0-11.0 mg/dl	0.323	2.58-3.55 mmol/L
Long-acting thyroid-stimulating hormone (LATS)	Serum	None	—	None
Luteinizing hormone (LH)	Serum			
Male		6-30 mIU/ml	0.23	1.4-6.9 mg/L
Female		Midcycle peak: 3 times baseline value		Midcycle peak: 3 times baseline value
		Premenopausal <30 mIU/ml		Premenopausal <5 times baseline value
		Postmenopausal >35 mIU/ml		Postmenopausal >5 times baseline value
Magnesium	Serum	1.3-2.1 mEq/L	0.5	0.7-1.1 mmol/L
Osmolality	Serum	280-295 mOsm/kg	1	280-295 mmol/L
Oxygen				
Pressure (P_{O_2})	Whole blood (arterial)	95-100 mm Hg	0.133	12.64-13.30 kPa
Saturation	Whole blood (arterial)	94%-100%	0.01	0.94-1.00
pH	Whole blood (arterial)	7.38-7.44	1	7.38-7.44
	Whole blood (venous)	7.36-7.41		7.36-7.41
	Serum or plasma (venous)	7.35-7.45		7.35-7.45
Phosphatase, alkaline	Serum	20-90 IU/L at 30° C (paranitrophenylphosphate in AMP buffer)	1	20-90 U/L at 30° C
Phosphorus, inorganic	Serum			
Adults		2.3-4.7 mg/dl	0.323	0.78-1.52 mmol/L
Children		4.0-7.0 mg/dl		1.29-2.26 mmol/L
Potassium	Plasma	3.8-5.0 mEq/L	1	3.8-5.0 mmol/L
Proteins	Serum			
Total		6.0-7.8 g/dl	10	60-78 g/L
Albumin		3.2-4.5 g/dl		32-45 g/L
Globulin		2.3-3.5 g/dl		23-35 g/L
Sodium	Plasma	136-142 mEq/L	1	136-142 mmol/L
Sulfate, inorganic	Serum	0.2-1.3 mEq/L	0.5	0.10-0.65 mmol/L
Testosterone	Serum or plasma			
Male		300-1200 ng/dl	0.035	10.0-42.0 nmol/L
Female		30-95 ng/dl		1.1-3.3 nmol/L
Transferases				
Aspartate amino transferase (AST or SGOT)	Serum	16-60 U/ml (Karmen) at 30° C	0.48	8-33 U/L at 37° C

Continued

Table 1—cont'd

Whole blood, serum, and plasma chemistry

Component	System	Typical reference intervals		
		Conventional units	Factor*	Recommended SI units†
Alanine amino transferase (ALT or SGPT)	Serum	8-50 U/ml (Karmen) at 30° C	0.48	4-36 U/L at 37° C
Triglycerides	Serum	10-190 mg/dl	0.011	0.11-2.09 mmol/L
Urea nitrogen	Serum	8-23 mg/dl	0.357	2.9-8.2 mmol/L
Urea clearance	Serum and urine			
Maximum		64-99 ml/min	0.0167	1.07-1.65 ml/sec
Standard		41-65 ml/min, or more than 75% of normal clearance		0.68-1.09 ml/sec or more than 0.75 of normal clearance
Uric acid	Serum			
Male		4.0-8.5 mg/dl	0.059	0.24-0.5 mmol/L
Female		2.7-7.3 mg/dl		0.16-0.43 mmol/L
Zinc	Serum	50-150 µg/dl	0.153	7.65-22.95 µmol/L

Table 2

Urine

Component	Type of urine specimen	Typical reference intervals		
		Conventional units	Factor	Recommended SI units
Acetone	Random	Negative	—	Negative
Albumin				
Qualitative	Random	Negative	—	Negative
Ammonia nitrogen	24 hr	20-70 mEq/24 hr		
Amylase	2 hr	35-260 Somogyi units/hr	0.185	6.5-48.1 U/hr
Arsenic	24 hr	<50 mg/L	0.013	<0.65 µmol/L
Calcium				
Qualitative (Sulkowitch)	Random	1+ turbidity	1	1+ turbidity
Quantitative	24 hr			
Average diet		100-240 mg/24 hr	0.025	2.50-6.25 mmol/24 hr
Low-calcium diet		<150 mg/24 hr		<3.75 mmol/24 hr
High-calcium diet		240-300 mg/24 hr		6.25-7.50 mmol/24 hr
Catecholamines	Random	0-14 µg/dl	10	0-140 µg/L
	24 hr	<100 µg/24 hr (varies with activity)	1	<100 µg/24 hr
Epinephrine		<10 ng/24 hr	5.46	<55 nmol/24 hr
Norepinephrine		<100 ng/24 hr	5.91	<590 nmol/24 hr
Total free catecholamines		4-126 µg/24 hr	1	4-126 µg/24 hr
Total metanephrines		0.1-1.6 mg/24 hr	1	0.1-1.6 mg/24 hr

Adapted from Henry JB: Todd-Sanford-Davidsohn clinical diagnosis and management by laboratory methods, ed 17, Philadelphia, 1984, WB Saunders Co.

Table 2—cont'd

Urine

Component	Type of urine specimen	Typical reference intervals		
		Conventional units	Factor	Recommended SI units
Chloride	24 hr	140-250 mEq/24 hr	1	140-250 mmol/24 hr
Copper	24 hr	0-50 μg/24 hr	0.016	0-0.48 μmol/24 hr
Creatine	24 hr			
Male		0-40 mg/24 hr	0.0076	0-0.30 mmol/24 hr
Female		0-100 mg/24 hr		0-0.76 mmol/24 hr
		Higher in children and during pregnancy	—	Higher in children and during pregnancy
Creatinine	24 hr			
Male		20-26 mg/kg/24 hr	0.0088	0.18-0.23 mmol/kg/24 hr
		1.0-2.0 g/24 hr	8.8	8.8-17.6 mmol/24 hr
Female		14-22 mg/kg/24 hr	0.0088	0.12-0.19 mmol/kg/24 hr
		0.8-1.8 g/24 hr	8.8	7.0-15.8 mmol/24 hr
Epinephrine	24 hr	0-20 μg/24 hr	0.0055	0.00-0.11 μmol/24 hr
Estrogens, total	24 hr			
Male		5-18 μg/24 hr	1	5-18 μg/24 hr
Female				
Ovulation		28-100 μg/24 hr		28-100 μg/24 hr
Luteal peak		22-80 μg/24 hr		22-80 μg/24 hr
At menses		4-25 μg/24 hr		4-25 μg/24 hr
Pregnancy		Up to 45,000 μg/24 hr		Up to 45,000 μg/24 hr
Postmenopausal		Up to 10 μg/24 hr		Up to 10 μg/24 hr
Fat, qualitative	Random	Negative	—	Negative
Fluoride	24 hr	<1 mg/24 hr	0.053	0.053 mmol/24 hr
Glucose, qualitative	Random	Negative	—	Negative
Lactose	24 hr	14-40 mg/24 hr	2.9	41-116 μmol/24 hr
Lead	24 hr	<100 μg/24 hr	0.0048	<0.48 μmol/24 hr
Magnesium	24 hr	6.0-8.5 mEq/24 hr	0.5	3.0-4.3 mmol/24 hr
Myoglobin				
Qualitative	Random	Negative	—	Negative
Quantitative	24 hr	<4 mg/L	1	<4 mg/L
Osmolaltity	Random	500-800 mOsm/kg water	1	500-800 mmol/kg
pH	Random	4.6-8.0	1	4.6-8.0
Phosphorus	Random	0.9-1.3 g/24 hr	32	29-42 mmol/24 hr
Potassium	24 hr	40-80 mEq/24 hr	1	40-80 mmol/24 hr
Protein, qualitative	Random	Negative	—	Negative
Sodium	24 hr	75-200 mEq/24 hr	1	75-200 mmol/24 hr
Specific gravity	Random			Relative density (U 20° C/water 20° C)
		1.016-1.022 (normal fluid intake)	1	1.016-1.022 (normal fluid intake)
		1.001-1.035 (range)		1.001-1.034 (range)
Sugars (excluding glucose)	Random	Negative	—	Negative
Urea nitrogen	24 hr	6-17 g/24 hr	0.0357	0.21-0.60 mol/24 hr
Uric acid	24 hr	250-750 mg/24 hr	0.0059	1.48-4.43 mmol/24 hr
Vanillylmandelic acid (VMA)	24 hr	1.5-7.5 mg/24 hr	5.05	7.6-37.9 μmol/24 hr
Zinc	24 hr	0.15-1.2 mg/24 hr	15.3	2.3-18.4 μmol/24 hr

Table 3
Hematology

Component	Typical reference intervals		
	Conventional units	Factor	Recommended SI units
Coagulation and hemostatic tests			
Fibrinogen split products	10 µg/ml		10 mg/L
Partial thromboplastin time (PTT)	Depends on phospholipid reagent used, typically 60-85 sec		
Activated PTT	Depends on activator and phospholipid reagents used, typically 20-35 sec		
Prothrombin time	Depends on thromboplastin reagent used, typically 9.5-12 sec		
Thrombin time	Depends on concentration of thrombin reagent used, typically 20-29 sec		
Complete blood count (CBC)			
Hematocrit			
Male	40%-54%	0.01	Volume fraction: 0.40-0.54
Female	38%-47%		0.38%-0.47%
Hemoglobin			
Male	13.5-18.0 g/dl	0.155	2.09-2.79 mmol/L
Female	12.0-16.0 g/dl		1.86-2.48 mmol/L
Red cell count			
Male	$4.6\text{-}6.2 \times 10^6/\mu L$	10^6	$4.6\text{-}6.2 \times 10^{12}/L$
Female	$4.2\text{-}5.4 \times 10^6/\mu L$		$4.2\text{-}5.4 \times 10^{12}/L$
White cell count	$4.5\text{-}11.0 \times 10^3/\mu L$	10^6	$4.5\text{-}11.0 \times 10^9/L$

White blood cell differential (adult)

	Mean percent	Range of absolute count		Mean number fraction*	Range of absolute count
Segmented neutrophils (or polymorphonuclear neutrophils [PMN])	56%	1800-7000/µL	10^6	0.56	$1.8\text{-}7.8 \times 10^9/L$
Bands	3%	0-700/µL	10^6	0.03	$0\text{-}0.70 \times 10^9/L$
Eosinophils	2.7%	0-450/µL	10^6	0.027	$0\text{-}0.45 \times 10^9/L$
Basophils	0.3%	0-200/µL	10^6	0.003	$0\text{-}0.20 \times 10^9/L$
Lymphocytes	34%	1000-4800/µL	10^6	0.34	$1.0\text{-}4.8 \times 10^9/L$
Monocytes	4%	0-800/µL	10^6	0.04	$0\text{-}0.80 \times 10^9/L$

Component	Conventional units	Factor	Recommended SI units
Platelet count	150,000-400,000/µL	10^6	$0.15\text{-}0.4 \times 10^{12}/L$
Sedimentation Rate (ESR)			
Men under 50 yrs	<50 mm/hr	1	<50 mm/hr
Men over 50 yrs	<20 mm/hr		<20 mm/hr
Women under 50 yrs	<20 mm/hr		<20 mm/hr
Women over 50 yrs	<30 mm/hr		<30 mm/hr

Adapted from Henry JB: Todd-Sanford-Davidsohn clinical diagnosis and management by laboratory methods, ed 17, Philadelphia, 1984. WB Saunders Co.

*All percentages are multiplied by 0.01 to give fraction.

Table 4
Some selected neonatal and pediatric values*

Component	Normal range	Conversion factor	Recommended SI units
Hematocrit	40%-50%	0.01	0.40-0.50
Hemoglobin	13.5-18.0 g/dl	10	135-180 g/L
RBC count	$4.5\text{-}6 \times 10^6/\mu L$	1	$4.6\text{-}6 \times 10^{12}/L$
WBC count	$4.5\text{-}10 \times 10^3/\mu L$	1	$4.5\text{-}10 \times 10^9/L$

Adapted from Hazinski MF: Nursing care of the critically ill child, St Louis, 1984, The CV Mosby Co.

*The International Committee for Standardization in Hematology recommends that the numbers remain the same but that the units change so that hemoglobin is expressed as grams per deciliter (g/dl), even though other measurements are expressed as units per liter (U/L).

INDEX

A

Acquired Immunodeficiency Syndrome Assessment Tool, 288-303
  development and refinement of, 288
  how to elicit appropriate data using, 291
  how to use, 288-289
  patient population and setting for, 288
Acquired immunodeficiency syndrome emphasis areas, 288, 289
Activity, focus questions related to, 28
Adolescent Assessment Tool, 357-371
  development and refinement of, 357
  how to elicit appropriate data using, 259, 361
  how to use, 358-359
  patient population and setting for, 357
Adolescent emphasis areas, 357-358
AIDS; *see* Acquired immunodeficiency syndrome emphasis areas
Ankle reflex, testing for, 30
Aortic insufficiency, 34
Aortic stenosis, 34
Assessment
  nursing models used to guide, 4-5
  of patients throughout the life span, 305-389
  of patients with major specialty dysfunctions, 127-303
  of patients with major systems dysfunctions, 57-126
  of rehabilitation patients, 391-436
Assessment Tool
  Acquired Immunodeficiency Syndrome, 288-303
  Adolescent, 357-371
  Cardiac Rehabilitation, 393-406
  Cardiovascular; *see* Cardiovascular Assessment Tool
  Critical Care, 179-197
  Endocrine, 108-126
  formulation of nursing diagnoses using, 12-13
  Gerontologic, 372-389
  Gynecologic, 145-160
  Labor-Delivery, 307-327
  Medical-Surgical, 129-144
  Neonatal, 328-342
  Neurologic, 75-95
  Oncologic, 272-287
  Orthopedic, 256-271
  Perioperative, 198-222
  Psychiatric, 161-178
  Pulmonary, 59-73
  Renal, 92-107
  Spinal Cord Injury Rehabilitation, 423-436
  Stroke Rehabilitation, 407-422

Assessment Tool—cont'd
  Transplant, 223-238
  Trauma, 239-255
  validity testing of, 11
Assessment variables in assessment tool, 10
  clustering of, 23

B

Biceps reflex, testing of, 30
Blood, whole, normal laboratory values for, 440-444
Brachioradialis reflex, testing for, 30

C

Cardiac Rehabilitation Assessment Tool, 393-406
  development and refinement of, 393
  how to elicit appropriate data using, 396
  how to use, 394, 396
  patient population and setting for, 393
Cardiac rehabilitation emphasis areas, 393, 394
Cardiovascular accident, 407
Cardiovascular Assessment Tool, 48-53
  adapting
    in practice setting, 45
    as screening tool, 45-47
  collecting sufficient data with, 46-47
  how to use, 11-13, 47
  as nursing data base prototype, 8, 10-11, 17-22
  patient population and setting for, 11, 45-46
  practical applications of, 40-55
  refining and testing of, 11
Cardiovascular emphasis areas, 11, 12
Cardiovascular Screening Tool, 45-47, 54-55
Care plan, sample, 41-44
Cerebrovascular problems, focus questions related to, 26
Choosing, 7
  in assessment tools; *see* Emphasis areas of assessment tools
  nursing diagnoses involving, 9, 438
Choosing pattern focus questions and parameters, 38-39
Circulation, focus questions related to, 31-35
Clinical assessment tools, 11
Clinical practice, refining and testing nursing data base prototype in, 11
Coma Scale, Glasgow, 31, 32
Comfort, focus questions related to, 27
Communicating, 7
  in assessment tools; *see* Emphasis areas of assessment tools
  nursing diagnoses involving, 8, 438

Communicating pattern focus questions and parameters, 24
Communication, focus questions related to, 24
Conceptual framework, 4
Conceptual model, 4
    to structure nursing data base, 4-5
Coping, focus questions related to, 38-39
Critical Care Assessment Tool, 179-197
    development and refinement of, 179
    how to elicit appropriate data using, 182
    how to use, 180, 182
    patient population and setting for, 179-180
Critical care emphasis areas, 180
Cultural orientation, focus questions related to, 24
Cultural practices, focus questions related to, 24
Current health problems, focus questions related to, 25

D

Data, appropriate, general focus questions and parameters for eliciting, 23-39
Data base
    medical, in nursing practice, 3-4
    nursing; *see* Nursing data base
Deep tendon reflexes, testing for, 30
Diagnoses, nursing; *see* Nursing diagnoses

E

Ejection sounds, 31, 33
Elimination, focus questions related to, 38
Emotional integrity/states, focus questions related to, 27-28
Emphasis areas of assessment tools, 11
    acquired immunodeficiency syndrome, 288, 289
    adolescent, 357-358
    cardiac rehabilitation, 393, 394
    cardiovascular, 11, 12
    critical care, 180
    endocrine, 108-109
    gerontologic, 372, 373
    gynecologic, 145, 146
    labor-delivery, 308
    medical-surgical, 130
    neonatal, 329
    neurologic, 76
    orthopedic, 256, 257
    pediatric, 344
    perioperative, 199, 200
    psychiatric, 161, 162
    pulmonary, 59-60
    renal, 92, 93
    spinal cord injury rehabilitation, 424
    stroke rehabilitation, 408
    transplant, 223, 224
    trauma, 240
Endocrine Assessment Tool, 108-126
    development and refinement of, 108
    how to elicit appropriate data using, 111-112
    how to use, 109, 111
    patient population and setting for, 108
Endocrine emphasis areas, 108-109
English, ability to read, write, and understand, focus questions related to, 24
Environmental maintenance, focus questions related to, 28-29
Exchanging, 7
    in assessment tools; *see* Emphasis areas
    nursing diagnoses involving, 8, 437-438
Exchanging pattern focus questions and parameters, 31-38

F

Feeling, 7
    in assessment tools; *see* Emphasis areas of assessment tools
    nursing diagnoses involving, 9, 439
Feeling pattern focus questions and parameters, 27-28
Financial support, focus questions related to, 24
Focus questions, 13
    with Acquired Immunodeficiency Syndrome Assessment Tool, 290
    with Adolescent Assessment Tool, 359-360
    with Cardiac Rehabilitation Assessment Tool, 395
    for choosing pattern, 38-39
    for communicating pattern, 24
    with Critical Care Assessment Tool, 181-182
    with Endocrine Assessment Tool, 110-111
    for exchanging pattern, 30-38
    for feeling pattern, 27-28
    general; *see* General focus questions and parameters
    with Gerontologic Assessment Tool, 374-375
    with Gynecologic Assessment Tool, 147
    for knowing pattern, 25-27
    with Labor-Delivery Assessment Tool, 309-310
    with Medical-Surgical Assessment Tool, 131
    for moving pattern, 28-29
    with Neonatal Assessment Tool, 330-331
    with Neurologic Assessment Tool, 77-78
    with Oncologic Assessment Tool, 274-275
    with Orthopedic Assessment Tool, 258
    with Pediatric Assessment Tool, 345-346
    for perceiving pattern, 29-30
    with Perioperative Assessment Tool, 201-203
    with Psychiatric Assessment Tool, 163-164
    with Pulmonary Assessment Tool, 61
    for relating pattern, 24-25
    with Renal Assessment Tool, 94-95
    with Spinal Cord Injury Rehabilitation Assessment Tool, 425
    with Stroke Rehabilitation Assessment Tool, 409
    with Transplant Assessment Tool, 225
    with Trauma Assessment Tool, 241-242
    for valuing pattern, 24
Friction rub, pericardial, 34

G

General focus questions and parameters
    applying, 39
    for eliciting appropriate data, 23-39
    using, 23
Gerontologic Assessment Tool, 372-389
    development and refinement of, 372
    how to elicit appropriate data using, 374-375
    how to use, 372-374
    patient population and setting for, 372
Gerontologic emphasis areas, 372, 373
Glasgow Coma Scale, 31, 32
Gynecologic Assessment Tool, 145-160
    development and refinement of, 145
    how to elicit appropriate data using, 146, 148
    how to use, 145-146
    patient population and setting for, 145
Gynecologic emphasis areas, 145, 146

H

Health maintenance, focus questions related to, 29
Heart, focus questions related to, 31-35
Heart murmurs, 33
    classification of, 34

Heart problems, focus questions related to, 25
Heart sounds, 31, 33
Hematology, normal laboratory values in, 446-447
Hospitalizations, previous, focus questions related to, 25
Human response patterns of unitary person, 7

I

Illness
    perception/knowledge of, focus questions related to, 26
    previous, focus questions related to, 25
Immune system, focus questions related to, 36
Intubation, focus questions related to, 24

J

Judgment, focus questions related to, 39

K

Kidney problems, focus questions related to, 25
Knee reflex, testing for, 30
Knowing, 7
    in assessment tools; *see* Emphasis areas of assessment tools
    nursing diagnoses involving, 9
Knowing pattern focus questions and parameters, 25-27
Knowledge of illness, focus questions related to, 26

L

Labor-Delivery Assessment Tool, 307-327
    development and refinement of, 307
    how to elicit appropriate data using, 310
    how to use, 308-309
    patient population and setting for, 307-308
Laboratory values, normal, selected, 440-447
Labor-delivery emphasis areas, 308
Language, focus questions related to, 24
Learning, readiness for, focus questions related to, 27
Life span, patients throughout, assessment of, 305-389
Liver problems, focus questions related to, 25
Lung problems, focus questions related to, 25

M

Major specialty dysfunctions, patients with, assessment of, 127-303
Major systems dysfunctions, patients with, assessing, 57-126
Meaningfulness, focus questions related to, 29
Medical data base in nursing practice, 3-4
Medical-Surgical Assessment Tool, 129-144
    development and refinement of, 129
    how to elicit appropriate data using, 131-132
    how to use, 130-131
    patient population and setting for, 129
Medical-surgical emphasis areas, 130
Medications, current, focus questions related to, 26
Memory, focus questions related to, 27
Midsystolic clicks, 33
Misconceptions, focus questions related to, 26-27
Mitral regurgitation, 34
Mitral stenosis, 34
Moving, 7
    in assessment tools; *see* Emphasis areas of assessment tools
    nursing diagnoses involving, 9, 438-439
Moving pattern focus questions and parameters, 28-29
Murmurs, heart, 33
    classification of, 34

N

Neonatal Assessment Tool, 328-342
    development and refinement of, 328

Neonatal Assessment Tool—cont'd
    how to elicit appropriate data using, 331-332
    how to use, 329-331
    patient population and setting for, 328-329
Neonatal emphasis areas, 329
Neurologic Assessment Tool, 75-95
    development and refinement of, 75
    how to elicit appropriate data using, 78
    how to use, 76, 78
    patient population and setting for, 75-76
Neurologic emphasis areas, 76
Normal laboratory values, selected, 404-447
North American Nursing Diagnosis Association (NANDA)
    formation of, 4
    nursing diagnoses of; *see* Nursing diagnoses
    and Unitary Person Framework, 6-7
Nursing, conceptual model of, to structure nursing data base, 4-5
Nursing care plan, sample, 41-44
Nursing data base
    conceptual model of nursing to structure, 4-5
    need for, 3-5
    traditional, 3-4
Nursing data base prototype
    Cardiovascular Assessment Tool as, 8, 10-11, 17-22
    developing, 1-55
        from Unitary Person Framework, 6-22
    overview of, 6-7
    refining and testing of, in clinical practice, 11
    Stage I, 15
    Stage II, 16
    Stage III, 17-22
    from Unitary Person Framework, benefits of, 13-14
Nursing diagnoses
    classification of, 7, 8-9
    definition of, 7
    formulation of, using assessment tools, 12-13
    framework for, 6-7
    and nursing care plan, 40
    qualifiers for, 10
Nursing diagnosis movement, 4-5
Nursing models used to guide assessment, 4-5
Nursing orders, 40
Nursing practice, medical data base in, 3-4
Nutrition, focus questions related to, 36-37

O

Occupation, focus questions related to, 25
Oncologic Assessment Tool, 272-287
    development and refinement of, 272
    how to elicit appropriate data using, 275
    how to use, 273, 275
    patient population and setting for, 272
Oncologic emphasis areas, 272, 273
Opening snaps, 33
Orders, nursing, 40
Orthopedic Assessment Tool, 256-271
    development and refinement of, 256
    how to elicit appropriate data using, 259
    how to use, 256-257, 259
    patient population and setting for, 256
Orthopedic emphasis areas, 256, 257
Outcome criteria, 40
Outcome Standards of Cancer Nursing Practice, 272
Outcomes, patient, 40
Oxygenation, focus questions related to, 35-36

P

Participation, focus questions related to, 39
Patient(s)
  with major specialty dysfunctions, assessment of, 127-303
  with major systems dysfunctions, assessment of, 57-126
  rehabilitation, assessment of, 391-436
  throughout the life span, assessment of, 305-389
Patient outcomes, 40
Pediatric Assessment Tool, 343-356
  development and refinement of, 343
  how to elicit appropriate data using, 345-346
  how to use, 344-345
  patient population and setting for, 343-344
Pediatric emphasis areas, 344
Perceiving, 7
  in assessment tools; *see* Emphasis areas of assessment tools
  nursing diagnoses involving, 9, 439
Perceiving pattern focus questions and parameters, 29-30
Perception of illness, focus questions related to, 26
Pericardial friction rub, 34
Perinatal Nurse Specialist Standards, 328
Perioperative Assessment Tool, 198-222
  development and refinement of, 198
  how to elicit appropriate data using, 204
  how to use, 199
  patient population and setting for, 198-199
Perioperative emphasis areas, 199, 200
Peripheral vascular problems, focus questions related to, 25
Physical integrity, focus questions related to, 35
Physical regulation, focus questions related to, 36
Plantar reflex, testing for, 30
Plasma chemistry, normal values for, 440-444
Practice setting, adapting Cardiovascular Assessment Tool in, 45
Previous illness/hospitalizations/surgeries, focus questions related to, 25
Psychiatric Assessment Tool, 161-178
  development and refinement of, 161
  how to elicit appropriate data using, 164
  how to use, 161-162, 164
  patient population and setting for, 161
Psychiatric emphasis areas, 161, 162
Pulmonary Assessment Tool, 59-73
  development and refinement of, 59
  how to elicit appropriate data using, 61-62
  how to use, 60
  patient population and setting for, 59
Pulmonary emphasis areas, 59-60
Pulmonary regurgitation, 34
Pulmonary stenosis, 34

Q

Quadruple rhythms, 31
Qualifiers, nursing diagnosis, 10
Questions, focus; *see* Focus questions

R

Readiness to learn, focus questions related to, 27
Recreation, focus questions related to, 28
Refining nursing data base prototype in clinical practice, 11
Reflexes, deep tendon, testing for, 30
Regurgitation, mitral, pulmonary, and tricuspid, 34
Rehabilitation patients, assessment of, 391-436
Relating, 7
  in assessment tools; *see* Emphasis areas of assessment tools
  nursing diagnoses involving, 8, 438
Relating pattern focus questions and parameters, 24-25

Reliability of research tool, 11
Religious practices, focus questions related to, 24
Religious preference, focus questions related to, 24
Renal Assessment Tool, 92-107
  development and refinement of, 92
  how to elicit appropriate data using, 95
  how to use, 92-93, 95
  patient population and setting for, 92
Renal emphasis areas, 92, 93
Research tools, 11
Response patterns, human, of unitary person, 7
Rest, focus questions related to, 28
Rheumatic fever, focus questions related to, 26
Risk factors for coronary artery disease, focus questions related to, 26
Role, focus questions related to, 24-25

S

Screening tool
  adapting Cardiovascular Assessment Tool as, 45-47
  Cardiovascular, 45-47, 54-55
  developing, 47
  purpose of, 45
Self-care, focus questions related to, 29
Self-concept, focus questions related to, 29
Sensory perception, focus questions related to, 30
Serum chemistry, normal values for, 440-444
Sexual relationships, focus questions related to, 25
Socialization, focus questions related to, 25
Specialty dysfunctions, major, patients with, assessment of, 127-303
Speech impairment, focus questions related to, 24
Spinal Cord Injury Rehabilitation Assessment Tool, 423-436
  development and refinement of, 423
  how to elicit appropriate data using, 425-426
  how to use, 424-425
  patient population and setting for, 423
Spinal cord injury rehabilitation emphasis areas, 424
Spiritual concerns, focus questions related to, 24
Standards of Cardiovascular Nursing Practice, 10, 393
Standards of Child and Adolescent Psychiatric and Mental Health Nursing Practice, 161
Standards of Maternal and Child Health Nursing Practice, 307, 343, 357
Standards of Neurological and Neurosurgical Nursing Practice, 75
Standards for the Nursing Care of the Critically Ill, 10, 179, 239
Standards of Perioperative Nursing Practice, 198
Standards for Psychiatric and Mental Health Nursing Practice, 161
Standards of Rehabilitation Nursing Practice, 407, 423
Stenosis, valve, 34
Stroke Rehabilitation Assessment Tool, 407-422
  development and refinement of, 407
  how to elicit appropriate data using, 410
  how to use, 408, 410
  patient population and setting for, 407-408
Stroke rehabilitation emphasis areas, 408
Surgery
  perception/knowledge of, focus questions related to, 26
  previous, focus questions related to, 25
Systems dysfunctions, major, patients with, assessment of, 57-126

T

Taxonomy I, 7, 8-9
  revised, 437-439
Taxonomy II, 7

Testing
  of nursing data base prototype in clinical practice, 11
  validity, of assessment tools, 11
Tests, perception/knowledge of, focus questions related to, 26
Theory, 4
Therapy, expectations of, focus questions related to, 26
Thyroid problems, focus questions related to, 26
Traditional nursing data base, 3-4
Transplant Assessment Tool, 223-238
  development and refinement of, 223
  how to elicit appropriate data using, 226
  how to use, 223-224, 226
  patient population and setting for, 223
Transplant emphasis areas, 223, 224
Trauma Assessment Tool, 239-255
  development and refinement of, 239
  how to elicit appropriate data using, 242-243
  how to use, 240-242
  patient population and setting for, 239-240
Trauma emphasis areas, 240
Triceps reflex, testing of, 30

Tricuspid regurgitation, 34
Tricuspid stenosis, 34

U
Unitary person, human response patterns of, 7
Unitary Person Framework, 6-7
  nursing data base prototype developed from, benefits of, 13-14
Urine, normal laboratory values for, 444-446

V
Validity of research tool, 11
Validity testing of assessment tools, 11
Valuing, 7
  in assessment tools; *see* Emphasis areas of assessment tools
  nursing diagnoses involving, 8, 438
Valuing pattern focus questions and parameters, 24
Vascular problems, peripheral, focus questions related to, 25

W
Whole blood chemistry, normal values for, 440-444

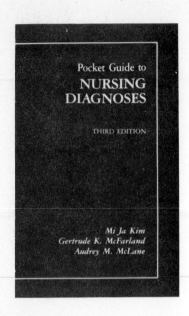
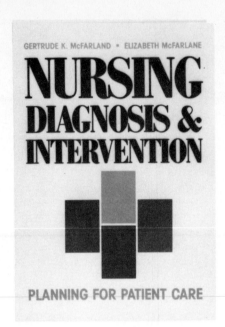
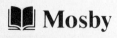